Contents

BASIC SKILLS FOR
NURSING ASSISTANTS
in LONG-TERM CARE

SHEILA A. SORRENTINO, RN, PhD
Curriculum and Health Care Consultant
Normal, Illinois

BERNIE GOREK, RNC, GNP, MA, NHA
Gerontology Consultant
Greeley, Colorado

With 438 Illustrations

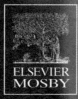

ELSEVIER
MOSBY

ELSEVIER
MOSBY

11830 Westline Industrial Drive
St. Louis, Missouri 63146

BASIC SKILLS FOR NURSING ASSISTANTS IN
LONG-TERM CARE   0-323-02203-0
Copyright © 2005, Elsevier Inc.

NOTICE

Nursing is an ever-changing field. Standard safety precautions must be followed, but as new research and clinical experience broaden our knowledge, changes in treatment and drug therapy may become necessary or appropriate. Readers are advised to check the most current product information provided by the manufacturer. It is the responsibility of the licensed provider, relying on experience and knowledge of the patient or resident, to determine the best treatment for each individual patient or resident. Neither the publisher nor the author assumes any liability for any injury and/or damage to persons or property arising from this publication.

International Standard Book Number 0-323-02203-0

Executive Editor: Susan R. Epstein
Senior Developmental Editor: Maria Broeker
Publishing Services Manager: John Rogers
Senior Project Manager: Kathleen L. Teal
Senior Designer: Kathi Gosche

Working together to grow
libraries in developing countries

www.elsevier.com | www.bookaid.org | www.sabre.org

ELSEVIER   BOOK AID International   Sabre Foundation

Printed in the United States of America

Last digit is the print number: 9 8 7 6 5 4 3 2 1

To my sister, Sandra, and her husband, Jack—for blessing our family with
Christopher and Kyle
To my brother, Tony, and his wife, Louise—for blessing our family with
Carly, Tony, and Mike
Sheila A. Sorrentino

To Emerson Charles—
Welcome to our family
Bernie Gorek

About the Authors

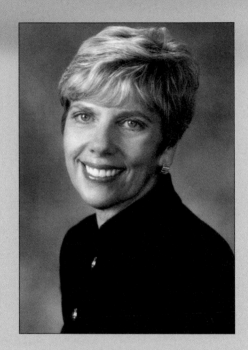

SHEILA A. SORRENTINO

Sheila A. Sorrentino is currently a curriculum and health care consultant focusing on career ladder nursing programs and effective delegation and partnering with assistive personnel in hospitals, long-term care centers, and home care agencies.

Dr. Sorrentino was instrumental in the development and approval of CNA-PN-ADN programs in the Illinois Community College System and has taught in nursing assistant, practical nursing, associate degree, and baccalaureate and higher degree programs. Her career includes experiences as a nursing assistant, staff nurse, charge nurse, head nurse, nursing educator, assistant dean, dean, and consultant.

A Mosby author since 1982, Dr. Sorrentino has written several textbooks for nursing assistants and other assistive personnel: *Mosby's Textbook for Nursing Assistants* (ed 6), *Mosby's Textbook for Long-Term Care Assistants* (ed 4), *Assisting With Patient Care* (ed 2), *Mosby's Essentials for Nursing Assistants* (ed 2), *Clinical Skills for Assistive Personnel,* and others. She was also

involved in the development of *Mosby's Nursing Assistant Skills Videos* and *Mosby's Nursing Skills Videos* (selected for the 2003 AJN Book of the Year Award for Electronic Media). An earlier version of *Nursing Assistant Skills Videos* won the 1992 International Medical Films Award on Caregiving.

Dr. Sorrentino has a bachelor of science degree in nursing, a master of arts in education, a master of science degree in community nursing, and a PhD in higher education administration. She is a member of Sigma Theta Tau and served as a member and chair of the Central Illinois Higher Education Health Care Task Force. She also served on the Iowa-Illinois Safety Council Board of Directors and the Board of Directors of Our Lady of Victory Nursing Center in Bourbonnais, Ill. In 1998, she received an alumni achievement award from Lewis University for outstanding leadership and dedication in nursing education. Her presentations at national conferences focus on delegation and other issues relating to assistive personnel.

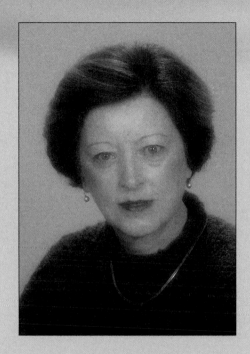

BERNIE GOREK

Bernie Gorek is a licensed nursing home administrator in Colorado and a gerontological consultant. She received her diploma in nursing from St. Mary's School of Nursing, Rochester, MN, a baccalaureate degree in Health Arts from The College of St. Francis, Joliet, IL, certification as a gerontological nurse practitioner from The University of Colorado, Denver, CO., and a Masters degree in Gerontology from The University of Northern Colorado, Greeley, CO., where she received the Dean's Citation for Excellence.

Bernie has had 24 years of experience in gerontological nursing: in a clinical role as a nurse practitioner and in nursing administration as Director of Community Health Services, Director of Nursing Services, and Director of Resident Care and Services at Bonell Good Samaritan Center in Greeley, CO. She

also has other experience as a nursing home administrator in Colorado and Wyoming.

She has been a leader in developing and implementing innovative programs for residents in independent living and long-term health care settings. She was instrumental in the development and implementation of a community nursing assistant training program. She has a Credential for Career and Technical Education from the Colorado State Board of Community Colleges and Occupational Education. She also consults for the School of Nursing at the University of Northern Colorado in various grant writing projects. Bernie is a respected speaker at the local, state, and national level. She served two terms as the president of The National Conference of Gerontological Nurse Practitioners.

Reviewers

Paula Hamilton, RN
Staff Development Coordinator
Evangelical Lutheran Good Samaritan Society
Sioux Falls, South Dakota

Julie Ann Harrah, RN
Instructor, Director of Staff Development
Heartland of Charleston
Charleston, West Virginia

Gloria Kas, RN, BSN
Nurse Aide Instructor
Norridge HealthCare and Rehabilitation Centre
Norridge, Illinois

Vickie L. Kepler, LVN, EMTB
Instructor
Kingsland Hills Care Center
Kingsland, Texas

Dee Robbins, RN
Instructor of Past Development
Lakeridge Care Center
Moses Lake, Washington

Acknowledgments

Many individuals and agencies have contributed to this new textbook for nursing assistants. We are especially grateful for and appreciate the efforts by:

- Jane DeBlois of OSF St. Joseph's Medical Center in Bloomington, Illinois for being a reliable and quick source of information.
- Bonnie McCrea, registered dietitian, President, McCrea and Associates Nutritional Management Systems, Inc., Ft. Collins, Colorado, for providing requested information in a timely, detailed, and professional manner
- Liz Burns, RN, BSN, Director of Nursing, Bonell Good Samaritan Center, Greeley, Colorado, for her professional expertise and her ongoing support.
- Zee Sala, physical therapist, Windsor, Colorado, for sharing her professional knowledge and practical insights.
- The artists at Graphic World in St. Louis, Missouri for their talented work.
- Paula Hamilton, Julie Harrah, Gloria Kas, Vickie Kepler, and Dee Robbins for reviewing the manuscript and for their candor and suggestions. They have contributed to the thoroughness and accuracy of this book.
- Betty Hazelwood, copy editor, for her attention to detail, questions, and humor. Once again, she made the copyediting process painless, efficient, and pleasant.
- And finally, to the talented and dedicated Elsevier/ Mosby staff, especially Suzi Epstein, Maria Broeker, Mary Jo Adams, and the members of John Roger's production team—Kathi Gosche and Kathy Teal. In her role as editor, Suzi once again gave guidance and support and kept the project on track. She also stressed the importance of taking care of self. Maria Broeker handled numerous details and manuscript needs. As always, what would we do without Maria? And Mary Jo provided clerical and secretarial assistance. And what would we do without Kathy Teal? Together Kathy and Maria produced a quality book that is user friendly and pleasing to the student. And Kathi Gosche created another unique and colorful book and cover design. As always, she made the book distinctive from the rest.
- And to all those who contributed to this effort in any way, we are sincerely grateful.

Sheila A. Sorrentino and *Bernie Gorek*

Instructor Preface

Basic Skills for Nursing Assistants in Long-Term Care follows the training requirements outlined in the Omnibus Budget Reconciliation Act of 1987 (OBRA). In doing so, it prepares students to function as nursing assistants in nursing centers. This new book serves the needs of students and instructors in community colleges, technical schools, high schools, and nursing centers. As students complete their education, the book is a valuable resource for competency test review. And as part of one's personal library, the book is a reference for the nursing assistant who seeks to review information for safe care.

Reflecting the spirit of OBRA, residents are presented as persons with dignity and value who have a past, a present, and a future. Caring, understanding, resident rights, and respect for residents as persons with dignity and value are attitudes conveyed throughout the book.

The nursing assistants of today and tomorrow must have a firm understanding of the legal principles affecting their role. Both federal and state laws directly and indirectly define their roles and limitations. Nursing assistant roles and functions also vary among centers. Therefore, emphasis is given to nursing assistant responsibilities and limitations, specifically in Chapter 1 which focuses on the legal and ethical aspects of the role including the reporting of elder abuse.

ORGANIZATIONAL STRATEGIES

These concepts, principles, and values serve as the guiding framework for this book:

- Awareness and understanding of the work setting and the individuals in that setting
- Respect for the resident as a physical, social, psychological, and spiritual being with basic needs and protected rights
- Respect for personal choice and dignity of person
- Appreciating the role of cultural heritage and religion in health and illness practices
- Understanding body structure and function and the changes with aging to give safe care and to safely perform procedures
- That learning proceeds from the simple to the complex
- Certain concepts and functions are foundational and central to other procedures—safety, body mechanics, and preventing infection
- That the nursing process is the basis for planning and delivering nursing care and that nursing assistants must follow the person's care plan

FEATURES AND DESIGN

Our vision included creating a book that fosters learning and respect for the resident, is very readable, and is user friendly. We want to gain and retain the student's attention. Therefore, the book is comprised of the following features and design elements:

- **Objectives**—tell what is presented in the chapter.
- **Illustrations**—the book contains 438 full-color photographs and line art.
- **Key Terms with definitions**—are at the beginning of each chapter.
- **Key Terms in bold print**—are throughout the text. The definition is presented in narrative in the text. Unlike other books, students do not have to turn to the margin for the definition, return to the text, and then try to understand the context of the term.
- **Boxes and tables**—list principles, guidelines, signs and symptoms, nursing measures, and other information. Body structure and function, changes with aging, and common health problems also are presented in a boxed format. Boxes and tables are efficient ways for instructors to highlight content. And they are useful study guides for students.
- **Icons**—in section headings alert the reader to an associated procedure. Procedure boxes contain the same icon.
- **Procedure boxes divided into *Pre-Procedure*, *Procedure*, and *Post-Procedure* steps**—labeling and color gradients also differentiate the sections. Including the Pre-Procedure and Post-Procedure steps, rather than referring the student to them as is done in other texts, serves to show the relationship between the content and the procedure and reinforces learning. Because procedures are not clustered at the end of the chapter as in other textbooks, the student does not have to hunt for the procedure or see the procedure out of context.
- **Quality of Life**—this section in the procedure boxes reminds the student, through the use of icons, of fundamental courtesies—knock before entering the room, address the person by name, and introduce one's self by name and title.
- **NNAAP™**—appears in the procedure box title bar for skills included in the National Nurse Aide Assessment Program (NNAAP™).
- **Delegation Guidelines**—nursing assistant functions and role limits depend on effective delegation. Building on the delegation principles presented in Chapter 1, *Delegation Guidelines* are presented as they relate to procedures. They

empower the student to seek information from the nurse and the care plan about critical aspects of the procedure and the observations to report and record. Step 1 of most procedures refers the student to the appropriate *Delegation Guidelines* box.

- **Safety Alerts**—focus the student's attention on the need to be safe and cautious when giving care. Step 1 of most procedures refers the student to the appropriate *Safety Alerts.*
- **Caring About Culture boxes**—serve to sensitize the student to cultural diversity and how culture influences health and illness practices.

- **Review Questions**—are found at the end of each chapter. A page number for the answer section is given.

May this book serve you and your students well. Our intent is to provide you and your students with the information needed to teach and learn safe and effective care during this time of dynamic change in health care.

Sheila A. Sorrentino, RN, BSN, MA, MSN, PhD

Bernie Gorek, RNC, GNP, MA, NHA

Student Preface

This book was designed for you. It was designed to help you learn. The book is a useful resource as you gain experience and expand your knowledge.

This preface gives some study guidelines and helps you use the book. When given a reading assignment, do you read from the first page to the last page without stopping? How much do you remember? You will learn more if you use a study system. A useful study system has these steps:

- Survey or preview
- Question
- Read and record
- Recite and review

PREVIEW

Before you start a reading assignment, preview or survey the assignment. This gives you an idea of what the assignment covers. It also helps you recall what you already know about the subject. Carefully look over the assignment. Preview the chapter title, headings, subheadings, and terms or ideas in bold print or italics. Also survey the objectives, key terms, boxes and review questions at the end of the chapter. Previewing only takes a few minutes. Remember, previewing helps you become familiar with the material.

QUESTION

After previewing, you need to form questions to answer while you read. Questions should relate to what might be asked on a test or how the information applies to giving care. Use the title, headings, and subheadings to form questions. Avoid questions that have one word answers. Questions that begin with what, how, or why are helpful. While reading, you may find that a question does not help you study. If so, just change the question. Remember, questioning sets a purpose for reading. So changing a question only makes this step more useful.

READ AND RECORD

Reading is the next step. Reading is more productive after determining what you already know and what you need to learn. Read to find answers to your questions. The purpose of reading is to:

- Gain new information
- Connect new information to what you know already

Break the assignment into smaller parts. Then answer your questions as you read each part. Also, mark important information—underline, highlight, or make notes. Underlining and highlighting remind you of what you need to learn. Go back and review the marked parts later. Making notes results in more immediate learning. To make notes, write down important information in the margins or in a notebook. Use words and statements to jog your memory about the material.

You need to remember what you read. To do so, work with the information. Organize information into a study guide. Study guides have many forms. Diagrams or charts show relationships or steps in a process. Note taking in outline format is also very useful. The following is a sample outline.

1. Main heading
   a. Second level
   b. Second level
      1. Third level
      ii. Third level
2. Main heading

RECITE AND REVIEW

Finally, recite and review. Use your notes and study guides. Answer the questions you formed earlier. Also answer other questions that came up when reading and answering the *Review Questions* at the end of a chapter. Answer all questions out loud (recite).

Reviewing is more about *when* to study rather than *what* to study. You already determined *what* to study during the preview, question, and reading steps. The best times to review are right after the first study session, one week later, and before a quiz or test.

This book was also designed to help you study. Special design features are described on the next pages.

We hope you enjoy learning and your work. You and your work are important. You and the care you give may be bright spots in a person's day!

Sheila A. Sorrentino and *Bernie Gorek*

- **Objectives** tell what is presented in the chapter.

- **Key Terms** are the important words and phrases in the chapter. Definitions are given for each term. The key terms introduce you to the chapter content. They are also a useful study guide.

- **Caring About Culture boxes** contain information to help you learn about the various practices of other cultures.

- **Bolded type** is used to highlight the key terms in the text. You again see the key term and read its definition. This helps reinforce your learning.

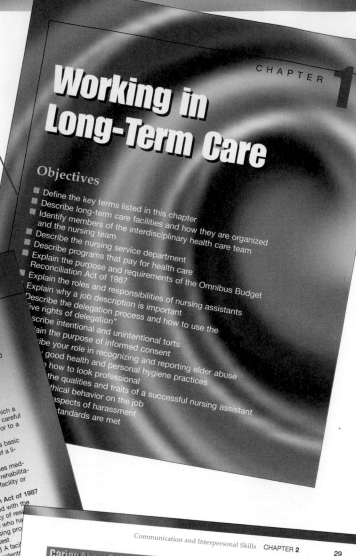

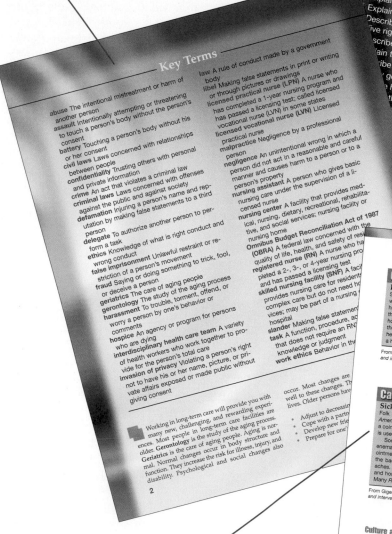

- **Delegation Guidelines** describe what information you need from the nurse and care plan before performing a procedure. They also tell you what observations to report and record.

- **Heading icons** alert you to associated procedures. Procedure boxes contain the same icon.

- **Procedure icons** in the title bar alert you to related content areas. Heading icons and procedure icons are the same.

- **Quality of Life icons** in the procedure boxes remind you to knock before entering the room, address the person by name, and introduce one's self by name and title. These simple courtesies show respect for the resident as a person.

- **Procedures** are written in a step-by-step format. They are divided into Pre-Procedure, Procedure, and Post-Procedure sections for easy studying.

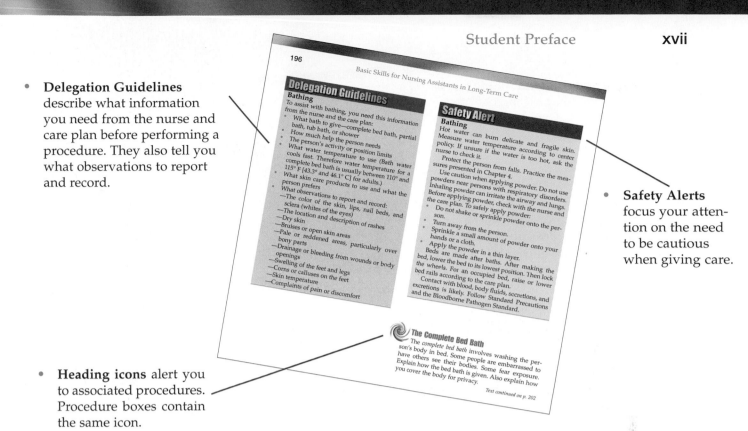

- **Safety Alerts** focus your attention on the need to be cautious when giving care.

- **NNAAP™** in the procedure title bar alerts you to those skills that are part of the National Nurse Aide Assessment Program (NNAAP™). *Note: All states do not participate in NNAAP™. Ask your instructor for a list of the skills tested in your state.*

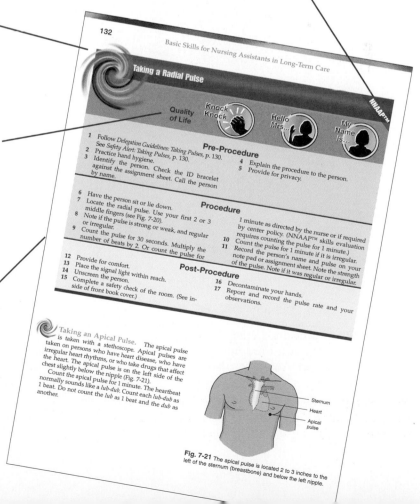

- **Color illustrations and photographs** visually present key ideas, concepts, or procedure steps. They help you apply and remember the written material.

- **Boxes and tables** contain important rules, principles, guidelines, signs and symptoms, nursing measures, and other information in a list format. They identify important information and are useful study guides.

- **Review Questions** are a useful study guide. They help you to review what you have learned. You can also use them to study for a test or the competency evaluation. Answers are given at the back of the book beginning on p. 388.

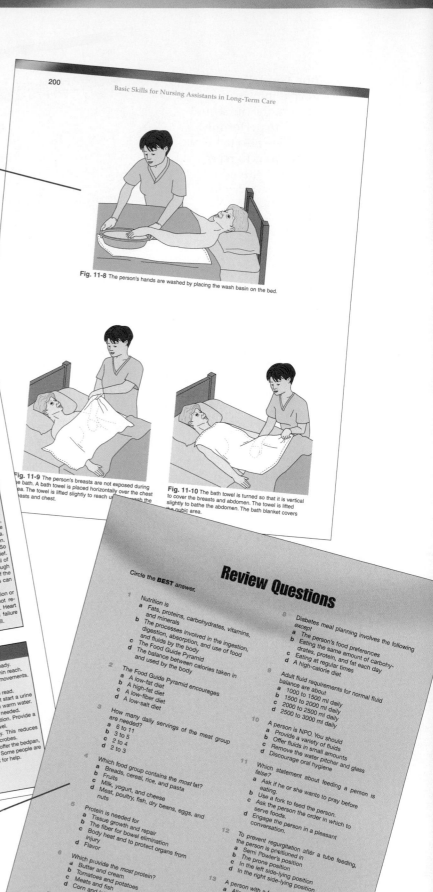

Contents

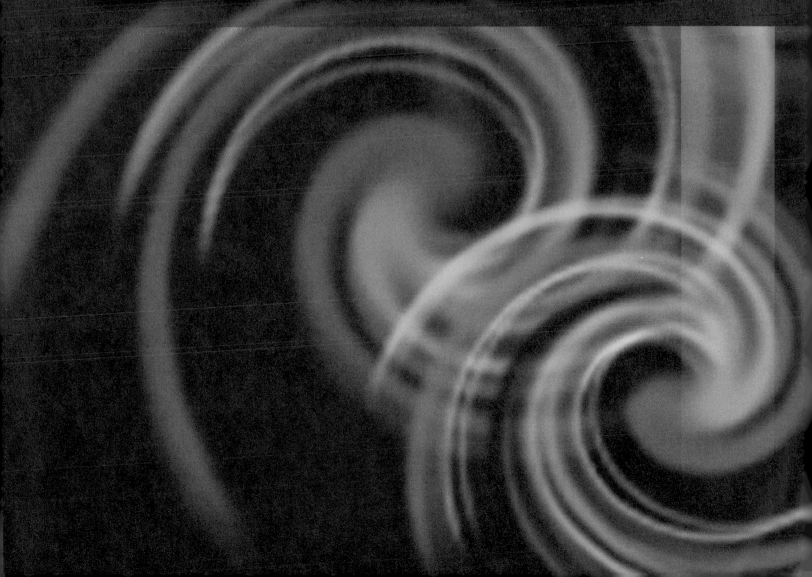

BASIC SKILLS FOR
NURSING ASSISTANTS
in LONG-TERM CARE

CHAPTER 1

Working in Long-Term Care

Objectives

- Define the key terms listed in this chapter
- Describe long-term care facilities and how they are organized
- Identify members of the interdisciplinary health care team and the nursing team
- Describe the nursing service department
- Describe programs that pay for health care
- Explain the purpose and requirements of the Omnibus Budget Reconciliation Act of 1987
- Explain the roles and responsibilities of nursing assistants
- Explain why a job description is important
- Describe the delegation process and how to use the "five rights of delegation"
- Describe intentional and unintentional torts
- Explain the purpose of informed consent
- Describe your role in recognizing and reporting elder abuse
- Identify good health and personal hygiene practices
- Describe how to look professional
- Describe the qualities and traits of a successful nursing assistant
- Describe ethical behavior on the job
- Explain the aspects of harassment
- Explain why standards are met

Key Terms

abuse The intentional mistreatment or harm of another person

assault Intentionally attempting or threatening to touch a person's body without the person's consent

battery Touching a person's body without his or her consent

civil laws Laws concerned with relationships between people

confidentiality Trusting others with personal and private information

crime An act that violates a criminal law

criminal laws Laws concerned with offenses against the public and against society

defamation Injuring a person's name and reputation by making false statements to a third person

delegate To authorize another person to perform a task

ethics Knowledge of what is right conduct and wrong conduct

false imprisonment Unlawful restraint or restriction of a person's movement

fraud Saying or doing something to trick, fool, or deceive a person

geriatrics The care of aging people

gerontology The study of the aging process

harassment To trouble, torment, offend, or worry a person by one's behavior or comments

hospice An agency or program for persons who are dying

interdisciplinary health care team A variety of health workers who work together to provide for the person's total care

invasion of privacy Violating a person's right not to have his or her name, picture, or private affairs exposed or made public without giving consent

law A rule of conduct made by a government body

libel Making false statements in print or writing or through pictures or drawings

licensed practical nurse (LPN) A nurse who has completed a 1-year nursing program and has passed a licensing test; called licensed vocational nurse (LVN) in some states

licensed vocational nurse (LVN) Licensed practical nurse

malpractice Negligence by a professional person

negligence An unintentional wrong in which a person did not act in a reasonable and careful manner and causes harm to a person or to a person's property

nursing assistant A person who gives basic nursing care under the supervision of a licensed nurse

nursing center A facility that provides medical, nursing, dietary, recreational, rehabilitative, and social services; nursing facility or nursing home

Omnibus Budget Reconciliation Act of 1987 (OBRA) A federal law concerned with the quality of life, health, and safety of residents

registered nurse (RN) A nurse who has completed a 2-, 3-, or 4-year nursing program and has passed a licensing test

skilled nursing facility (SNF) A facility that provides nursing care for residents who need complex care but do not need hospital services; may be part of a nursing center or a hospital

slander Making false statements orally

task A function, procedure, activity, or work that does not require an RN's professional knowledge or judgment

work ethics Behavior in the workplace

Working in long-term care will provide you with many new, challenging, and rewarding experiences. Most people in long-term care facilities are older. **Gerontology** is the study of the aging process. **Geriatrics** is the care of aging people. Aging is normal. Normal changes occur in body structure and function. They increase the risk for illness, injury, and disability. Psychological and social changes also occur. Most changes are slow. Most people adjust well to these changes. They lead happy, meaningful lives. Older persons have to:

- Adjust to decreasing strength and loss of health
- Cope with a partner's death
- Develop new friends and relationships
- Prepare for one's own death

BOX 1-1 Myths and Facts About Aging	
Myth	**Fact**
All old people are the same.	Each person is unique. People age in different ways. Culture, religion, education, income, and life experiences affect aging. People develop throughout life.
Aging means illness and disability.	Older persons are at risk for health problems and disabilities. However, most are healthy. Not smoking, good nutrition, and exercise can reverse or slow many changes blamed on aging.
Older persons lose interest in sex.	Aging does not mean that sexual activity and expression must end. Many older people enjoy a fulfilling sex life. Sexuality is important throughout life. Intimacy, love, and companionship are needed.
Older people are lonely and isolated.	Most older people have frequent contact with their children. Most older parents live within 10 minutes of their children. Most see a child at least once a week and take part in family activities. Regular contact with sisters and brothers is common. They can provide support and companionship. Many older persons have jobs, do volunteer work, and enjoy hobbies.
Mental function declines with age.	Older persons may receive and process information more slowly than younger people. However, people learn until very late in life. Many 90-year-olds have high levels of mental function.
Most older persons live in nursing centers.	Only 5.2 percent of older persons live in nursing centers. Most live in their own homes.
Old people are crabby and rude.	Some old people are crabby and rude. So are people of all ages. Older persons who are crabby and rude were probably crabby and rude when younger.

There are many myths about aging and older persons. A *myth* is a widely believed story that is not true. To provide good care, you need to know the facts about older persons and aging. See Box 1-1 for some common myths and facts.

LONG-TERM CARE FACILITIES

Before admission to a long-term care facility, many people need hospital care. Hospital services include emergency care, surgery, nursing care, x-ray procedures and treatments, and laboratory testing. Services also include respiratory, physical, occupational, and speech therapies.

Some people cannot care for themselves at home. But they do not need hospital care. Long-term care facilities can help them. Medical, nursing, dietary, recreational, rehabilitative, and social services are provided.

Persons in long-term care facilities are called *residents*. They are not patients. The facility is their temporary or permanent home. Long-term care facilities are designed to meet the needs of older or disabled residents. Some residents return home when well enough. Others need nursing care until death. Long-term care facilities meet the needs of:

- *Alert, oriented residents*—Some residents know who they are, where they are, the year, and the time of day. They have physical problems. The level of disability affects the amount of care required. Some require complete care. Others need help with daily activities.
- *Confused and disoriented residents*—These residents are mildly to severely confused and disoriented. Some simply have trouble remembering where the dining room is or the month and year. Others are more confused and disoriented—they do not know who or where they are. Sometimes the problem is short term. For other residents, the confusion and disorientation are permanent and become worse (Chapter 18.)

- *Complete care residents*—Some residents are disabled, confused, and disoriented. They cannot meet their own needs, and they cannot tell you what they need. They need to be kept clean, safe, and comfortable.
- *Short-term residents*—Some residents need to recover from fractures, acute illnesses, or surgery. The goal is to help these residents regain strength and mobility so they can return to former living situations. Some people cared for at home are admitted to nursing centers for short stays. This is *respite care*. The home caregiver can take a vacation, tend to business matters, or simply rest.
- *Lifelong residents*—Birth defects and childhood injuries and diseases can cause disabilities. Mental retardation and Down syndrome are common causes. A disability occurring before 22 years of age is called a *developmental disability*. It may be a physical impairment, intellectual impairment, or both. The person has limited function in at least three of these areas: self-care, understanding or expressing language, learning, mobility, self-direction, independent living, and financial support of one's self. The person needs lifelong assistance, support, and special services. Some nursing centers admit developmentally disabled children and adults.
- *Mentally ill residents*—Some people have disturbances in coping or adjusting to stress (Chapter 17). Their behavior and function are affected. In severe cases, self-care and independent living are impaired. Some residents have physical and mental illnesses.
- *Terminally ill residents*—Terminally ill residents may have advanced cancer; advanced liver, kidney, respiratory, or heart disease; or AIDS. Some are alert and oriented; others are comatose. Comatose residents cannot respond to verbal stimuli but may still feel pain. Some residents have severe pain. Terminally ill residents may need hospice care.

Nursing Centers

A **nursing center** provides medical, nursing, dietary, recreational, rehabilitative, and social services. *Nursing facility* and *nursing home* are other names. A licensed nursing staff is required.

Skilled Nursing Facilities.   Some nursing centers provide more complex care. A **skilled nursing facility (SNF)** provides nursing care for residents who need complex care but do not need hospital services. It may be part of a nursing center or a hospital. The person has severe health problems. Many residents are admitted to SNFs directly from hospitals. They need rehabilitation or time to recover from illness or surgery. Often they return home after a short stay. Others become permanent nursing center residents.

Hospices.   A **hospice** is an agency or program for persons who are dying. Such persons no longer respond to treatments aimed at cures. Usually the person has less than 6 months to live.

The physical, emotional, social, and spiritual needs of the person and family are met. The focus is on comfort, not cure. Hospitals, nursing centers, and home care agencies provide hospice care.

Alzheimer's Units (Dementia Care Units). An Alzheimer's unit is designed for residents with Alzheimer's disease and other dementias (Chapter 18). Persons affected suffer increasing memory loss and confusion until they cannot take care of simple personal needs. They often wander about and may become agitated or combative. The unit usually is closed off from the rest of the center. The closed unit provides a setting where residents can wander safely.

Other Facilities

A *board and care home (residential care facility)* is in a home setting. Or it is part of a nursing center. *Supportive care* is given on a 24-hour basis that meets the person's basic needs. A safe setting and supervision are provided but not 24-hour nursing care. Residents can usually tend to grooming, dressing, and bathroom needs with little help. Services include 3 meals a day, housekeeping, laundry, and transportation. There is a 24-hour caregiver and an emergency call system. Residents receive help with personal care and drug reminders. The caregiver may be a nursing assistant.

An *assisted living facility* provides housing, personal care, support services, health care, and social activities in a home-like setting. Some are part of retirement communities or nursing centers. Residents have a room or an apartment. They usually need help with bathing, dressing, elimination, meals, or taking drugs. Services include 3 meals a day, housekeeping, laundry, transportation, and social and recreational activities. The person has access to health and medical services.

Organization

Nursing centers usually are owned by an individual or a corporation. Some are owned by county health departments. The owners must make sure that safe care is provided. Local, state, and federal rules must be followed.

Each center has an administrator. Department directors report to the administrator. Most nursing centers have nursing, therapy, and food service departments (Fig. 1-1). Human resources, finance, social services, and activity departments are common.

Nursing Department. The director of nursing (DON) is an RN. The DON is responsible for the entire nursing staff and the care given. Nurse managers (RNs) assist the DON. They manage and carry out nursing department functions.

Nurse managers are responsible for a work shift or a certain function. Examples include staff development, restorative nursing, infection control, or continuous quality improvement. Shift supervisors coordinate resident care for each shift.

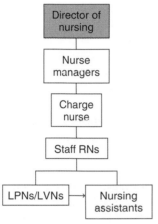

Fig. 1-1 Organization of the nursing department.

Each unit usually has an RN as the charge nurse. In some states, LPNs/LVNs can be charge nurses. The charge nurse is responsible for all resident care and the actions of nursing staff on a unit. Staff RNs report to the charge nurse. LPNs/LVNs report to staff RNs or to the charge nurse. You report to the nurse supervising your work.

Nursing education or staff development personnel do the following:

- Plan and present educational programs
- Provide the nursing team with new and changing information
- Instruct the nursing team on the use of new equipment
- Educate and train nursing assistants
- Conduct new employee orientation programs

THE INTERDISCIPLINARY HEALTH CARE TEAM

The **interdisciplinary health care team** is a variety of health workers who work together to provide for the person's total care. Their skills and knowledge focus on the person's total care (Box 1-2). The goal is to provide quality care. The person is the focus of care.

Many staff members are involved in the care of one person. Coordinated care is important. An RN usually coordinates the person's care.

BOX 1-2 The Interdisciplinary Health Care Team

- Activities director—assesses, plans, and implements recreational needs
- Assistive personnel—assist nurses in giving nursing care; supervised by a licensed nurse (see "Nursing assistant")
- Audiologist—tests hearing; prescribes hearing aids; works with hearing-impaired persons
- Cleric (clergyman; clergywoman)—assists with spiritual needs
- Dietitian—assesses and plans for nutritional needs; teaches good nutrition, food selection, and preparation
- Licensed practical/vocational nurse (LPN/LVN)—provides direct nursing care, including the administration of drugs, under the direction of an RN
- Medical records and health information technician—maintains medical records; transcribes medical reports, files records, completes required reports
- Medical technologist (MT)—performs laboratory tests
- Nurse practitioner—works with other health care providers to plan and provide care; does physical examinations, health assessments, and health education
- Nursing assistant—assists nurses and gives nursing care; supervised by a licensed nurse
- Occupational therapist (OT)—assists persons to learn or retain skills needed to perform activities of daily living; designs adaptive equipment for activities of daily living

- Pharmacist—fills drug orders written by doctors; monitors and evaluates drug interactions; consults with doctors and nurses about drug actions and interactions
- Physical therapist (PT)—assists persons with musculoskeletal problems; focuses on restoring function and preventing disability
- Physician (doctor)—diagnoses and treats diseases and injuries
- Podiatrist—prevents, diagnoses, and treats foot disorders
- Radiographer/radiologic technologist—takes x-rays and processes film for viewing
- Registered nurse (RN)—assesses, makes nursing diagnoses, plans, implements, and evaluates nursing care; supervises LPNs/LVNs and nursing assistants
- Respiratory therapist—assists in the treatment of lung and heart disorders; gives respiratory treatments and therapies
- Social worker—helps residents and families with social, emotional, and environmental issues affecting illness and recovery; coordinates community agencies to assist residents and families
- Speech-language pathologist—evaluates speech and language and treats persons with speech, voice, hearing, communication, and swallowing disorders

The Nursing Team

The *nursing team* involves the individuals who provide nursing care—RNs, LPNs/LVNs, and nursing assistants. Each has different roles and responsibilities. All focus on the physical, social, emotional, and spiritual needs of the person and family.

Registered Nurses.

A **registered nurse (RN)** has completed a 2-, 3-, or 4-year nursing program and has passed a licensing test.

* Community college programs—2 years
* Hospital-based diploma programs—2 or 3 years
* College or university programs—4 years

The graduate nurse takes a licensing test offered by a state board of nursing. The nurse receives a license and becomes *registered* when the test is passed. RNs must have a license recognized by the state in which they work.

RNs assess, make nursing diagnoses, plan, implement, and evaluate nursing care (Chapter 9). They develop care plans for each person and provide care. They also delegate nursing care and tasks to the nursing team. They make sure that the nursing team follows the care plans. They evaluate how the care plans and nursing care affect each person. RNs teach persons how to improve health and independence. They also teach the family.

RNs carry out the doctor's orders. They may delegate them to LPNs/LVNs or nursing assistants. RNs do not diagnose diseases or illnesses. They do not prescribe treatments or drugs. However, RNs can study to become clinical nurse specialists or nurse practitioners. These RNs have diagnosing and prescribing functions.

Licensed Practical Nurses and Licensed Vocational Nurses.

A **licensed practical nurse (LPN)** has completed a 1-year nursing program and has passed a licensing test. Hospitals, community colleges, vocational schools, and technical schools offer programs. Some programs are 10 months long; others take 18 months. Some high schools offer 2-year programs.

Graduates take a licensing test for practical nursing. When the test is passed, the nurse receives a license and the title of *licensed practical nurse*. Some states use the term **licensed vocational nurse (LVN)**. Like RNs, practical or vocational nurses must have a license to work.

LPNs/LVNs are supervised by RNs, licensed doctors, and licensed dentists. They have fewer responsibilities and functions than RNs do. They need little supervision when the person's condition is stable and care is simple. They assist RNs in caring for acutely ill persons and with complex procedures.

Nursing Assistants.

Nursing assistants give basic nursing care under the supervision of an RN or a licensed nurse. *Nurse's aide, nursing attendant,* and *health care assistant* are other titles. Nursing assistants provide much of the care given in nursing centers. To work in a nursing center, nursing assistants must have formal training and pass a competency evaluation.

PAYING FOR HEALTH CARE

Health care is a major focus of society. The goals are to provide health care to everyone and to reduce care costs. Cost-cutting efforts include managed care and prospective payment systems. You need to know the following:

* *Private insurance* is bought by individuals and families. The insurance company pays for some or all health care costs.
* *Group insurance* is bought by groups for individuals. Many employers and organizations provide health insurance for employees and members under group coverage.
* *Medicare* is a federal health insurance program for persons 65 years of age or older. Some younger people with certain disabilities are covered. Medicare has two parts. Part A pays for some hospital, SNF, hospice, and home care costs. Part B helps pay for doctors' services, outpatient hospital care, physical and occupational therapists, some home health care, and many other services. Part B is voluntary. The person pays a monthly premium.
* *Medicaid* is a health care payment program. It is sponsored by federal and state governments. Benefits, rules, and eligibility requirements vary from state to state. Older, blind, and disabled people are usually eligible. So are families with low incomes. There is no insurance premium. The amount paid for each covered service is limited.

Prospective Payment Systems

Prospective payment systems limit the amounts paid by insurers, Medicare, and Medicaid. Prospective means *before* care. The amount paid for services is determined before the person enters the hospital, SNF, or rehabilitation center. If treatment costs are less than the amount paid, the center keeps the extra money. If costs are greater, the center takes the loss. *Diagnosis-related groups (DRGs)* help reduce Medicare and Medicaid costs for hospital care. *Resource utilization groups (RUGs)* are for SNF payments. *Case mix groups (CMGs)* are used to decide payments to rehabilitation centers.

Managed Care

Managed care deals with health care delivery and payment:

- *Health maintenance organization (HMO)*—provides health care services for a prepaid fee. For the fee, persons receive needed services offered by the HMO. Some need just an annual physical exam. Others require hospital care. Whatever services are used, the cost is covered by the prepaid fee. HMOs focus on preventing disease and maintaining health. Keeping someone healthy costs far less than treating illness.
- *Preferred provider organization (PPO)*—is a group of doctors and hospitals. They provide health care at reduced rates. Usually the arrangement is made between the PPO and an employer or an insurance company. Those insured are given reduced rates for the services used. The person can choose any doctor or hospital in the PPO.

Insurers contract with doctors and hospitals for reduced rates or discounts. The insured person uses doctors and agencies providing the lower rates. If others are used, care is covered only in part or not at all. The person pays for costs not covered by insurance.

Managed care limits the choice of where to go for health care. It also limits the care that doctors provide. Many states require managed care for Medicaid and Medicare coverage.

THE OMNIBUS BUDGET RECONCILIATION ACT OF 1987

The **Omnibus Budget Reconciliation Act of 1987 (OBRA)** is a federal law concerned with the quality of life, health, and safety of residents. It applies to all 50 states.

The law requires each state to have a nursing assistant training and competency evaluation program. It must be completed by nursing assistants working in nursing centers and hospital long-term care units.

The Training Program

OBRA requires at least 75 hours of instruction. Some states require more hours. The training program includes the knowledge and skills needed to give basic nursing care. Sixteen hours is supervised practical training. It occurs in a laboratory or clinical setting. The student performs nursing care and procedures on another person. A nurse supervises this practical training.

Competency Evaluation

The competency evaluation has a written test and a skills test (Appendix A, p. 391). The written test has multiple-choice questions. For the skills test, you perform skills learned in your training program.

You take the competency evaluation after your training program. Your instructor tells you where the tests are given and helps you complete the application. The required fee is sent with your application.

If you listen, study hard, and practice safe care, you should do well. If the first attempt was not successful, you can retest. OBRA allows at least 3 attempts to successfully complete the evaluation.

Nursing Assistant Registry

Each state must have a nursing assistant registry. It is an official record of persons who successfully completed a state-approved nursing assistant training and competency evaluation program. The registry has information about each nursing assistant:

- Full name, including maiden name and any married names
- Last known home address
- Registration number and its expiration date
- Date of birth
- Last known employer, date hired, and date employment ended
- Date the competency evaluation was passed
- Information about abuse, neglect, or dishonest use of property. It includes the nature of the offense and supporting evidence. If a hearing was held, the date and its outcome are included. The person has the right to include a statement disputing the finding. All information stays in the registry for at least 5 years.

Any health care agency can access registry information. You also receive a copy of your registry information. The copy is provided when the first entry is made and when information is changed or added. You can correct wrong information.

Other OBRA Requirements

Retraining and a new competency evaluation program are required for nursing assistants who have not worked for 2 consecutive years (24 months). It does not matter how long someone worked as a nursing assistant. What matters is how long that person did *not* work. States can require:

- A new competency evaluation
- Both retraining and a new competency evaluation

Regular in-service education and performance reviews also are required. Nursing centers must provide educational programs to nursing assistants. Their work must be evaluated. These requirements help ensure that nursing assistants have current knowledge and skills to give safe, effective care.

<table>
<tr><td>

BOX 1-3 **Rules for Nursing Assistants**

- You are an assistant to the nurse.
- A nurse assigns and supervises your work.
- You report observations about the person's physical or mental status to the nurse. Report changes at once.
- The nurse decides what should be done for a person. The nurse decides what should not be done for a person. You do not make these decisions.
- Review directions with the nurse before going to the person.
- Perform no function or task that you are not trained to do.
- Perform no function or task that you are not comfortable doing without a nurse's supervision.
- Perform only those functions and tasks that your state and job description allow.

</td></tr>
</table>

ROLES AND RESPONSIBILITIES

OBRA and state laws give direction to what you can do. To protect persons from harm, you must understand what you can do, what you cannot do, and the legal limits of your role.

RNs supervise your work. In some states, LPNs/LVNs can do so. Often you function without a nurse in the room. At other times you help nurses give care. The rules in Box 1-3 will help you understand your role.

Generally, you assist nurses in meeting the hygiene, safety, comfort, nutrition, exercise, and elimination needs of residents. You also observe residents and measure their temperatures, pulses, respirations, and blood pressures.

Box 1-4 describes the procedures and tasks that you never perform. State laws differ. You must know what you can do in the state in which you are working. State laws and rules limit nursing assistant functions. Nursing assistant job descriptions reflect those laws and rules.

Job Description

The *job description* is a list of responsibilities and functions the center expects you to perform (Fig. 1-2). Always request a written job description when you apply for a job. Ask questions about it during your job interview. Before accepting a job, tell the employer what functions you did not learn. Also advise the employer of functions you cannot do for moral or religious reasons. Clearly understand what is

<table>
<tr><td>

BOX 1-4 **Role Limits for Nursing Assistants**

- ***Never give drugs.*** Licensed nurses give drugs. They cannot delegate this responsibility to you. Some states allow nursing assistants to give drugs under certain conditions. To do so, you must complete a state-required medication training program. The function must be in your job description. You must have the necessary supervision.
- ***Never insert tubes or objects into body openings or remove them from the body unless allowed by your state and job description.*** Exceptions to this rule are those procedures that you will study and practice during your training.
- ***Never take oral or telephone orders from doctors.*** Politely give your name and title, and ask the doctor to wait. Promptly find a nurse to speak with the doctor.
- ***Never perform procedures that require sterile technique.*** With sterile technique, all objects in contact with the person's body are free of microorganisms. You can assist a nurse with a sterile procedure. However, you will not perform the procedure yourself.
- ***Never tell the person or family the person's diagnosis or medical or surgical treatment plans.*** This is the doctor's responsibility. Nurses may clarify what the doctor has said.
- ***Never diagnose or prescribe treatments or drugs for anyone.*** Only doctors can diagnose and prescribe.
- ***Never supervise other nursing assistants or assistive personnel.*** This is a nurse's responsibility. You will not be trained to supervise others. Supervising others can have serious legal consequences.
- ***Never ignore an order or request to do something that you cannot do or that is beyond your legal limits.*** Promptly explain to the nurse why you cannot carry out the order or request. The nurse assumes you are doing what you were told to do unless you explain otherwise. You cannot neglect the person's care.

</td></tr>
</table>

expected before taking a job. Do not take a job that requires you to:

- Act beyond the legal limits of your role
- Function beyond your training limits
- Perform acts that are against your morals or religion

No one can force you to do something beyond the legal limits of your role. Jobs may be threatened for refusing to follow a nurse's orders. Often staff members obey out of fear. That is why you must know your roles and responsibilities. You also need to know the functions you can safely perform, the things you should never do, and your job description.

POSITION DESCRIPTION/PERFORMANCE EVALUATION

Job Title: Certified Nursing Assistant (CNA),   Supervised by: Licensed Nurse
Skilled Nursing Facility

Prepared by: _____   Date: _____   Approved by: _____   Date: _____

Job Summary: Provides direct and indirect resident care activities under the direction of an RN or LPN. Assists residents with activities of daily living, provides for personal care and comfort, and assists in the maintenance of a safe and clean environment for an assigned group of residents.

DUTIES AND RESPONSIBILITIES:

E=Exceeds the Standard   M=Meets the Standard   NI=Needs Improvement

Demonstrates Competency in the Following Areas:	E	M	NI
Assists in the preparation for admission of residents.	2	1	0
Assists in and accompanies residents in the admission, transfer, and discharge procedures.	2	1	0
Provides morning care, which may include bed bath, shower or whirlpool, oral hygiene, combing hair, back massage, dressing resident, changing bed linen, cleaning overbed table and bedside stand, straightening room, and other general care as necessary throughout the day.	2	1	0
Provides evening care, which includes hand/face washing as needed, oral hygiene, back massage, peri-care, freshening linen, cleaning overbed table, straightening room, and other general care as needed.	2	1	0
Notifies RN/LPN when resident complains of pain.	2	1	0
Provides post-mortem care and assists in transporting bodies to the morgue.	2	1	0
Assists nurses in treatment procedures.	2	1	0
Provides general nursing care such as positioning residents, lifting and turning residents, applying/utilizing special equipment, assisting in use of bedpan or commode, and ambulating the residents.	2	1	0
Performs all aspects of resident care in an environment that optimizes resident safety and reduces the likelihood of medical/health care errors.	2	1	0
Takes and records temperature, pulse, respiration, weight, blood pressure, and intake-output.	2	1	0
Makes rounds with outgoing shift. Knows whereabouts of assigned residents.	2	1	0
Makes rounds with oncoming shift to ensure the unit is left in good condition.	2	1	0
Adheres to policies and procedures of the center and the Department of Nursing.	2	1	0
Participates in socialization activities on the unit.	2	1	0
Turns and positions residents as ordered and/or as needed, making sure no rough surfaces are in direct contact with the body. Lifts and turns with proper and safe body mechanics and with available resources.	2	1	0
Checks for reddened areas or skin breakdown and reports to RN or LPN.	2	1	0
Ensures residents are dressed properly and assists, as necessary. Ensures that clothing is properly stored in bedside stand or on hangers in closet. Ensures that all residents are clean and dry at all times.	2	1	0
Checks unit for adequate linen. Cleans linen cart. Provides clean linen and clothing. Makes beds.	2	1	0
Treats residents and their families with respect and dignity.	2	1	0
Follows center policies and procedures when caring for persons who are restrained.	2	1	0
Prepares residents for meals. Serves and removes food trays. Assists with meals or feeds residents, if necessary.	2	1	0
Distributes drinking water and other nourishments to residents.	2	1	0

Fig. 1-2 Nursing assistant job description. This job description is used also to evaluate job performance. (Modified from Medical Consultants Network, Inc., Denver, Colo.)   *Continued*

POSITION DESCRIPTION/PERFORMANCE EVALUATION—cont'd

	E	M	NI
Performs general care activities for residents in isolation.	2	1	0
Answers residents' signal lights promptly. Anticipates residents' needs, and makes rounds to assigned residents.	2	1	0
Assists residents with handling and care of clothing and other personal property (including dentures, glasses, contact lenses, hearing aids, and prosthetic devices).	2	1	0
Transports residents to and from various departments, as requested.	2	1	0
Reports and, when appropriate, records any changes observed in condition or behavior of residents and unusual incidents.	2	1	0
Participates in and contributes to Resident Care Conferences.	2	1	0
Follows directions, both oral and written, and works cooperatively with other staff members.	2	1	0
Establishes and maintains interpersonal relationships with residents, family members, and other center personnel while assuring confidentiality of resident information.	2	1	0
Has the ability to acquire knowledge of and develop skills in basic nursing procedures and simple charting.	2	1	0
Attends inservice education programs, as assigned, to learn new treatments, procedures, skills, etc.	2	1	0
Maintains personal health in order to prevent absence from work due to health problems.	2	1	0

Professional Requirements:

	E	M	NI
Meets dress code standards. Appearance is neat and clean.	2	1	0
Completes annual education requirements.	2	1	0
Maintains regulatory requirements.	2	1	0
Meets center's standards for attendance.	2	1	0
Consistently completes and maintains assigned duties.	2	1	0
Wears identification while on duty.	2	1	0
Practices careful, efficient, and nonwasteful use of supplies and linen. Follows established charge procedure for resident charge items.	2	1	0
Attends annual review and department inservices, as scheduled.	2	1	0
Attends at least 75% of staff meetings. Reads and returns all monthly staff meeting minutes.	2	1	0
Represents the center in a positive and professional manner.	2	1	0
Actively participates in the Continuous Quality Improvement (CQI) activities.	2	1	0
Complies with all center policies regarding ethical business practices.	2	1	0
Communicates the mission, ethics, and goals of the center, as well as the focus statement of the department.	2	1	0
Possesses a genuine interest and concern for older and disabled persons.	2	1	0

TOTAL POINTS _____ _____ _____

Regulatory Requirements:

• High School graduate or equivalent

• Current Certified Nursing Assistant (CNA) certification.

• Current Basic Cardiac Life Support for Healthcare Providers certification within three (3) months of hire date

Fig. 1-2 Nursing assistant job description. This job description is used also to evaluate job performance. (Modified from Medical Consultants Network, Inc., Denver, Colo.)   *Continued*

Language Skills:

• Ability to read and communicate effectively in English

• Additional languages preferred

Skills:

• Basic computer knowledge

Physical Demands:

• For physical demands of position, including vision, hearing, repetitive motion, and environment, see following description

  Reasonable accommodations may be made to enable individuals with disabilities to perform the essential functions of the position without compromising care.

I have received, read, and understand the Position Description/Performance Evaluation above.

Name/Signature   Date Signed

Fig. 1-2, cont'd For legend see facing page.

DELEGATION

In nursing, a **task** is a function, procedure, activity, or work that does not require an RN's professional knowledge or judgment. **Delegate** means to authorize another person to perform a task. The person must be competent to perform the task in a given situation. For example, you know how to give a bed bath. However, Mr. Jones is a new resident. The RN wants to spend time with him and assess his nursing needs. The RN gives the bath.

Who Can Delegate

RNs can delegate tasks to LPNs/LVNs and nursing assistants. In some states, LPNs/LVNs can delegate tasks to nursing assistants.

The delegating nurse must make sure that the task was completed safely and correctly. If the RN delegates, the RN is responsible for the delegated task. If the LPN/LVN delegates, the LPN/LVN is responsible for the delegated task. The RN also supervises LPNs/LVNs. Therefore the RN also is legally accountable for the tasks that LPNs/LVNs delegate to nursing assistants. The RN is accountable for all nursing care.

Nursing assistants cannot delegate. You cannot delegate any task to other nursing assistants. You can ask someone to help you. But you cannot ask or tell someone to do your work.

Delegation Process

Delegated tasks must be within the legal limits of what you can do. The nurse must know:

• What tasks your state allows nursing assistants to perform
• The tasks in your job description
• What you were taught in your education program
• What skills you learned
• How your skills were evaluated
• About your work experiences

The nurse discusses these areas with you. The nurse needs to learn about you, your abilities, and your concerns. You may be a new employee or new to the nursing unit. Or the nurse may be new. In any case, the nurse needs to know about you. You need to know about the nurse.

Center policies and your job description state the tasks that nurses can delegate to you. The person's needs, the task, and the staff member doing the task must fit. The nurse can decide to delegate the task to you. Or the nurse can decide not to delegate the task. The person's needs and the task may require a nurse's knowledge, judgment, and skill.

Delegation decisions should result in good care. A person's health and safety are at risk with poor delegation decisions.

The Five Rights of Delegation. The National Council of State Boards of Nursing's five rights of delegation sum up the delegation process:

- *The right task*—Can the task be delegated? Is the nurse allowed to delegate the task? Is the task in your job description?
- *The right circumstances*—What are the person's physical, mental, emotional, and spiritual needs at this time?
- *The right person*—Do you have the training and experience to safely perform the task for this person?
- *The right directions and communication*—The nurse must give clear directions. The nurse tells you what to do and when to do it. The nurse tells you what observations to make and when to report back. The nurse allows questions and helps you set priorities.
- *The right supervision*—The nurse guides, directs, and evaluates the care you give. The nurse demonstrates tasks as necessary and is available to answer questions. The less experience you have with a task, the more supervision you need. Also, the person's circumstances affect the supervision needed. The nurse assesses how the task affected the person and how well you performed the task. The nurse tells you what you did well and what you can do to improve your work. This is to help you learn and give better care.

Your Role in Delegation

You must perform delegated tasks safely. This protects the person from harm. Use the "five rights of delegation" to accept or refuse a task (Box 1-5).

Accepting a Task. When you agree to perform a task, you are responsible for your own actions. What you do or fail to do can harm the person. *You must complete the task safely.* Ask for help when you are unsure or have questions about a task. Report to the nurse what you did and the observations you made.

Refusing a Task. You have the right to say "no." Sometimes refusing to follow the nurse's directions is your right and duty. You should refuse to perform a task when:

- The task is beyond the legal limits of your role.
- The task is not in your job description.
- You were not prepared to perform the task.
- The task could harm the person.
- The person's condition has changed.
- You do not know how to use the supplies or equipment.
- Directions are unethical, illegal, or against center policies.
- Directions are unclear or incomplete.
- A nurse is not available for supervision.

Use common sense. This protects you and the person. Ask yourself if what you are doing is safe for the person.

> ### BOX 1-5   The Five Rights of Delegation for Nursing Assistants
>
> **The Right Task**
>
> - Does your state allow you to perform the task?
> - Were you trained to do the task?
> - Do you have experience performing the task?
> - Is the task in your job description?
>
> **The Right Circumstances**
>
> - Do you have experience performing the task given the person's condition and needs?
> - Do you understand the purpose of the task for the person?
> - Can you perform the task safely under the current circumstances?
> - Do you have the equipment and supplies to safely complete the task?
> - Do you know how to use the equipment and supplies?
>
> **The Right Person**
>
> - Are you comfortable performing the task?
> - Do you have concerns about performing the task?
>
> **The Right Directions and Communication**
>
> - Did the nurse give clear directions and instructions?
> - Did you review the task with the nurse?
> - Do you understand what the nurse expects?
>
> **The Right Supervision**
>
> - Is a nurse available to answer questions?
> - Is a nurse available if the person's condition changes or if problems occur?

Modified from the NCSBN web site (www.ncsbn.org) and used with permission from the National Council of State Boards of Nursing, Inc., Chicago. Copyright 1995.

Never ignore an order or request to do something. Tell the nurse about your concerns. You must not refuse a task because you do not like it or do not want to do it. You must have sound reasons. Otherwise, you place the person at risk for harm. You also risk losing your job.

ETHICAL AND LEGAL ASPECTS

Ethics is knowledge of what is right conduct and wrong conduct. It involves morals and choices or judgments about what should or should not be done. An ethical person behaves and acts in the right way. He or she does not cause a person harm.

Ethical behavior also involves not being *prejudiced* or *biased*. To be prejudiced or biased means to make judgments and have views before knowing the facts. Judgments and views usually are based on one's values and standards. They are based in the person's culture, religion, education, and experiences. The person's situation may be very different from your own. For example:

- A person has many tattoos and body piercings. You do not like tattoos or body piercings.
- An 80-year-old man does not want lifesaving measures. You believe that everything should be done to save life.

Codes of ethics are rules or standards of conduct. Nursing organizations have codes of ethics for RNs and LPNs/LVNs. The rules of conduct in Box 1-6 can guide your thinking and behavior.

Legal Aspects

A **law** is a rule of conduct made by a government body. The U.S. Congress and state legislatures make laws. Enforced by the government, laws protect the public welfare.

Criminal laws are concerned with offenses against the public and against society. An act that violates a criminal law is called a **crime**. A person found guilty of a crime is fined or sent to prison. Murder, robbery, rape, and kidnapping are some crimes.

Civil laws are concerned with relationships between people. Examples include contracts and nursing practice. A person found guilty of breaking a civil law usually has to pay a sum of money to the injured person.

Tort comes from a French word meaning *wrong*. Torts are part of civil law. Torts are committed against a person or the person's property. Torts are intentional or unintentional.

Unintentional Torts.   **Negligence** is an unintentional wrong. The negligent person did not act in a reasonable and careful manner. As a result, harm was caused to a person or to a person's property. The person did not mean or intend to cause harm. The person did not do what a reasonable and careful person would have done. Or he or she did what a reasonable and careful person would not have done.

Malpractice is negligence by a professional person. A person has professional status because of training, education, and the service provided. Nurses, doctors, dentists, and pharmacists are examples.

You are legally responsible (*liable*) for your own actions. What you do or do not do can lead to a lawsuit if a person or property is harmed. A nurse may have you do something beyond the legal limits of your role. The nurse is liable as your supervisor. However, you are responsible for your actions. Sometimes refusing to follow the nurse's directions is your right and duty.

BOX 1-6	Rules of Conduct for Nursing Assistants
<ul><li>Respect each person as an individual.</li><li>Perform no act that is not within the legal limits of your role.</li><li>Perform only those acts that you have been prepared to do.</li><li>Take no drug without the prescription and supervision of a doctor.</li><li>Carry out the directions and instructions of the nurse to your best possible ability.</li></ul>	<ul><li>Complete each task safely.</li><li>Be loyal to your employer and co-workers.</li><li>Act as a responsible citizen at all times.</li><li>Know the limits of your role and knowledge.</li><li>Keep the person's information confidential.</li><li>Protect the person's privacy.</li><li>Consider the person's needs to be more important than your own.</li><li>Perform no action that will cause the person harm.</li></ul>

Intentional Torts. Intentional torts are acts meant to be harmful.

- **Defamation** is injuring a person's name or reputation by making false statements to a third person. **Libel** is making false statements in print or writing or through pictures or drawings. **Slander** is making false statements orally.
- **Assault** is intentionally attempting or threatening to touch a person's body without the person's consent. The person fears bodily harm.
- **Battery** is touching a person's body without his or her consent. The person must consent to any procedure, treatment, or other act that involves touching the body. The person has the right to withdraw consent at any time.
- **False imprisonment** is the unlawful restraint or restriction of a person's movement. It can be a threat of restraint or actual physical restraint. Preventing a person from leaving the center also is false imprisonment.
- **Invasion of privacy** is violating a person's right not to have his or her name, picture, or private affairs exposed or made public without giving consent. Only staff involved in the person's care should see, touch, or examine his or her body. The Health Insurance Portability and Accountability Act of 1996 (HIPAA) protects the privacy and security of a person's health information. *Protected health information* refers to identifying information and information about the person's health care. Failure to comply with HIPAA rules can result in fines, penalties, and criminal action including jail time. You must follow center policies and procedures. Direct any questions about the person or the person's care to the nurse. Also follow the center's rules for telephone and computer use. See Box 1-7 for measures to protect privacy.
- **Fraud** is saying or doing something to trick, fool, or deceive a person. The act is fraud if it does or could cause harm to a person or the person's property. Telling a person or family that you are a nurse is fraud. So is giving wrong or incomplete information on a job application.

BOX 1-7	**Protecting the Right to Privacy**

- Keep all information about the person confidential.
- Cover the person when he or she is being moved in hallways.
- Screen the person as in Figure 1-3. Close the door when giving care. Also close drapes and window shades.
- Expose only the body part involved in care or a procedure.
- Do not discuss the person or the person's treatment with anyone except the nurse supervising your work.
- Ask visitors to leave the room when care is given.
- Do not open the person's mail.
- Allow the person to visit with others in private.
- Allow the person to use the telephone in private.

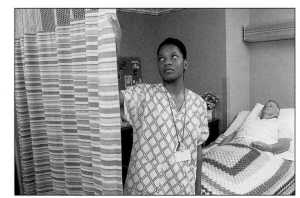

Fig. 1-3 Pulling the curtain around the bed helps protect the person's privacy.

Informed Consent. A person has the right to decide what will be done to and who can touch his or her body. The doctor is responsible for informing the person about all aspects of treatment. Consent is informed when the person clearly understands all aspects of treatment.

Persons under legal age (usually 18 years of age) cannot give consent. Nor can mentally incompetent persons. Such persons are unconscious, sedated, or confused or have certain mental health problems. Informed consent is given by a responsible party—a husband, wife, daughter, son, or a legal representative.

You are never responsible for obtaining written consent. However, you can witness the signing of a consent. To be a witness, you must be present when the person signs the consent.

ELDER ABUSE

Abuse is the intentional mistreatment or harm of another person. Abuse is a crime. Abuse causes physical harm, pain, or mental anguish. The abuser is usually a family member or a caregiver. Elder abuse can take these forms:

- *Physical abuse*—grabbing, hitting, slapping, kicking, pinching, hair-pulling, or beating. It also includes punishment inflicted directly on the body. Beatings, lashings, and whippings are examples. Neglect is also physical abuse. The person is deprived of needed health care or treatment. Neglect is also failure to provide food, clothing, hygiene, and other needs. In health care, neglect includes but is not limited to:

  —Leaving persons lying or sitting in urine or feces
  —Isolating persons in their rooms or other areas
  —Failing to answer signal lights

- *Verbal abuse*—using oral or written words or statements that speak badly of, sneer at, criticize, or condemn the person. It includes unkind gestures.
- *Involuntary seclusion*—confining the person to a certain area. People have been locked in rooms, bathrooms, closets, basements, attics, and other spaces.
- *Financial abuse*—the person's money is stolen or used by another person. It is also misusing a person's property.
- *Mental abuse*—humiliation, harassment, ridicule, and threats of punishment. It includes being deprived of needs such as food, clothing, care, a home, or a place to sleep.
- *Sexual abuse*—the person is harassed about sex or is attacked sexually. The person may be forced to perform sexual acts out of fear of punishment or physical harm.

The abused person may show only some of the signs in Box 1-8. OBRA and state laws require the reporting of elder abuse. If abuse is suspected, it must be reported. Where and how to report suspected abuse vary among states. You may suspect that a person is being abused. If so, discuss the matter and your observations with the nurse. Give as much information as possible. The nurse contacts health team members as needed. The nurse also contacts community agencies that investigate elder abuse. They act at once if the problem is life-threatening. Sometimes the help of police or the courts is necessary.

BOX 1-8   Signs of Elder Abuse

- Living conditions are unsafe, unclean, or inadequate.
- Personal hygiene is lacking. The person is unclean. Clothes are dirty.
- Weight loss—there are signs of poor nutrition and inadequate fluid intake.
- Assistive devices are missing or broken—eyeglasses, hearing aids, dentures, cane, walker.
- Frequent injuries—conditions behind the injuries are strange or seem impossible.
- Old and new injuries—bruises, welts, scars, and punctures.
- Complaints of pain or itching in the genital area.
- Bleeding and bruising in the genital area.
- Burns on the feet, hands, or buttocks. Cigarettes and cigars cause small, circle-like burns.
- Pressure ulcers (Chapter 15) or contractures (Chapter 19).
- The person seems very quiet or withdrawn.
- The person seems fearful, anxious, or agitated.
- The person does not seem to want to talk or answer questions.
- The person is restrained. Or the person is locked in a certain area for long periods.
- The person cannot reach toilet facilities, food, water, and other necessary items.
- Private conversations are not allowed. The caregiver is present during all conversations.
- The person seems anxious to please the caregiver.
- Drugs are not taken properly. Drugs are not purchased. Or too much or too little of the drug is taken.
- Visits to the emergency room may be frequent.
- The person may change doctors often. Some people do not have a doctor.

OBRA does not allow nursing centers to employ persons who were convicted of abuse, neglect, or mistreatment of persons in any health care agency. Before hiring a person, the center must thoroughly check the applicant's work history. All references must be checked. Efforts must be made to find out about any criminal prosecutions.

The employer also checks the nursing assistant registry for any findings about abuse, neglect, or mistreatment of residents. It is checked also for misusing or stealing a resident's property.

The center must take certain actions if abuse is suspected within the center:

- The incident is reported at once to the administrator and to other officials as required by federal and state laws.
- All claims of abuse are thoroughly investigated.
- The center must prevent further potential for abuse while the investigation is in progress.
- Investigation results are reported to the center administrator and to other officials as required by federal and state laws within 5 days of the incident.
- Corrective actions are taken if the claim is found to be true.

WORK ETHICS

Work ethics deals with behavior in the workplace. Your conduct reflects your choices and judgments. Work ethics involves how you look, what you say, how you behave, and how you treat and work with others.

Personal Health, Hygiene, and Appearance

Residents and families expect the health team to look and act healthy. Therefore your personal health, appearance, and hygiene need careful attention.

Your Health.   You must be physically and mentally healthy to function at your best:

- *Diet*—Good nutrition involves eating a balanced diet (Chapter 14).
- *Sleep and rest*—Most adults need about 7 hours of sleep daily.
- *Body mechanics*—You will bend, carry heavy objects, and lift, move, and turn persons. You need to use your muscles correctly (Chapter 4).
- *Exercise*—Regular exercise is needed for muscle tone, circulation, and weight control.
- *Your eyes*—You will read instructions and take measurements. Wrong readings can cause the person harm. Have your eyes checked. Wear needed glasses or contact lenses. Provide enough light when reading or doing fine work.
- *Smoking*—Smoking causes lung, heart, and circulatory disorders. Smoke odors stay on your breath, hands, clothing, and hair. Hand washing and good personal hygiene are needed.
- *Drugs*—Some drugs affect thinking, feeling, behavior, and function. Working under the influence of drugs affects the person's safety. Take only those drugs ordered by a doctor. Take them in the prescribed way.
- *Alcohol*—Alcohol is a drug that affects thinking, balance, coordination, and mental alertness. Never report to work under the influence of alcohol. Do not drink alcohol while working.

Your Hygiene.   Personal hygiene needs careful attention. Bathe daily. Use a deodorant or antiperspirant to prevent body odors. Brush your teeth after meals. Use a mouthwash to prevent breath odors. Shampoo often. Style hair in an attractive and simple way. Keep fingernails clean, short, and neatly shaped.

Foot care prevents odors and infection. Bathe your feet daily. Dry thoroughly between the toes. Cut toenails straight across after bathing or soaking them.

Menstrual hygiene is important. Change tampons or sanitary napkins often, especially if flow is heavy. Wash your genital area with soap and water at least twice a day. Also practice good hand washing.

Your Appearance.   Good health and personal hygiene practices help you look and feel well. Follow the practices in Box 1-9. They help you look neat, clean, and professional (Fig. 1-4).

What Employers Look for.   If you had your own business, whom would you want to hire? Your answer helps you better understand the employer's point of view. Employers want employees who:

- Are dependable
- Are well-groomed
- Have the needed job skills and training
- Have values and attitudes that fit with the center (Box 1-10)

You must be at work on time and when scheduled. Undependable people cause everyone problems.

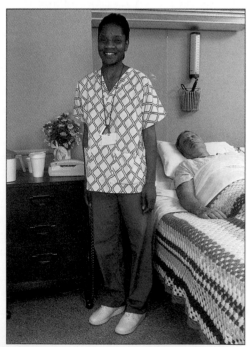

Fig. 1-4 The nursing assistant is well groomed. Her uniform and shoes are clean. Her hair has a simple style and is out of her face and off of her collar. No jewelry is worn.

BOX 1-9 Practices for a Professional Appearance

- Practice good hygiene.
- Wear uniforms that fit well. They are modest in length and style. Follow the center's dress code.
- Keep uniforms clean, pressed, and mended. Sew on buttons. Repair zippers, tears, and hems.
- Wear a clean uniform daily.
- Wear your name badge or photo ID at all times when on duty.
- Wear undergarments that are clean and fit properly. Change them daily. Do not wear colored undergarments. They can be seen through white and light-colored uniforms.
- Cover tattoos. They may offend others.
- Do not wear jewelry. Wedding and engagement rings may be allowed. Rings and bracelets can scratch a person. Confused or combative persons can easily pull on jewelry.
- Do not wear jewelry in pierced eyebrows, nose, lips, or tongue while on duty.
- Follow the center's dress code for earrings. Usually small, simple earrings are allowed. For multiple ear piercings, usually only one pair of earrings is allowed. The pair is worn in the earlobes, not ear cartilage.
- Wear a wristwatch with a second hand.
- Wear clean stockings and socks that fit well. Change them daily.
- Wear shoes that fit properly, are comfortable, and give needed support. Do not wear sandals or open-toed shoes.
- Clean and polish shoes often. Wash and replace laces as needed.
- Keep fingernails clean, short, and neatly shaped. Long nails can scratch a person.
- Do not wear nail polish or fake nails. Chipped nail polish and fake nails may provide a place for microorganisms to grow.
- Have a simple, attractive hair style. Hair is off your collar and away from your face. Use simple pins, combs, barrettes, and bands to keep long hair up and in place.
- Keep beards and mustaches clean and trimmed.
- Use makeup that is modest in amount and moderate in color. Avoid a painted and severe look.
- Do not wear perfume, cologne, or after-shave lotion. They may offend, nauseate, or cause breathing problems in residents.

BOX 1-10 Qualities and Traits for Good Work Ethics

- *Caring.* Have concern for the person. Help make the person's life happier, easier, or less painful.
- *Dependable.* Report to work on time and when scheduled. Perform delegated tasks. Keep obligations and promises.
- *Considerate.* Respect the person's physical and emotional feelings. Be gentle and kind toward residents, families, and co-workers.
- *Cheerful.* Greet and talk to people in a pleasant manner. Do not be moody, bad tempered, or unhappy while at work.
- *Empathetic.* Empathy is seeing things from the person's point of view—putting yourself in the person's position. How would you feel if you had the person's problem?
- *Trustworthy.* Residents and staff members have confidence in you. They believe you will keep information confidential. They trust you not to gossip about residents or the health team.
- *Respectful.* The person has rights, values, beliefs, and feelings. They may differ from yours. Do not judge or condemn the person. Treat the person with respect and dignity at all times. Also show respect for the health team.
- *Courteous.* Be polite and courteous to residents, families, visitors, and co-workers (p. 19).
- *Conscientious.* Be careful, alert, and exact in following instructions. Give thorough care. Do not lose or damage the person's property.
- *Honest.* Accurately report the care given, your observations, and any errors.
- *Cooperative.* Willingly help and work with others. Take that "extra step" during busy and stressful times.
- *Enthusiastic.* Be eager, interested, and excited about your work. Your work is important.
- *Self-aware.* Know your feelings, strengths, and weaknesses. You need to understand yourself before you can understand the person.

Other staff members take on extra work. Fewer people give care. Quality of care suffers. You want co-workers to work when scheduled. Otherwise, you have extra work. You have less time to spend with the residents. Likewise, co-workers also expect you to work when scheduled.

Applicants who look good communicate many things to the employer. You have only one chance to make a good first impression. A well-groomed person is likely to get the job. A sloppy person, with wrinkled or dirty clothes and body or breath odors, is not likely to get the job.

Employers need to know that you can do required job skills. The employer requests proof of required training. Proof of training includes:

- A certificate of course completion
- A high school, college, or technical school transcript
- An official grade report (report card)

Give the employer only a *copy* of your certificate, transcript, or grade report. Never give the original to the employer. Keep it for future use. The employer may want a transcript sent directly from the school or college.

On the Job

How you look, how you behave, and what you say affect everyone in the center. Practice good work ethics—work when scheduled, be cheerful and friendly, perform delegated tasks, help others, and be kind to others.

Personal Hygiene and Appearance.   Home and social attire is often improper at work. You cannot wear jeans, halter tops, tank tops, or short skirts. Clothing must not be tight, revealing, or sexual. Females cannot show cleavage, the tops of breasts, or upper thighs. Males must avoid tight pants and exposing their chests. Only the top shirt button is open. Follow the center's dress code and the practices in Box 1-9.

Attendance.   Report to work when scheduled and on time. Call the center if you will be late or cannot go to work. Follow the center's attendance policies in the employee handbook.

Be *ready to work* when your shift starts. Store your coat, purse, backpack, and other items before your shift starts. Use the restroom when you arrive at the center. Plan to arrive on your nursing unit a few minutes early. This gives you time to greet others and settle yourself.

Attendance also means staying the entire shift. Prepare for childcare emergencies. You may need to work overtime. You need to prepare to stay longer if necessary.

Your Attitude.   A good attitude is needed. Show that you enjoy your work. Listen to others. Be willing to learn. Stay busy, and use your time well.

Always think before you speak. These statements signal a bad attitude:

"That's not my resident."
"I can't. I'm too busy."
"I didn't do it."
"It's not my fault."
"It's not my turn."

"Nobody told me."
"That's not my job."
"You didn't tell me that you needed it right away."
"I work harder than anyone else."
"No one appreciates what I do."

Gossip.   To *gossip* means to spread rumors or talk about the private matters of others. Gossiping is unprofessional and hurtful. To avoid being a part of gossip:

- Remove yourself from a group or situation where gossip is occurring.
- Do not make or repeat any comment that can hurt a person, family member, co-worker, or the center.
- Do not make or repeat any comment that you do not know to be true.
- Do not talk about residents, visitors, families, co-workers, or the center at home or in social settings.

Confidentiality.   The person's information is private and personal. **Confidentiality** means trusting others with personal and private information. The person's information is shared only among health team members involved in his or her care. The person has the right to privacy and confidentiality (Chapter 6). Center and co-worker information also is confidential.

Avoid talking about residents, the center, or co-workers when others are present. Share information only with the nurse. Do not talk about residents, the center, or co-workers in hallways, elevators, dining areas, or outside the center. Others may overhear you.

Avoid eavesdropping. To *eavesdrop* means to listen in or overhear what others are saying. It invades a person's privacy.

Many centers have intercom systems. They allow for communication between the bedside and the nurses' station (Chapter 4). Be careful what you say over the intercom. It is like a loudspeaker. Others nearby can hear what you are saying.

Speech and Language.   Speech and language used in home and social settings may be improper at work. Words used with family and friends may offend residents, visitors, and co-workers. Remember the following:

- Do not swear or use foul, vulgar, or abusive language.
- Do not use slang.
- Control the volume and tone of your voice. Speak softly and gently.
- Speak clearly. The person may have a hearing problem (Chapter 2).
- Do not shout or yell.
- Do not fight or argue with the person, family, or co-workers.

Courtesies.   *Courtesies* are polite or helpful comments or acts. They require little time or energy:

- Address others by Miss, Mrs., Ms., Mr., or Doctor. Use a first name only if the person asks you to do so.
- Say "please." Begin or end each request with "please."
- Say "thank you" whenever someone does something for you.
- Apologize whenever you make a mistake or hurt someone.
- Hold doors, including elevator doors, open for others.
- Let residents, families, and visitors enter elevators first.
- Help others willingly when asked.

Personal Matters.   Personal matters cannot interfere with the job. Otherwise care is neglected. You could lose your job for tending to personal matters at work. To keep personal matters out of the workplace:

- Make personal phone calls only during meals and breaks. Use pay phones or your wireless phone.
- Do not let family and friends visit you on the unit. If they must see you, arrange for them to meet you for a meal or break.
- Make appointments (doctor, dentist, lawyer, beauty, and others) for your days off.
- Do not use center computers, printers, fax machines, photocopiers, or other equipment for your personal use.
- Do not take center supplies (pens, paper, and others) for your personal use.
- Do not discuss personal problems at work.
- Do not sell things or engage in fund-raising at work. Do not sell your child's candy or raffle tickets to co-workers.
- Do not have personal pagers or wireless phones turned on while at work.

Meals and Breaks.   Meal breaks are usually 30 minutes. Other breaks are usually for 15 minutes. Meals and breaks are scheduled so that some staff members are always on the unit. Staff remaining on the unit cover for the staff on break.

Leave for and return from breaks on time. That way other staff can have their turn. Do not take longer than allowed. Tell the nurse when you leave and return to the unit.

Planning Your Work.   You will give care and perform routine tasks on the nursing unit. You must complete some things by a certain time. Others are done by the end of the shift. Plan your work to give safe, thorough care and to make good use of your time (Box 1-11).

BOX 1-11   Planning Your Work

- Discuss priorities with the nurse.
- Know the routine of your shift and nursing unit.
- List care or procedures that are on a schedule.
- Judge how much time you need for each person, procedure, and task.
- Identify which tasks and procedures can be done while the person is eating, visiting, or involved in activities or therapies.
- Plan care around mealtimes, visiting hours, and therapies. Also consider daily recreation and social activities.
- Identify when you will need help from a co-worker. Ask a co-worker to help you. Give the time when you will need help.
- Schedule equipment or rooms for the person's use.
- Review procedures. Gather needed supplies beforehand.
- Do not waste time. Stay focused on your work.
- Do not leave a messy work area. Make sure rooms and utility areas are neat and orderly.
- Be a self-starter. Have initiative. Ask others if they need help, follow unit routines, stock supply areas, and clean utility rooms. Stay busy.

HARASSMENT

Harassment means to trouble, torment, offend, or worry a person by one's behavior or comments. Harassment can be sexual. Or it can involve age, race, ethnic background, religion, or disability. You must respect others. Do not offend others by your gestures, remarks, or use of touch. Do not offend others with jokes or pictures. Harassment is not legal in the workplace.

Sexual Harassment

Sexual harassment involves unwanted sexual behaviors by another. The behavior may be a sexual advance. Or it may be a request for a sexual favor. Some comments or touch is sexual. The behavior affects the person's work and comfort. In extreme cases, the person's job is threatened if sexual favors are not granted.

Victims of sexual harassment may be men or women. Men harass women or men. Women harass men or women. You might feel that you are being harassed. If so, report the matter to your supervisor and the human resource officer.

Be careful about what you say or do. Even innocent remarks and behaviors can be viewed as harassment. Employee orientation programs address harassment. You might not be sure about your own or another person's remarks or behaviors. If so, discuss the matter with the nurse. You cannot be too careful.

MEETING STANDARDS

Nursing centers must meet certain standards. Standards are set by the federal and state governments. They also are set by accrediting agencies. Standards relate to center policies and procedures, budget and finances, and quality of care. A center must meet standards for:

- *Licensure.* A license is issued by the state. A center must have a license to operate and provide care.
- *Certification.* This is required to receive Medicare and Medicaid funds.
- *Accreditation.* This is voluntary. It signals quality and excellence.

The Survey Process

Surveys are done to see if the center meets set standards. A survey team will:

- Review policies and procedures
- Review medical records
- Interview staff, residents, and families
- Observe how care is given
- Check for cleanliness and safety
- Review budgets and finances
- Make sure the staff meets state requirements (Are doctors and nurses licensed? Are nursing assistants on the state registry?)

The survey team decides if the center meets the standards. If standards are met, the center receives a license, certification, or accreditation.

Sometimes problems are found. A problem is called a *deficiency*. The center is given time to correct it. Usually 30 to 60 days are given. However, the amount of time given depends on the seriousness of the deficiency. The center can be fined for uncorrected or serious deficiencies. Or it can lose its license, certification, or accreditation.

Your Role

You have an important role in meeting standards and in the survey process. You must:

- Provide quality care
- Protect the person's rights
- Provide for the person's and your own safety
- Help keep the center clean and safe
- Conduct yourself in a professional manner
- Have good work ethics
- Follow center policies and procedures
- Answer surveyor questions honestly and completely

Review Questions

Circle the **BEST** answer.

1. A health care program for persons who are dying is called a
   - a Hospice
   - b Nursing center
   - c Skilled nursing facility
   - d Hospital

2. Who is responsible for the entire nursing staff and safe nursing care?
   - a The case manager
   - b The director of nursing
   - c The nursing supervisor
   - d An RN

3. You are a member of
   - a The interdisciplinary health care team and the nursing team
   - b The interdisciplinary health care team and the medical team
   - c The nursing team and the medical team
   - d An HMO and a PPO

4. The nursing team includes the following *except*
   - a RNs
   - b Doctors
   - c Nursing assistants
   - d LVNs/LPNs

Review Questions

5 These statements are about paying for health care. Which is *false?*
- **a** PPOs provide health care at reduced rates.
- **b** HMOs provide health care for a prepaid fee.
- **c** Medicare and Medicaid are for anyone in need.
- **d** DRGs and RUGs affect Medicare payments.

6 You perform a task not allowed by your state. Which is *true?*
- **a** If an RN delegated the task, there is no legal problem.
- **b** You could be found guilty of practicing nursing without a license.
- **c** Performing the task is allowed if it is in your job description.
- **d** If you complete the task safely, there is no legal problem.

7 An RN asks you to give a drug. Which is *true?*
- **a** Nursing assistants do not give drugs.
- **b** The RN must supervise your work.
- **c** You must know how the drug works.
- **d** You must know why the person needs the drug.

8 A task is in your job description. Which is *false?*
- **a** The nurse must always delegate the task to you.
- **b** The nurse delegates the task to you if the person's circumstances are right.
- **c** The nurse must make sure you have the necessary education and training.
- **d** You must have clear directions before you perform the task.

9 A nurse delegates a task to you. You must
- **a** Complete the task
- **b** Decide to accept or refuse the task
- **c** Delegate the task if you are busy
- **d** Ignore the request if you do not know what to do

10 You are responsible for
- **a** Completing tasks safely
- **b** Delegation
- **c** The "five rights of delegation"
- **d** Delegating tasks to nursing assistants

11 You can refuse to perform a task for these reasons *except*
- **a** The task is beyond the legal limits of your role
- **b** The task is not in your job description
- **c** You do not like the task
- **d** A nurse is not available to supervise you

12 You decide to refuse a task. What should you do?
- **a** Delegate the task to someone else
- **b** Communicate your concerns to the nurse
- **c** Ignore the request
- **d** Talk to the nurse's supervisor

13 Codes of ethics are
- **a** Federal laws
- **b** State laws
- **c** About right conduct and wrong conduct
- **d** Rules stating what you can and cannot do

14 Which is *not* a crime?
- **a** Negligence
- **c** Robbery
- **b** Murder
- **d** Rape

15 These statements are about negligence. Which is *false?*
- **a** It is an unintentional tort.
- **b** The negligent person did not act in a reasonable manner.
- **c** Harm was caused to a person or a person's property.
- **d** A prison term is likely.

16 The intentional attempt or threat to touch a person's body without the person's consent is
- **a** Assault
- **c** Defamation
- **b** Battery
- **d** False imprisonment

17 The illegal restraint of a person's freedom of movement is
- **a** Assault
- **c** Defamation
- **b** Battery
- **d** False imprisonment

Review Questions

18 Which will *not* protect the person's right to privacy?
a Informed consent
b Screening the person when giving care
c Exposing only the body part involved in the treatment or procedure
d Asking visitors to leave the room when care is given

19 A person asks if you are a nurse. You answer "yes." This is
a Negligence   c Libel
b Fraud   d Slander

20 Who obtains the person's informed consent?
a The doctor   c The LPN/LVN
b The RN   d The nursing assistant

21 Which is *not* a sign of elder abuse?
a Stiff joints and joint pain
b Old and new bruises
c Poor personal hygiene
d Frequent injuries

22 You suspect a person was abused. What should you do?
a Tell the family.   c Tell the nurse.
b Call a state   d Ask the person if he
  agency.   or she was abused.

23 To perform your job well you need the following *except*
a Adequate sleep and rest
b Regular exercise
c To use drugs and alcohol
d Good nutrition

24 Good hygiene for work involves the following *except*
a Bathing daily
b Using a deodorant or antiperspirant
c Brushing teeth after meals
d Keeping fingernails long and polished

25 You are getting ready for work. You should do the following *except*
a Press and mend your uniform
b Wear your name badge or photo ID
c Wear jewelry
d Style hair so it is up and off the collar

26 A co-worker tells you that a doctor and nurse are dating. This is
a Gossip
b Eavesdropping
c Confidential information
d Sexual harassment

27 Which is *not* a courteous act?
a Saying "please" and "thank you"
b Expecting others to open doors for you
c Saying "I'm sorry"
d Complimenting others

28 You are on your meal break. Which is *false?*
a You can make personal phone calls.
b Family members can meet you.
c You can take a few extra minutes if necessary.
d The nurse needs to know that you are off the unit.

29 You are planning your work. You should do the following *except*
a Discuss priorities with the nurse
b Ask others if they need help
c Stay busy
d Plan care so that you can watch the person's TV

30 Which is *not* harassment?
a Using touch to comfort a person.
b Joking about a person's religion.
c Asking for a sexual favor.
d Imitating a person's disability.

31 Which process is voluntary for health care agencies?
a Licensure
b Certification
c Accreditation
d Surveys

Answers to these questions are on p. 388.

CHAPTER 2

Communication and Interpersonal Skills

Objectives

- Define the key terms listed in this chapter
- Explain why health team members need to communicate
- Describe the rules for good communication
- Explain the purpose, parts, and information found in the medical record
- Describe the legal and ethical aspects of medical records
- Describe the rules for answering phones
- Explain how to deal with conflict
- Identify the parts that make up the whole person
- Explain Abraham Maslow's theory of basic needs
- Explain how culture and religion influence health and illness
- Describe how to use verbal and nonverbal communication
- Explain the methods and barriers to good communication
- Explain how to communicate with persons with disabilities
- Explain why family and visitors are important to the person

aphasia The inability (a) to speak (*phasia*)

body language Messages sent through facial expressions, gestures, posture, hand and body movements, gait, eye contact, and appearance

chart The medical record

communication The exchange of information—a message sent is received and interpreted by the intended person

culture The characteristics of a group of people—language, values, beliefs, habits, likes, dislikes, customs—passed from one generation to the next

disability A lost, absent, or impaired physical or mental function

expressive aphasia Difficulty expressing or sending out thoughts

expressive-receptive aphasia Difficulty expressing or sending out thoughts and difficulty receiving information

medical record A written account of a person's condition and response to treatment and care; chart

need Something necessary or desired for maintaining life and mental well-being

nonverbal communication Communication that does not use words

receptive aphasia Difficulty receiving information

religion Spiritual beliefs, needs, and practices

verbal communication Communication that uses written or spoken words

---

Communication is the exchange of information—a message sent is received and interpreted by the intended person. You need to communicate with the health team and with residents and families. For good communication, follow these rules. Otherwise communication does not occur.

- Use words that mean the same thing to the sender and the receiver of the message. Avoid words with more than one meaning.
- Use familiar words. Do not use terms unfamiliar to the person and family.
- Be brief and concise. Do not add unrelated or unneeded information. Stay on the subject. Avoid wandering in thought. Do not get wordy.
- Give information in a logical and orderly manner. Organize your thoughts. Present them step-by-step.
- Give facts, and be specific. You report a pulse rate of 110. It is more specific and factual than saying the "pulse is fast."

COMMUNICATING WITH THE HEALTH TEAM

The health team shares information about the person with each other. They communicate through oral reports and written records. (See Chapter 9 for your role in reporting and recording.)

The Medical Record

The **medical record (chart)** is a written account of a person's condition and response to treatment and care. The record is permanent and is a legal document. It can be used as evidence in a court of law of the person's problems, treatment, and care.

Health team members involved in a person's care can review the chart. If you have access, you have an ethical and legal duty to keep the person's information confidential. If you are not involved in a person's care, you have no right to review that person's chart. To do so is an invasion of privacy.

The following parts of the medical record relate to your work:

- *Admission sheet*—is completed when the person is admitted to the center. It has identifying information about the person—legal name, birth date, age, gender (male or female), current address, and marital status. Use it to fill out other forms that require the same information.
- *Progress notes*—describe the care given and the person's response (Fig. 2-1). They are used to record information about special treatments and drugs, teaching and counseling, and procedures performed by the doctor. Nurses chart about a change in the person's condition, unusual events, or problems. Summaries of care address the person's progress toward goals and response to care.
- *Flow sheets*—are used to record frequent measurements or observations. Flow sheets are used for vital signs and daily weight measurements (Fig. 2-2). The activities-of-daily-living (ADL) flow sheet is used to record the person's everyday activities (Fig. 2-3, p. 26). Flow sheets are used also for recording intake and output (Chapter 7).

Date	Time	Nursing Margin	Other Depts Margin	
3-19	1700	Out with family for dinner. Jane Doe, LPN	———	
	1930	Returned from outing accompanied by her son. States she had a pleasant time. Mary Smith, CNA	———	
3-20	0900	In bed. Complains of headache. T. 98.4 orally, radial pulse 72 and regular, respiration 18 and unlabored. BP 134/84 left arm lying down. Alice Jones, RN notified of resident complaint and vital signs. Ann Adams, CNA	———	
	0910	In bed resting. States she has had a headache for about 1/2 hour. Denies nausea and dizziness. No other complaints. PRN Tylenol given. Instructed resident to use signal light if headache worsens or other symptoms occur. Alice Jones, RN	———	
	0945	Resting quietly. Denies headache at this time. T. 98.4 orally, radial pulse 70 and regular, respirations 18 and unlabored. BP 132/84 left arm lying down. Alice Jones, RN	———	

Fig. 2-1 Progress note. (Modified from Evangelical Lutheran Good Samaritan Society, Sioux Falls, SD.)

Date	Time	Weight	T	P	R	BP				Signatures
10/19	0700	126	98.4	72	20	142/84				Mary Smith CNA
10/26	0715	125	98.6	72	18	140/84				Jane Doe LPN
11/2	0715	126	98.6	70	18	144/82				Mary Smith CNA

Fig. 2-2 Vital signs and daily weight flow sheet. (Modified from Evangelical Lutheran Good Samaritan Society, Sioux Falls, SD.)

Activities-of-Daily-Living Flow Sheet

JAN   FEB   (MAR)   APR   MAY   JUN   JUL   AUG   SEP   OCT   NOV   DEC

ORDER/INSTRUCTION	TIME	1	2	3	4	5	6	7	8	9	10	11	12	13	14	15	16	17	18	19	20	21	22	23	24	25	26	27	28	29	30	31
Bowel Movements L = Large M = Medium S = Small IC = Incontinent	11-7	M																														
	7-3			L																												
	3-11																															
Bladder Elimination I = Independent IC = Incontinent FC = Foley catheter	11-7	I	I	I	I																											
	7-3	I	I	I	I																											
	3-11	I	IC	I	I																											
Weight Bearing Status TT = Toe touch AT = As tol. P = Partial F = Full NWB = No wt. bearing	11-7	AT	AT	AT	AT																											
	7-3	AT	AT	AT	AT																											
	3-11	AT	AT	AT	AT																											
Transfer Status ML = Mech lift SBA = Stand By Assist; Assist of 1 or 2	11-7	SBA	SBA	SBA	SBA																											
	7-3	SBA	SBA	SBA	SBA																											
	3-11	SBA	SBA	SBA	A-1																											
Activity A = Ambulate GC = Gerichair T = Turn every 2 hrs. W/C = Wheelchair	11-7	T	T	T	T																											
	7-3	A	A	A	A																											
	3-11	A	A	A	A																											
Safety LT = Lap tray BR = Bed rails BA = Bed alarm SB = Seat belt	11-7																															
	7-3																															
	3-11																															
Feeding Status I = Independent S = Set up F = Staff feed SP = Swallow precautions TL = Thickened liquids	Breakfast	S	S	S	S																											
	Lunch	S	S	S	S																											
	Supper	S	S	S	S																											
Amount of food taken in %	Breakfast	75	100	100	75																											
	Lunch	75	75	100	75																											
	Supper	50	50	50	75																											
Bath and Shampoo every Monday & Thursday on 7-3 shift T = Tub S = Shower B = Bed bath	11-7																															
	7-3		T																													
	3-11																															
Oral Care Own/Dentures/None I = Independent S = Set up A = Assist	11-7	S	S	S	S																											
	7-3	S	S	S	S																											
	3-11	S	S	S	S																											
Dressing I = Independent S = Set up A = Assist T = Total care	11-7	A	A	S	S																											
	7-3																															
	3-11	A	A	A																												
Grooming: Washing Face and Hands Combing Hair I = Independent S = Set up A = Assist T = Total care	11-7	A	A	A	A																											
	7-3	A	A	A	A																											
	3-11	A	A	A	A																											
Trim Fingernails weekly	11-7																															
	7-3		✓																													
	3-11																															
Lotion Arms and Legs twice daily	11-7																															
	7-3	✓	✓	✓	✓																											
	3-11	✓	✓	✓	✓																											
Shave Men daily Shave Women every 3 days	11-7																															
	7-3	✓			✓																											
	3-11																															
Amount snacks taken in %	AM	100	75	100	50																											
	PM	100	100	75	75																											
	HS	50	75	75	75																											
Intake and Output	11-7																															
	7-3																															
	3-11																															
Vital Signs Every Week	11-7																															
	7-3		✓																													
	3-11																															
Weight Every Week	11-7		✓																													
	7-3																															
	3-11																															

Fig. 2-3 Some of the items on an activities-of-daily-living flow sheet.

The Comprehensive Care Plan

Planning involves setting priorities and goals. Priorities reflect what is most important for the person. Goals are aimed at the person's highest level of well-being and function: physical, emotional, social, spiritual. OBRA requires that the health team be involved in planning the person's care. The care plan is called a *comprehensive care plan*. OBRA requires one for each resident. It identifies the person's strengths, problems, goals for care, and actions to take.

Phone Communications

You may have to answer phones at the nurses' station or in the person's room. Good phone communication skills are needed. The caller cannot see you. But you give much information by your tone of voice, how clearly you speak, and your attitude. You must be professional and courteous and practice good work ethics. Follow the center's policy and the guidelines in Box 2-1.

Dealing With Conflict

People bring their values, attitudes, opinions, experiences, and expectations to the work setting. Differences often lead to conflict—a clash between opposing interests and ideas. People disagree and argue. There are misunderstandings and unrest.

Conflicts arise over issues or events. Work schedules, absences, and the amount and quality of work performed are examples. The problems must be worked out. Otherwise, unkind words or actions may occur. The work setting becomes unpleasant. Care is affected.

To resolve a conflict, you need to identify the real problem. This is part of *problem solving*. The problem solving process involves these steps:

- Step 1: Define the problem. *A nurse ignores me.*
- Step 2: Collect information. The information must be about the problem. Do not include unrelated information. *The nurse does not look at me. The nurse does not talk to me. The nurse does not respond when I call her by name. The nurse does not ask me to help with tasks that require two people. The nurse talks to other staff members.*
- Step 3: Identify possible solutions. *Ignore the nurse. Talk to my supervisor. Talk to co-workers about the problem. Change jobs.*
- Step 4: Select the best solution. *Talk to my supervisor.*
- Step 5: Carry out the solution. *See below.*
- Step 6: Evaluate the results. *See below.*

Communication and good work ethics help prevent and resolve conflicts. Identify and solve problems before they become major issues. These guidelines can help you deal with conflict:

BOX 2-1   Guidelines for Answering Phones

- Answer the call after the first ring if possible. Be sure to answer by the fourth ring.
- Do not answer the phone in a rushed or hasty manner.
- Give a courteous greeting. Give your name, title, and department. For example: "Good morning. Three center. Jack Parks, nursing assistant."
- Write the following information when taking a message:
  —The caller's name and telephone number (include area code and extension number)
  —The date and time
  —The message
- Repeat the message and phone number back to the caller.
- Ask the caller to "Please hold" if necessary. First find out who is calling. Then ask if the caller can hold. Do not put callers with an emergency on hold.
- Do not lay the phone down or cover the receiver with your hand when not speaking to the caller. The caller may overhear confidential conversations.
- Return to a caller on hold within 30 seconds. Ask if the caller can wait longer or if the call can be returned.
- Do not give confidential information to any caller. Information about residents and employees is confidential. Refer such calls to a nurse.
- Transfer the call if appropriate:
  —Tell the caller that you are going to transfer the call.
  —Give the name of the department if appropriate.
  —Give the caller the phone number in case the call gets disconnected or the line is busy.
- End the conversation politely. Thank the person for calling, and say good-bye.
- Give the message to the appropriate person.

- Ask your supervisor for some time to talk privately. Explain the problem. Give facts and specific examples. Ask for advice in solving the problem.
- Approach the person with whom you have a conflict. Ask to talk privately. Be polite and professional.
- Agree on a time and place to talk.
- Talk in a private setting. No one should see or hear you and the other person.
- Explain the problem and what is bothering you. Give facts and specific behaviors. Focus on the problem. Do not focus on the person.
- Listen to the person. Do not interrupt.
- Identify ways to solve the problem. Offer your thoughts. Ask for the co-worker's ideas.
- Set a date and time to review the matter.
- Thank the person for meeting with you.
- Carry out the solutions.
- Review the matter as scheduled.

COMMUNICATING WITH THE RESIDENT

The resident is the most important person in the center. Each person has value. Each person has fears, needs, and rights. Each has suffered losses—loss of a home, family members, friends, and body functions.

The Whole Person

The whole person has physical, social, psychological, and spiritual parts. The parts are woven together and cannot be separated (Fig. 2-4).

Each part relates to and depends on the others. As a social being, a person speaks and communicates with others. Physically, the brain, mouth, tongue, lips, and throat structures must function for speech. Communication is also psychological. It involves thinking and reasoning.

To consider only the physical part is to ignore the person's ability to think, make decisions, and interact with others. It also ignores the person's experiences, life-style, culture, joys, sorrows, and needs.

Needs

A **need** is something necessary or desired for maintaining life and mental well-being. According to Abraham Maslow, a famous psychologist, basic needs must be met for a person to survive and function. These needs are arranged in order of importance (Fig. 2-5). Lower-level needs must be met before the higher-level needs. Basic needs, from the lowest level to the highest level, are:

- *Physical needs*—Oxygen, food, water, elimination, rest, and shelter are needed for life. They are needed to survive. A person dies within minutes without oxygen. Without food or water, a person feels weak and ill within a few hours. The kidneys and intestines must function. Otherwise toxic wastes build up in the blood. This can cause death. Without enough rest and sleep, a person becomes very tired. Without shelter, the person is exposed to extremes of heat and cold.
- *Safety and security needs*—These relate to feeling safe from harm, danger, and fear. Many persons do not feel safe and secure when admitted to a nursing center. They are not in their usual, secure home setting. They are in a strange place with strange routines. Strangers care for them. Some become scared and confused. Some fear pain and discomfort.
- *Love and belonging needs*—These relate to love, closeness, affection, and meaningful relationships. Some people become weaker or die from the lack of love and belonging. This is seen in older persons who have outlived family and friends.

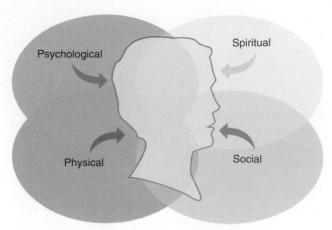

Fig. 2-4 The person is a physical, psychological, social, and spiritual being. The parts overlap and cannot be separated.

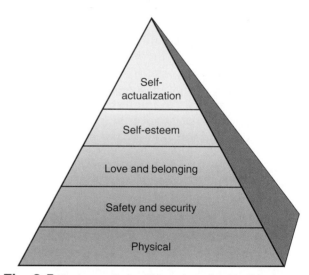

Fig. 2-5 Basic needs for life as described by Maslow. (From Maslow, Abraham H: *Motivation and personality*, © 1954, 1987. © 1970 by Abraham H. Maslow. Modified by permission of Prentice-Hall, Inc., Upper Saddle River, NJ.)

- *Self-esteem needs*—Self-esteem means to think well of oneself and to see oneself as useful and having value. People often lack self-esteem when ill, injured, older, or disabled.
- *Self-actualization needs*—Self-actualization means experiencing one's potential. It involves learning, understanding, and creating to the limit of a person's capacity. This is the highest need. Rarely, if ever, is it totally met. Most people constantly try to learn and understand more. This need can be postponed and life will continue.

Caring About Culture

Health Care Beliefs

Some *Mexican Americans* believe that illness is caused when hot and cold are not in balance. The ill person has had prolonged exposure to hot or cold. If cold caused the illness, the person is treated with "hot" therapies. If hot caused the illness; the person is treated with "cold" therapies. For example, if cold caused a headache, hot herbs are applied to the person's temples. If hot caused a headache, cold herbs are applied.

From Giger JN, Davidhizar RE: *Transcultural nursing: assessment and intervention*, ed 4, St Louis, 2004, Mosby.

Caring About Culture

Sick Care Practices

Folk practices are common among some *Vietnamese Americans.* They include *cao gio*—rubbing the skin with a coin to treat the common cold. Skin pinching *(bat gio)* is used for headaches and sore throats.

Some *Russian Americans* add herbs to drinks and enemas to treat stomach acidity. For headaches, an ointment is placed behind the ears and temples and at the back of the neck. There are treatments for backaches. One involves making a dough of dark rye flour and honey. The dough is placed on the spinal column. Many *Russian Americans* think that massage is useful.

From Giger JN, Davidhizar RE: *Transcultural nursing: assessment and intervention*, ed 4, St Louis, 2004, Mosby.

Culture and Religion

Culture is the characteristics of a group of people—language, values, beliefs, habits, likes, dislikes, and customs. They are passed from one generation to the next. The person's culture influences health beliefs and practices. Culture also affects behavior during illness.

People come from many cultures, races, and nationalities. Their family practices and food choices may differ from yours. So might their hygiene habits and clothing styles. Some speak a foreign language. Some cultures have beliefs about the causes and cures of illness. (See *Caring About Culture: Health Care Beliefs.*) They may perform rituals to rid the body of disease. (See *Caring About Culture: Sick Care Practices.*) Many have beliefs and rituals about dying and death (Chapter 10). Culture also is a factor in communication.

Religion relates to spiritual beliefs, needs, and practices. A person's religion influences health and illness practices. Religions may have beliefs and practices about daily living, behaviors, relationships with others, diet, healing, days of worship, medicine, and death.

Many people find comfort and strength from religion during illness. They may want to pray and observe religious practices. Nursing centers offer religious services. Assist the person to attend services as needed.

The care plan reflects the person's culture and religion. You must respect and accept the person's culture and religion. A person may not follow all beliefs and practices of his or her culture or religion. Some people do not practice a religion. Each person is unique. Do not judge the person by your standards.

Effective Communication

For effective communication between you and the person, you must:

- Follow the rules of communication (p. 24).
- Understand and respect the resident as a person.
- View the person as a physical, psychological, social, and spiritual human being.
- Appreciate the person's problems and frustrations.
- Respect the person's rights (Chapter 6).
- Respect the person's religion and culture.
- Give the person time to process (understand) information.
- Repeat information as often as needed. Repeat exactly what you said. Do not give the person a new message to process.
- Ask questions to see if the person understood you.
- Be patient. People with memory problems may ask the same question many times. Do not say that you are repeating information.

Verbal Communication. Words are used in **verbal communication.** Words are spoken or written. Most verbal communication involves the spoken word. Follow these rules:

- Face the person.
- Control the loudness and tone of your voice.
- Speak clearly, slowly, and distinctly.
- Do not use slang or vulgar words.
- Repeat information as needed.
- Ask one question at a time. Wait for the answer.
- Do not shout, whisper, or mumble.
- Be kind, courteous, and friendly.

Nonverbal Communication. **Nonverbal communication** does not use words. Messages are sent with gestures, facial expressions, posture, body movements, touch, and smell. Nonverbal messages more

Caring About Culture

Touch Practices

Touch practices vary among cultural groups. Touch is used often in *Mexico*. Some people believe that using touch while complimenting a person is important. It is thought to neutralize the power of the evil eye *(mal de ojo)*. Touch also is important in the *Philippine* culture.

Persons from the *United Kingdom* tend not to use touch. Touch is socially acceptable in *Poland*.

In *India*, men shake hands with other men. Men do not shake hands with women. Similar practices occur in *Vietnam*.

People from *China* do not like being touched by strangers. A nod or slight bow is given during introductions.

From D'Avanzo CE, Geissler EM: *Pocket guide to cultural health assessment*, ed 3, St Louis, 2003, Mosby.

Caring About Culture

Facial Expressions of Americans

- Coldness—there is a constant stare. Face muscles do not move.
- Fear—eyes are wide open. Eyebrows are raised. The mouth is tense with the lips drawn back.
- Anger—eyes are fixed in a hard stare. Upper lids are lowered. Eyebrows are drawn down. Lips are tightly compressed.
- Tiredness—eyes are rolled upward.
- Disapproval—eyes are rolled upward.
- Disgust—eyes are narrowed. The upper lip is curled. There are nose movements.
- Embarrassment—eyes are turned away or down. The face is flushed. The person pretends to smile. He or she rubs the eyes, nose, or face. He or she twitches hair, beard, or mustache.
- Surprise—there is a direct gaze with raised eyebrows.

From Giger JN, Davidhizar RE: *Transcultural nursing: assessment and intervention*, ed 4, St Louis, 2004, Mosby.

Caring About Culture

Facial Expressions of Other Cultures

Italian, Jewish, African-American, and *Spanish-speaking* persons smile readily. They use many facial expressions and gestures for happiness, pain, or displeasure. *Irish, English,* and *Northern European* persons tend to have less facial expression.

In some cultures, facial expressions mean the opposite of what the person is feeling. For example, *Asians* may conceal negative emotions with a smile.

From Giger JN, Davidhizar RE: *Transcultural nursing: assessment and intervention*, ed 4, St Louis, 2004, Mosby.

accurately reflect a person's feelings than words do. They are usually involuntary and hard to control. A person may say one thing but act another way. Watch the person's eyes, hand movements, gestures, posture, and other actions.

Touch. Touch is a very important form of nonverbal communication. It conveys comfort, caring, love, affection, interest, trust, concern, and reassurance. Touch means different things to different people. The meaning depends on age, gender (male or female), experiences, and culture. (See *Caring About Culture: Touch Practices.*)

Some people do not like to be touched. However, touch can show caring and warmth. Stroking or holding a hand can comfort a person. Touch should be gentle. It should not be hurried, rough, or sexual. To use touch, follow the person's care plan.

Body Language. People send messages through their **body language:**

- Facial expressions (See *Caring About Culture: Facial Expressions of Americans.* Also see *Caring About Culture: Facial Expressions of Other Cultures.*)
- Gestures
- Posture
- Hand and body movements
- Gait
- Eye contact
- Appearance (dress, hygiene, jewelry, perfume, cosmetics, tattoos, and so on)

Slumped posture may mean the person is not happy or feeling well. A person may deny pain. However, he or she protects the affected body part by standing, lying, or sitting in a certain way. Many messages are sent through body language.

Your actions, movements, and facial expressions send messages. So do how you stand, sit, walk, and look at a person. Your body language should show interest and enthusiasm. It should show caring and respect for the person. Often you will need to control your body language. Control reactions to odors from fluids, excretions, or the person's body. Many odors are beyond the person's control.

COMMUNICATION METHODS

Certain methods help you communicate with others. They result in better relationships. Information also is gained for the nurse to better plan to meet the person's needs.

Listening

Listening means to focus on verbal and nonverbal communication. You use sight, hearing, touch, and smell. You focus on what the person is saying. You observe nonverbal clues. They can support what the

person says. Or they can show other feelings. For example, Mr. Kerr says, "I don't want to go home. I want to stay here so my daughter won't have to care for me." You see tears, and he looks away from you. His verbal says happy. His nonverbal shows sadness.

Listening requires that you care and have interest. Follow these guidelines:

- Face the person.
- Have good eye contact with the person. (See *Caring About Culture: Eye Contact Practices.*)
- Lean toward the person. Do not sit back with your arms crossed.
- Respond to the person. Nod your head. Say "uh huh," "mmm," and "I see." Repeat what the person says. Ask questions.
- Avoid the communication barriers (p. 32).

Direct Questions

Direct questions focus on certain information. You ask the person something you need to know. Some direct questions have "yes" or "no" answers. Others require that the person give more information. For example:

You: Mr. Kerr, do you want to shave this morning?
Mr. Kerr: Yes.
You: Mr. Kerr, when would you like to do that?
Mr. Kerr: Could we start in 15 minutes? I want to call my son first.

You: Yes, we can start in 15 minutes. Did you have a bowel movement today?
Mr. Kerr: No.
You: You said you didn't eat well this morning. Can you tell me what you ate?
Mr. Kerr: I had toast and coffee. I just don't feel like eating.

Open-Ended Questions

Open-ended questions lead or invite the person to share thoughts, feelings, or ideas. The person chooses what to talk about. He or she controls what is talked about and the information given. Answers require more than a "yes" or "no." For example:

"What do you like about living with your daughter?"
"Tell me about your grandson."
"What was your wife like?"

Clarifying

Clarifying lets you make sure that you understand the message. You can ask the person to repeat the message, say you do not understand, or restate the message. For example:

"Could you say that again?"
"I'm sorry, I don't understand what you mean."
"You want Mrs. Parks to have a bed bath, not a shower."

Silence

Silence is a very powerful way to communicate. Sometimes you do not need to say anything. This is true during sad times. Just being there shows you care. At other times, silence gives time to think, organize thoughts, or choose words. Silence is useful when making decisions. It also helps when the person is upset and needs to regain control. Silence on your part shows caring and respect for the person's situation and feelings.

Sometimes pauses or long silences are uncomfortable. You do not need to talk when the person is silent. The person may need silence. (See *Caring About Culture: The Meaning of Silence.*)

Caring About Culture

Communicating With Persons From Other Cultures

- Ask the nurse about the beliefs and values of the person's culture. Learn as much as you can about the person's culture.
- Do not judge the person by your own attitudes, values, beliefs, and ideas.
- Follow the person's care plan. It includes the person's cultural beliefs and customs.
- Do the following when communicating with foreign-speaking persons:
  —Convey comfort by your tone of voice and body language.
  —Do not speak loudly or shout. It will not help the person understand English.
  —Speak slowly and distinctly.
  —Keep messages short and simple.
  —Be alert for words the person seems to understand.
  —Use gestures and pictures.
  —Repeat the message in other ways.
  —Avoid using medical terms and abbreviations.
  —Be alert for signs that the person is pretending to understand. Nodding and answering "yes" to all questions are signs that the person does not understand what you are saying.

Modified from Geissler EM: *Pocket guide to cultural assessment,* ed 2, St Louis, 1998, Mosby.

COMMUNICATION BARRIERS

Communication barriers prevent the sending and receiving of messages. Communication fails. You must avoid these barriers:

- *Using unfamiliar language.* You and the person must use and understand the same language. If not, messages are not accurately interpreted.
- *Cultural differences.* The person may attach different meanings to verbal and nonverbal communication. (See *Caring About Culture: Communicating With Persons From Other Cultures.*)
- *Changing the subject.* Someone changes the subject when the topic is uncomfortable. Avoid changing the subject whenever possible.
- *Giving opinions.* Opinions involve judging values, behavior, or feelings. Let others express feelings and concerns without adding your opinion. Do not make judgments or jump to conclusions.
- *Talking a lot when others are silent.* Talking too much is usually because of nervousness and discomfort with silence.
- *Failure to listen* Do not pretend to listen. It shows lack of interest and caring. This causes poor responses. You can miss complaints of pain, discomfort, or other symptoms that you must report to the nurse. You also can miss important information from the nurse.

- *Pat answers.* "Don't worry." "Everything will be okay." "Your doctor knows best." These make the person feel that you do not care about his or her concerns, feelings, and fears.
- *Illness and disability.* See "Residents With Disabilities" section.

RESIDENTS WITH DISABILITIES

A **disability** is a lost, absent, or impaired physical or mental function. Some illnesses, injuries, and birth defects affect speech, hearing, vision, cognitive function, and body movements. Verbal and nonverbal communication is affected.

The written word is used when a person cannot speak or hear. The nurse and care plan tell you how to communicate with the person. The devices shown in Figure 2-6 are often used. The person also may have poor vision. When writing messages:

- Keep them brief and concise.
- Use a black felt pen on white paper.
- Print in large letters.

Some persons can hear but cannot speak or read. Ask questions that have "yes" or "no" answers. The person can nod, blink, or use other gestures for "yes" and "no." Follow the care plan.

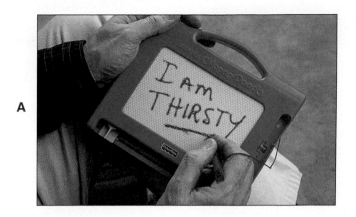

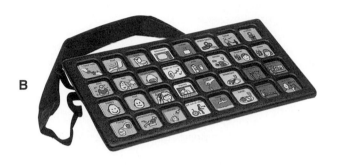

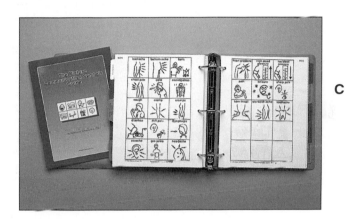

Fig. 2-6 Communication aids. **A,** Magic Slate. **B,** Electronic talking aid. **C,** Communication binder. (**B,** Courtesy Mayer-Johnson Co., Solana Beach, Calif.)

Persons With Ear Disorders

The ear functions in hearing and speech (Box 2-2, p. 34). How you pronounce words and voice volume depend on how you hear yourself. Hearing loss may result in slurred speech. Words may be pronounced wrong. Some people have monotone speech or drop word endings. It may be hard to understand what they say. Do not assume or pretend that you understand what a person says. Otherwise serious problems can result. Follow the guidelines in Box 2-3 on p. 35.

Hearing-impaired persons may wear hearing aids or read lips. They watch facial expressions, gestures, and body language. Follow the measures in Box 2-4 on p. 35 to help the person hear or lip-read (speech-read). Some people learn sign language (Fig. 2-8, p. 36).

Some people have *hearing assistance* dogs (hearing guide dogs). The dog alerts the person to sounds. Examples include phones, doorbells, smoke detectors, alarm clocks, sirens, or oncoming cars.

Hearing Aids. A hearing aid makes sounds louder (Fig. 2-9). It does not correct or cure the hearing problem. Hearing ability does not improve. The person hears better because the device makes sounds louder. Background noise and speech are louder.

Sometimes hearing aids do not seem to work properly. Try these simple measures:

- Check if the hearing aid is *on.* It has an *on* and *off* switch.
- Check the battery position.
- Insert a new battery if needed.
- Clean the earmold if necessary.

Hearing aids are costly. Handle and care for them properly. Report lost or damaged hearing aids to the nurse at once. *Check with the nurse before washing a hearing aid. Also follow the manufacturer's instructions.* Remove the battery at night. When not in use, turn the hearing aid off.

Text continued on p. 36

BOX 2-2   Hearing

Structure and Function

The ear functions in hearing (Fig. 2-7). It is divided into the *external ear, middle ear,* and *inner ear.*

The external ear (outer part) is called the *pinna* or *auricle.* Sound waves are guided through the external ear into the *auditory canal.* Glands in the auditory canal secrete a waxy substance called *cerumen.* The auditory canal extends about 1 inch to the *eardrum.* The eardrum *(tympanic membrane)* separates the external and middle ear.

The middle ear is a small space. It contains the *eustachian tube* and three small bones called *ossicles.* The eustachian tube connects the middle ear and the throat. Air enters the eustachian tube so that there is equal pressure on both sides of the eardrum. The ossicles amplify sound received from the eardrum. They transmit the sound to the inner ear.

The inner ear consists of the *semicircular canals* and the cochlea. The cochlea looks like a snail shell. It contains fluid. The fluid carries sound waves from the middle ear to the *auditory nerve.* The auditory nerve then carries the message to the brain.

Changes With Aging

Changes occur in the auditory nerve. Eardrums atrophy (shrink). High-pitched sounds are hard to hear. Severe hearing loss occurs if these changes progress. A hearing aid may be needed. It must be clean and correctly placed in the ear.

Wax secretion decreases. Wax becomes harder and thicker. It is easily impacted (wedged in the ear). This can cause hearing loss. A doctor or nurse removes the wax.

Common Disorders

- *Otitis media*—Otitis media is infection *(itis)* of the middle *(media)* ear *(ot).* It is acute or chronic. Chronic otitis media can damage the tympanic membrane (eardrum) or the ossicles. Permanent hearing loss can occur. Fluid builds up in the ear. Pain (earache) and hearing loss occur. So do fever and ringing in the ears *(tinnitus).*
- *Meniere's disease*—Meniere's disease is a chronic disease of the inner ear. The increased fluid causes pressure in the middle ear. Tinnitus, hearing loss, and vertigo occur. *Vertigo* means dizziness. Whirling and spinning sensations are felt. Severe dizziness causes nausea and vomiting. Attacks last a few minutes or many hours.
- *Hearing loss*—Hearing loss means difficulty hearing normal conversations. Losses range from mild to severe. Deafness is the most severe form. *Deafness* is hearing loss in which it is impossible for the person to understand speech through hearing alone. Temporary hearing loss can occur from ear wax (cerumen). Symptoms of hearing loss include:
  —Speaking too loudly
  —Leaning forward to hear
  —Turning and cupping the better ear toward the speaker
  —Answering questions or responding inappropriately
  —Asking for words to be repeated

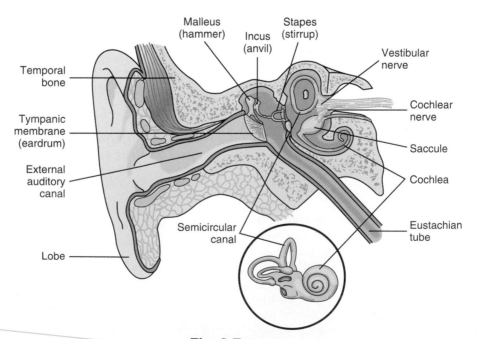

Fig. 2-7 The ear.

BOX 2-3 | **Communicating With the Speech-Impaired Person**

- Listen and give the person your full attention.
- Ask the person questions to which you know the answer. This helps you learn how the person speaks.
- Determine the subject being discussed. This helps you understand main points.
- Ask the person to repeat or rephrase statements if necessary.

- Repeat what the person has said. Ask if your understanding is correct.
- Ask the person to write down key words or the message.
- Watch the person's lip movements.
- Watch facial expressions, gestures, and body language for clues about what is being said.

BOX 2-4 | **Communicating With the Hearing-Impaired Person**

- Gain attention. Alert the person to your presence. Raise an arm or hand or lightly touch the person's arm. Do not startle or approach the person from behind.
- Position yourself at the person's level. If the person is sitting, you sit. If the person is standing, you stand.
- Face the person when speaking. Do not turn or walk away while you are talking. Do not talk to the person from the doorway or another room.
- Make sure the person is wearing his or her hearing aid. Make sure it is turned on and working.
- Stand or sit in good light. Shadows and glares affect the person's ability to see your face clearly.
- Make sure the person is wearing needed eyeglasses or contact lenses. This helps the person see your face for speech-reading. NOTE: Eyeglasses and contact lenses must be clean for clear vision.
- Speak clearly, distinctly, and slowly.
- Speak in a normal tone of voice. Do not shout.
- Adjust the pitch of your voice as needed. Ask the person if he or she can hear you better:
  —If the person does not wear a hearing aid, lower the pitch if you are a female. Women's voices are higher-pitched and are harder to hear than lower-pitched male voices.
  —If the person wears a hearing aid, raise the pitch slightly.

- Do not cover your mouth, smoke, eat, or chew gum while talking. Mouth movements are affected.
- Keep your hands away from your face. The person must be able to clearly see your face.
- Stand or sit on the side of the better ear.
- State the topic of conversation first.
- Tell the person when you are changing the subject. State the new subject of conversation.
- Use short sentences and simple words.
- Use gestures and facial expressions to give useful clues.
- Write out important names and words.
- Say things in another way if the person does not seem to understand.
- Keep conversations and discussions short. This avoids tiring the person.
- Repeat and rephrase statements as needed.
- Be alert to the messages you send by your facial expressions, gestures, and body language.
- Reduce or eliminate background noises. For example, turn off radios, stereos, TVs, air conditioners, and fans.

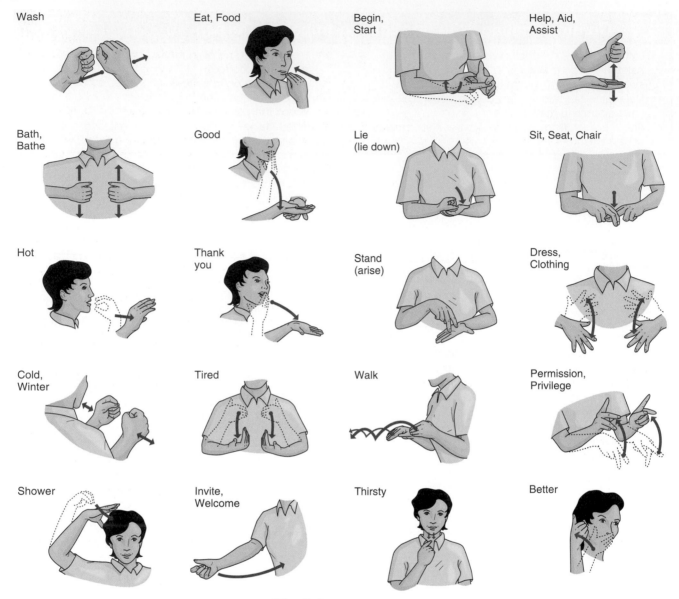

Wash

Eat, Food

Begin, Start

Help, Aid, Assist

Bath, Bathe

Good

Lie (lie down)

Sit, Seat, Chair

Hot

Thank you

Stand (arise)

Dress, Clothing

Cold, Winter

Tired

Walk

Permission, Privilege

Shower

Invite, Welcome

Thirsty

Better

Fig. 2-8 Sign language.

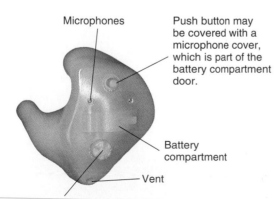

Microphones

Push button may be covered with a microphone cover, which is part of the battery compartment door.

Battery compartment

Vent

On/Off switch/Volume control

Fig. 2-9 A hearing aid. (Courtesy Siemens Hearing Instrument, Piscataway, NJ.)

Persons With Eye Disorders

Problems range from mild vision loss to complete blindness. Vision loss is sudden or gradual in onset. One or both eyes are affected. See Box 2-5.

Eyeglasses and contact lenses can correct many vision problems. Some people wear glasses for reading or seeing at a distance (Fig. 2-11, p. 38). Others wear them for all activities. Contact lenses are usually worn while awake.

Blindness. Some people are totally blind. Others sense some light but have no usable vision. Still others have some usable vision but cannot read newsprint. Moving about, daily activities, reading braille, and using a guide dog (Seeing Eye dog) all require training.

BOX 2-5   Vision

Structure and Function

The eye is a delicate organ that is easily injured. Bones of the skull, eyelids and eyelashes, and tears protect the eyes from injury. Eye structures are shown in Figure 2-10. The eye has three layers:

- The *sclera,* the white of the eye, is the outer layer. It is made of tough connective tissue.
- The *choroid* is the second layer. Blood vessels, the *ciliary muscle,* and the iris make up the choroid. The iris gives the eye its color. The opening in the middle of the iris is the *pupil.* Pupil size varies with the amount of light entering the eye. The pupil constricts (narrows) in bright light and dilates (widens) in dim or dark places.
- The *retina* is the inner layer of the eye. Receptors for vision and the nerve fibers of the optic nerve are in the retina.

Light enters the eye through the *cornea.* The cornea is the transparent part of the outer layer that lies over the eye. Light rays pass to the *lens,* which lies behind the pupil. The light is then reflected to the retina and carried to the brain by the optic nerve.

The *aqueous chamber* separates the cornea from the lens. The chamber is filled with a fluid called *aqueous humor.* The fluid helps the cornea keep its shape and position. The *vitreous body* is behind the lens. The vitreous body is a gelatin-like substance that supports the retina and maintains the eye's shape.

Changes With Aging

Eyelids thin and wrinkle. Tear secretion is less.

The pupil becomes smaller and responds less to light. Vision is poor at night or in dark rooms. The eye takes longer to adjust to lighting changes. Vision problems occur when going from a dark to a bright room. They also occur when going from a bright to a dark room.

Clear vision is reduced. Eyeglasses are needed. The lens of the eye yellows. Therefore greens and blues are harder to see.

Older persons become more farsighted. The lens becomes more rigid with age. It is harder for the eye to shift from far to near vision and from near to far vision. These changes increase the risk of falls and accidents (Chapter 4).

Common Disorders

- *Glaucoma*—Fluid pressure within the eye increases. This damages the optic nerve. Vision loss with eventual blindness occurs. Onset is gradual or sudden. Peripheral vision is lost. The person sees through a tunnel. Blurred vision, halos around lights, and sensitivity to glares occur. Treatment involves drug therapy and possibly surgery. The goal is to prevent further damage to the optic nerve. Prior damage cannot be reversed.
- *Cataract*—The lens of the eye becomes cloudy (opaque). Light cannot enter the eye. Cataract comes from the Greek word that means *waterfall.* Trying to see is like looking through a waterfall. Vision blurs and dims. Print and colors look faded. The person is sensitive to light and glares. A cataract can occur in one or both eyes. Aging is the most common cause. Surgery is the only treatment. The lens is removed. A plastic lens is put in the eye. Vision returns to near normal.

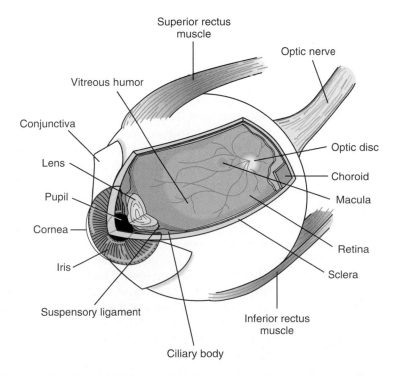

Fig. 2-10 The eye.

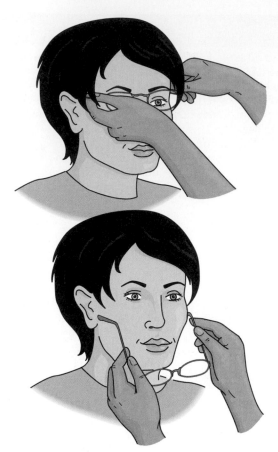

Fig. 2-11 Removing eyeglasses. Remove eyeglasses by holding the frames in front of both ears. Lift the frames from the ears, and bring the glasses down away from the face.

BOX 2-6 Communicating With a Blind Person

- Ask the person how much he or she can see. Do not assume the person is totally blind or that the person has some vision.
- Face the person when speaking. Speak slowly and clearly.
- Use a normal tone of voice. Do not shout or speak loudly. Blindness does not mean the person has hearing loss.
- Identify yourself. Give your name, title, and reason for being there. Do not touch the person until you have indicated your presence.
- Identify others. Explain where each person is located and what the person is doing.
- Address the person by name. This tells the person that you are directing a comment or question to him or her.
- Do not avoid using the words "see," "look," or "read."
- Give step-by-step explanations of procedures as you perform them. Indicate when the procedure is over.
- Offer assistance. Simply say "May I help you?" Respect the person's answer.
- Give specific directions. Say "right behind you," "on your left," or "in front of you." Avoid phrases like "over here" or "over there."
- Keep the signal light within the person's reach.
- Provide a radio, compact disks or audiotapes, audio books, television, and braille books.
- Tell the person when you are leaving the room.

Braille is a writing system that uses raised dots. Dots are arranged for each letter of the alphabet. The first 10 letters also represent 0 through 9. Braille is read with the fingers.

Blind persons learn to move about using a white cane with a red tip or a Seeing Eye dog. Both are used worldwide by persons who are blind. The dog sees for the person. The dog is aware of danger and guides the person through traffic.

Treat the blind person with respect and dignity—not with pity. Most blind people adjust well and lead independent lives. Some were blind for a long time. Others for a short time. Follow the practices in Box 2-6.

Persons With Aphasia

Aphasia is the inability (*a*) to speak (*phasia*). *Stroke* is a common cause. With a stroke, blood supply to part of the brain is suddenly interrupted. Brain cells in the area do not get oxygen and nutrients. Brain damage occurs. Functions controlled by that part of the brain are lost or impaired.

There are two basic types of aphasia. **Expressive aphasia** is difficulty expressing or sending out thoughts. Thinking is clear. There are problems speaking, spelling, counting, gesturing, or writing. The person thinks one thing but says another. For example, the person thinks about food but asks for a book. People are called the wrong names even when names are known. Some people produce sounds and no words. The person may cry or swear for no reason.

Receptive aphasia relates to difficulty receiving information. The person has trouble understanding what is said or read. People and common objects are not recognized. The person may not know how to use a fork, toilet, cup, TV, phone, or other items.

With *expressive* aphasia, messages are not sent. With *receptive* aphasia, messages are not interpreted. Some people have both types. This is called **expressive-receptive aphasia.**

The person has many emotional needs. Frustration, depression, and anger are common. Communication is needed to function and relate to others. The person wants to communicate but cannot. You need to be patient and kind.

Person Who Are Comatose

People who are comatose are unconscious. They cannot respond to others. Often they can hear and feel touch and pain. Assume that a comatose person can hear and understand you. Use touch and give care gently. Practice these measures:

- Knock before entering the person's room.
- Tell the person your name, the time, and the place every time you enter the room.
- Give care on the same schedule every day.
- Explain what you are going to do. Explain care measures step-by-step as you do them.
- Tell the person when you are finishing care.
- Use touch to communicate care, concern, and comfort (p. 30).
- Tell the person what time you will be back to check on him or her.
- Tell the person when you are leaving the room.

THE FAMILY AND VISITORS

Family and friends help meet safety and security, love and belonging, and self-esteem needs. They offer support and comfort. They lessen loneliness. Some also help with the person's care. (See *Caring About Culture: Family Roles in Sick Care*.) The presence or absence of family or friends can affect recovery and quality of life.

The person has the right to visit with family and friends in private and without any unnecessary interruptions. You may need to give care when visitors are there. Do not expose the person's body in front of them. Politely ask them to leave the room. Show them where to wait. Promptly tell them when they can return.

Treat family and visitors with courtesy and respect. They have concerns about the person's condition and care. They need support and understanding. However, do not discuss the person's condition with them. Refer their questions to the nurse.

Visiting rules depend on center policy and the person's age and condition. Dying persons can usually have family present all the time. Know your center's policies and each person's needs.

A visitor may upset or tire a person. Report your observations to the nurse. The nurse will speak with the visitor about the person's needs.

Caring About Culture

Family Roles in Sick Care

In *Vietnam*, all family members are involved in the person's care. A similar practice is common in *China*. Family members bathe, feed, and comfort the person. However, women in *Mexico* cannot give care at home if it involves touching the genitals of adult men.

From D'Avanzo CE, Geissler EM: *Pocket guide to cultural health assessment*, ed 3, St Louis, 2003, Mosby.

Review Questions

Circle the **BEST** answer.

1   To communicate, you should
   a   Use medical terms
   b   Give long answers
   c   Present information as it comes to your mind
   d   Give facts and be specific

2   Mrs. Barr is discharged from the center. Her medical record is
   a   Destroyed to protect privacy
   b   Sent home with her
   c   Permanent
   d   On computer

3   These statements are about medical records. Which is *false?*
   a   The record is used to communicate information about the person.
   b   The record is a written account of the person's illness and response to treatment.
   c   The record can be used as evidence of the care given.
   d   Anyone working in the center can read the medical record.

4   A person is weighed daily. The measurement is recorded on the
   a   Admission sheet   c   Flow sheet
   b   Activities-of-daily-   d   Progress notes
      living record

Review Questions

5 Where does the nurse describe the nursing care given?
   a Admission sheet
   b Nursing history
   c Graphic sheet
   d Progress notes

6 How should you answer a resident's phone?
   a "Good morning. Mrs. Barr's room."
   b "Good morning. Third floor."
   c "Hello."
   d "Good morning. Mrs. Barr's room. Joan Bates, nursing assistant, speaking."

7 A co-worker is often late for work. This means extra work for you. To resolve the conflict you should
   a Explain the problem to your supervisor
   b Tell other nursing assistants how you feel about the problem
   c Ignore that co-worker
   d Refuse to work with that co-worker

8 Mrs. Jones is blind. You focus on her
   a Care plan
   b Physical, safety and security, and esteem needs
   c As a physical, psychological, social, and spiritual person
   d Cultural and religious needs

9 Which basic needs are the *most* essential?
   a Self-actualization needs
   b Self-esteem needs
   c Love and belonging needs
   d Safety and security needs

10 Mrs. Jones says "What are they doing to me?" What basic needs are not being met?
   a Physical needs
   b Safety and security needs
   c Love and belonging needs
   d Self-esteem needs

11 Mr. Kerr has a garden behind the nursing center's garage. This relates to
   a Self-actualization
   b Self-esteem
   c Love and belonging
   d Safety and security

12 Which is *false?*
   a Culture influences health and illness practices.
   b Culture and religion influence food practices.
   c Religious and cultural practices are allowed in nursing centers.
   d A person must follow all beliefs and practices of his or her religion or culture.

13 Which is *false?*
   a Verbal communication uses the written or spoken word.
   b Verbal communication is the truest reflection of a person's feelings.
   c Messages are sent by facial expressions, gestures, posture, and body movements.
   d Touch means different things to different people.

14 To communicate with Mrs. Long, you should
   a Use medical words and phrases
   b Change the subject often
   c Give your opinions
   d Be quiet when she is silent

15 Which might mean that you are *not* listening?
   a You sit facing the person.
   b You have good eye contact with the person.
   c You sit with your arms crossed.
   d You ask questions.

16 Which is a direct question?
   a "Do you feel better now?"
   b "What are your plans for home."
   c "What will you do when you get home?"
   d "You said that you can't work."

Review Questions

17 Which promotes communication?
a "Don't worry."
b "Everything will be just fine."
c "This is a good hospital."
d "Why are you crying?"

18 Mr. Brown has hearing loss. When talking to him, you should do the following *except*
a Speak clearly, distinctly, and slowly
b Sit or stand where there is good light
c Shout
d Stand or sit on the side of the better ear

19 A person has a speech problem. You should
a Pretend to understand so the person is not embarrassed
b Write key words and shout
c Ask the person to repeat or rephrase statements when necessary
d Ask only a few questions at a time

20 A person has a hearing aid. The hearing aid
a Corrects the hearing problem
b Makes sounds louder
c Makes speech clearer
d Lowers background noise

21 A person's hearing aid does not seem to be working. First, you should
a See if it is turned on
b Wash it with soap and water
c Have it repaired
d Remove the batteries

22 Braille involves
a A white cane with a red tip for walking
b Raised dots arranged for letters of the alphabet
c Using a Seeing Eye dog
d Audio books

23 Mrs. Hart is blind. You should do the following *except*
a Identify yourself
b Shout when speaking to her
c Explain procedures step-by-step
d Ask how much she can see

24 Receptive aphasia means that the person has trouble
a Talking
b Writing
c Understanding messages
d Using gestures

25 Mrs. Parker is comatose. Which action is *false?*
a Assume that she can hear and feel touch.
b Explain what you are going to do.
c Use listening and silence to communicate.
d Tell her when you are leaving the room.

26 A visitor seems to tire a person. What should you do?
a Ask the person to leave
b Tell the nurse
c Stay in the room to observe the person and visitor
d Find out the visitor's relationship to the person

Answers to these questions are on p. 388.

CHAPTER 3

Preventing Infection

Objectives

- Define the key terms listed in this chapter
- Identify what microbes need to live and grow
- List the signs and symptoms of infection
- Explain the chain of infection
- Describe the changes in the immune system that occur with aging
- Describe aseptic practices
- Explain how to care for equipment and supplies
- Explain Standard Precautions, Transmission-Based Precautions, and the Bloodborne Pathogen Standard
- Perform the procedures described in this chapter

asepsis Being free of disease-producing microbes

biohazardous waste Items contaminated with blood, body fluids, secretions, and excretions; *bio* means life, and *hazardous* means dangerous or harmful

carrier A human or animal that is a reservoir for microbes but does not have signs and symptoms of infection

clean technique Medical asepsis

communicable disease A disease caused by pathogens that spread easily; a contagious disease

contagious disease Communicable disease

contamination The process of becoming unclean

disinfection The process of destroying pathogens

infection A disease resulting from the invasion and growth of microbes in the body

infection control Methods to prevent the spread of infection

medical asepsis Practices used to remove or destroy pathogens and to prevent their spread from one person or place to another person or place; clean technique

microbe A microorganism

microorganism A small *(micro)* living plant or animal *(organism)* seen only with a microscope; a microbe

non-pathogen A microbe that does not usually cause an infection

pathogen A microbe that is harmful and can cause an infection

sterile The absence of *all* microbes

sterilization The process of destroying *all* microbes

Infection is a major safety and health hazard. Minor infections cause short illnesses. Some infections are serious and can cause death. Older and disabled persons are at risk. The health team uses methods to prevent the spread of infection. Called **infection control,** such methods protect residents, visitors, and staff from infection.

MICROORGANISMS

A **microorganism (microbe)** is a small *(micro)* living plant or animal *(organism)*. It is seen only with a microscope. Microbes are everywhere—in the mouth, nose, respiratory tract, stomach, and intestines. They are on the skin and in the air, soil, water, and food. They are on animals, clothing, and furniture.

Some microbes are harmful and can cause infections. They are called **pathogens. Non-pathogens** are microbes that do not usually cause an infection.

Microbes need a *reservoir (host)* to live and grow. People, plants, animals, the soil, food, and water are reservoirs. Microbes need *water* and *nourishment* from the reservoir. Most need *oxygen* to live. Others cannot live where there is oxygen. A *warm* and *dark* environment is needed. Most microbes grow best at body temperature. They are destroyed by heat and light.

INFECTION

An **infection** is a disease resulting from the invasion and growth of microbes in the body. A *local infection* is in a body part. A *systemic infection* involves the whole body. The person has some or all of the signs and symptoms in Box 3-1 on p. 44.

The chain of infection (Fig. 3-1, p. 44) begins with a *source*—a pathogen. The pathogen needs a *reservoir* where it can grow and multiply. Humans and animals are reservoirs. If they do not have signs and symptoms of infection, they are **carriers**. Carriers can pass the pathogen to others. To leave the reservoir, the pathogen needs a *portal of exit*. Exits are the respiratory, gastrointestinal, urinary, and reproductive tracts, breaks in the skin, and the blood.

After leaving the reservoir, the pathogen must be *transmitted* to another host (Fig. 3-2, p. 44). The pathogen enters the body through a *portal of entry*. Portals of entry and exit are the same. A *susceptible host* (a person at risk for infection) is needed for the microbe to grow and multiply.

The human body can protect itself from infection. Being able to resist infection relates to age, nutrition, stress, fatigue, and health. Drugs, disease, and injury also are factors. See Box 3-2 on p. 45.

Text continued on p. 46

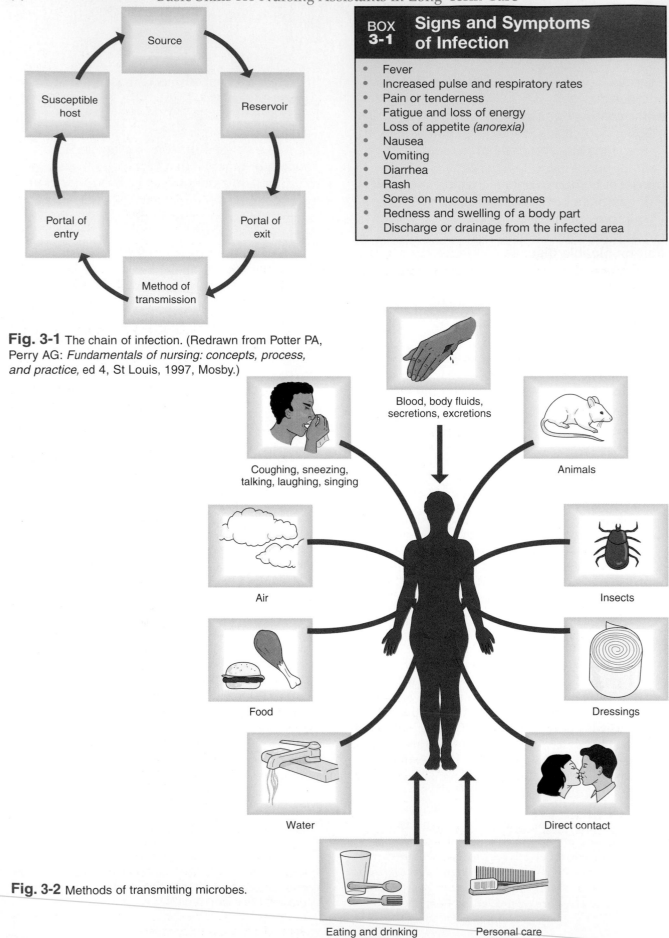

Fig. 3-1 The chain of infection. (Redrawn from Potter PA, Perry AG: *Fundamentals of nursing: concepts, process, and practice,* ed 4, St Louis, 1997, Mosby.)

BOX 3-1	Signs and Symptoms of Infection

- Fever
- Increased pulse and respiratory rates
- Pain or tenderness
- Fatigue and loss of energy
- Loss of appetite (*anorexia*)
- Nausea
- Vomiting
- Diarrhea
- Rash
- Sores on mucous membranes
- Redness and swelling of a body part
- Discharge or drainage from the infected area

Fig. 3-2 Methods of transmitting microbes.

BOX
3-2

The Immune System

Structure and Function

The immune system protects the body from disease and infection. Abnormal body cells can grow into tumors. Sometimes the body produces substances that cause the body to attack itself. Microorganisms (bacteria, viruses, and other germs) can cause an infection. The immune system defends against threats inside and outside the body.

The immune system gives the body immunity. *Immunity* means that a person has protection against a disease or condition. The person will not get or be affected by the disease.

Changes With Aging

With aging, the immune system weakens and declines in function. Therefore older persons are at risk for infections, cancer, and other diseases. Some can be life-threatening.

Common Disorders

- *Pneumonia*—is an inflammation and infection of lung tissue. Affected tissues fill with fluid. The person is very ill. Fever, chills, painful cough, chest pain on breathing, and a rapid pulse occur. Sputum is thick and green, yellowish, or rust colored. Drugs are ordered for infection and pain. Fluid intake is increased because of fever and to thin mucous secretions so they are easier to cough up. IV fluids and oxygen may be needed. The person needs plenty of rest. The semi-Fowler's position eases breathing. Mouth care is important. Frequent linen changes are needed because of fever.
- *Tuberculosis (TB)* –is a bacterial infection. It affects the lungs. It also can occur in the kidneys and bones. If untreated, death can occur. TB is spread by airborne droplets with coughing, sneezing, speaking, and singing. An active infection may not occur for many years. Signs and symptoms are tiredness, loss of appetite, weight loss, fever, and night sweats. Coughing and sputum production increase over time. Chest pain occurs. Drugs for TB are given. The mouth and nose are covered with tissues when coughing or sneezing. Tissues are placed in a biohazard bag. Hand washing after contact with sputum is essential.
- *Cystitis*—is a bladder *(cyst)* infection *(itis)* caused by bacteria. Urinary frequency and urgency are common. So is pain on urination. Urine may contain blood and pus and have a foul odor. Antibiotics are ordered. Fluids are encouraged—usually 2000 ml per day. Untreated cystitis can lead to pyelonephritis.
- *Pyelonephritis*—is an inflammation *(itis)* of the kidney *(nephr)* pelvis *(pyelo)*. Infection is the most common cause. Cloudy urine may contain pus, mucus, and blood. Chills, fever, back pain, and nausea and vomiting occur. So do the signs and symptoms of cystitis. Treatment involves antibiotics and fluids.
- *Hepatitis*—is an inflammation of the liver. It can be mild or cause death. Signs and symptoms include loss of appetite, weakness, fatigue, nausea, and vomiting. Fever, rash, dark urine, jaundice (yellow skin color), and light-colored bowel movements occur. Treatment involves bedrest, a healthy diet, and no alcohol. Recovery takes about 8 weeks. There are five types of hepatitis:
  —*Hepatitis A* is spread by the fecal-oral route. The virus is ingested when eating or drinking contaminated food or water. It is ingested also when eating or drinking from a contaminated vessel. Causes include poor sanitation, crowded living conditions, poor nutrition, and poor hygiene. Anal sex and IV drug abuse also are causes.
  —*Hepatitis B* is caused by the hepatitis B virus (HBV). It is present in the blood and body fluids (saliva, semen, vaginal secretions) of infected persons. It is spread by contaminated blood products, IV drug use, and sexual contact, especially anal sex. (For the HBV vaccine, see p. 61.)
  —*Hepatitis C* is spread by blood contaminated with the virus. A person may have the virus but no symptoms. Serious liver disease and damage may show up years later. Even without symptoms, the person can transmit the disease. The virus is spread by blood contaminated with the virus, IV drug use, inhaling cocaine through contaminated straws, contaminated needles used for tattooing and body piercing, and high-risk sexual activity.
  —*Hepatitis D* and *Hepatitis E*—Hepatitis D occurs in persons infected with the hepatitis B virus (HBV). It is spread the same way as HBV. Hepatitis E occurs in countries with contaminated water supplies. It is spread by the fecal-oral route.
- *Acquired immunodeficiency syndrome (AIDS)*—is caused by the human immunodeficiency virus (HIV). It attacks the immune system. The person's ability to fight other diseases is affected. AIDS has no vaccine and no cure at present. It is a life-threatening disease. The virus is spread through certain body fluids—blood, semen, vaginal secretions, and breast milk. The virus is transmitted mainly by:
  —Unprotected anal, vaginal, or oral sex with an infected person ("Unprotected" is without a new latex or polyurethane condom.)
  —Needle and syringe sharing among IV drug users
  —HIV-infected mothers before or during childbirth
  —HIV-infected mothers through breast-feeding
  Signs and symptoms include loss of appetite, weight loss, fever, cough, night sweats, and diarrhea. The person is tired, has skin rashes, and has swollen glands. White patches in the mouth and purple blotches or bumps on the skin also occur. Dementia can occur (Chapter 18). Some persons infected with HIV are symptom-free for 8 to 10 years. However, they carry the virus. They can spread it to others. You may care for persons with AIDS or those who are HIV carriers. This includes older persons. A person may have the HIV virus but no symptoms. In some persons, HIV is not yet diagnosed.

Continued

BOX 3-2   The Immune System—cont'd

- *Sexually transmitted diseases (STDs)*—are spread by oral, vaginal, or anal sex. At least one partner must have an STD. Some people do not have signs and symptoms or are not aware of an infection. Others know but do not seek treatment because of embarrassment. Using condoms helps prevent the spread of STDs, especially HIV and AIDS. Some STDs are also spread through skin breaks, by contact with infected body fluids (blood, semen, saliva), or by contaminated blood or needles.
- *Pediculosis (lice)*—is the infestation with lice. (*Infestation* means being in or on a host.) Lice are parasites. Lice bites cause severe itching in the affected area. *Pediculosis capitis* is the infestation of the scalp *(capitis)* with lice. *Pediculosis pubis* is the infestation of the pubic *(pubis)* hair with lice. Head and pubic lice attach their eggs to hair shafts. *Pediculosis corporis* is the infestation of the body *(corporis)* with lice. Lice eggs attach to clothing and furniture. Lice easily spread to others through clothing, furniture, bed linen, and sexual contact. They also are spread by sharing combs and brushes. Medicated shampoos, lotions, and creams are used to treat lice. Thorough bathing is needed. So is washing clothing and linen in hot water. Report signs of lice to the nurse at once.
- *Scabies*—is a skin disorder caused by a female mite. A *mite* is a very small spider-like organism. The female mite burrows into the skin and lays eggs. When the eggs hatch, the females produce more eggs. The skin becomes infested with mites. The person has a rash and intense itching. Common sites are between the fingers, around the wrists, in the underarm area, on the thighs, and in the genital area. The other sites include the breasts, waist, and buttocks. Scabies is highly contagious. It is transmitted to others by close contact. Persons living in crowded living settings are at risk. So are persons with weakened immune systems. Special creams are ordered to kill the mites. The person's room is cleaned. Clothing and linens are washed in hot water.
- *Drug resistant organisms*—are organisms that are able to resist the effects of antibiotics. Antibiotics are drugs that kill microbes that cause infections. Some microbes can change their structures. This makes them more difficult to kill. They can survive in the presence of antibiotics. Therefore the infections they cause are difficult to treat. There are two main causes of drug-resistant organisms—doctors prescribing antibiotics when they are not needed (over-prescribing) and people not taking antibiotics for the amount of time prescribed. Two common types of drug resistant organisms are:
  - *Methicillin-resistant Staphylococcus aureus (MRSA)*—*Staphylococcus aureus* (commonly called "staph") is normally found in the nose and on the skin. It can cause serious wound infections and pneumonia. This microbe has become resistant to methicillin, a type of penicillin.
  - *Vancomycin-resistant Enterococcus (VRE)*—*Enterococcus* is normally found in the intestines and is present in feces. It can be transmitted to others by contaminated hands, toilet seats, care equipment, and other items that the hands touch. When not in its natural site (the intestines), it can cause an infection. It can cause urinary tract, wound, pelvic, and other infections. This microbe is resistant to many antibiotics.

ASEPSIS

Asepsis is being free of disease-producing microbes. Microbes are everywhere. Measures are needed to achieve asepsis. **Medical asepsis (clean technique)** is the practices used to:

- Remove or destroy pathogens. The number of pathogens is reduced.
- Prevent pathogens from spreading from one person or place to another person or place.

Contamination is the process of becoming unclean. An item or area is *clean* when it is free of pathogens. The item or area is contaminated if pathogens are present. **Sterile** means the absence of *all* microbes—pathogens and non-pathogens. A sterile item or area is contaminated when pathogens or non-pathogens are present.

Common Aseptic Practices

Aseptic practices break the chain of infection. To prevent the spread of microbes:

- Wash your hands:
  - After urinating or having a bowel movement
  - After changing tampons or sanitary pads
  - After contact with your own or another person's blood, body fluids, secretions, or excretions. This includes saliva, vomitus, urine, feces, vaginal discharge, mucus, semen, wound drainage, pus, and respiratory secretions
  - After coughing, sneezing, or blowing your nose
  - Before and after handling, preparing, or eating food
- Cover your nose and mouth when coughing, sneezing, or blowing your nose.
- Bathe, wash hair, and brush your teeth regularly.
- Wash fruits and raw vegetables before eating or serving them.
- Wash cooking and eating utensils with soap and water after use.
- Practice the measures in Box 3-3.

BOX 3-3   Aseptic Measures

Controlling Reservoirs (Hosts—You or the Person)

- Provide for the person's hygiene needs (Chapter 11).
- Wash contaminated areas with soap and water. Feces, urine, and blood can contain microbes. So can body fluids, secretions, and excretions.
- Use leak-proof plastic bags for soiled tissues, linen, and other materials.
- Keep tables, counters, wheelchair trays, and other surfaces clean and dry.
- Label bottles with the person's name and the date the bottle was opened.
- Keep bottles and fluid containers tightly capped or covered.
- Keep drainage containers below the drainage site.
- Empty drainage containers and dispose of drainage following center policy. Usually drainage containers are emptied every shift. Follow the nurse's instructions.

Controlling Portals of Exit

- Cover your nose and mouth when coughing or sneezing.
- Provide the person with tissues to use when coughing or sneezing.
- Wear personal protective equipment as needed (p. 52).

Controlling Transmission

- Make sure all persons have their own linens and personal care items. This includes wash basins, bedpans, urinals, commodes, and eating and drinking utensils.
- Do not take equipment from one person's room to use for another person. Even if the item is unused, do not take it from one room to another.
- Hold equipment and linens away from your uniform (Fig. 3-3, p. 48).
- Practice hand hygiene (p. 48):
  —Before and after contact with every person
  —Whenever your hands are soiled
  —After contact with blood, body fluids, secretions, or excretions
  —After removing gloves
  —Before assisting with any sterile procedure
- Assist the person with hand washing:
  —Before and after eating
  —After elimination
  —After changing tampons, sanitary napkins, or other personal hygiene products
  —After contact with blood, body fluids, secretions, or excretions

- Do not shake linens or equipment.
- Clean from the cleanest area to the dirtiest. This prevents soiling a clean area.
- Clean away from your body. Do not dust, brush, or wipe toward yourself. Otherwise you transmit microbes to your skin, hair, and clothing.
- Flush urine and feces down the toilet. Avoid splatters and splashes.
- Pour contaminated liquids directly into sinks or toilets. Avoid splashing onto other areas.
- Do not sit on a person's bed. You will pick up microbes. You will transfer them to the next surface that you sit on.
- Do not use items that are on the floor. The floor is contaminated.
- Clean tubs, showers, and shower chairs after each use. Follow the center's disinfection procedures.
- Clean bedpans, urinals, and commodes after each use. Follow the center's disinfection procedures.
- Report pests—ants, spiders, mice, and so on.

Controlling Portals of Entry

- Provide for good skin care (Chapters 11 and 15). This promotes intact skin.
- Provide for good oral hygiene (Chapter 11). This promotes intact mucous membranes.
- Do not let the person lie on tubes or other items. This protects the skin from injury.
- Make sure linens are dry and wrinkle-free (Chapter 8). This protects the skin from injury.
- Turn and reposition the person as directed by the nurse. This protects the skin from injury.
- Assist with or clean the genital area after elimination (Chapter 11). Wipe and clean from the urethra (the cleanest area) to the rectum (the dirtiest area). This helps prevent urinary tract infections.
- Make sure drainage tubes are properly connected. Otherwise microbes can enter the drainage system.

Protecting the Susceptible Host

- Follow the care plan to meet hygiene needs. This protects the skin and mucous membranes.
- Follow the care plan to meet nutrition and fluid needs. This helps prevent infection.
- Assist with coughing and deep-breathing exercises as directed. This helps prevent respiratory infections.

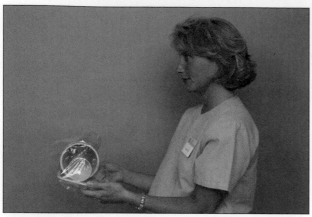

Fig. 3-3 Hold equipment away from your uniform.

Hand Hygiene

Hand hygiene is the easiest and most important way to prevent the spread of infection. Easily contaminated, your hands can spread microbes to other persons or items. Practice hand hygiene before and after giving care. See Box 3-4 for the rules of hand hygiene.

Safety Alert

Hand Hygiene

You use your hands for almost every task. They can pick up microbes from one person, place, or thing. They transfer them to other people, places, and things. That is why hand hygiene is so very important. You must practice hand hygiene before and after giving care.

BOX 3-4   Rules of Hand Hygiene

- Wash your hands (with soap and water) when they are visibly dirty or soiled with blood, body fluids, secretions, or excretions.
- Wash your hands (with soap and water) before eating and after using a restroom.
- Wash your hands (with soap and water) if exposure to the anthrax spore is suspected or proven.
- Use an alcohol-based hand rub to decontaminate your hands if they are not visibly soiled. (If an alcohol-based hand rub is not available, wash your hands with soap and water.) Follow this rule in the following clinical situations:
  —Before having direct contact with a person
  —After contact with the person's intact skin (for example, after taking a pulse or blood pressure or after lifting and moving a person)
  —After contact with body fluids or excretions, mucous membranes, non-intact skin, and wound dressings if hands are not visibly soiled
  —When moving from a contaminated body site to a clean body site during care activities
  —After contact with objects (including equipment) in the person's care setting
  —After removing gloves
- Follow these rules for washing your hands with soap and water. See procedure: *Hand Washing*, p. 50:
  —Wash your hands under warm running water. Do not use hot water.
  —Stand away from the sink. Do not let your hands, body, or uniform touch the sink. The sink is contaminated (Fig. 3-4).
  —Keep your hands and forearms lower than your elbows. Your hands are dirtier than your elbows and forearms. If you hold your hands and forearms up, dirty water runs from hands to elbows. Those areas become contaminated.
  —Rub your palms together to work up a good lather (Fig. 3-5). The rubbing action helps remove microbes and dirt.
  —Pay attention to areas often missed during hand washing—thumbs, knuckles, sides of the hands, little fingers, and under the nails.
  —Clean fingernails by rubbing the tips against your palms (Fig. 3-6).
  —Use a nail file or orange stick to clean under fingernails (Fig. 3-7). Microbes easily grow under the fingernails.
  —Wash your hands for at least 15 seconds. Wash your hands longer if they are dirty or soiled with blood, body fluids, secretions, or excretions. Use your judgment.
  —Dry your hands starting at the fingers. Work up to your forearms. You will dry the cleanest area first.
  —Use a clean paper towel for each faucet to turn water off (Fig. 3-8). Faucets are contaminated. The paper towels prevent clean hands from becoming contaminated again.
- Follow these rules when decontaminating your hands with an alcohol-based hand rub:
  —Apply the product to the palm of one hand. Follow the manufacturer's instructions for the amount to use.
  —Rub your hands together.
  —Make sure you cover all surfaces of your hands and fingers.
  —Continue rubbing your hands together until your hands are dry.
- Apply hand lotion or cream after hand hygiene. This prevents skin chapping and drying. Skin breaks can occur in chapped and dry skin. Skin breaks are portals of entry for microbes.

Modified from Centers for Disease Control and Prevention, *Guideline for hand hygiene in health-care settings*, Morbidity and Mortality Report, October 25, 2002, Vol 51. No. RR–16.

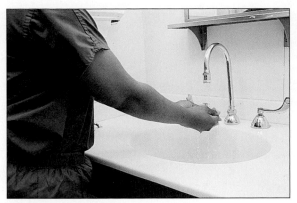

Fig. 3-4 The uniform does not touch the sink. Soap and water are within reach. Hands are lower than the elbows.

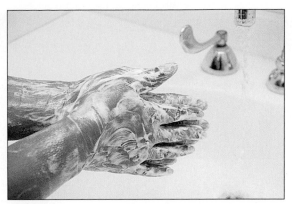

Fig. 3-5 The palms are rubbed together to work up a good lather.

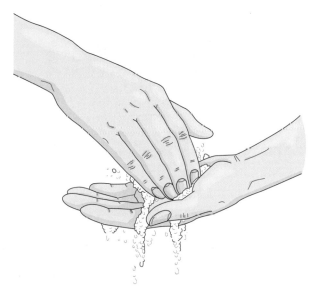

Fig. 3-6 The finger tips are rubbed against the palms to clean under the fingernails.

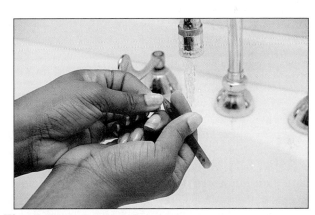

Fig. 3-7 A nail file is used to clean under the fingernails.

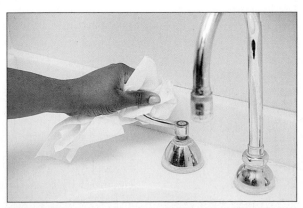

Fig. 3-8 A paper towel is used to turn off the faucet.

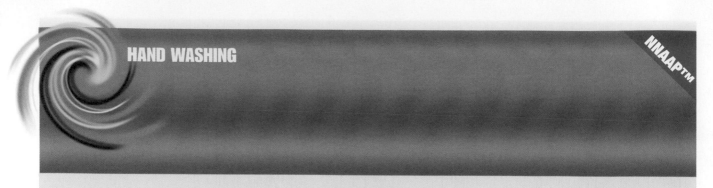

HAND WASHING

Procedure

1   See *Safety Alert: Hand Hygiene*, p. 48.
2   Make sure you have soap, paper towels, an orange stick or nail file, and a wastebasket. Collect missing items.
3   Push your watch up 4 to 5 inches. Also push up uniform sleeves.
4   Stand away from the sink so your clothes do not touch the sink. Stand so the soap and faucet are easy to reach (see Fig. 3-4).
5   Turn on and adjust the water until it feels warm.
6   Wet your wrists and hands. Keep your hands lower than your elbows.
7   Apply about 1 teaspoon of soap to your hands.
8   Rub your palms together and interlace your fingers to work up a good lather (see Fig. 3-5). This step should last at least 15 seconds.
9   Wash each hand and wrist thoroughly. Clean well between the fingers.
10 Clean under the fingernails. Rub your finger tips against your palms (see Fig. 3-6).
11 Clean under fingernails with a nail file or orange stick (see Fig. 3-7). This step is done for the first hand washing of the day and when your hands are highly soiled.
12 Rinse your wrists and hands well. Water flows from the arms to the hands.
13 Repeat steps 7 through 12, if needed.
14 Dry your wrists and hands with paper towels. Pat dry starting at your fingertips.
15 Discard the paper towels.
16 Turn off faucets with clean paper towels. This prevents you from contaminating your hands (see Fig. 3-8). Use a clean paper towel for each faucet.
17 Discard paper towels.

Supplies and Equipment

Many care items are disposable. Single-use items are discarded after one use. A person uses multi-use items many times. They include bedpans, urinals, wash basins, water pitchers, and drinking cups. Do not "borrow" them for another person. Non-disposable items are cleaned, disinfected, and then sterilized.

Cleaning.   Cleaning reduces the number of microbes present. It also removes organic matter—blood, body fluids, secretions, and excretions. To clean equipment:

- Wear personal protective equipment (gloves, mask, gown, and protective eyewear) if items are contaminated with blood, body fluids, secretions, or excretions.
- Rinse the item in cold water to remove organic matter. Heat causes organic matter to become thick, sticky, and hard to remove.
- Wash the item with soap and hot water.
- Scrub thoroughly. Use a brush if necessary.
- Rinse the item in warm water.

- Dry the item.
- Disinfect or sterilize the item.
- Disinfect equipment and the sink used in the cleaning procedure.
- Discard personal protective equipment.
- Practice hand hygiene.

Disinfection and Sterilization.   **Disinfection** is the process of destroying pathogens. Reusable items are cleaned with chemical disinfectants. Such items include blood pressure cuffs, commodes and bedpans, counter tops, wheelchairs, stretchers, and furniture.

Chemical disinfectants can burn and irritate the skin. Wear utility gloves or rubber household gloves to protect your hands. These gloves are *waterproof*. Do not wear disposable gloves. Follow center procedures for handling hazardous substances.

Sterilization is the process of destroying *all* microbes. Very high temperatures are used. Items are sterilized by the manufacturer or the center's supply department.

ISOLATION PRECAUTIONS

Blood, body fluids, secretions, and excretions can transmit pathogens. Sometimes barriers are needed to keep pathogens within a certain area. Usually the area is the person's room. This requires isolation procedures.

The Centers for Disease Control and Prevention (CDC) has guidelines for Standard Precautions and Transmission-Based Precautions. They prevent the spread of **communicable** or **contagious diseases.** They are diseases caused by pathogens that are spread easily. Examples include measles, mumps, chickenpox, and sexually transmitted diseases. Some respiratory, gastrointestinal, wound, skin, and blood infections also are highly contagious.

Isolation precautions are based on *clean* and *dirty*. *Clean* areas or objects are free of pathogens. They are not contaminated. *Dirty* areas or objects are contaminated with pathogens. If a *clean* area or object has contact with something *dirty,* the clean item is now dirty. *Clean* and *dirty* also depend on how the pathogen is spread.

Standard Precautions

Standard Precautions (Box 3-5) reduce the risk of spreading pathogens and known and unknown infections. *Standard Precautions are used for all persons.* They prevent the spread of infection from:

- Blood
- All body fluids, secretions, and excretions (except sweat) even if blood is not visible
- Non-intact skin (skin with open breaks)
- Mucous membranes

BOX 3-5   Standard Precautions

Hand Hygiene*

- Wash your hands after touching blood, body fluids, secretions, excretions, and contaminated items.
- Decontaminate your hands right away after removing gloves.
- Decontaminate your hands between resident contacts.
- Practice hand hygiene whenever needed to avoid spreading microbes to other persons or areas.
- Decontaminate your hands between tasks and procedures on the same person. This prevents cross-contamination of different body sites.
- Use soap for routine hand washing. (The nurse tells you when other agents are needed. The nurse also tells you what to use.)

Gloves

- Wear gloves when touching blood, body fluids, secretions, and excretions.
- Wear gloves when touching contaminated items.
- Put on clean gloves just before touching mucous membranes and non-intact skin.
- Change gloves between tasks and procedures on the same person.
- Change gloves after contacting matter that may be highly contaminated.
- Remove gloves promptly after use.
- Remove gloves before touching uncontaminated items and surfaces.
- Remove gloves before going to another person.
- Decontaminate your hands at once after removing gloves. This prevents the transfer of microbes to other persons or areas.

Masks, Eye Protection, and Face Shields

- Wear masks, eye protection, and face shields during procedures and tasks that are likely to cause splashes or sprays of blood, body fluids, secretions, and excretions. They protect the mucous membranes of the mouth, eyes, and nose from splashes or sprays (Fig. 3-9, p. 52).

Gowns

- Wear a gown during tasks that are likely to cause splashes or sprays of blood, body fluids, secretions, or excretions. The gown protects the skin and prevents soiling of clothing.
- Remove a soiled gown as soon as possible.
- Decontaminate your hands after gown removal. This prevents spreading microbes to other persons or areas.

Care Equipment

- Handle used care equipment carefully. Equipment may be soiled with blood, body fluids, secretions, and excretions. Prevent skin and mucous membrane exposure and clothing contamination. Also prevent the transfer of microbes to other persons and areas.
- Do not use reusable items for another person. The item must be cleaned and disinfected or sterilized.
- Discard disposable (single-use) items properly.

*Modified to comply with *Guideline for hand hygiene in health-care settings,* Centers for Disease Control and Prevention, October 25, 2002.

Continued

BOX 3-5   Standard Precautions—cont'd

Environmental Control

- Follow center procedures for the routine care, cleaning, and disinfection of surfaces. This includes environmental surfaces, bed rails, bedside equipment, and other surfaces.

Linens

- Follow center policy for linen that is soiled with blood, body fluids, secretions, or excretions. The policy describes how to handle, transport, and process soiled linen.
- Prevent skin and mucous membrane exposures and clothing contamination when handling linens.
- Prevent the transfer of microbes to other persons and areas when handling linens.

Occupational Health and Bloodborne Pathogens

- Prevent injuries when handling needles, scalpels, and other sharp instruments or devices.
- Prevent injuries when handling sharp instruments after procedures.

- Prevent injuries when cleaning instruments.
- Prevent injuries when disposing of needles.
- Never recap used needles. Do not handle them with both hands. Do not use any method that involves directing the needle point toward any body part. Follow center policy for handling and disposing of needles.
- Do not remove used needles from disposable syringes by hand.
- Do not bend, break, or otherwise handle used needles by hand.
- Place used syringes and needles, scalpel blades, and other sharp items in puncture-resistant containers.
- Use barrier devices for rescue breathing (Chapter 5).

Resident Placement

- A private room is used if the person:
  —Contaminates the area
  —Does not or cannot assist in maintaining hygiene or environmental control
- Follow the nurse's instructions if a private room is not available.

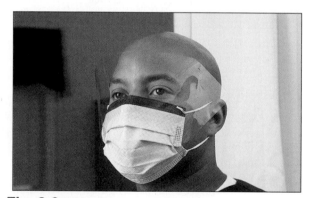

Fig. 3-9 Protective eyewear protects the eyes and mucous membranes of the mouth and nose.

Delegation Guidelines

Transmission-Based Precautions

Some people require Transmission-Based Precautions. Review the type used with the nurse. You also need this information from the nurse and the care plan:

- What agent to use for hand hygiene
- What personal protective equipment to use
- What special safety measures are needed

Transmission-Based Precautions

Some infections also require Transmission-Based Precautions (Box 3-6). The type used depends on how the infection is spread.

Protective Measures

Isolation Precautions involve wearing gloves, a gown, a mask, or protective eyewear. Removing linens, trash, and equipment from the room may require double bagging. Follow center procedures for Isolation Precautions when collecting specimens and transporting persons.

Safety Alert

Transmission-Based Precautions

Transmission-Based Precautions protect everyone—residents, visitors, staff, and you. If you are careless, everyone's safety is at risk.

BOX 3-6   **Transmission-Based Precautions**

Airborne Precautions

For known or suspected infections involving microbes transmitted by airborne droplets—measles, chickenpox, tuberculosis (TB)

Practices:
- Standard Precautions are followed.
- A private room is preferred.
- Keep the room door closed and the person in the room.
- Wear respiratory protection (tuberculosis respirator) when entering the room of a person with known or suspected TB.
- Do not enter the room of a person with known or suspected measles or chickenpox if you are susceptible to these diseases.
- Wear respiratory protection (mask) if you must enter the room of a person with known or suspected measles or chickenpox if you are susceptible to these diseases. (Respiratory protection is not needed for persons immune to measles or chickenpox.)
- Limit moving and transporting the person from the room. The person wears a mask if moving or transporting from the room is necessary.

Droplet Precautions

For known or suspected infections involving microbes transmitted by droplets produced by coughing, sneezing, talking, or procedures—meningitis, pneumonia, epiglottitis, diphtheria, pertussis (whooping cough), influenza, mumps, rubella, streptococcal pharyngitis, or scarlet fever.

Practices:
- Standard Precautions are followed.
- A private room is preferred.
- Wear a mask when working within 3 feet of the person. (Wear a mask on entering the room if required by center policy.)

- Limit moving and transporting the person from the room. The person wears a mask if moving or transporting from the room is necessary.

Contact Precautions

For known or suspected infections involving microbes transmitted by:
- Direct contact with the person (hand or skin-to-skin contact that occurs during care)
- Indirect contact (touching surfaces or care items in the person's room)—gastrointestinal, respiratory, skin, or wound infections

Practices:
- Standard Precautions are followed.
- A private room is preferred.
- Wear gloves when entering the room.
- Change gloves after having contact with infective matter that may contain high concentrations of microbes.
- Remove gloves before leaving the person's room.
- Practice hand hygiene immediately after removing gloves. The nurse tells you what agent to use.
- Do not touch potentially contaminated surfaces or items after removing gloves and hand hygiene.
- Wear a gown on entering the room if you will have substantial contact with the person, surfaces, or items in the room.
- Wear a gown on entering the room if the person is incontinent or has diarrhea, an ileostomy, a colostomy, or wound drainage not contained by a dressing.
- Remove the gown before leaving the person's room. Make sure your clothing does not contact potentially contaminated surfaces in the person's room.
- Limit moving or transferring the person from the room. Maintain precautions if the person is moved or transferred from the room.

Gloves. Small skin breaks on the hands and fingers are common. They are portals of entry for microbes. Disposable gloves protect you from pathogens in the person's blood, body fluids, secretions, and excretions. They also protect the person from microbes on your hands.

Wear gloves whenever contact with blood, body fluids, secretions, excretions, mucous membranes, and non-intact skin is likely. Contact may be direct. Or contact may be with contaminated items or surfaces.

Do not tear gloves when putting them on. Carelessness, long fingernails, and rings can tear gloves. Blood, body fluids, secretions, and excretions can enter the glove through the tear. This contaminates the hand. Remember the following:

- Gloves are easier to put on when your hands are dry.
- You need a new pair for every person.

- Remove and discard torn, cut, or punctured gloves at once. Practice hand hygiene. Then put on a new pair.
- Wear gloves once. Discard them after use.
- Put on clean gloves just before touching mucous membranes or non-intact skin.
- Put on new gloves whenever gloves become contaminated with blood, body fluids, secretions, or excretions. A task may require more than one pair of gloves.
- Change gloves when moving from a contaminated body site to a clean body site.
- Make sure gloves cover your wrists or the cuffs of a gown (Fig. 3-10, p. 54).
- Remove gloves so the inside part is on the outside. The inside is clean.
- Decontaminate your hands after removing gloves.

Safety Alert

Gloves

Some gloves are made of latex (a rubber product). Latex allergies are common. They can cause skin rashes. Asthma and shock are more serious problems. Report skin rashes and breathing problems to the nurse at once.

If you have a latex allergy, wear latex-free gloves. Some residents are allergic to latex. This information is on the care plan and your assignment sheet.

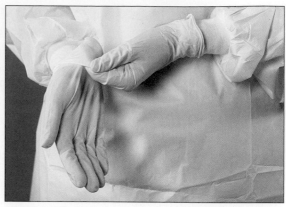

Fig. 3-10 The gloves cover the cuffs of the gown.

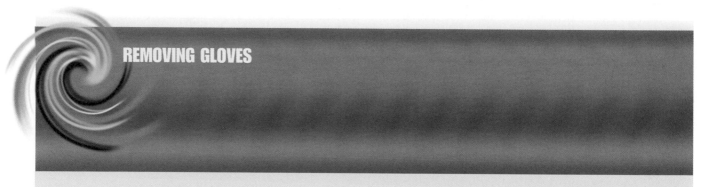

REMOVING GLOVES

Procedure

1 See *Safety Alert: Gloves.*
2 Make sure that glove touches only glove.
3 Grasp a glove just below the cuff (Fig. 3-11, A). Grasp it on the outside.
4 Pull the glove down over your hand so it is inside out (Fig. 3-11, B).
5 Hold the removed glove with your other gloved hand.
6 Reach inside the other glove. Use the first two fingers of the ungloved hand (Fig. 3-11, C).
7 Pull the glove down (inside out) over your hand and the other glove (Fig. 3-11, D).
8 Discard the gloves. Follow center policy.
9 Decontaminate your hands.

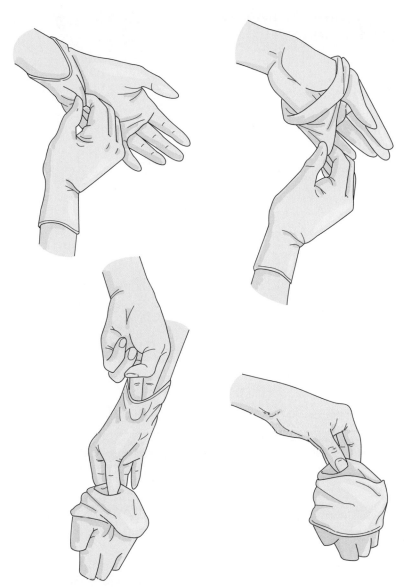

Fig. 3-11 Removing gloves. **A,** Grasp the glove below the cuff. **B,** Pull the glove down over the hand. The glove is inside out. **C,** Insert the fingers of the ungloved hand inside the other glove. **D,** Pull the glove down and over the hand and glove. The glove is inside out.

Masks and Respiratory Protection.

Masks prevent the spread of microbes from the respiratory tract. They are used for Airborne and Droplet Precautions.

Masks are disposable. A wet or moist mask is contaminated. Breathing can cause masks to become wet or moist. Apply a new mask when contamination occurs.

A mask fits snugly over your nose and mouth. Practice hand hygiene before putting on a mask. When removing a mask, touch only the ties. The front of the mask is contaminated.

Tuberculosis respirators (Fig. 3-12) are worn when caring for persons with tuberculosis (TB) (see Box 3-2). They are worn for Airborne Precautions.

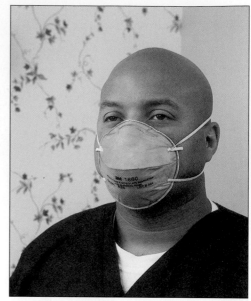

Fig. 3-12 Tuberculosis respirator.

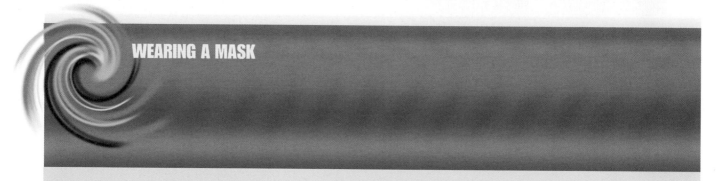

WEARING A MASK

Procedure

1 Practice hand hygiene.
2 Pick up the mask by its upper ties. Do not touch the part that will cover your face.
3 Place the mask over your nose and mouth (Fig. 3-13, A).
4 Place the upper strings above your ears. Tie them at the back of your head (Fig. 3-13, B).
5 Tie the lower strings at the back of your neck (Fig. 3-13, C). The lower part of the mask is under your chin.
6 Pinch the metal band around your nose. The top of the mask must be snug over your nose. If you wear glasses, the mask must be snug under the bottom of the glasses.
7 Decontaminate your hands. Put on gloves.

8 Provide care. Avoid coughing, sneezing, and unnecessary talking.
9 Change the mask if it becomes moist or contaminated.
10 Remove the mask as follows:
   a Remove the gloves.
   b Decontaminate your hands.
   c Untie the lower strings.
   d Untie the top strings.
   e Hold the top strings. Remove the mask.
   f Bring the strings together. The inside of the mask folds together (Fig. 3-13, D). Do not touch the inside of the mask.
11 Discard the mask. Follow center policy.
12 Decontaminate your hands.

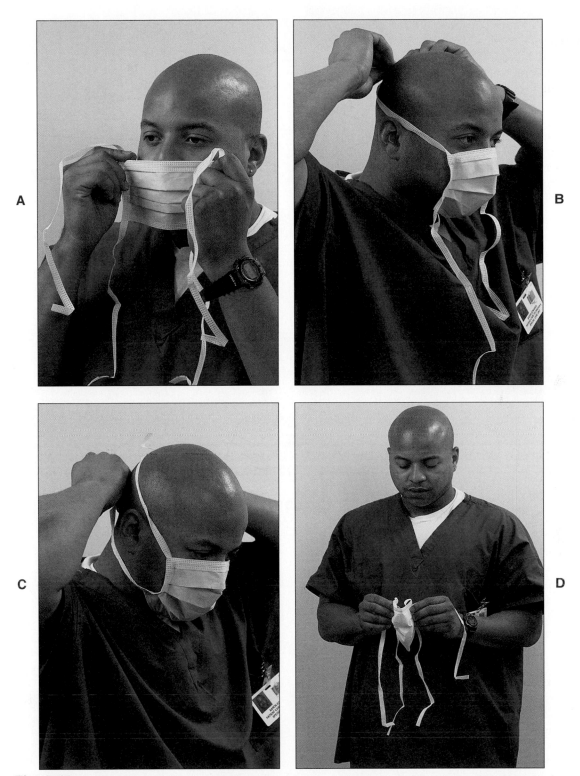

Fig. 3-13 Donning a mask. **A,** The mask covers the nose and mouth. **B,** The upper strings are tied at the back of the head. **C,** The lower strings are tied at the back of the neck. **D,** The inside of the mask is folded together after removal.

Gowns. Gowns protect your clothes, wrists, and arms from contact with blood, body fluids, secretions, or excretions. They also protect against splashes and sprays.

Gowns must completely cover clothing. The long sleeves have tight cuffs. The gown opens at the back. It is tied at the neck and waist. The inside and neck are *clean*. The outside and waist strings are *contaminated*.

Gowns are used once. A wet gown is contaminated. It is removed and a dry one put on. Disposable gowns are made of paper. They are discarded after use.

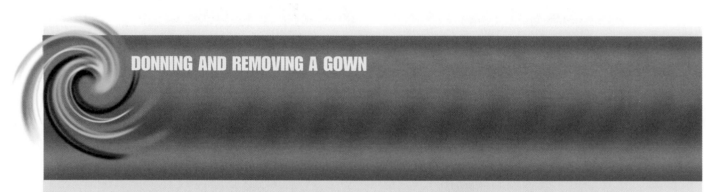

DONNING AND REMOVING A GOWN

Procedure

1 Remove your watch and all jewelry.
2 Roll up uniform sleeves.
3 Practice hand hygiene.
4 Put on a mask and eyewear if required. (See procedure: *Wearing a Mask*, p. 56.)
5 Hold a clean gown out in front of you. Let it unfold. Do not shake the gown.
6 Put your hands and arms through the sleeves (Fig. 3-14, A).
7 Make sure the gown covers the front of your uniform. It should be snug at the neck.
8 Tie the strings at the back of the neck (Fig. 3-14, B).
9 Overlap the back of the gown. Make sure it covers your uniform. The gown should be snug, not loose (Fig. 3-14, C).
10 Tie the waist strings at the back.
11 Put on the gloves.
12 Provide care.
13 Remove and discard the gloves. Decontaminate your hands.
14 Remove and discard the mask.
15 Remove the gown:
   a Untie the waist strings.
   b Untie the neck strings. Do not touch the outside of the gown.
   c Pull the gown down from the shoulder.
   d Turn the gown inside out as it is removed. Hold it at the inside shoulder seams, and bring your hands together (Fig. 3-14, D).
16 Roll up the gown away from you. Keep it inside out.
17 Discard the gown. Follow center policy.
18 Remove and discard the eyewear.
19 Decontaminate your hands.
20 Open the door using a paper towel. Discard it as you leave.

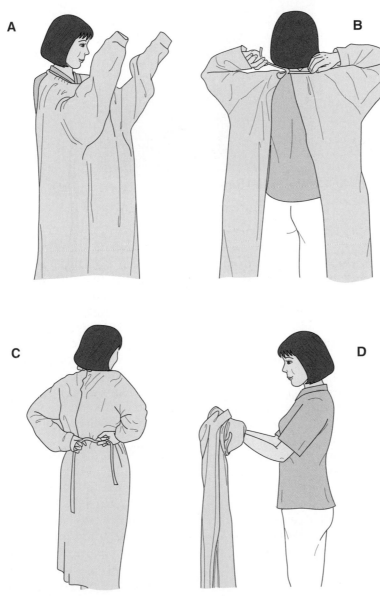

Fig. 3-14 Gowning. **A,** The arms and hands are put through the sleeves. **B,** The strings are tied at the back of the neck. **C,** The gown is overlapped in the back to cover the entire uniform. **D,** The gown is turned inside out as it is removed.

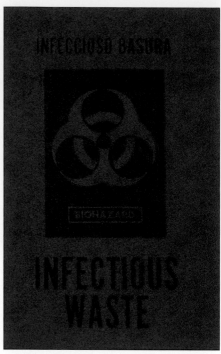

Fig. 3-15 *BIOHAZARD* symbol.

Eyewear and Face Shields.   Goggles and face shields protect your eyes, mouth, and nose from splashing or spraying of blood, body fluids, secretions, or excretions (see Fig. 3-9). Splashes and sprays can occur when giving care, cleaning items, or disposing of fluids.

Discard disposable eyewear after use. Reusable eyewear is cleaned before reuse. It is washed with soap and water. Then a disinfectant is used.

Bagging Items.   Leak-proof plastic bags are used to remove items from the person's room. They have the *BIOHAZARD* symbol, usually black lettering on a red background (Fig. 3-15). **Biohazardous waste** is items contaminated with blood, body fluids, secretions, or excretions. (*Bio* means life. *Hazardous* means dangerous or harmful.)

Bag and transport linens following center policy. All linen bags need a *BIOHAZARD* symbol. Melt-away bags are common. They dissolve in hot water. Do not overfill the bag. Tie the bag securely. Then place it in a laundry hamper lined with a biohazard plastic bag.

Trash is placed in a container labeled with the *BIO-HAZARD* symbol. Follow center policy for bagging and transporting trash, equipment, and supplies. Usually one bag is needed. Double bagging involves two bags. Double bagging is not needed unless the outside of the bag is soiled.

Meeting Basic Needs

The person has love, belonging, and self-esteem needs. Often they are unmet when Transmission-Based Precautions are used. The person may feel lonely, unwanted, and rejected. Self-esteem suffers. The person knows the disease can be spread to others. He or she may feel dirty and undesirable. Remember, the pathogen is undesirable, not the person.

Masks and eyewear change how you look. Always let the person see your face before you put on personal protective equipment. Tell the person who you are and what you are going to do.

BLOODBORNE PATHOGEN STANDARD

The Bloodborne Pathogen Standard protects workers from exposure to the AIDS virus (human immunodeficiency virus [HIV]) and the hepatitis virus (see Box 3-2). It is a regulation of the Occupational Safety and Health Administration (OSHA).

HIV and the hepatitis B virus (HBV) are bloodborne pathogens. They exit the body through blood. HIV and HBV are spread to others by blood or other potentially infectious materials (OPIM). OPIM are contaminated with blood or with a body fluid that may contain blood. Such body fluids include semen and vaginal secretions. OPIM include needles, linens, dressings, and other care items.

Staff receive free training upon employment and yearly. Training is also required for new or changed tasks involving exposure to bloodborne pathogens.

Hepatitis B Vaccination

The hepatitis B vaccine produces immunity against hepatitis B. You can receive the hepatitis B vaccination within 10 working days of being hired. The center pays for it. You can refuse the vaccination. If so, you must sign a statement refusing the vaccine. You can receive the vaccine at a later time.

Methods of Control

All tasks involving blood or OPIM are done in ways to limit splatters, splashes, and sprays. Producing droplets also is avoided. Follow these OSHA required measures:

- Do not eat, drink, smoke, apply cosmetics or lip balm, or handle contact lenses in areas of occupational exposure.
- Do not store food or drinks where blood or OPIM are kept.
- Practice hand hygiene after removing gloves.
- Wash hands as soon as possible after skin contact with blood or OPIM.
- Never recap, bend, or remove needles by hand. If such actions are required, use mechanical means (forceps) or a one-handed method.
- Never shear or break contaminated needles.
- Discard sharps (needles, instruments, and broken glass) in containers that are puncture-resistant and leak-proof. Containers are color-coded red and have the *BIOHAZARD* symbol. Containers must be upright and not allowed to overfill.

Personal Protective Equipment (PPE).   This includes gloves, goggles, face shields, masks, laboratory coats, gowns, shoe covers, and surgical caps. Blood or OPIM must not pass through them. They protect your clothes, undergarments, skin, eyes, and mouth.

PPE is free to employees. The center cleans, launders, repairs, replaces, or discards PPE. You must safely handle and use PPE. Follow these OSHA required measures:

- Remove PPE before leaving the work area.
- Remove PPE when a garment becomes contaminated.
- Place used PPE in marked areas or containers when being stored, washed, decontaminated, or discarded.
- Wear gloves when you expect contact with blood or OPIM.
- Wear gloves when handling or touching contaminated items or surfaces.
- Replace worn, punctured, or contaminated gloves.
- Never wash or decontaminate disposable gloves for reuse.
- Discard utility gloves that show signs of cracking, peeling, tearing, or puncturing. Utility gloves are decontaminated for reuse if the process will not ruin them.

Equipment.   Contaminated equipment is cleaned and decontaminated. Decontaminate work surfaces with a proper disinfectant:

- Upon completing tasks
- At once when there is obvious contamination
- After any spill of blood or OPIM
- At the end of the work shift when surfaces became contaminated since the last cleaning

Use a brush and dustpan or tongs to clean up broken glass. Never pick up broken glass with your hands, not even with gloves. Discard broken glass into a puncture-resistant container.

Laundry.   OSHA requires these measures for contaminated laundry:

- Handle it as little as possible.
- Wear gloves or other needed PPE.
- Bag contaminated laundry where it was used.
- Mark laundry bags or containers with the *BIOHAZARD* symbol for laundry sent offsite.
- Place wet contaminated laundry in leak-proof containers before transport. The containers are color-coded in red or labeled with the *BIOHAZARD* symbol.

Exposure Incidents

An *exposure incident* is any eye, mouth, other mucous membrane, non-intact skin, or parenteral contact with blood or OPIM. *Parenteral* means piercing the mucous membranes or the skin barrier. Piercing occurs through needle-sticks, human bites, cuts, and abrasions.

Report exposure incidents at once. Medical evaluation and follow-up are free. This includes required tests. Your blood is tested for HBV and HIV. If you refuse testing, the blood sample is kept for at least 90 days. Testing is done later if you change your mind. You are told of test results and about any medical conditions that may need treatment. You receive a written opinion of the medical evaluation within 15 days after its completion.

The *source individual* is the person whose blood or body fluids are the source of an exposure incident. His or her blood is tested for HIV or HBV. State laws vary about releasing the results. The center informs you about laws affecting the source's identity and test results.

Review Questions

Circle **T** if the statement is true or **F** if the statement is false.

1   **T F**   A pathogen can cause an infection.
2   **T F**   An item is sterile if non-pathogens are present.
3   **T F**   You hold your hands and forearms up during hand washing.
4   **T F**   Unused items in a person's room are used for another person.
5   **T F**   You received the hepatitis B vaccine. You will develop the disease.

Circle the **BEST** answer.

6   Most pathogens need the following to grow *except*
   a   Water
   b   Light
   c   Oxygen
   d   Nourishment

7   Signs and symptoms of infection include the following *except*
   a   Fever, nausea, vomiting, rash, and/or sores
   b   Pain or tenderness, redness, and/or swelling
   c   Fatigue, loss of appetite, and/or a discharge
   d   A wound and/or bleeding

8   Which is *not* a portal of exit?
   a   Respiratory tract
   b   Blood
   c   Reproductive system
   d   Intact skin

9   When cleaning equipment, you
   a   Rinse the item in hot water before cleaning
   b   Wash the item with soap and cold water
   c   Disinfect the item first
   d   Work from clean to dirty areas

10   Isolation precautions
   a   Prevent infection
   b   Destroy pathogens
   c   Keep pathogens within a certain area
   d   Destroy all microbes

11   Standard Precautions
   a   Are used for all persons
   b   Prevent the spread of pathogens through the air
   c   Require gowns, masks, gloves, and eyewear
   d   Require HIV testing

12   You wear utility gloves for contact with
   a   Blood
   b   Body fluids
   c   Secretions and excretions
   d   Cleaning solutions

13   A mask
   a   Can be reused
   b   Is clean on the inside
   c   Is contaminated when moist
   d   Should fit loosely for breathing

14   Contaminated work surfaces are cleaned at the following times *except*
   a   After completing a task
   b   When there is obvious contamination
   c   After blood is spilled
   d   After removing gloves

15   The Bloodborne Pathogen Standard involves the following *except*
   a   Wearing gloves
   b   Discarding sharp items into a *BIOHAZARD* container
   c   Storing food and blood in different places
   d   Eating and drinking in areas of occupational exposure

16   You were exposed to a bloodborne pathogen. Which is *true?*
   a   You do not have to report the incident.
   b   You pay for required tests.
   c   You can refuse HBV and HIV testing.
   d   The source individual can refuse testing.

Answers to these questions are on p. 388.

CHAPTER 4

Safety

Objectives

- Define the key terms listed in this chapter
- Describe how aging and common health problems affect the musculoskeletal system
- Describe accident risk factors
- Explain how to use good body mechanics
- Explain how to accurately identify a person before giving care
- Explain how to use the call system
- Describe how to prevent falls, burns, poisoning, and equipment accidents
- Explain how to handle hazardous substances
- Identify the sources and equipment used in oxygen therapy
- Describe safety measures for oxygen use and fire prevention
- Explain what to do during a fire
- Give examples of natural and human-made disasters
- Explain how to protect yourself from workplace violence
- Describe your role in risk management
- Perform the procedures described in this chapter

base of support The area on which an object rests

body alignment The way the head, trunk, arms, and legs are aligned with one another; posture

body mechanics Using the body in an efficient and careful way

coma A state of being unaware of one's surroundings and being unable to react or respond to people, places, or things

hazardous substance Any chemical in the workplace that can cause harm

incident Any event that has harmed or could harm a resident, staff member, or visitor

workplace violence Violent acts directed toward persons at work or while on duty

---

Safety is a basic need. Residents are at great risk for falls and other accidents. Musculoskeletal injuries can occur (Box 4-1). Some accidents and injuries cause death. The health team must keep residents safe. The goal is to lower their risk of accidents and injuries without limiting mobility and independence. Common sense and simple safety measures can prevent most accidents. The care plan lists other safety measures needed by the person.

ACCIDENT RISK FACTORS

Some people cannot protect themselves. They rely on others for safety. Certain factors increase the risk of injury:

- *Age*—Body changes occur from aging. Older persons have decreased strength and move slowly. Some are unsteady or have tremors or shaking. If balance is affected, they may fall easily. They also have sensory changes—sensitivity to heat and cold, impaired vision and hearing, and a dulled sense of smell. Reflexes are slower. Changes in the cardiovascular system may cause the blood pressure to drop with position changes. This causes dizziness and weakness. Fainting can occur.
- *Awareness of surroundings*—**Coma** is a state of being unaware of one's surroundings and being unable to react or respond to people, places, or things. The person in a coma relies on others for protection. Confusion, forgetfulness, poor judgment, memory problems, and disorientation may occur in other persons (Chapter 18). They also rely on others for protection.

- *Impaired vision*—Poor vision can lead to falls. A person may not see equipment, furniture, or cords. Some have problems reading labels on cleaners and other containers. They may eat or drink such things as perfume, lotion, or cleaning agents.
- *Impaired hearing*—Persons with impaired hearing have problems hearing explanations and instructions. They may not hear warning signals or fire alarms. Some cannot hear approaching meal carts, drug carts, stretchers, or wheelchairs.
- *Impaired smell and touch*—Illness and aging affect smell and touch. The person may not detect smoke or gas odors. When touch is reduced, burns are a risk. There are problems sensing heat and cold. Some people have a decreased pain sense. They may be injured and not know it.
- *Impaired mobility*—Some diseases, injuries, and surgeries affect mobility. Weakness is common. Some people have problems moving. A person may be aware of danger but cannot move to safety. Some persons cannot walk or propel wheelchairs.
- *Drugs*—Drugs have side effects. They include loss of balance, drowsiness, and lack of coordination. Reduced awareness, confusion, and disorientation also can occur.

BOX 4-1　The Musculoskeletal System

Structure and Function

The bones, joints, and muscles are the major structures of the musculoskeletal system.

Bones

Bones are hard, rigid structures. *Long bones* (leg bones) bear the body's weight. *Short bones* allow skill and ease in movement. Bones in the wrists, fingers, ankles, and toes are short bones. *Flat bones* include the ribs, skull, pelvic bones, and shoulder blades. They protect the organs. *Irregular bones* are the vertebrae in the spinal column. They allow movement and flexibility.

Joints

A *joint* is the point at which two or more bones meet (Fig. 4-1, p. 66). Bones are held together at the joint by strong bands of tissue called *ligaments.* Joints allow movement. A *ball-and-socket joint* allows movement in all directions. The hip and shoulder joints are ball-and-socket joints. A *hinge joint* allows movement in one direction. The elbow and knee are hinge joints. A *pivot joint* allows turning from side to side. The skull is connected to the spine by a pivot joint.

Muscles

The human body has more than 500 muscles. *Voluntary muscles* can be consciously controlled. Muscles that are attached to bones *(skeletal muscles)* are voluntary. Arm muscles do not work unless you move your arm. Likewise for leg muscles.

Involuntary muscles work automatically and cannot be consciously controlled. They control the action of the stomach, intestines, blood vessels, and other body organs. *Cardiac muscle* is in the heart. It is an involuntary muscle.

Strong, tough connective tissues called *tendons* connect muscles to bones. When muscles contract (shorten), tendons at each end of the muscle cause the bone to move.

Changes With Aging

Muscle cells decrease in number. Muscles atrophy (shrink). They decrease in strength. Bones lose strength, become brittle, and break easily. Joints become stiff and painful.

Vertebrae shorten. Hip and knee joints flex (bend) slightly. These changes cause gradual loss of height and strength. Mobility also decreases.

Activity, exercise, and diet help prevent bone loss and loss of muscle strength. Walking is good exercise. Exercise groups and range-of-motion exercises are helpful (Chapter 19). A diet high in protein, calcium, and vitamins is needed.

Protect the person from injury and prevent falls. Turn and move the person gently and carefully. Some persons need help and support getting out of bed and with walking.

Common Disorders

* *Arthritis*—*Arthritis* means joint *(arth)* inflammation *(itis).* Pain and decreased mobility occur in the affected joints. There are two basic types of arthritis:

　—*Osteoarthritis (degenerative joint disease)* occurs from aging, joint injury, and obesity. Finger and thumb joints are often affected (Fig. 4-2, p. 66). So are the hips, knees, and spine. These joints bear the body's weight. The person has joint stiffness, pain, swelling, and tenderness. Joint stiffness occurs with rest and lack of motion. Pain occurs with weight-bearing and joint motion. Cold weather and dampness seem to increase symptoms. Treatment involves drugs to decrease swelling and relieve pain. Heat applications relieve pain and stiffness. Sometimes cold applications are used to relieve pain or numb the area.

　—*Rheumatoid arthritis (RA)* is an inflammatory disease. It causes joint pain, swelling, and stiffness. RA occurs on both sides of the body. For example, if the right wrist is involved, so is the left wrist. The wrist and finger joints closest to the hand are often affected. Neck, shoulder, elbow, hip, knee, ankle, and foot joints can be affected. Joints are tender, warm, and swollen. Fatigue and fever are common. Symptoms can last for many years. Other body parts may be affected. Some people have flare-ups and then feel better. In others, the disease is active most of the time. Drugs are ordered for pain relief and to reduce inflammation. Heat or local cold applications may be ordered. Some persons need joint replacement surgery.

* *Osteoporosis*—Bones *(osteo)* become porous and brittle *(porosis).* They are fragile and break easily. Spine, hip, and wrist fractures are common. Older persons and women after menopause are at risk. The lack of estrogen after menopause causes bone changes. So do low levels of dietary calcium. Back pain, gradual loss of height, and stooped posture occur. Even slight activity can cause a fracture—turning in bed, getting up from a chair, or coughing. Prevention is important. The diet must contain enough calcium and vitamin D. Often doctors order calcium and vitamin supplements. Estrogen is ordered for some women. Exercise and strength training (lifting weights) are helpful.

* *Fractures*—A *fracture* is a broken bone. Tissues around the fracture (muscles, blood vessels, nerves, and tendons) are injured. Fractures are open or closed (Fig. 4-3, p. 66). With a closed fracture (simple fracture), the bone is broken but the skin is intact. With an open fracture (compound fracture), the broken bone has come through the skin. Hip fractures are common in older persons (Fig. 4-4, p. 66). Fractures cause pain and tenderness, swelling, limited movement, loss of function, deformity (abnormal position), bruising and skin color changes, and bleeding. For healing, bone ends are brought into normal position. A cast, traction, splint, walking boot, or other device is used to keep the bone ends in place.

* *Sprains and strains*—A *sprain* is an injury to a ligament. The ligament is torn or stretched. The ankles and knees are common sites. With a *strain,* a muscle is torn or stretched. Sprains and strains cause pain, swelling, and loss of function. Treatment involves cold applications, pain-relief drugs, an elastic bandage to the part, and elevating the part on pillows. A splint prevents movement of the part.

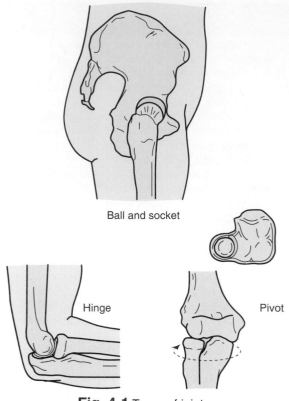

Ball and socket

Hinge   Pivot

Fig. 4-1 Types of joints.

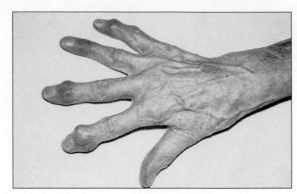

Fig. 4-2 Bony growths called *Heberden's nodes* occur in the finger joints. (From Kamal A, Brocklehurst JC: *A color atlas of geriatric medicine,* ed 2, St Louis, 1991, Mosby.)

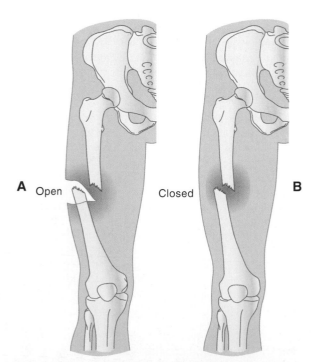

A Open   Closed   **B**

Fig. 4-3 A, Open fracture. **B,** Closed fracture. (From Thibodeau GA, Patton KT: *The human body in health & disease,* ed 3, St Louis, 2002, Mosby.)

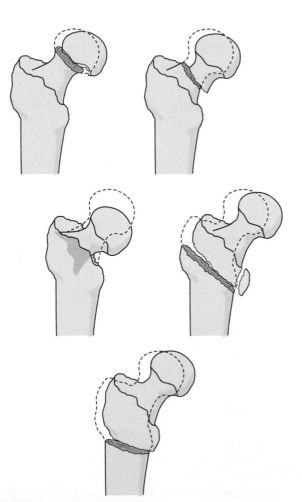

Fig. 4-4 Hip fractures. (From Phipps WJ, and others: *Medical-surgical nursing: health and illness perspectives,* ed 7, St Louis, 2003, Mosby.)

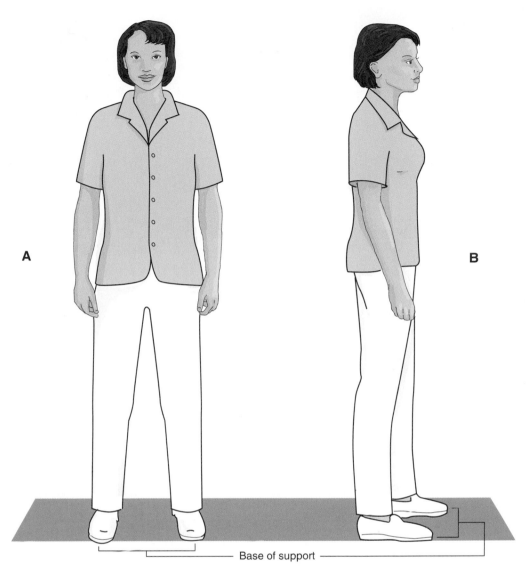

Fig. 4-5 A, Anterior (front) view of an adult in good body alignment. The feet are apart for a wide base of support. **B,** Lateral (side) view of an adult with good posture and alignment.

Base of support

BODY MECHANICS

Body mechanics means using the body in an efficient and careful way. Good posture, balance, and the strongest and largest muscles are used. Fatigue, muscle strain, and injury result when the body is not used or positioned properly.

Body alignment *(posture)* is the way the head, trunk, arms, and legs are aligned with one another. Good alignment lets the body move and function with strength and efficiency. Standing, sitting, and lying down require good alignment.

Base of support is the area on which an object rests. A good base of support is needed for balance (Fig. 4-5). Stand with your feet apart for a wider base of support and more balance.

Your strongest and largest muscles are in the shoulders, upper arms, hips, and thighs. Use these muscles to lift and move heavy objects. Otherwise, you place strain and exertion on smaller and weaker muscles. This causes fatigue and injury. *Back injuries are a major risk.* For good body mechanics:

- Bend your knees and squat to lift a heavy object (Fig. 4-6, p. 68). Do not bend from your waist. That places strain on small back muscles.
- Hold items close to your body and base of support (see Fig. 4-6). This involves upper arm and shoulder muscles. Holding objects away from your body places strain on small muscles in your lower arms.

All activities require good body mechanics. Follow the rules in Box 4-2 on p. 68.

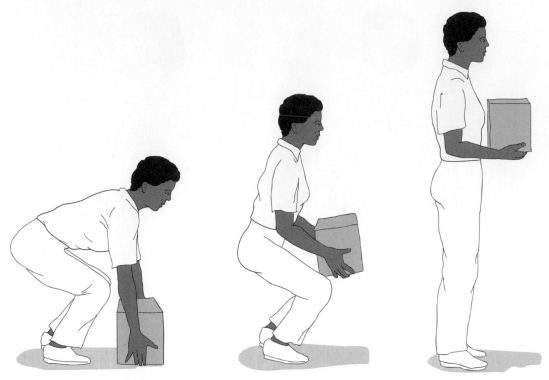

Fig. 4-6 Picking up a box using good body mechanics.

BOX 4-2   Rules for Body Mechanics

- Keep your body in good alignment with a wide base of support.
- Use the stronger and larger muscles in your shoulders, upper arms, thighs, and hips.
- Keep objects close to your body when you lift, move, or carry them (see Fig. 4-6).
- Avoid unnecessary bending and reaching. Raise the bed so it is close to your waist. Adjust the overbed table so it is at your waist level.
- Face your work area. This prevents unnecessary twisting.
- Push, slide, or pull heavy objects whenever you can, rather than lifting them.
- Widen your base of support when pushing or pulling. Move your front leg forward when pushing. Move your rear leg back when pulling (Fig. 4-7).
- Use both hands and arms to lift, move, or carry heavy objects.

- Turn your whole body when changing the direction of your movement. Move and turn your feet in the direction of the turn, instead of twisting your body.
- Work with smooth and even movements. Avoid sudden or jerky motions.
- *Get help from a co-worker if the person cannot assist with turning or moving.*
- *Get help from a co-worker to move heavy objects or persons. Do not lift or move them by yourself.*
- Bend your hips and knees to lift heavy objects from the floor (see Fig. 4-6). Straighten your back as the object reaches thigh level. Your leg and thigh muscles work to raise the item off the floor and to waist level.
- Do not lift objects higher than chest level. Do not lift above your shoulders. Use a step stool to reach an object higher than chest level.

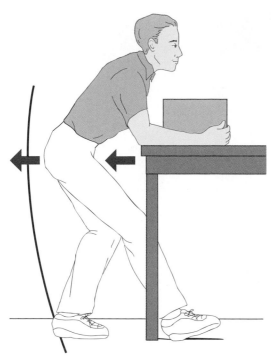

Fig. 4-7 Move your rear leg back when pulling an item.

Safety Alert

Body Mechanics

Use good body mechanics to protect yourself and others from injury. Do not work alone. Have a co-worker help you lift, move, turn, or transfer a person.

Ergonomics

Ergonomics is the science of designing the job to fit the worker. (*Ergo* means work; *nomos* means law.) The task, work station, equipment, and tools are changed to reduce stress on the worker's body. The goal is to prevent a serious and disabling work-related musculoskeletal disorder (MSD).

MSDs are injuries and disorders of the muscles, tendons, ligaments, joints, and cartilage. They also involve the nervous system. The arms and back are often affected. Back injuries are a major threat. MSDs are painful. They can develop slowly over weeks, months, and years. Or they can occur from one event. Pain, numbness, tingling, stiff joints, difficulty moving, and muscle loss can occur.

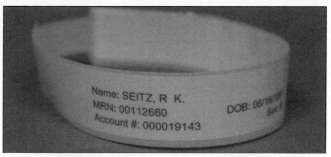

Fig. 4-8 Identification bracelet.

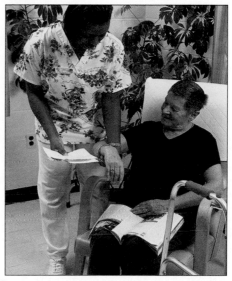

Fig. 4-9 The ID bracelet is compared against the assignment sheet to accurately identify the person.

IDENTIFYING THE PERSON

Each person has different treatments, therapies, and activity limits. Life and health are threatened if the wrong care is given.

Residents may have identification (ID) bracelets (Fig. 4-8). The bracelet has the person's name, room and bed number, birth date, age, center name, and other identifying information.

You use the ID bracelet to identify the person before giving care. The assignment sheet states what care to give. To identify the person:

- Compare identifying information on the assignment sheet with that on the ID bracelet (Fig. 4-9). Carefully check the person's full name. Some people have the same first and last names.
- Call the person by name when checking the ID bracelet. This is a courtesy given as you touch the person and before giving care. Just calling the person by name is not enough to identify him or her. Confused, disoriented, drowsy, hearing-impaired, or distracted persons may answer to any name.

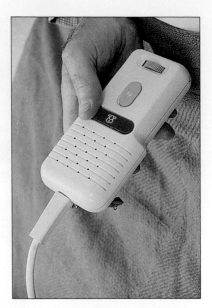

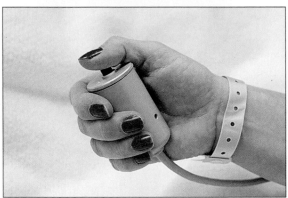

Fig. 4-10 The signal light button is pressed when help is needed. *NOTE:* There are different types of signal lights.

Some residents choose not to wear ID bracelets. This is noted on the person's care plan. Follow center policy and the care plan to identify the person.

Some centers have a photograph ID system. Others use color-coded ID bracelets for residents with special needs. Some apply colored dots to the ID bracelet. For example, pink may indicate diabetes. Green may mean a high risk for falls.

Residents at risk for leaving the center may wear bracelets with magnetic sensors. If the person goes through an outside door, the bracelet sets off an alarm. Center staff are alerted and can lead the person to safety.

Whatever the ID system used, learn to use it safely.

THE CALL SYSTEM

The call system lets the person signal for help. The signal light is at the end of a long cord (Fig. 4-10). It attaches to the bed or chair. Always keep the signal light within the person's reach—in the room, bathroom, and shower or tub room.

To get help, the person presses a button at the end of the signal light. The signal light connects to a light above the room door and to a light panel or intercom system at the nurses' station (Fig. 4-11). These tell the nursing team that the person needs help. The staff member turns off the signal light at the bedside when responding to the call for help.

In bathrooms, usually the signal light is next to the toilet. Pressing a button or pulling a cord turns on the signal light. When the bathroom signal light is used, the light flashes above the room door and at the nurses' station. The sound at the nurses' station is different from signal lights in rooms. These differences alert the nursing team that the person is in the bathroom. Someone must respond at once when a person needs help in a bathroom.

Some people cannot use signal lights. Examples are persons who are confused or in a coma. Check the care plan for special communication measures. Check these persons often. Make sure their needs are met.

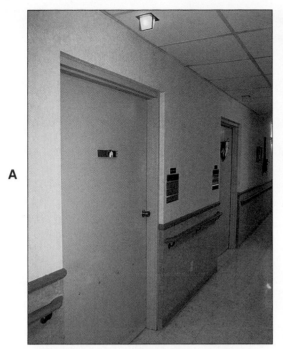 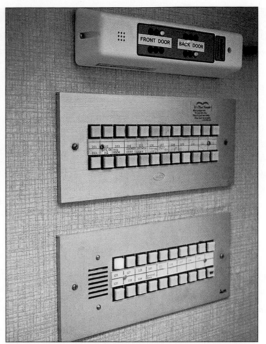

Fig. 4-11 A, Light above the room door. **B,** Light panel and intercom at the nurses' station.

For the person's safety, you must:

- Keep the signal light within the person's reach. Even if the person cannot use the signal light, keep it within reach for use by visitors and staff. They may need to signal for help.
- Place the signal light on the person's strong side.
- Remind the person to signal when help is needed.
- Answer signal lights promptly. The person signals when help is needed. The person may have an urgent need to use the bathroom. You can prevent falls and embarrassing problems by promptly helping the person to the bathroom.
- Answer bathroom and shower or tub room signal lights at once.

PREVENTING FALLS

The risk of falling increases with age. Persons over the age of 65 are at high risk. A history of falls increases the risk of falling again. Most falls occur in the evening, between 1800 (6:00 PM) and 2100 (9:00 PM). Falls also are more likely during shift changes.

Nursing centers have fall prevention programs for persons at risk (Box 4-3). The safety measures in Box 4-4 on p. 72 are part of fall prevention programs. The care plan also lists measures for the person's risk factors.

BOX 4-3	**Factors Increasing the Risk of Falls**

- A history of falls
- Weakness and being unsteady
- Drowsiness and slow reaction time
- Poor vision
- Confusion, disorientation, memory problems, poor judgment
- Decreased mobility
- Foot problems
- Shoes that fit poorly
- Elimination needs (including frequent urination and incontinence)
- Dizziness and lightheadedness
- Joint pain and stiffness
- Muscle weakness
- Low blood pressure
- Balance problems
- Fainting
- Depression
- Strange setting
- Equipment (IV poles, drainage tubes and bags, wheelchairs, walkers, canes, crutches, and others)
- Improper use of wheelchairs, walkers, canes, and crutches
- Not answering signal lights

BOX 4-4   Safety Measures to Prevent Falls

Basic Needs

- Fluid needs are met.
- Glasses and hearing aids are worn as needed.
- Help is given with elimination needs. It is given at regular times and whenever requested. Assist the person to the bathroom. Or provide the bedpan, urinal, or commode.
- The bedpan, urinal, or commode is kept within reach if the person can use the device without help.
- The person is properly positioned at all times. Use pillows, wedge pads, or seats as the nurse and care plan direct (Chapter 16).
- Correct procedures are used for transfers (Chapter 16).

Bathrooms and Shower/Tub Rooms

- Tubs and showers have nonslip surfaces or nonslip bath mats.
- Safety rails and grab bars are in showers. They are by tubs and toilets.
- Shower chairs are used (Chapter 11).
- Safety measures for tub baths and showers are followed (Chapter 11).

Floors

- Scatter, area, and throw rugs are not used.
- Loose floor boards and tiles are reported. Report frayed rugs and carpets.
- Floors and stairs are free of clutter, cords, and other items.
- Floors are free of spills. Wipe up spills at once. Put a "wet floor" sign by the wet area.
- Floors are free of excess furniture and equipment.
- Furniture is placed for easy movement and is not rearranged.
- Equipment and supplies are kept on one side of the hallway.

Beds and Other Equipment

- The bed is in the lowest horizontal position, except when giving bedside care. The distance from the bed to the floor is reduced if the person falls or gets out of bed.
- Bed rails are used according to the care plan.
- Wheelchairs, walkers, and canes fit properly. Another person's equipment is not used.
- Crutches, canes, and walkers have nonskid tips.
- Correct equipment is used for transfers (Chapter 16). Follow the care plan.
- Wheel locks on beds, wheelchairs, and stretchers are in working order. They are locked for transfers.
- Wheelchair and stretcher safety measures are followed (p.•••).

- Rooms, hallways, stairways, and bathrooms have good lighting.
- Night-lights are in bedrooms, hallways, and bathrooms.
- The person can reach the bedside phone, lamp, and personal belongings.
- Linens are checked for sharp objects and for the person's property (dentures, eyeglasses, hearing aids, and so on).

Shoes and Clothing

- Nonskid footwear is worn. Socks, bedroom slippers, and long shoelaces are avoided.
- Clothing fits properly. Clothing is not loose. It does not drag on the floor. Belts are tied or secured in place.

Signal Lights and Alarms

- The person is taught how to use the signal light (p. 70).
- The signal light is always within the person's reach. This includes when in bathrooms and tub/shower rooms.
- The person is asked to call for assistance when help is needed:
  —When getting in or out of bed or a chair
  —With walking
  —With getting to or from the bathroom or commode
  —With getting on or off the bedpan
- Signal lights are answered promptly. The person may need help right away. He or she may not wait for help.
- Bed and chair alarms are used. They sense when the person tries to get up.
- Bed and chair alarms are responded to at once.

Other

- The person is checked often.
- Frequent checks are made on persons with poor judgment or memory.
- Tasks and procedures are explained before and while performing them.
- The person uses handrails when walking.
- Nonslip strips are on the floor next to the bed and in the bathroom. They are intact.
- Caution is used when turning corners, entering corridor intersections, and going through doors. You could injure a person coming from the other direction.
- Pull (do not push) wheelchairs, stretchers, carts, and other wheeled equipment through doorways. This allows you to lead the way and to see where you are going.
- A safety check is made of the room after visitors leave (see the inside front cover). They may have lowered a bed rail, removed the signal light, or moved a walker out of reach. Or they may have brought an item that could harm the person.

Safety Alert

Preventing Falls

Some people are blind. Besides the measures in Box 4-4, other safety measures are needed to protect them from falling:

- Orient the person to the room. Describe the layout, location, and purpose of furniture and equipment.
- Let the person move about and touch and locate furniture and equipment.
- Do not leave the person in the middle of a room. Make sure he or she can reach a wall or furniture.
- Keep doors open or shut, never partly open.
- Offer assistance. Simply say "May I help you?" Respect the person's answer.
- Assist the person in walking. Walk slightly ahead of him or her and offer an arm (Fig. 4-12). Tell the person which arm is offered. Never push, pull, or guide the person in front of you. Walk at a normal pace.
- Tell the person when you are coming to a curb or steps. State if you will step up or down.
- Tell the person about doors, turns, furniture, and other obstructions.
- Give specific directions. Say "right behind you," "on your left," or "in front of you." Avoid phrases such as "over here" or "over there."

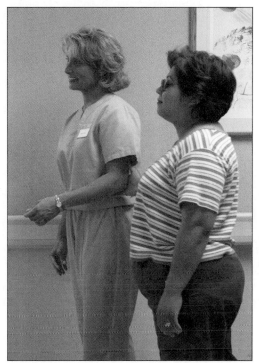

Fig. 4-12 The blind person walks slightly behind the nursing assistant. She takes the nursing assistant's arm.

The Falling Person

A person may start to fall when standing or walking. The person may be weak, lightheaded, or dizzy. Fainting may occur.

Do not try to prevent the fall. Instead, ease the person to the floor. This lets you control the direction of the fall. You can also protect the person's head. Do not let the person move or get up before the nurse checks for injuries. Calmly explain that the nurse will check for injuries.

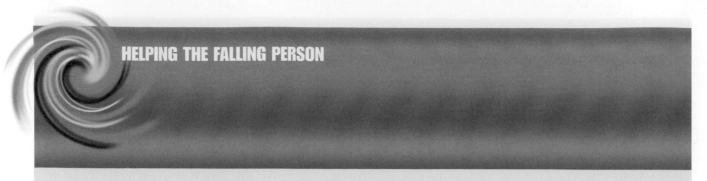

HELPING THE FALLING PERSON

Procedure

1 Stand with your feet apart. Keep your back straight.

2 Bring the person close to your body as fast as possible. Use the gait belt (Chapter 16). Or wrap your arms around the person's waist. You can also hold the person under the arms (Fig. 4-13, A).

3 Move your leg so the person's buttocks rest on it (Fig. 4-13, B). Move the leg near the person.

4 Lower the person to the floor. The person slides down your leg to the floor (Fig. 4-13, C). Bend at your hips and knees as you lower the person.

5 Call a nurse to check the person. Stay with the person.

6 Help the nurse return the person to bed. Get other staff to help if needed.

7 Report the following to the nurse:
- How the fall occurred
- How far the person walked
- How activity was tolerated before the fall
- Complaints before the fall
- How much help the person needed while walking

8 Complete an incident report (p. 90).

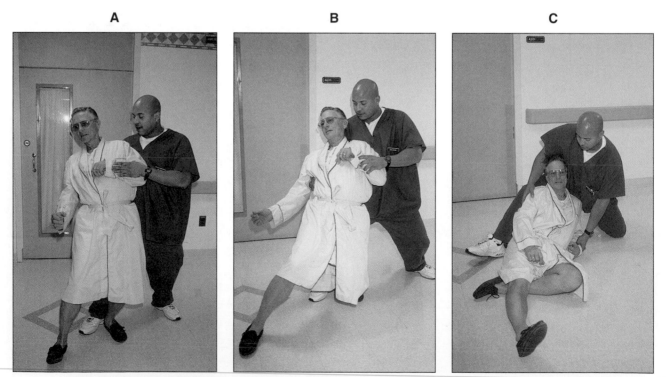

Fig. 4-13 A, The falling person is supported. **B,** The person's buttocks rest on the nursing assistant's leg. **C,** The person is eased to the floor on the nursing assistant's leg.

Bed Rails

Bed rails (side rails) on hospital beds are raised and lowered. They lock in place with levers, latches, or buttons. Bed rails are half, three quarters, or the full length of the bed. When half-length rails are used, each side may have two rails. One is for the upper part of the bed, the other for the lower part.

The nurse and care plan tell you when to raise bed rails. They are needed by persons who are unconscious or sedated with drugs. Some confused or disoriented people need them. If a person needs bed rails, keep them up at all times except when giving bedside care.

Bed rails present hazards. The person can fall when trying to climb over them. Or the person cannot get out of bed to use the bathroom. Entrapment is a risk (Fig. 4-14). That is, a person can get caught, trapped, or entangled in bed rail bars or bed rail gaps. Injury or death can occur if the person's head, neck, chest, arm, or leg is trapped. Persons at greatest risk:

- Are confused or disoriented
- Are restrained (Chapter 20)
- Are small in size
- Have poor muscle control

Bed rails prevent the person from getting out of bed. They are considered restraints. Bed rails cannot be used unless they are needed to treat a person's medical symptoms. Some people feel safer with bed rails up. Others use them to change positions in bed. The person or legal representative must give consent for raised bed rails. The need for bed rails must be carefully noted in the person's medical record and care plan.

The procedures in this book include using bed rails. This helps you learn how to use them correctly.

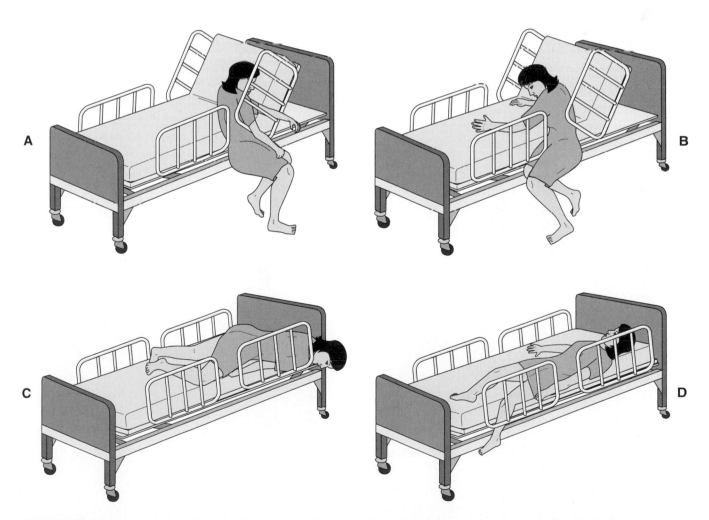

Fig. 4-14 Entrapment is a safety risk with bed rails. **A,** The person is trapped between the bed rail bars. **B,** The person is trapped between the bed rail gaps. **C,** The person is trapped between the bed rail and the headboard. **D,** The person is caught between the mattress and the bed rail.

The nurse, the care plan, and your assignment sheet tell you which people use bed rails. If a person does not use bed rails, omit the "raise or lower bed rails" steps.

If a person uses bed rails, check the person often. Report to the nurse that you checked the person. If you are allowed to chart, record when you checked the person and your observations.

Safety Alert

Bed Rails

You will raise the bed to give care. Follow these safety measures to prevent the person from falling:
- If the person uses bed rails, always raise the far bed rail if you are working alone. Raise both bed rails if you need to leave the bedside for any reason.
- If the person does not use bed rails, ask a co-worker to help you. The co-worker stands on the far side of the bed. This protects the person from falling off the bed.
- Never leave the person alone when the bed is raised.

Hand Rails and Grab Bars

Hand rails are in hallways, stairways, and bathrooms (Fig. 4-15). They give support to persons who are weak or unsteady when walking. They also provide support for sitting down on or getting up from a toilet. Grab bars are along bathtubs and in showers. They are used for getting in and out of the tub or shower.

Wheel Locks

Bed legs have wheels. They let the bed move easily. Each wheel has a lock to prevent the bed from moving (Fig. 4-16). Wheels are locked at all times except when moving the bed. Make sure bed wheels are locked:

- When giving bedside care
- When you transfer a person to and from the bed

Wheelchair and stretcher wheels also are locked during transfers. You or the person can be injured if the bed, wheelchair, or stretcher moves.

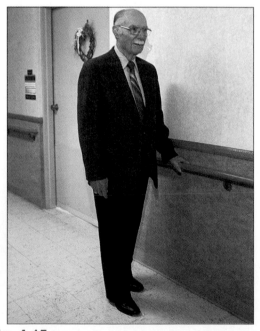

Fig. 4-15 Hand rails provide support when walking.

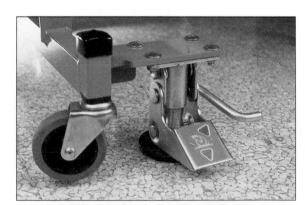

Fig. 4-16 Lock on a bed wheel.

Wheelchair and Stretcher Safety

Wheelchair use is common in nursing centers (Fig. 4-17). Some people use the handrims to propel their chairs. Others use their feet to move the chair. Some wheelchairs are propelled by motors. The person uses hand, chin, mouth, or other controls. If the person cannot propel the wheelchair, another person pushes it using the handgrips/push handles.

Stretchers are used to transport persons who cannot use wheelchairs. They cannot sit up or must lie down.

Follow the safety measures in Box 4-5 on p. 78 when using wheelchairs and stretchers. The person can fall from the chair or stretcher. Or the person can fall during transfers to and from the chair or stretcher.

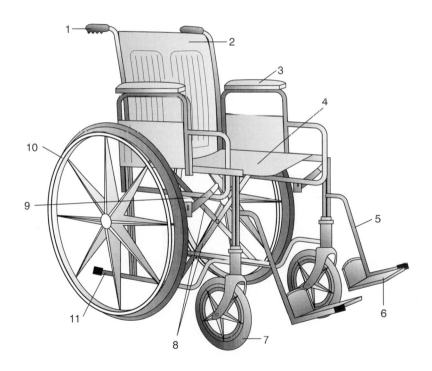

1. Handgrip/push handle
2. Back upholstery
3. Armrest
4. Seat upholstery
5. Front rigging
6. Footplate
7. Caster
8. Crossbrace
9. Wheel lock/brake
10. Wheel and handrim
11. Tipping lever

Fig. 4-17 Parts of a wheelchair.

BOX 4-5 Wheelchair and Stretcher Safety

Wheelchair Safety

- Check the wheel locks. Make sure you can lock and unlock them.
- Check for flat or loose tires. A wheel lock will not work on a flat or loose tire.
- Make sure that wheel spokes are intact. Damaged, broken, or loose spokes can interfere with moving the wheelchair or locking the wheels.
- Make sure casters point forward. This keeps the wheelchair balanced and stable.
- Position the person's feet on the footplates.
- Make sure the person's feet are on the footplates before pushing or repositioning the chair. The person's feet must not touch or drag on the floor when the chair is moving.
- Push the chair forward when transporting the person. Do not pull the chair backward.
- Lock both wheels before you transfer a person to or from the wheelchair.
- Follow the care plan for keeping the wheels locked when not moving the wheelchair. Locking the wheels prevents the chair from moving if the person wants to move to or from the chair.
- Do not let the person stand on the footplates.
- Do not let the footplates fall back onto the person's legs.
- Make sure the person has needed wheelchair accessories—safety belt, pouch, tray, lapboard, cushion.
- Remove the armrests (if removable) when the person transfers to the bed, commode, tub, or car.
- Remove the armrests (if removable) when lifting the person from the chair (Chapter 16).
- Swing the front rigging out of the way for transfers to and from the wheelchair. Some footplates detach for transfers.
- Clean the wheelchair according to center policy.
- Ask a nurse or physical therapist to show you how to propel wheelchairs up steps and ramps and over curbs.
- Follow measures to prevent equipment accidents (p. 82).

Stretcher Safety

- Ask 2 co-workers to help with the transfer (Chapter 16).
- Lock the stretcher wheels before the transfer.
- Fasten the safety straps when the person is properly positioned on the stretcher.
- Ask a co-worker to help with the transport.
- Raise the side rails. Keep them up during the transport.
- Make sure the person's arms and hands do not dangle through the side rail bars.
- Stand at the head of the stretcher. Your co-worker stands at the foot of the stretcher.
- Move the stretcher feet first (Fig. 4-18).
- Do not leave the person alone.
- Follow measures to prevent equipment accidents (p. 82).

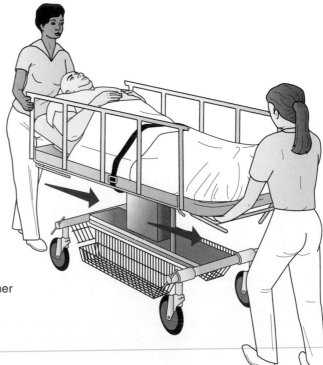

Fig. 4-18 A person is transported by stretcher. The stretcher is moved feet first.

PREVENTING BURNS

Smoking, spilled hot food and liquids, electrical appliances, and very hot bath water are common causes of burns. These safety measures can prevent burns:

- Assist with eating and drinking as needed.
- Turn on cold water first, then hot water. Turn off hot water first, then cold water.
- Measure bath water temperature (Chapter 11). Check for "hot spots" in bath water. Move your hand back and forth.
- Do not let the person use heating pads or electric blankets.
- Be sure people smoke only in smoking areas. Do not allow smoking in bed.
- Do not leave smoking materials at the bedside. They are left at the bedside if the person is trusted to smoke alone in smoking areas. Follow the care plan.
- Supervise the smoking of persons who cannot protect themselves.
- Do not allow smoking where oxygen is used or stored (p. 84).
- Follow the safety measures for using electrical equipment (p. 84).

Heat and Cold Applications

Heat applications are often used for musculoskeletal problems (see Box 4-1). However, heat and cold applications also can cause burns. Doctors order them to promote healing and comfort. They also reduce tissue swelling. Heat and cold have opposite effects on body function. Severe injuries and changes in body function can occur.

Heat Applications.   Heat applications relieve pain, relax muscles, and decrease joint stiffness. They also promote healing and reduce tissue swelling.

When heat is applied to the skin, blood vessels in the area dilate. *Dilate* means to expand or open wider. Blood flow increases. Tissues have more oxygen and nutrients for healing. Excess fluid is removed from the area faster. The skin is red and warm.

High temperatures can cause burns. Pain, excessive redness, and blisters are danger signs. Report these signs at once. Older and fair-skinned people have fragile skin that is easily burned. Persons with problems sensing heat or pain are also at risk. Nervous system damage, loss of consciousness, and circulatory disorders affect sensation. So do confusion and some drugs.

Persons with metal implants are at risk. Metal conducts heat. Deep tissues can be burned. Pacemakers and joint replacements are made of metal. Do not apply heat in the implant area.

Moist and Dry Heat Applications. With a *moist heat application,* water is in contact with the skin. Water conducts heat. Moist heat has greater and faster effects than dry heat. Heat penetrates deeper with a moist application. To prevent injury, moist heat applications have lower (cooler) temperatures than dry heat applications. Moist heat applications include:

- Hot compresses (Fig. 4-19, A, p. 80)—A *compress* is a soft pad applied over a body area. It is usually made of cloth.
- Hot soaks (Fig. 4-19, B, p. 80)—A body part is put into water.
- Sitz baths (Fig. 4-19, C, p. 80)—The perineal and rectal areas are immersed in warm or hot water. (*Sitz* means *seat* in German.)
- Hot packs (Fig. 4-19, D, p. 80)—A *pack* involves wrapping a body part.

With *dry heat applications,* water is not in contact with the skin. A dry heat application stays at the desired temperature longer. Dry heat does not penetrate as deeply as moist heat. Because water is not used, dry heat needs higher (hotter) temperatures to achieve the desired effect. Therefore burns are still a risk. Hot packs and the aquathermia pad (Aqua-K, K-Pad) are dry heat applications (Fig. 4-20, p. 80). The aquathermia pad is an electric device used for dry heat. Tubes inside the pad are filled with distilled water. Heated water flows to the pad through a hose. Another hose returns water to the heating unit. The water is reheated and returned back into the pad.

Cold Applications.   Cold applications reduce pain, prevent swelling, and decrease circulation and bleeding.

Cold has the opposite effect of heat. When cold is applied to the skin, blood vessels constrict. *Constrict* means to narrow. Blood flow decreases. Less oxygen and nutrients are carried to the tissues. Cold applications are useful right after injury. Decreased blood flow reduces the amount of bleeding. Less fluid collects in the tissues. Cold has a numbing effect on the skin. This helps reduce or relieve pain in the part.

Complications include pain, burns, and blisters. Burns and blisters occur from intense cold. They also occur when dry cold is in direct contact with the skin.

Older and fair-skinned persons have fragile skin. They are at great risk for complications. So are persons with mental or sensory impairments.

Moist and Dry Cold Applications. Moist cold applications penetrate deeper than dry ones. Therefore moist applications are not as cold as dry applications.

The cold compress is a moist cold application (see Fig. 4-19, A). Dry cold applications include ice bags, ice collars, and ice gloves (Fig. 4-21, p. 81). Cold packs can be moist or dry applications (see Fig. 4-19, *D*).

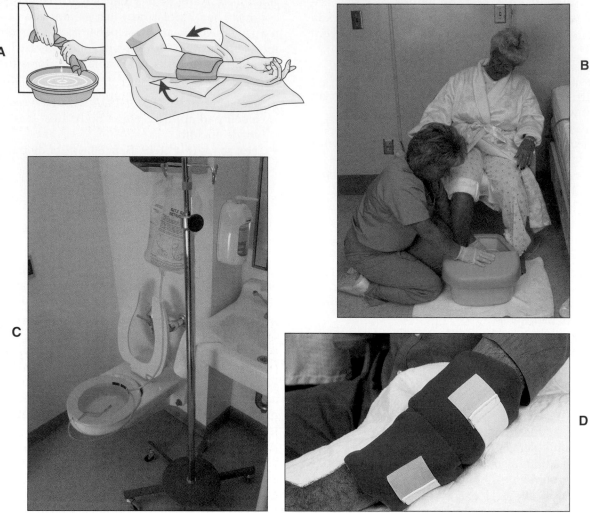

Fig. 4-19 Moist heat applications. **A,** Hot compress. **B,** Hot soak. **C,** Sitz bath. **D,** Hot pack.

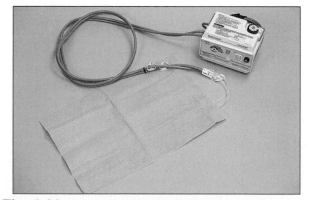

Fig. 4-20 The aquathermia pad is a dry heat application.

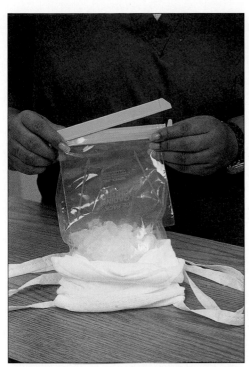

Fig. 4-21 The ice bag is a dry cold application.

Delegation Guidelines

Applying Heat and Cold

Before applying heat and cold, you need this information from the nurse and care plan:

- The type of application
- How to cover the application
- The application site
- What temperature to use
- How long to leave the application in place
- What observations to report and record:
  —Complaints of pain, numbness, or burning
  —Excessive redness
  —Blisters
  —Pale, white, or gray skin
  —Cyanosis (bluish skin color)
  —Shivering
  —Time, site, and length of the application
- What observations to report at once

Safety Alert

Applying Heat and Cold

Before applying heat and cold, make sure that:
- Your state allows you to perform the procedure
- The procedure is in your job description
- You have the necessary training
- You are familiar with the equipment
- You review the procedure with the nurse
- A nurse is available to answer questions and to supervise you

Protect the person from injury during heat and cold applications. Practice the rules in Box 4-6 to prevent burns and other complications.

BOX 4-6	Rules for Applying Heat and Cold

- Know how to use the equipment.
- Ask the nurse what the temperature of the application should be:
  —Heat: cooler temperatures are needed for persons at risk.
  —Cold: warmer temperatures are needed for persons at risk.
- Measure the temperature of moist applications. Use a bath thermometer. Or follow center policy for measuring temperature.
- Know the precise site of the application. Ask the nurse to show you the site.
- Cover dry heat or cold applications before applying them. Use a flannel cover, towel, or pillowcase. Follow center policy.
- Observe the skin every 5 minutes for signs of complications. See *Delegation Guidelines: Applying Heat and Cold.*
- Do not let the person change the temperature of the application.
- Ask the nurse how long to leave the application in place. Carefully watch the time. Heat and cold are applied for no longer than 15 to 20 minutes.
- Follow the rules of electrical safety when using electrical appliances to apply heat (p. 82).
- Provide for privacy. Properly drape and screen the person. Expose only the body part where you will apply heat or cold.
- Place the signal light within the person's reach.

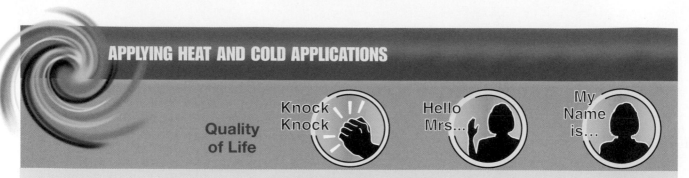

APPLYING HEAT AND COLD APPLICATIONS

Quality of Life · Knock Knock · Hello Mrs... · My Name is...

Pre-Procedure

1　Follow *Delegation Guidelines: Applying Heat and Cold*, p. 81. *See Safety Alert: Applying Heat and Cold*, p. 81.
2　Explain the procedure to the person.
3　Practice hand hygiene.

4　Collect needed equipment.
5　Identify the person. Check the ID bracelet against the assignment sheet. Call the person by name.
6　Provide for privacy.

Procedure

7　Prepare the application. Follow center procedures and the manufacturer's instructions.
8　Place a dry application in a cover.
9　Place the application on the affected part. Note the time.
10　Secure the application in place with ties, tape, or rolled gauze. Do not use pins.
11　Unscreen the person. Place the signal light within reach.

12　Raise or lower bed rails. Follow the care plan.
13　Check the person every 5 minutes. Check for signs and symptoms of complications (see *Delegation Guidelines: Applying Heat and Cold*, p. 81). Remove the application if any occur. Tell the nurse at once.
14　Remove the application at the specified time. (If bed rails are up, lower the near one for this step.)

Post-Procedure

15　Provide for comfort.
16　Unscreen the person.
17　Place the signal light within reach.
18　Raise or lower bed rails. Follow the care plan.
19　Complete a safety check of the room. (See inside of front book cover.)
20　Clean the sitz bath with disinfectant solution. Wear utility gloves.

21　Clean and return reusable items to their proper place. Follow center policy for soiled linen. Wear gloves for this step.
22　Discard the gloves. Decontaminate your hands.
23　Report and record your observations.

PREVENTING POISONING

Poisoning from poor vision or confusion is a major hazard in older persons. Make sure residents cannot reach plants and hazardous materials (p. 84). Follow center procedures for storing personal items (for example, mouthwash, lotion, deodorant). These items are harmful when swallowed.

PREVENTING EQUIPMENT ACCIDENTS

All equipment is unsafe if broken, not used correctly, or not working properly. Inspect all equipment before use. Check glass and plastic items for cracks, chips, and sharp or rough edges. They can cause cuts, stabs, or scratches. Follow the Bloodborne Pathogen Standard (Chapter 3). Do not use or give damaged items to residents. Take the item to the nurse. The nurse will have you do one of the following:

• Discard the item following center policy
• Tag the item and send it for repair following center policy

Electrical items must work properly and be in good repair. Check for frayed cords (Fig. 4-22) and overloaded electrical outlets (Fig. 4-23). They can cause fires and electrical shocks. An electrical shock can burn the skin, muscles, nerves, and other tissues.

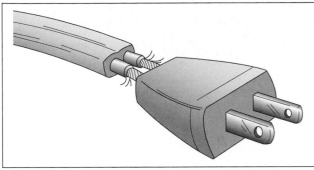

Fig. 4-22 A frayed electrical cord.

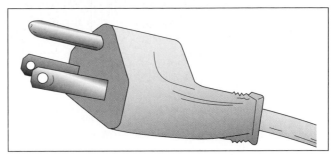

Fig. 4-24 A three-pronged plug.

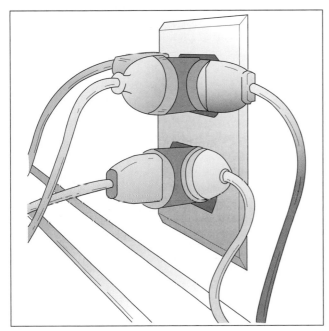

Fig. 4-23 An overloaded electrical outlet.

It can affect the heart and cause death. Practice these safety measures:

- Follow center policies and procedures and the manufacturer's instruction.
- Read and follow all caution and warning labels.
- Do not use electrical items owned by the person until they are safety checked by the maintenance department.
- Do not use an unfamiliar item. Ask for needed training. Also ask a nurse to supervise you the first time you use the item.
- Use equipment only for its intended purpose.
- Use three-pronged plugs for all electrical items (Fig. 4-24).

- Practice bed safety:
  —Plug the power cord into a wall outlet. Do not use extension cords or electrical strips.
  —Check the power cord for damage or fraying.
  —Make sure the bed moves up and down freely.
  —Make sure the bed controls work properly.
  —Report any unusual sounds or odors. Also report if the bed is not working properly.
- Use electrical appliances correctly. Unplug them when not in use.
- Make sure the item works before you begin.
- Place a "do not use" tag on broken items. Complete a repair request form and explain the problem.
- Tell the nurse about broken items.
- Do not try to repair broken items.
- Keep electrical items away from water. Wipe up spills right away.
- Do not touch electrical items if you are wet, your hands are wet, or you are standing in water.
- Do not cover power cords (including the bed's power cord) with carpets, rugs, or other coverings.
- Turn off equipment before unplugging it. Sparks occur when electrical items are unplugged while turned on.
- Hold onto the plug (not the cord) when removing it from an outlet.
- Do not use water to put out an electrical fire. If possible, turn off or unplug the item.
- Do not touch a person who is experiencing an electrical shock. If possible, turn off or unplug the item. Call for help at once.

An incident report (p. 90) is completed if a resident, visitor, or staff member has an equipment-related accident. The Safe Medical Devices Act requires that centers report equipment-related illnesses, injuries, and deaths.

HANDLING HAZARDOUS SUBSTANCES

The Occupational Safety and Health Administration (OSHA) has standards and guidelines for handling hazardous substances. A **hazardous substance** is any chemical in the workplace that can cause harm. Fire, explosions, and health problems can occur. The center provides hazardous substance training for employees. The center also provides eyewash and total body wash stations in areas where hazardous substances are used. Hazardous substances include:

- Drugs used in cancer therapy (chemotherapy, anti-cancer drugs)
- Gases used for anesthesia and to sterilize equipment
- Oxygen
- Disinfectants and cleaning solutions
- Radiation used for x-rays and cancer treatments
- Mercury (found in thermometers and blood pressure devices)

Labeling

Hazardous substance containers need warning labels (Fig. 4-25). The manufacturer applies the labels. Warning labels identify:

- The type of hazard
- Safety precautions including needed personal protective equipment (Chapter 3)
- How to use the substance safely
- Storage and disposal information

If a warning label is removed or damaged, do not use the substance. Take the container to the nurse, and explain the problem. Do not leave the container unattended.

Material Safety Data Sheets

Every hazardous substance has a material safety data sheet (MSDS). It gives detailed information about the substance. Check the MSDS before using a hazardous substance, cleaning up a leak or spill, or disposing of the substance. Tell the nurse about a leak or spill right away. Do not leave a leak or spill unattended.

OXYGEN SAFETY

Air has some oxygen. Disease, injury, and surgery often interfere with breathing. The amount of oxygen in the blood may be less than normal. If so, the doctor orders oxygen therapy.

Oxygen is treated as a drug. The doctor orders the amount of oxygen to give, the device to use, and when to give it. *You do not give oxygen.* The nurse and respiratory therapist start and maintain oxygen therapy. You assist the nurse in providing safe care.

Oxygen Sources

Oxygen is supplied as follows:

- *Wall outlet*—Oxygen is piped into each person's unit (Fig. 4-26).
- *Oxygen tank*—The oxygen tank is placed at the bedside. Small tanks are used during emergencies and transfers (Fig. 4-27).
- *Oxygen concentrator*—The machine removes oxygen from the air (Fig. 4-28).
- *Liquid oxygen system*—A portable unit is filled from a stationary unit (Fig. 4-29). The portable unit can be worn over the shoulder. This allows the person to be mobile.

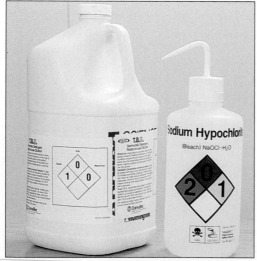

Fig. 4-25 Warning labels on hazardous substances.

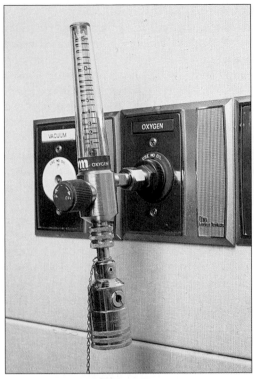

Fig. 4-26 Wall oxygen outlet.

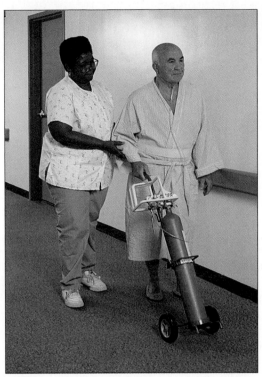

Fig. 4-27 A portable oxygen tank is used when walking.

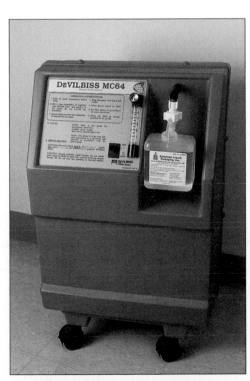

Fig. 4-28 Oxygen concentrator.

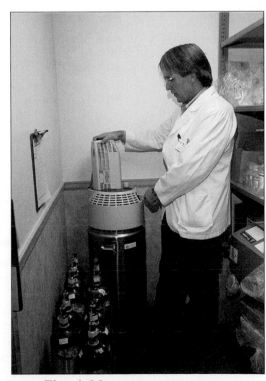

Fig. 4-29 Liquid oxygen system.

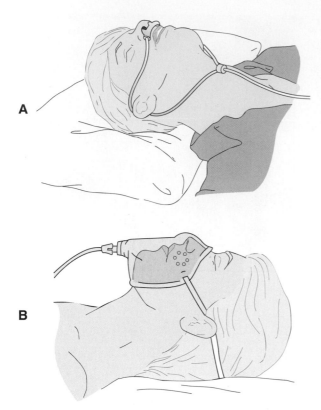

Fig. 4-30 A, Nasal cannula. **B,** Simple mask.

Oxygen Devices

The doctor orders the device used to give oxygen. These devices are common:

- *Nasal cannula* (Fig. 4-30, A)—The prongs are inserted into the nostrils. A band goes over the ears and under the chin to keep the device in place. It allows eating and drinking. Tight prongs can irritate the nose. Pressure on the ears and cheekbones is possible.
- *Simple mask* (Fig. 4-30, B)—It covers the nose and mouth. Talking is hard to do with a mask. Listen carefully. Moisture can build up under masks. Keep the face clean and dry to prevent irritation from the mask. Masks are removed for eating. Usually oxygen is given by cannula during meals.

Oxygen Flow Rates

The *flow rate* is the amount of oxygen given. It is measured in liters per minute (L/min). The doctor orders 2 to 15 liters of oxygen per minute.

The nurse and care plan tell you the person's flow rate. When giving care and checking the person, always check the flow rate. Tell the nurse at once if it is too high or too low. A nurse or respiratory therapist will adjust the flow rate. Some states and centers let nursing assistants adjust flow rates. Know your center's policy.

Oxygen Administration Set-Up

Oxygen is a dry gas. If not humidified (made moist), oxygen dries the airway's mucous membranes. Distilled water is added to the humidifier to create water vapor (Fig. 4-31). Oxygen picks up water vapor as it flows into the system. Bubbling in the humidifier means water vapor is being produced. Low flow rates (1 to 2 L/min) by cannula usually do not need humidification.

When giving care and checking the person, note the amount of water in the humidifier. Tell the nurse if the water level is low. Follow center procedures for adding water.

Safety Measures

You assist the nurse with oxygen therapy. You do not give oxygen. You do not adjust the flow rate unless allowed by your state and center.

Oxygen is a hazardous substance (p. 84). It is needed to start and maintain a fire. Practice these safety measures:

- Place "Oxygen" and "No Smoking" signs in the room and on the room door.
- Remove smoking materials from the room—cigarettes, cigars, pipes, matches, and lighters.
- Remind the person and visitors not to smoke in the room.
- Remove materials from the room that ignite easily—alcohol, nail polish remover, oils, greases.
- Follow safety measures to prevent equipment accidents (p. 83).
- Use cotton blankets, gowns, and pajamas. Wools and synthetic fabrics can cause static electricity.
- Turn off the oxygen if a fire occurs.
- Tell the nurse if the oxygen source (tank, liquid oxygen system) is low. Check the gauge or dial on the device.
- Make sure the oxygen source (tank, oxygen concentrator, liquid oxygen system) is secured properly. Follow center procedures.

FIRE SAFETY

Fire is a constant danger. The entire health team must prevent fires. They must act quickly if a fire occurs. Three things are needed for a fire:

- A spark or flame
- A material that will burn
- Oxygen

Fire prevention measures were described in relation to burns, equipment-related accidents, and oxygen use. Other measures are listed in Box 4-7.

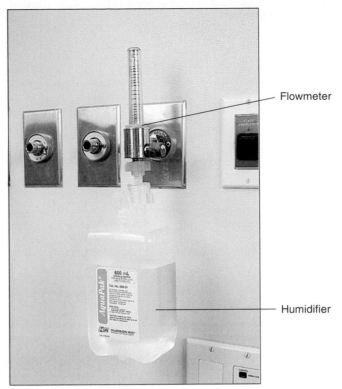

Fig. 4-31 Oxygen administration system with humidifier. Note that the flowmeter shows the flow rate.

BOX 4-7	Fire Prevention Measures

- Follow the safety measures for oxygen use.
- Smoke only where allowed to do so. Do not smoke in resident rooms.
- Be sure all ashes, cigars, cigarettes, and other smoking materials are out before emptying ashtrays.
- Provide ashtrays to persons who are allowed to smoke.
- Empty ashtrays into a metal container partially filled with sand or water. Do not empty ashtrays into plastic containers or wastebaskets lined with paper or plastic bags.
- Supervise persons who smoke. This is very important for persons who are confused, disoriented, or sedated.
- Follow safety practices when using electrical items (p. 83).
- Store flammable liquids in their original containers.
- Do not light matches or lighters or smoke around flammable liquids or materials.

What To Do During a Fire

Know your center's policies and procedures for fire emergencies. Know where to find fire alarms, fire extinguishers, and emergency exits. Remember the word *RACE:*

- *R*—for *rescue.* Rescue persons in immediate danger. Move them to a safe place.
- *A*—for *alarm.* Sound the nearest fire alarm. Notify the switchboard operator.
- *C*—for *confine.* Close doors and windows to confine the fire. Turn off oxygen or electrical items used in the general area of the fire.
- *E*—for *extinguish.* Use a fire extinguisher if a small fire has not spread to a larger area.

Clear equipment from all normal and emergency exists. *Do not use elevators.*

Using a Fire Extinguisher. Different extinguishers are used for different kinds of fires: oil and grease fires, electrical fires, and paper and wood fires. A general procedure for using a fire extinguisher follows.

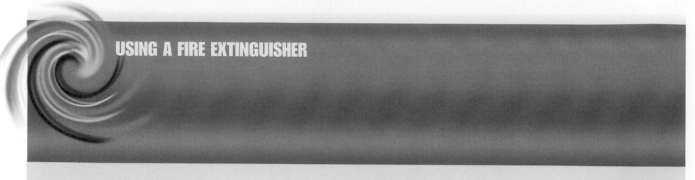

USING A FIRE EXTINGUISHER

1　Pull the fire alarm.
2　Get the nearest fire extinguisher.
3　Carry it upright.
4　Take it to the fire.
5　Remove the safety pin (Fig. 4-32, A).

6　Direct the hose at the base of the fire (Fig. 4-32, B).
7　Push the top handle down (Fig. 4-32, C).
8　Sweep the hose slowly back and forth at the base of the fire.

A
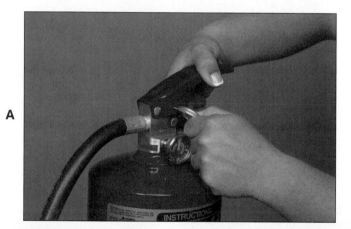

B
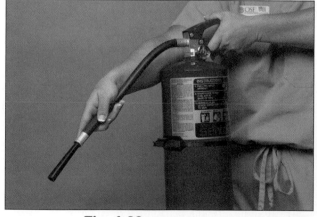

C
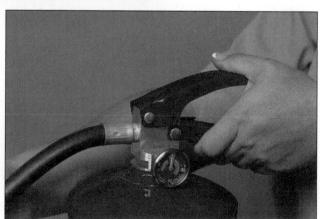

Fig. 4-32 Using a fire extinguisher. **A,** Remove the safety pin. **B,** Direct the hose at the base of the fire. **C,** Push the top handle down.

DISASTERS

A *disaster* is a sudden catastrophic event. Many people are injured and killed. Property is destroyed. Natural disasters include tornadoes, hurricanes, blizzards, earthquakes, volcanic eruptions, floods, and some fires. Human-made disasters include auto, bus, train, and airplane accidents. They also include fires, bombings, nuclear power plant accidents, riots, explosions, gas or chemical leaks, and wars.

The center has procedures for disasters that could occur in your area. Follow them to keep residents, visitors, and staff safe. A disaster may damage the center. The disaster plan includes policies and procedures to evacuate the center.

Bomb Threats

Centers have polices and procedures for bomb threats. You must follow them if a caller makes a bomb threat or if you find an item that looks or sounds strange. Often bomb threats are sent by phone. However, they can be sent by mail, e-mail, messenger, or other means. Or the person can leave a bomb in the center.

WORKPLACE VIOLENCE

Workplace violence is violent acts directed toward persons at work or while on duty. It includes:

- Murders
- Beatings and use of weapons—firearms, bombs, or knives
- Kidnapping
- Robbery
- Threats—obscene phone calls; threatening oral, written, or body language; and harassment of any nature (being followed, sworn at, or shouted at)

According to OSHA, nurses and nursing assistants are at risk for workplace violence. They have the most contact with residents and visitors. Risk factors include:

- People with visible or concealed weapons
- Acutely disturbed and violent persons
- Alcohol and drug abuse
- Mentally ill persons who do not follow a treatment program
- Pharmacies have drugs, and are a target for robberies
- Gang members and substance abusers are residents or visitors
- Upset, agitated, and disturbed family and visitors
- Long waits for services

- Being alone with residents during care or transport to other areas
- Low staff levels during meals, emergencies, and at night
- Poor lighting in hallways, rooms, parking lots, and other areas
- Lack of training in recognizing and managing potentially violent situations

OSHA has guidelines for violence prevention programs. The goal is to prevent or reduce staff exposure to situations that can cause death or injury. Worksite hazards are identified. Prevention measures are developed and followed. The staff receives safety and health training.

Practice these measures when dealing with agitated or aggressive persons:

- Stand away from the person. Judge the length of the person's arms and legs. Stand far enough away so the person cannot hit or kick you.
- Stand close to the door. Do not become trapped in the room.
- Know where to find panic buttons, signal lights, alarms, closed-circuit monitors, and other security devices.
- Keep your hands free.
- Stay calm. Talk to the person in a calm manner. Do not raise your voice or argue, scold, or interrupt the person.
- Do not touch the person.
- Tell the person that you will get a nurse to speak to him or her.
- Leave the room as soon as you can. Make sure the person is safe.
- Tell the nurse or security officer about the matter.
- Complete an incident report according to center policy (p. 90).

RISK MANAGEMENT

Risk management involves identifying and controlling risks and safety hazards affecting the center. It also involves meeting state and federal requirements. The intent is to protect everyone in the center (residents, visitors, and staff) and all property from harm or danger.

Personal Belongings

The person's belongings must be kept safe. Often they are sent home with the family. A personal belongings list is completed. Each item is listed and described. The staff member and person sign the completed list.

A valuables envelope is used for money and jewelry. Each jewelry item is listed and described on the envelope. Describe what you see. For example, describe a ring as having a white stone with four prongs in a yellow setting. Do not assume the stone is a diamond in a gold setting. For valuables:

- Count money with the person.
- Put money and each jewelry item in the envelope with the person watching. Sign the envelope like the personal belongings list.
- Give the envelope to the nurse. The nurse puts it in a safe or gives it to the family.

Dentures, eyeglasses, contact lenses, hearing aids, and watches are kept at the bedside. Items kept at the bedside are listed in the person's record. Some people keep money for newspapers and gift shop items. The amount is noted in the person's record. Clothing and shoes are labeled with the person's name. So are radios, blankets, and other items brought from home.

Reporting Incidents

An **incident** is any event that has harmed or could harm a resident, staff member, or visitor. It includes accidents and errors in giving care. See Box 4-8 for examples.

Report accidents and errors at once. This includes:

- Accidents involving residents, visitors, or staff.
- Errors in care. This includes giving the wrong care, giving care to the wrong person, or not giving care.
- Broken, damaged, or lost items owned by the person. Dentures, hearing aids, eyeglasses, clothing, and money are examples.
- Hazardous substance accidents.
- Workplace violence incidents.

An *incident report* is completed as soon as possible after the incident. It includes:

- Names of those involved
- Date and time of the accident or error
- Location of the accident or error
- A complete description of what happened
- Names of witnesses
- Any other requested information

BOX 4-8	Common Incidents

- A resident's dentures are lost. They are found broken in the laundry.
- A confused resident is found sleeping in bed with another resident.
- An agitated resident strikes another resident.
- A resident wanders away from the center. The person is found many hours later sitting on the porch of a house four blocks from the center.
- A resident is found asleep in the front seat of a visitor's car.
- A visitor slips on a wet floor and falls.
- While dusting, a housekeeper drops and breaks a resident's clock.
- A resident is found sitting on the floor beside the bed.
- A nurse gives the wrong drug to a resident.
- A resident receives a burn while taking a bath.
- A resident drops a hearing aid in the toilet.
- While resisting staff efforts to assist with dressing, a resident receives a skin tear.
- A nursing assistant wears a ring with a large stone. A resident is scratched during care.
- A confused and agitated resident bites a staff member.
- A nurse leaves a needle on the resident's bed. A nursing assistant receives a needle-stick injury when making the bed.
- A resident is given the wrong meal tray. The error is found after the resident is done eating.
- A maintenance staff member leaves tools in a resident's room. The resident is injured on the tools.
- A resident is bruised from a restraint.
- A resident falls in the hallway.
- A resident was not repositioned for 6 hours. A pressure ulcer develops.
- A nursing assistant receives an electrical shock from an electric bed.
- A resident's dentures are dropped and broken.
- Visitors are shouting in the hallway. Security is called.
- A resident reports missing money or jewelry.

Incident reports are reviewed by risk management and a committee of health care workers. They look for patterns and trends of accidents or errors. For example, are falls occurring on the same shift and on the same unit? Are lost or missing items being reported on the same shift or same unit? There may be new policies or procedures to prevent future incidents.

Review Questions

Circle **T** if the statement is true or **F** if the statement is false.

1 **T F** To correctly identify a person, call him or her by name.

2 **T F** Falls are more common during the evening.

3 **T F** Older persons are at risk for accidents because of changes in the body.

4 **T F** Needing to urinate is a major cause of falls.

5 **T F** Socks and bedroom slippers help prevent falls.

6 **T F** Good lighting helps prevent falls.

7 **T F** Bed rails are always raised when the bed is raised.

8 **T F** The signal light must always be within the person's reach.

9 **T F** Hazardous substances must have warning labels.

10 **T F** Many people are injured and killed and property is destroyed in a disaster.

11 **T F** Smoking is allowed where oxygen is used.

Circle the **BEST** answer.

12 These actions are about body mechanics. Which is *false*?
a Hold objects away from your body when lifting, moving, or carrying them.
b Face the direction you are working to prevent twisting.
c Push, pull, or slide heavy objects.
d Use both hands and arms to lift, move, or carry heavy objects.

13 Which is *not* a risk factor for accidents?
a Wearing eyeglasses
b Hearing impairment
c Memory problems
d Being over 65 years of age

14 A person in a coma
a Has suffered an electrical shock
b Is confused and disoriented
c Is not aware of his or her surroundings
d Has stopped breathing

15 Mrs. Ford often tries to get up without help. You should do the following *except*
a Remind her to use the signal light
b Check on her often
c Help her to the bathroom at regular intervals
d Keep her bed rails up

16 To prevent falls, you should do the following *except*
a Wipe up spills right away
b Turn on night-lights
c Encourage the use of hand rails and grab bars
d Keep bed rails up

17 These statements are about bed rails. Which is *true*?
a The person can get caught in bed rails.
b Bed rails are kept up when the person is in bed.
c OBRA requires the use of bed rails.
d Bed rails allow the person to get out of bed.

18 Mr. Wallace uses a wheelchair. Which measure is *unsafe*?
a The wheels are locked for transfers.
b He can stand on the footplates
c The wheels are locked when he transfers from the wheelchair to bed.
d The casters point forward.

19 Stretcher safety involves the following *except*
a Locking the wheels for transfers
b Fastening the safety straps
c Raising the side rails
d Moving the stretcher head first

20 The greatest threat from heat applications is
a Infection
b Burns
c Chilling
d Dizziness

21 Who has the greatest risk of complications from local heat applications?
a A 10-year-old boy
b A teenager
c A 40-year-old woman
d An older person

Review Questions

22 Mrs. Parks is using an aquathermia pad. Which is *false?*
a It is a dry heat application.
b You observe the skin under the pad every 5 minutes.
c Electrical safety precautions are practiced.
d Pins secure the pad in place.

23 Heat and cold applications are left in place no longer than
a 20 minutes
b 30 minutes
c 45 minutes
d 60 minutes

24 To prevent equipment accidents, you should
a Fix broken items
b Use two-pronged plugs
c Check glass and plastic items for damage
d Complete an incident report

25 Mr. Wallace is a new resident. You need to shave him. Before using his electric shaver
a You need to inspect it
b The maintenance staff needs to do a safety check
c You need to check for a frayed cord
d You need an outlet

26 You are using equipment. Which is *unsafe?*
a Following the manufacturer's instructions
b Keeping electrical items away from water and spills
c Pulling on the cord to remove a plug from an outlet
d Turning off electrical items after using them

27 You spilled a hazardous substance. You should do the following *except*
a Read the material safety data sheet
b Cover the spill, and go tell the nurse
c Wear any needed personal protective equipment to clean up the spill
d Complete an incident report

28 When assisting with oxygen therapy, you can
a Turn the oxygen on and off
b Start the oxygen
c Decide what device to use
d Check the flow rate

29 The following are needed to start a fire *except*
a A spark or flame
b A material that will burn
c Oxygen
d Carbon monoxide

30 The fire alarm sounds. The following are done *except*
a Turning off oxygen
b Using elevators
c Closing doors and windows
d Moving residents to a safe place

31 A person is agitated and aggressive. You should do the following *except*
a Stand away from the person
b Stand close to the door
c Use touch to show you care
d Talk to the person without raising your voice

32 You gave Mrs. Ford the wrong treatment. Which is *true?*
a Report the error at the end of the shift.
b Take action only if Mrs. Ford was injured.
c You committed a crime.
d You must complete an incident report.

Answers to these questions are on p. 388.

CHAPTER 5

Basic Emergency Care

Objectives

- Define the key terms listed in this chapter
- Describe the general rules of emergency care
- Identify the signs of cardiac arrest and obstructed airway
- Describe the signs, symptoms, and emergency care for hemorrhage
- Identify the signs, symptoms, and emergency care for shock
- Describe the types of seizures and how to care for a person during a seizure
- Identify the common causes and emergency care for fainting
- Identify the emergency care for vomiting and aspiration
- Describe the signs, symptoms, and emergency care for stroke
- Perform the procedures described in this chapter

aspiration Breathing fluid or an object into the lungs

cardiac arrest The heart and breathing stop suddenly and without warning

convulsion A seizure

fainting The sudden loss of consciousness from an inadequate blood supply to the brain; syncope

hemorrhage The excessive loss of blood in a short time

seizure Violent and sudden contractions or tremors of muscle groups; convulsion

shock Results when organs and tissues do not get enough blood

---

Emergencies can occur anywhere. Sometimes you can save a life if you know what to do. You are encouraged to take a first aid course and a basic life support course. These courses prepare you to give emergency care.

Each emergency is different. The rules in Box 5-1 apply to any emergency.

Safety Alert

Emergency Care
Contact with blood, body fluids, secretions, and excretions is likely. Follow Standard Precautions and the Bloodborne Pathogen Standard to the extent possible. Practice hand hygiene as soon as possible.

BASIC LIFE SUPPORT

When the heart and breathing stop, the person is clinically dead. Blood and oxygen are not circulated through the body. Brain and other organ damage occurs within minutes. Sometimes death is expected (Chapter 10). However, **cardiac arrest** is when the heart and breathing stop suddenly and without warning. The three major signs of cardiac arrest are: *no response, no breathing,* and *no pulse.* The skin is cool, pale, and gray. The person is not coughing or moving. Basic life support (BLS) procedures support breathing and circulation.

Safety Alert

Basic Life Support
The basic life support procedures in this chapter are given as information. They do not replace certification training. You need a basic life support course for health care providers.

The discussion and procedures that follow assume that the person does not have injuries from trauma. If injuries are present, special measures are needed to position the person and open the airway. Such measures are learned during a BLS certification course.

 Cardiopulmonary Resuscitation for Adults

Cardiopulmonary resuscitation (CPR) must be started at once when a person is in cardiac arrest. It provides oxygen to the brain and heart until advanced emergency care is given. The ABCs of CPR are: **A**irway, **B**reathing, and **C**irculation.

Airway.   The airway is often obstructed (blocked) during cardiac arrest. The person's tongue falls toward the back of the throat and blocks the airway. The head-tilt/chin-lift maneuver opens the airway (Fig. 5-1):

* Position the person supine (on his or her back) on a hard, flat surface.

BOX 5-1 General Rules of Emergency Care

- Know your limits. Do not do more than you are able. Do not perform an unfamiliar procedure. Do what you can under the circumstances.
- Call or send for help.
- Stay calm. This helps the person feel more secure.
- Know where to find emergency equipment and supplies.
- Follow Standard Precautions and the Bloodborne Pathogen Standard to the extent possible.
- Check for life-threatening problems. Check for breathing, a pulse, and bleeding.
- Keep the person lying down or as you found him or her. Moving the person could make an injury worse.
- Perform necessary emergency measures.
- Do not remove clothes unless you have to. If you must remove clothing, tear or cut garments along the seams.
- Keep the person warm. Cover the person with a blanket.
- Reassure the conscious person. Explain what is happening.
- Do not give the person food or fluids.
- Keep bystanders away. They invade privacy, and tend to stare, give advice, and comment about the person's condition. The person may think the situation is worse than it really is.
- Measure blood pressure, pulse, and respirations every 5 minutes (Chapter 7).
- Report and record the following:
  —The time of the emergency
  —What happened
  —Your observations (Chapter 9)
  —What you did to help the person
  —The person's response to the help given
  —Blood pressure, pulse, and respiration measurements
  —The names of witnesses to the emergency

- Kneel or stand at the person's side.
- Place the palm of one hand on the forehead.
- Tilt the head back by pushing down on the forehead with your palm.
- Place the fingers of the other hand under the bony part of the chin.
- Lift the chin as you tilt the head backward with your other hand.

When the airway is open, check for vomitus, loose dentures, or other objects. These can obstruct the airway. Remove dentures and wipe vomitus away with your index and middle fingers. Wear gloves, or cover your fingers with a cloth.

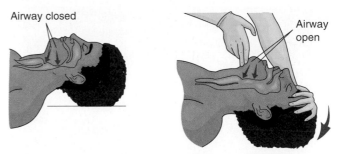

Fig. 5-1 The head-tilt/chin-lift maneuver opens the airway. One hand is on the person's forehead. Pressure is applied to tilt the head back. The chin is lifted with the fingers of the other hand

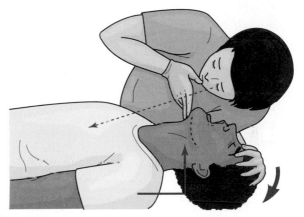

Fig. 5-2 Determining adequate breathing. *Look* to see if the chest rises and falls. *Listen* for the escape of air. *Feel* for the flow of air on your cheek.

Breathing. Check for adequate breathing (Fig. 5-2). Take no more than 10 seconds to:

- Maintain an open airway.
- Place your ear over the person's mouth and nose.
- *Look* to see if the chest rises and falls.
- *Listen* for the escape of air.
- *Feel* for the flow of air.

Rescue breathing involves inflating the person's lungs. To give *mouth-to-mouth breathing* (Fig. 5-3, p. 96):

- Keep the airway open.
- Pinch the person's nostrils shut to prevent the escape of air. Use your thumb and index finger of the hand on the forehead.
- Take a deep breath.
- Place your mouth tightly over the person's mouth.
- Blow air into the person's mouth slowly. You should see the chest rise as the lungs fill with air. You should also hear air escape when the person exhales.
- Remove your mouth from the person's mouth. Then take in a quick, deep breath.

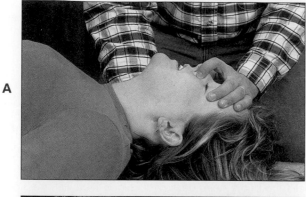

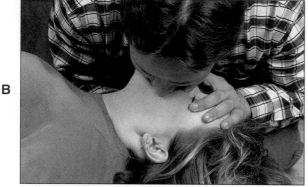

Fig. 5-3 Mouth-to-mouth breathing. **A,** The person's airway is opened. The nostrils are pinched shut. **B,** The person's mouth is sealed by the rescuer's mouth.

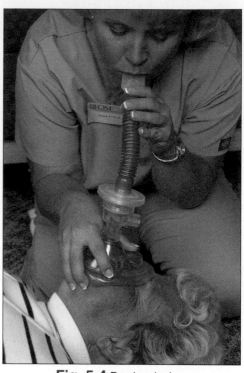

Fig. 5-4 Barrier device.

For *mouth-to-barrier device breathing*, a barrier device is placed over the person's mouth and nose. It prevents contact with the person's mouth and blood, body fluids, secretions, or excretions (Fig. 5-4). The seal must be tight.

When you start CPR, give 2 breaths first. Allow exhalation after each breath. Then give 10 to 12 breaths per minute. Give 2 breaths after every 15 chest compressions.

Circulation.   Chest compressions force blood through the circulatory system. Before starting chest compressions, check for a pulse. Use the carotid artery on the side near you. To find the carotid pulse, place 2 fingers on the person's trachea (windpipe). Then slide your fingertips down off the trachea to the groove of the neck (Fig. 5-5). While checking for a pulse, look to see if the person has started breathing or is coughing or moving.

The heart lies between the sternum (breastbone) and the spinal column. When pressure is applied to the sternum, the sternum is depressed. This compresses the heart between the sternum and spinal column (Fig. 5-6). The person must be supine and on a hard, flat surface. Proper hand position is needed (Fig. 5-7).

To give chest compressions, your arms are straight. Your shoulders are directly over your hands (Fig. 5-8). Exert firm downward pressure to depress the sternum about 1½ to 2 inches in the adult. Then release pressure without removing your hands from the chest. Give compressions in a regular rhythm at a rate of 100 per minute.

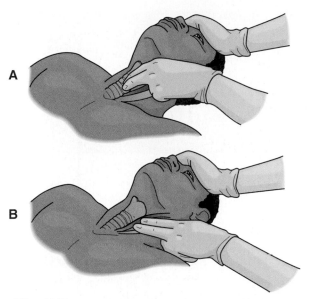

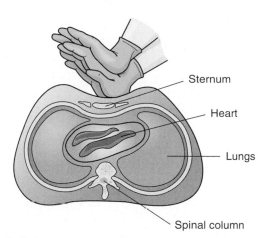

Fig. 5-5 Locating the carotid pulse. **A,** Two fingers are placed on the trachea. **B,** The fingerstips are moved down into the groove of the neck to the carotid pulse.

Fig. 5-6 The heart lies between the sternum and spinal column. The heart is compressed when pressure is applied to the sternum.

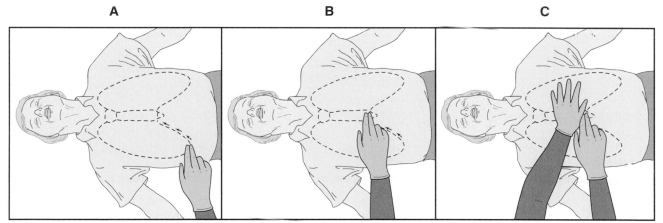

Fig. 5-7 Proper hand position for CPR. **A,** Find the rib cage. **B,** Move your fingers along the rib cage to the notch. **C,** Place the heel of your hand next to your index finger.

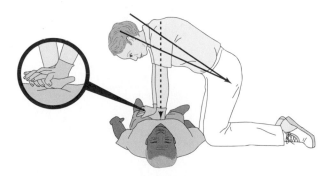

Fig. 5-8 To give chest compressions, the arms are straight and shoulders are over the hands.

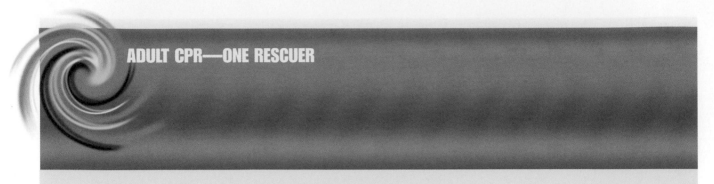

ADULT CPR—ONE RESCUER

Procedure

1 Check if the person is responding. Tap or gently shake the person, call the person by name, and shout "Are you OK?"
2 Call for help.
3 Position the person supine. Logroll the person so there is no twisting of the spine (Chapter 16). Place the person's arms alongside the body.
4 Open the airway. Use the head-tilt/chin-lift method.
5 Check for breathing. *Look* to see if the chest rises and falls. *Listen* for the escape of air. *Feel* for the flow of air on your cheek.
6 Give 2 slow breaths if the person is not breathing or is not breathing adequately. Each breath takes 2 seconds. Let the person's lungs deflate between breaths.
7 Check for a carotid pulse and for breathing, coughing, and moving. This should take 5 to 10 seconds. Use one hand to keep the airway open with the head-tilt/chin-lift method. Start chest compressions if there are no signs of circulation.
8 Give 100 chest compressions per minute. Give 15 compressions and then 2 slow breaths:

a Establish a rhythm and count out loud. (Try: "1 and, 2 and, 3 and, 4 and, 5 and, 6 and, 7 and, 8 and, 9 and, 10 and, 11 and, 12 and, 13 and, 14 and, 15.")
b Open the airway. Give 2 slow breaths.
c Repeat this step until 4 cycles of 15 compressions and 2 breaths are given.
9 Check for a carotid pulse. Also check for breathing, coughing, and moving.
10 Continue with 15 compressions and 2 slow breaths if the person has no signs of circulation. Start with chest compressions. Check for circulation every few minutes.
11 Do the following if the person has signs of circulation:
a Check for breathing.
b Position the person in the recovery position (p. 102) if the person is breathing.
c Monitor breathing and circulation.
12 Do the following if the person has signs of circulation but breathing is absent:
a Give 1 rescue breath every 5 seconds. Give 10 to 12 breaths per minute.
b Monitor circulation.

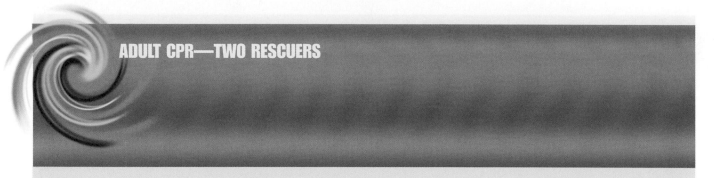

ADULT CPR—TWO RESCUERS

Procedure

1 Check if the person is responding. Tap or gently shake the person, call the person by name, and shout "Are you OK?" One rescuer calls for help.

2 Open the airway, and check for breathing. Use the head-tilt/chin-lift method.

3 Give 2 slow rescue breaths if the person is not breathing or if breathing is inadequate. Let the lungs deflate between breaths.

4 Check for a pulse using the carotid artery. Check for breathing, coughing, and moving.

5 Perform 2 person CPR (Fig. 5-9) if there are no signs of circulation:

  a One rescuer gives 100 chest compressions per minute. Count out loud in a rhythm. (Try: "1 and, 2 and, 3 and, 4 and, 5 and, 6 and, 7 and, 8 and, 9 and, 10 and, 11 and, 12 and, 13 and, 14 and, 15.")

  b The other rescuer gives 2 slow breaths after every 15 compressions. Pause for the breaths. Continue chest compressions after the breaths.

6 One rescuer does the following after 4 cycles of 15 compressions and 2 breaths:

  a Gives 2 slow breaths.

  b Checks for circulation—carotid pulse, breathing, coughing, and moving.

7 Continue with 15 compressions and 2 slow breaths if the person has no signs of circulation. Start with chest compressions.

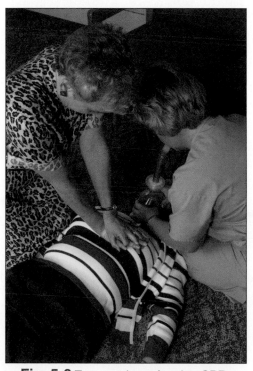

Fig. 5-9 Two people performing CPR.

Foreign-Body Airway Obstruction in Adults

Foreign-body airway obstruction (FBAO) *(choking)* can lead to cardiac arrest. Air cannot pass through the air passages to the lungs. The body does not get oxygen.

Foreign bodies can cause airway obstruction. This often occurs during eating. A large, poorly chewed piece of meat is the most common cause. Laughing and talking while eating also are causes. Older persons are at risk for choking. Weakness, poorly fitting dentures, difficulty swallowing *(dysphagia)*, and chronic illnesses are common causes.

The choking person usually clutches his or her throat. The *Heimlich maneuver* is used to relieve FBAO. Abdominal thrusts are given with the person standing, sitting, or lying down. The finger sweep is used with the Heimlich maneuver when an adult becomes unconscious.

The Heimlich maneuver is not effective in very obese persons or pregnant women. Chest thrusts are used (Box 5-2).

BOX 5-2 Obstructed Airway: Chest Thrusts for Obese or Pregnant Persons

The Victim Is Sitting or Standing

1 Stand behind the person.
2 Place your arms under the person's underarms. Wrap your arms around the person's chest.
3 Make a fist. Place the thumb side of the fist on the middle of the sternum (breastbone).
4 Grasp the fist with your other hand.
5 Give backward chest thrusts until the object is expelled or the person becomes unconscious.

The Victim Is Lying Down or Unconscious

1 Position the person supine.
2 Kneel next to the person.
3 Position your hands as for external chest compressions.
4 Give chest thrusts until the object is expelled or the person becomes unconscious.

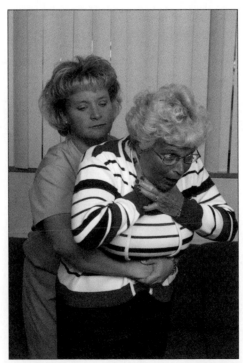

Fig. 5-10 The choking person clutches at the throat. Abdominal thrusts are given with the person standing.

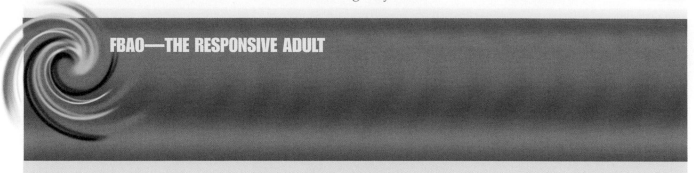

FBAO—THE RESPONSIVE ADULT

Procedure

1 Ask the person if he or she is choking.
2 Ask if the person can cough or speak.
3 Give abdominal thrusts (Fig. 5-10):
  a Stand behind the person.
  b Wrap your arms around the person's waist.
  c Make a fist with one hand.
  d Place the thumb side of the fist against the abdomen. The fist is in the middle above the navel and below the end of the sternum (breastbone).
  e Grasp your fist with your other hand.
  f Press your fist and hand into the person's abdomen with a quick, upward thrust.
  g Repeat thrusts until the object is expelled or the person loses consciousness.
4 Lower the unresponsive person to the floor or ground. Position the person supine.
5 Call for help.
6 Do a finger sweep to check for a foreign object:
  a Open the person's mouth. Use the tongue–jaw lift method (Fig. 5-11, A):
    (1) Grasp the tongue and lower jaw with your thumb and fingers.
    (2) Lift the lower jaw upward.
  b Insert your other index finger into the mouth along the side of the cheek and deep into the throat (Fig. 5-11, B). Your finger should be at the base of the tongue.
  c Form a hook with your index finger.
  d Try to dislodge and remove the object. Do not push it deeper into the throat.
  e Grasp and remove the object if it is within reach.
7 Open the airway with the head-tilt/chin-lift method.
8 Give 1 or 2 rescue breaths.
9 Reposition the person's head if the chest did not rise. Give 1 or 2 rescue breaths.
10 Give up to 5 abdominal thrusts (see procedure: *FBAO—The Unresponsive Adult*, p. 102).
11 Repeat steps 6 through 10 (finger sweeps, rescue breathing, and abdominal thrusts) until rescue breathing is effective. Start CPR if necessary.

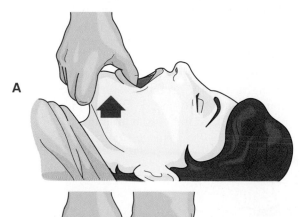

Fig. 5-11 Tongue—jaw lift maneuver. **A,** Grasp the person's tongue and lift the jaw forward with one hand. **B,** Use the index finger of the other hand to check for a foreign object.

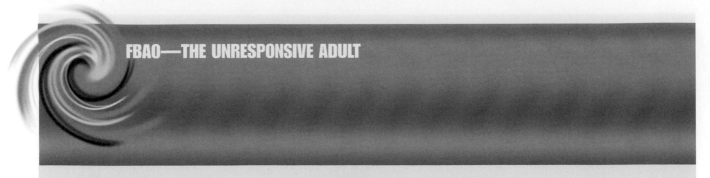

FBAO—THE UNRESPONSIVE ADULT

Procedure

1 Check to see if the person is responding.
2 Call for help.
3 Logroll the person to the supine position with his or her face up. Arms are at the sides.
4 Open the airway. Use the head-tilt/chin-lift method.
5 Check for breathing.
6 Give 1 or 2 slow rescue breaths. Reposition the person's head and open the airway if the chest does not rise. Give 1 or 2 rescue breaths.
7 Give 5 abdominal thrusts (Fig. 5-12) if you cannot ventilate the person:
   a Straddle the person's thighs.

b Place the heel of one hand against the abdomen. It is in the middle above the navel and below the end of the sternum (breastbone).
c Place your second hand on top of your first hand.
d Press both hands into the abdomen with a quick, upward thrust. Give 5 thrusts.
8 Do a finger sweep to check for a foreign object. See step 6 in procedure: *FBAO—The Responsive Adult,* p. 101.
9 Repeat steps 6 through 8 until rescue breathing is effective. Start CPR if necessary.

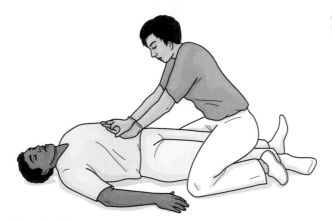

Fig. 5-12 Abdominal thrusts with the person lying down. The rescuer straddles the thighs.

The Unresponsive Adult. You may find an adult who is unresponsive. You did not see the person lose consciousness, and you do not know the cause. Do not assume the cause is choking. Check for unresponsiveness and start rescue breathing. Abdominal thrusts are done if you cannot ventilate the person. Then use the finger-sweep maneuver.

Recovery Position

The recovery position is a side-lying position (Fig. 5-13). It is used when the person is breathing and has a pulse but is not responding. Logroll the person into the recovery position. Keep the head, neck, and spine straight. Then keep the person in good alignment. A hand supports the head. This position keeps the airway open and prevents aspiration (p. 105). *Do not use this position if the person might have neck injuries or other trauma.*

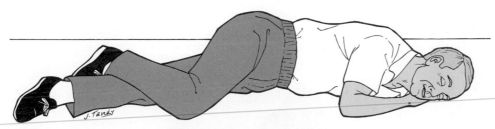

Fig. 5-13 Recovery position.

Automated External Defibrillators

Ventricular fibrillation (VF, V-fib) is an abnormal heart rhythm. It causes cardiac arrest. Rather than beating in a regular rhythm, the heart shakes and quivers like a bowl of Jell-O. The heart does not pump blood. The heart, brain, and other organs do not receive blood and oxygen.

A *defibrillator* is used to deliver a shock to the heart. The shock stops the VF. This allows the return of a regular heart rhythm. Defibrillation as soon as possible after the onset of VF increases the person's chance of survival.

Automatic external defibrillators (AEDs) are found in hospitals, nursing centers, dental offices, and other health care agencies. They are on airplanes and in airports, health clubs, malls, and many other public places. A basic life support course teaches health care providers how to use them. Remember, the goal is early defibrillation.

HEMORRHAGE

If a blood vessel is torn or cut, bleeding occurs. **Hemorrhage** is the excessive loss of blood in a short time. If the bleeding is not stopped, the person will die.

You cannot see internal hemorrhage. Bleeding occurs inside the body into tissues and body cavities. Pain, shock (p. 104), vomiting blood, coughing up blood, and loss of consciousness signal internal hemorrhage. There is little you can do for internal bleeding. Call for help, and keep the person warm, flat, and quiet until help arrives. Do not give fluids.

If not hidden by clothing, external bleeding is usually seen. Bleeding from an artery occurs in spurts. There is a steady flow of blood from a vein. To control external bleeding:

* Follow the rules in Box 5-1.
* Have the person lie down.
* Do not remove any objects that have pierced or stabbed the person.
* Place a sterile dressing directly over the wound. Use any clean material (handkerchief, towel, cloth, or sanitary napkin) if there is no sterile dressing.
* Apply pressure with your hand directly over the bleeding site (Fig. 5-14). Do not release the pressure until the bleeding stops.
* If direct pressure does not control bleeding, apply pressure over the artery above the bleeding site (Fig. 5-15, p. 104). Use your first three fingers. For example, if bleeding is from the lower arm, apply pressure over the brachial artery. Continue to apply pressure to the wound with your other hand.
* Bind the wound when bleeding stops. Tape or tie the dressing in place. You can tie the dressing with such things as clothing, a scarf, a necktie, or a belt.

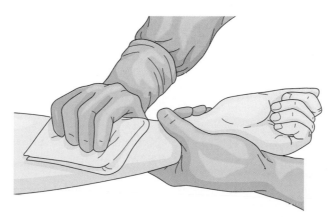

Fig. 5-14 Direct pressure is applied to the wound to stop bleeding. The hand is placed over the wound.

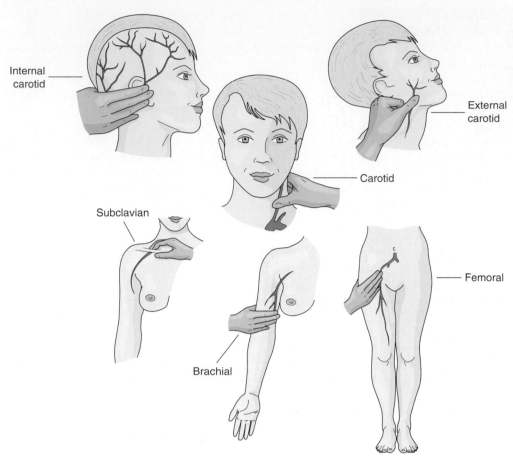

Fig. 5-15 Pressure points to control bleeding.

SHOCK

Shock results when organs and tissues do not get enough blood. Blood loss, heart attack (myocardial infarction), burns, and severe infection are causes. Signs and symptoms include low or falling blood pressure, rapid and weak pulse, and rapid respirations. The person is thirsty and has cold, moist, and pale skin. Confusion and loss of consciousness occur as shock worsens.

Shock is possible with any illness or injury. Follow the rules in Box 5-1 to prevent and treat shock.

SEIZURES

Seizures (convulsions) are violent and sudden contractions or tremors of muscle groups. They are caused by an abnormality in the brain. Causes include head injury, high fever, brain tumors, poisoning, seizure disorders, and nervous system infections. Lack of blood flow to the brain can also cause seizures. The major types of seizures are *partial seizures* and *generalized seizures*.

Only a part of the brain is involved with a partial seizure. A body part may jerk. Or the person has hearing or vision problems or stomach discomfort. Consciousness is not lost.

With generalized seizures, the whole brain is involved. The *generalized tonic-clonic (grand mal)* seizure has two phases. In the tonic phase, the person loses consciousness. If standing or sitting, the person falls to the floor. The body is rigid because all muscles contract at once. The clonic phase follows. Muscle groups contract and relax. This causes jerking and twitching movements. Urinary and fecal incontinence may occur (Chapter 13). A deep sleep is common after the seizure. Confusion and headache may occur on awakening.

The *generalized absence (petit mal) seizure* usually lasts a few seconds. There is loss of consciousness, twitching of the eyelids, and staring.

You cannot stop a seizure. However, you can protect the person from injury:

- Follow the rules in Box 5-1.
- Do not leave the person alone.
- Lower the person to the floor. This protects the person from falling.
- Place a folded blanket, towel, cushion, pillow, or other soft item under the person's head (Fig. 5-16). Or cradle the person's head in your lap. This prevents the person's head from striking the floor.
- Turn the person onto his or her side. Make sure the head is turned to the side.
- Loosen tight jewelry and clothing (ties, scarves, collars, necklaces) around the neck.
- Move furniture, equipment, and sharp objects away from the person.
- Do not give the person food or fluids.
- Do not try to restrain body movements during the seizure.
- Do not put any object or your fingers between the person's teeth. The person can bite down on your fingers during the seizure.

FAINTING

Fainting *(syncope)* is the sudden loss of consciousness from an inadequate blood supply to the brain. Hunger, fatigue, fear, and pain are common causes. So are standing in one position for a long time and being in a warm, crowded room. Dizziness, perspiration, and blackness before the eyes are warning signals. The person looks pale. The pulse is weak. Respirations are shallow if consciousness is lost. Emergency care includes the following:

- Follow the rules in Box 5-1.
- Have the person sit or lie down before fainting occurs.
- If sitting, the person bends forward and places the head between the knees (Fig. 5-17).
- If the person is lying down, raise the legs.
- Loosen tight clothing (belts, ties, scarves, collars, and so on).
- Keep the person lying down if fainting has occurred. Raise the legs.
- Do not let the person get up until symptoms have subsided for about 5 minutes.
- Help the person to a sitting position after recovery from fainting. Observe for fainting.

VOMITING AND ASPIRATION

Vomiting signals illness or injury. It can be life-threatening. Aspirated vomitus can obstruct the airway. **Aspiration** is breathing fluid or an object into the lungs. Vomiting large amounts of blood can lead to shock. These measures are needed:

- Follow the rules in Box 5-1.

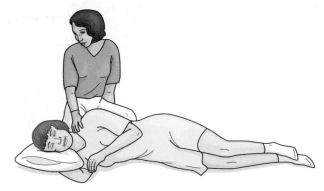

Fig. 5-16 A pillow protects the person's head during a seizure.

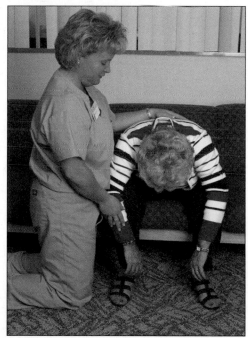

Fig. 5-17 The person bends forward and lowers her head between her knees to prevent fainting.

- Turn the person's head well to one side. This prevents aspiration.
- Place a kidney basin under the person's chin.
- Move vomitus away from the person.
- Provide oral hygiene. This helps remove the bitter taste of vomitus.
- Eliminate odors.
- Change linens as necessary.
- Observe vomitus for color, odor, and undigested food. If it looks like coffee grounds, it contains digested blood. This signals bleeding. Report your observations.
- Measure, report, and record the amount of vomitus. Note the amount on the intake and output record (Chapter 7).
- Save a specimen for laboratory study.
- Dispose of vomitus after the nurse observes it.

STROKE

Stroke (cerebrovascular accident) occurs when the brain is suddenly deprived of its blood supply (Chapter 19). Usually only part of the brain is affected. A stroke may be caused by:

* A thrombus—a blood clot in a blood vessel in the brain
* An embolus—a blood clot that travels to a blood vessel in the brain
* Hemorrhage—a blood vessel in the brain ruptures, causing bleeding in the brain

Signs of stroke vary. They depend on the size and location of brain injury. Loss of consciousness or semiconsciousness, rapid pulse, labored respirations, elevated blood pressure, and hemiplegia are signs of stroke. The person may have slurred speech or *aphasia* (the inability to speak). Loss of vision in one eye, unsteadiness, and falling also are signs. Seizures may occur.

Emergency care includes the following:

* Follow the rules in Box 5-1.
* Position the person in the recovery position on the affected side (see Fig. 5-13). The affected side is limp, and the cheek appears puffy.
* Elevate the head without flexing the neck.
* Loosen tight jewelry and clothing (belts, ties, scarves, collars, and so on).
* Keep the person quiet and warm.
* Reassure the person.
* Provide rescue breathing and CPR if necessary.
* Provide emergency care for seizures if necessary.

Review Questions

Circle the **BEST** answer.

1   When giving emergency care, you should
   a Be aware of your own limits
   b Move the person
   c Give the person fluids
   d Perform needed emergency measures

2   Cardiac arrest is
   a The same as stroke
   b The sudden stopping of heart action and breathing
   c The sudden loss of consciousness
   d When organs and tissues do not get enough blood

3   Which is *not* a sign of cardiac arrest?
   a No pulse
   b No breathing
   c A sudden drop in blood pressure
   d Unconsciousness

4   CPR involves the following *except*
   a Compressing the chest $1\frac{1}{2}$ to 2 inches with two hands
   b Counting respirations for 30 seconds
   c Blowing air into the person's mouth
   d Checking for a carotid pulse

5   You are doing adult CPR alone. Which is *false?*
   a Give 2 breaths after every 15 compressions
   b Check for a pulse after 1 minute
   c Give 1 breath after every fifth compression
   d Count out loud

6   The most common cause of FBAO in adults is
   a A loose denture
   b Meat
   c Marbles
   d Candy

Review Questions

7 Chest thrusts are used for FBOA in an adult. Which is *false*?
- **a** The person can be standing, sitting, or lying down.
- **b** A fist is made with one hand.
- **c** The thrusts are given inward and upward at the lower end of the sternum.
- **d** The hands are over the sternum.

8 Poking motions are used with a finger sweep.
- **a** True
- **b** False

9 A person is hemorrhaging from the left forearm. The first action is to
- **a** Lower the body part
- **b** Apply pressure to the brachial artery
- **c** Apply direct pressure to the wound
- **d** Cover the person

10 A person in shock needs
- **a** Rescue breathing
- **b** To be kept lying down
- **c** Clothes removed
- **d** The recovery position

11 A person is having a seizure. You need to
- **a** Protect the person's head
- **b** Control bleeding
- **c** Open the airway with your fingers
- **d** Apply direct pressure

12 A person is about to faint. Which is *false?*
- **a** Take the person outside for fresh air.
- **b** Have the person sit or lie down.
- **c** Loosen tight clothing.
- **d** Raise the legs if the person is lying down.

13 A person is vomiting. You need to
- **a** Position the person supine
- **b** Turn his or her head to the side
- **c** Raise the feet and legs
- **d** Give rescue breathing

14 A person is having a stroke. Emergency care includes the following *except*
- **a** Positioning the person on the affected side
- **b** Giving the person sips of water
- **c** Loosening tight clothing
- **d** Keeping the person quiet and warm

Answers to these questions are on p. 388.

CHAPTER 6

Promoting Residents' Rights and Independence

Objectives

- Define the key terms listed in this chapter
- Identify the losses experienced by nursing center residents
- Describe residents' rights as required by OBRA
- Explain how you can promote the resident's rights
- Explain how to promote a resident's independence
- Identify the OBRA environment requirements that promote independence
- Explain how social activities promote independence
- Describe how the nursing team can promote a person's sexuality
- Explain the purpose of the Patient Self-Determination Act
- Describe the role of a long-term care ombudsman

advance directive A document stating a person's wishes about health care when that person cannot make his or her own decisions

ombudsman Someone who supports or promotes the needs and interests of another person

sexuality The physical, psychological, social, cultural, and spiritual factors that affect a person's feelings and attitudes about his or her sex

---

Today, 1 of every 8 Americans is 65 years old or older. The U.S. Government reported that there were 34,500,000 older people in 1999. That is 3,300,000 more people than in 1990.

Most older people live in a family setting—with a partner, child, or other family. Some live alone or with friends. Others live in nursing centers. The need for nursing center care increases with aging. When nursing center care is needed, the person suffers many losses:

- Loss of identify as a productive member of family and community
- Loss of possessions (home, household items, and a car are examples)
- Loss of independence
- Loss of real-world experiences (shopping, traveling, cooking, driving, hobbies)
- Loss of health and mobility

These losses can cause the person to feel useless, powerless, and hopeless. The health team helps residents cope with loss and improve their quality of life. This is done by promoting their rights and independence.

PROMOTING RESIDENTS' RIGHTS

OBRA requires that nursing centers provide care in a manner and in a setting that maintains or improves each person's quality of life, health, and safety. Resident rights are a major part of OBRA.

Nursing center residents have rights as United States citizens. They also have rights relating to their everyday lives and care in a nursing center. Nursing centers must protect and promote their rights. The center cannot interfere with their rights. Some residents are not competent (not able). They cannot exercise their rights. A responsible party (spouse or adult child) or legal representatives does so for them.

Nursing centers must inform residents of their rights. This is done orally and in writing before or during admission to the center. It is given in the language the person uses and understands. The following resident rights relate to your work.

Information

The person has the right to all of his or her records. They include the medical record, contracts, incident reports, and financial records. The request for a record can be oral or written.

The person has the right to be fully informed of his or her total health condition. Information is given in language the person can understand. Interpreters are used as needed. Sign language or other aids are used for those with hearing losses.

The person must also have information about his or her doctor. This includes the doctor's name, specialty, and how to contact the doctor.

Report any request for information to the nurse. You *do not* give the information described above to the person or family.

Refusing Treatment

The person has the right to refuse treatment. If a person does not give consent or refuses treatment, it cannot be given. The center must find out what the person is refusing and why. If a person refuses a certain treatment, the center must provide all other services.

Advance directives are part of the right to refuse treatment (p. 114). They include living wills or instructions about life support.

Tell the nurse if a person refuses care measures. Care plan changes may be needed.

Privacy and Confidentiality

Residents have the right to personal privacy. This includes using the bathroom in private. Privacy is maintained for all personal care measures. The person's body is not exposed unnecessarily. Only staff directly involved in the person's care are present. The person must give consent for others to be present.

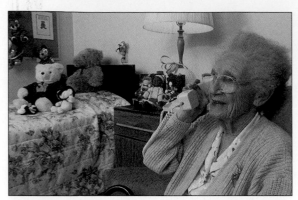

Fig. 6-1 Resident talking privately on a telephone.

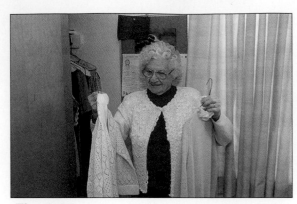

Fig. 6-2 Resident choosing what clothing to wear.

Residents have the right to visit with others in private—in areas where others cannot see or hear them. If requested, the center must provide private space. Offices, chapels, dining rooms, and meeting rooms are used as needed.

The right to privacy also involves mail and phone calls (Fig. 6-1). The person has the right to send and receive mail without others interfering. No one can open mail the person sends or receives without his or her consent. Mail is given to the person within 24 hours of delivery to the center.

Information about the person's care, treatment, and condition is kept confidential. So are medical and financial records.

Personal Choice

Residents can choose their own doctors. They also help plan and decide about their care and treatment. They have the right to choose activities, schedules, and care based on their preferences. They can decide when to get up and go to bed, what to wear, how to spend time, and what to eat (Fig. 6-2). They can choose friends and visitors inside and outside the center. Allow personal choice whenever safely possible.

Disputes and Grievances

Residents have the right to voice concerns, questions, and complaints about treatment or care. The problem may involve another person. It may be about treatment or care that was not given. The center must promptly try to correct the matter. No one can punish the person in any way for voicing the dispute or grievance.

Work

The person does not work for care, care items, or other things or privileges. The person is not required to perform services for the center.

However, the person *can* work or perform services if he or she wants to. A person may want to garden, repair or build things, sew, mend, or cook. Other persons need work for rehabilitation or activity reasons. The desire or need for work is part of the person's care plan.

Participation in Resident and Family Groups

Residents have the right to form and take part in resident and family groups. Families have the right to meet with other families. These groups can discuss concerns, suggest center improvements, and plan activities. They can support and comfort group members.

Residents have the right to take part in social, cultural, religious, and community events. They have the right to be helped in getting to and from events of their choice.

Care and Security of Personal Possessions

Residents have the right to keep and use personal items. This includes clothing and some furnishings. Treat the person's property with care and respect. The items may not have value to you but are important to the person. They also relate to personal choice, dignity, and quality of life.

The center must protect the person's property. Items are labeled with the person's name. The center must investigate reports of lost, stolen, or damaged items.

Protect yourself and the center from being accused of stealing a person's property. Do not go through a person's closet, drawers, purse, or other space without the person's knowledge and consent. A nurse may ask you to inspect closets and drawers. If so, have another worker with you and the person or legal representative. They are witnesses to your activities.

BOX 6-1   OBRA-Required Actions to Promote the Resident's Dignity and Privacy

Courteous and Dignified Interactions

- Use the right tone of voice.
- Use good eye contact.
- Stand or sit close enough as needed.
- Use the person's proper name and title.
- Gain the person's attention before interacting with him or her.
- Use touch if the person approves.
- Respect the person's social status.
- Listen with interest to what the person is saying.
- Do not yell, scold, or embarrass the person.

Courteous and Dignified Care

- Groom hair, beards, and nails as the person wishes.
- Assist with dressing in the right clothing for time of day and personal choice.
- Promote independence and dignity in dining.
- Respect private space and property.
- Assist with walking and transfers without interfering with independence.
- Assist with bathing and hygiene preferences without interfering with independence:
  - Neat and clean appearance
  - Clean shaven or groomed beard
  - Nails trimmed and clean
  - Dentures, hearing aids, eyeglasses, and other prostheses used correctly

  - Clean clothing
  - Clothing properly fitted and fastened
  - Shoes, hose, and socks properly applied and fastened
  - Extra clothing for warmth as needed such as sweater or lap blanket

Privacy and Self-Determination

- Drape properly during care and procedures to avoid exposure and embarrassment.
- Drape properly in chair.
- Use curtains or screens during care and procedures.
- Close the door to the room during care and procedures.
- Knock on the door before entering. Wait to be asked in.
- Close the bathroom door when person uses the bathroom.

Maintain Personal Choice and Independence

- Person smokes in designated areas.
- Person takes part in activities according to interests.
- Person is involved in scheduling activities and care.
- Person gives input into care plan about preferences and independence.
- Person is involved in room or roommate change.

Freedom from Abuse, Mistreatment, and Neglect

Residents have the right to be free from verbal, sexual, physical, mental, or financial abuse (Chapter 1). They also have the right to be free from involuntary seclusion. *Involuntary seclusion* is:

- Separating a person from others against his or her will
- Keeping the person confined to a certain area
- Keeping the person away from his or her room without consent

No one can abuse, neglect, or mistreat a resident. This includes center staff, volunteers, staff from other agencies or groups, other residents, family members, visitors, and legal representatives. Nursing centers must investigate suspected or reported cases of abuse. Nursing centers cannot employ persons who were convicted of abusing, neglecting, or mistreating others.

Freedom From Restraint

Residents have the right not to have body movements restricted. Restraints and certain drugs can restrict body movements. Some drugs are restraints because they affect mood, behavior, and mental function. Sometimes residents are restrained to protect them from harming themselves or others. A doctor's order is needed for restraint use. Restraints are not used for staff convenience or to discipline a person. Restraints are discussed in Chapter 20.

Quality of Life

Nursing centers must care for residents in a manner that promotes dignity and self-esteem. It must also promote physical, psychological, and mental well-being. Protecting resident rights promotes quality of life. It shows respect for the person.

The person is spoken to in a polite and courteous manner (Chapter 2). Good, honest, and thoughtful care also enhances quality of life. Box 6-1 lists OBRA-required actions that promote dignity and privacy.

Activities.   Nursing centers provide activity programs that allow personal choice. They must promote physical, intellectual, social, spiritual, and emotional well-being. Many centers provide religious services for spiritual health. You assist residents to and from activity programs. You may need to help them with activities.

Environment. The center's environment must promote quality of life. It must be clean, safe, and as homelike as possible (Chapter 8). Letting the person have personal items enhances quality of life. It allows personal choice and promotes a homelike setting.

PROMOTING INDEPENDENCE

To promote and enhance quality of life, residents must be as independent as possible. They make decisions and meet their own needs to the extent possible.

The measures in Box 6-2 help promote independence. OBRA has certain environment requirements that promote independence and safety (Box 6-3). Resident independence is also promoted through:

- Social relationships
- Expressing sexuality
- Making advance directives
- Ombudsmen programs
- Restorative care and rehabilitation (Chapter 19)

BOX 6-2   Measures to Promote Independence

General Measures

- Focus on the person.
- Treat each person and his or her body with dignity and respect.
- Know what you can and cannot do as a nursing assistant. Do not cause the person harm.
- Practice within the legal limits of your role.
- Work when scheduled. Arrive at work on time.
- Complete assignments thoroughly and safely.
- Understand the reasons for the person's care.
- Be pleasant and courteous.
- Help the person make the room as homelike as possible.
- Make sure that dentures, eye glasses, hearing aids, canes, walkers, wheelchairs, and other devices are in place.
- Make sure the person has special equipment or eating utensils.
- Handle the person's property carefully and with respect. Protect personal items from loss or damage.
- Explain what you are going to do. Obtain the person's consent before you proceed.
- Explain procedures step-by-step.

Privacy and Confidentiality

- Provide factual, concise, and understandable information to the nurse.
- Share information about the person only with health team members involved in the person's care.
- Do not give information to the person's family, friends, or other visitors.
- Share your observations and ideas about the person's care with the health team.
- Ask visitors to leave the room before you give care.
- Screen the person properly.
- Expose only the body part involved in the procedure.
- Close doors, curtains, and drapes. Close window shades and blinds.
- Learn as much as you can about a person's religious and cultural beliefs and practices.
- Focus on the person's abilities. Do not focus on disabilities.
- Report signs and symptoms of abuse, mistreatment, and neglect.
- Offer to take residents to their friends' rooms or to activities.

- Respect the person's choice for quiet and time alone. Do not force the person to attend activities.
- Encourage residents to talk about their losses. They may find that other residents have similar losses.
- Allow privacy during elimination (Chapter 13).

Sexuality

- Do not judge or gossip about a person's sexuality or sexual relationships.
- See "Sexuality" on the next page.

Safety

- Know the common safety hazards and the causes of accidents.
- Know which residents need extra protection.
- Keep the signal light within the person's reach.
- Practice safety measures (Chapter 4).
- Use safety devices as needed.
- Encourage residents to use hand rails, walkers, or canes.
- Assist residents as needed.
- Identify the person before giving care. Follow center policies.
- Prevent infection. Practice hand hygiene, and follow Standard Precautions and the Bloodborne Pathogen Standard.
- Practice good body mechanics (Chapter 4).
- Use bed rails according to the care plan.
- Complete a safety check before leaving the room. (See the inside front cover.)

Personal Choice

- Let the person choose such things as bed positions, chair or wheelchair placement, and when to get up or go back to bed. Check with the nurse and care plan to make sure the person's choices are safe.
- Let the person help with lifting, moving, and transferring procedures to the extent possible.
- Let the person choose how to arrange and where to place personal items.
- Let the person choose when the bed is made and which bed linens to use.
- Let the person choose when and how hygiene and grooming are done.
- Share the person's food likes and dislikes with the nurse.
- Let the person choose when and where to walk. The person may want to go outside.

<table>
<tr><td>

BOX 6-3   OBRA Environment Requirements

- Dining areas are large enough and comfortable for the residents.
- Dining areas allow the use of wheelchairs, walkers, and other walking aids.
- Dining areas are equipped to meet the physical and social needs of residents.
- Recreation, program, and activity areas are large enough and comfortable for the residents.
  - There is enough space to store supplies and projects.
- Furnishings are sound and functional.
  - Chairs vary in size to meet residents' needs.
  - Wheelchairs can fit under dining room tables.
- Non-smoking areas are identified by signs.
- The space is well-ventilated.
- There is good air movement.
- Temperature, humidity, and odor levels are acceptable.
- Handrails are secured to the walls in hallways.
- The area is free of pests (roaches, ants, flies, mice, rats, and so on).
- Toilet facilities are in or near each resident room.
- Resident rooms and toilet and bathing facilities are equipped with a call system. The call system functions properly.
- Lighting levels are adequate and comfortable.

</td></tr>
</table>

Caring About Culture

Foreign-Born Persons

Some older persons speak and understand a foreign language. Communication occurs with family and friends who speak the same language. They also share cultural values and practices. These relatives and friends may move away or die. The person may not have anyone to talk to. He or she may not be understood by others. The person feels greater loneliness and isolation.

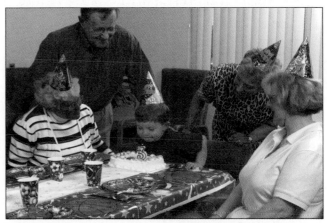

Fig. 6-3 An older woman takes part in family activities.

Social Relationships

Social relationships change throughout life (see *Caring About Culture: Foreign-Born Persons*). Children grow up and leave home. They have their own families. Many live far away from parents. Older family and friends die, move away, or are disabled. Life partners die.

Yet most older people have regular contact with children, grandchildren, family, and friends. Grandchildren can bring great love and joy. Family times help prevent loneliness. They help the older person feel useful and wanted (Fig. 6-3).

Sexuality

Sexuality is the physical, psychological, social, cultural, and spiritual factors that affect a person's feelings and attitudes about his or her sex. Sexuality affects how a person behaves, thinks, dresses, and responds to others.

Love, affection, and intimacy are needed throughout life. Attitudes and sex needs change as a person grows older. Life circumstances change. These include death of a partner, divorce, injury, illness, and aging. However, sexual relationships are important to older persons (Fig. 6-4, p. 114). They love and fall in love, hold hands, embrace, and have sex.

The nursing team allows and promotes the meeting of sexual needs. The measures in Box 6-4, p. 114 may be part of the person's care plan.

Married couples in nursing centers are allowed to share the same room. This is an OBRA requirement. They can share the same bed if their conditions permit.

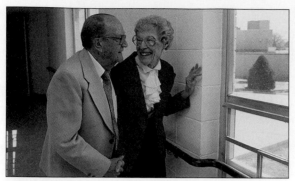

Fig. 6-4 Relationships develop in nursing centers.

BOX 6-4 Promoting Sexuality

- Let the person practice grooming routines. Assist as needed. For women, this includes applying makeup, nail polish, lotion, and cologne. Many women shave their legs and underarms and pluck eyebrows. Men may use after-shave lotion and cologne. Hair care is important to men and women.
- Let the person choose clothing. Hospital gowns embarrass both men and women. Street clothes are worn if the person's condition permits.
- Protect the right to privacy. Do not expose the person. Drape and screen the person.
- Accept the person's sexual relationships. The person may not share your sexual attitudes, values, or practices. The person may have a homosexual, pre-marital, or extramarital relationship. Do not judge or gossip about relationships.
- Allow privacy. You can usually tell when people want to be alone. If the person has a private room, close the door for privacy. Some centers have *Do Not Disturb* signs for doors. Let the person and partner know how much time they have alone. For example, remind them about meal times, drugs, or treatments. Tell other staff members that the person wants time alone.
- Knock before you enter any room. Wait to be invited in. This is a simple courtesy that shows respect for privacy.
- Consider the person's roommate. Privacy curtains provide little privacy. Arrange for privacy when the roommate is out of the room. Sometimes room-mates offer to leave for a while. If the roommate cannot leave, the nurse finds other private areas.
- Allow privacy for masturbation. It is a normal form of sexual expression and release. Close the privacy curtain and the door. Knock before you enter any room, and wait to be invited in. This saves you and the person embarrassment. Sometimes con-fused persons masturbate in public areas. Lead the person to a private area. Or distract him or her with an activity.

The Patient Self-Determination Act

The Patient Self-Determination Act and OBRA give persons the right to accept or refuse treatment. They also give the right to make advance directives. An **advance directive** is a document stating a person's wishes about health care when that person cannot make his or her own decisions. Advance directives usually forbid certain care if there is no hope of re-covery. Living wills and durable power of attorney are common advance directives:

- *Living will*—a document about measures that sup-port or maintain life when death is likely. Tube feedings, ventilators, and CPR are examples. A living will may instruct doctors:
  —Not to start measures that prolong dying
  —To remove measures that prolong dying
- *Durable power of attorney for health care*—gives the power to make care decisions to another person. Usually this is a family member, friend, or lawyer. When a person cannot make care decisions, the person with durable power of attorney can do so.

Ombudsman Program

The Older Americans Act is a federal law. It requires a Long-Term Care Ombudsman Program in every state. An **ombudsman** is someone who supports or promotes the needs and interests of another person. Long-term care ombudsmen are employed by a state agency. Some are volunteers. They do not work at a nursing center. They act on behalf of the residents.

Ombudsmen protect the health, safety, welfare, and rights of residents. They:

- Investigate and resolve complaints
- Provide services to assist residents
- Provide information about long-term care services
- Monitor nursing center care
- Monitor nursing center conditions
- Provide support to resident and family groups
- Educate residents, families, and the public about long-term care issues and concerns

Nursing centers must post the names, addresses, and phone numbers of local and state ombudsmen. This information must be posted where residents can easily see it.

A resident or family member may share a concern with you. You must know state and center policies and procedures for contacting an ombudsman. Ombudsman services are useful when:

- There is concern about a person's care or treat-ment
- Someone interferes with a person's rights, health, safety, or welfare

Review Questions

Circle the **BEST** answer.

1 Residents' rights are aimed at
   a Promoting quality of life
   b Promoting independence
   c Promoting health and well-being
   d Promoting health

2 Mr. Hall asks you about the cost of his care. What should you do?
   a Give him his medical record.
   b Give him his financial record.
   c Tell Mr. Hall that you will ask the nurse to talk to him.
   d Tell him that such information is confidential.

3 Mr. Hall refuses to have his bed made. What should you do?
   a Make the bed.
   b Tell the nurse.
   c Make the bed when he is out of the room.
   d Ask him to make the bed.

4 Mr. Hall's son has arrived for a visit. What should you do?
   a Let them visit in private.
   b Tell the nurse.
   c Stay within hearing distance.
   d Make notes of their conversation.

5 Mrs. Smith received 3 cards and a letter today. What should you do?
   a Tell the nurse.
   b Open her mail.
   c Read her mail.
   d Give her the mail.

6 Mr. Hall's son asks you about his father's care. What should you do?
   a Answer his questions.
   b Refer him to the nurse.
   c Tell him that care matters are confidential.
   d Give him Mr. Hall's medical record.

7 You are assisting Mrs. Smith with hair care. Who decides how to style her hair?
   a Mrs. Smith
   b The nurse
   c You
   d The ombudsman

8 Mrs. Smith does not like the food served. Which statement is *true?*
   a She has to eat the food served.
   b She can voice her concerns.
   c She has to work for different food.
   d She has to prepare her own food.

9 Mr. Hall wants to form a group to watch football on Sunday afternoons. He has the right to do this.
   a True
   b False

10 Residents have the right to the following *except*
   a To be free from restraints
   b To attend activities of their choice
   c To free care
   d To keep personal items

11 Mr. Hall's son is visiting. As you walk past the room, you see Mr. Hall being slapped by his son. What should you do?
   a Nothing. Family matters are private.
   b Call an ombudsman.
   c Tell the nurse.
   d Close the room door to provide for privacy.

12 The following cause loneliness in older persons *except*
   a Death of a life partner
   b Death of family and friends
   c Family times
   d Children moving away

13 Sexuality is important to
   a Small children
   b Teenagers and young adults
   c Middle-aged adults
   d Persons of all ages

Review Questions

14 Mr. and Mrs. Green live in a nursing center. Which will *not* promote their sexuality?
a Allowing their normal grooming routines
b Having them wear hospital gowns
c Allowing them privacy
d Accepting their relationship

15 Two nursing center residents are holding hands. Nursing staff should keep them apart.
a True
b False

16 Mr. and Mrs. Green want some time alone. The nursing team can do the following *except*
a Close the room door
b Put a *Do Not Disturb* sign on the door
c Tell other staff that Mr. and Mrs. Green want some time alone
d Close the privacy curtain so no one can hear them

17 Mr. Cole is masturbating in the dining room. You should do the following *except*
a Cover him and take him quietly to his room
b Scold him
c Provide privacy
d Tell the nurse

18 An advance directive states a person's wishes about health care when that person cannot make his or her own decisions
a True
b False

19 You need to call a resident by his or her
a Room and bed number
b Nickname
c Proper name and title
d Diagnosis

20 You need to enter a resident's room. What should you do?
a Walk right in.
b Knock before entering. Wait to be invited in.
c Call the person by name before entering.
d See if the roommate is there.

21 Which does *not* promote independence?
a Obtaining the person's consent before giving care
b Properly screening the person
c Focusing on the person's disabilities
d Letting the person choose what to wear

22 Which does *not* promote the resident's independence?
a Keeping bed rails up
b Using safety devices as needed
c Keeping the signal light within reach
d Practicing good body mechanics

Answers to these questions are on p. 388.

CHAPTER 7

Measurements

Objectives

- Define the key terms listed in this chapter
- Explain why vital signs are measured
- List the factors affecting vital signs
- Identify the normal ranges for each temperature site
- Know when to use each temperature site
- Identify the pulse sites
- Describe normal respirations
- Describe the practices followed when measuring blood pressure
- Explain how to prepare the person for height and weight measurements
- Explain why intake and output are measured
- Identify the fluids counted as intake and the fluids counted as output
- Explain how to assist with pain assessment
- Perform the procedures described in this chapter

blood pressure The amount of force exerted against the walls of an artery by the blood

body temperature The amount of heat in the body that is a balance between the amount of heat produced and the amount lost by the body

diastolic pressure The pressure in the arteries when the heart is at rest

hypertension Systolic pressures that remain above (hyper) 140 mm Hg and diastolic pressures that remain above 90 mm Hg

hypotension When the systolic blood pressure is below (hypo) 90 mm Hg and the diastolic pressure is below 60 mm Hg

pulse The beat of the heart felt at an artery as a wave of blood passes through the artery

pulse rate The number of heartbeats or pulses felt in 1 minute

respiration Breathing air into (inhalation) and out of (exhalation) the lungs

sphygmomanometer A cuff and measuring device used to measure blood pressure

systolic pressure The amount of force needed to pump blood out of the heart into the arterial circulation

vital signs Temperature, pulse, respirations, and blood pressure

You assist the nurse with making observations about the person. Some observations involve measurements. You measure **vital signs** (temperature, pulse, respirations, and blood pressure), height and weight, and intake and output. You also assist with assessing pain.

VITAL SIGNS

A person's vital signs vary within certain limits. They are affected by sleep, activity, eating, weather, noise, exercise, drugs, anger, fear, anxiety, pain, and illness. Vital signs show even minor changes in a person's condition. They tell about a person's response to treatment and signal life-threatening events.

Accuracy is essential when you measure, report, and record vital signs. If unsure of your measurements, promptly ask the nurse to take them again. Unless otherwise ordered, take vital signs with the person lying or sitting. Report the following at once:

- Any vital sign that is changed from a prior measurement
- Vital signs above the normal range
- Vital signs below the normal range

Body Temperature

Body temperature is the amount of heat in the body. It is a balance between the amount of heat produced and the amount lost by the body. Heat is produced as cells use food for energy. It is lost through the skin, breathing, urine, and feces. Body temperature stays fairly stable. It is lower in the morning and higher in the afternoon and evening. Body temperature is affected by age, weather, exercise, emotions, stress, and illness.

Thermometers are used to measure temperature. It is measured using the Fahrenheit (F) and Centigrade or Celsius (C) scale. Sites for measuring temperature are the mouth, rectum, ear (tympanic membrane), and axilla (underarm). Each site has a normal range (Table 7-1).

Oral temperatures are *not* taken if the person:

- Is an infant or a child younger than 6 years
- Is unconscious
- Has a sore mouth or has had surgery or an injury to the face, neck, nose, or mouth
- Is receiving oxygen or breathes through the mouth
- Has a nasogastric tube
- Is delirious, restless, confused, or disoriented
- Is paralyzed on one side of the body
- Has a convulsive (seizure) disorder

Rectal temperatures are taken when the oral route cannot be used. Rectal temperatures are *not* taken if the person has:

- Diarrhea
- A rectal disorder or injury
- Heart disease
- Had rectal surgery
- Confusion or is agitated

The tympanic membrane site has fewer microbes than the mouth or rectum. Therefore the risk of spreading infection is reduced. This site is *not* used if the person has an ear disorder or ear drainage.

The axillary site is less reliable than the other sites. It is used when the other sites cannot be used.

Older persons have lower body temperatures than younger adults. An oral temperature of 98.6° F may signal an elevated temperature (fever) in an older person.

TABLE 7-1	Normal Body Temperatures	
Site	Baseline	Normal Range
Rectal	99.6° F (37.5° C)	98.6° to 100.6° F (37.0° to 38.1° C)
Oral	98.6° F (37° C)	97.6° to 99.6° F (36.5° to 37.5° C)
Tympanic membrane	98.6° F (37° C)	98.6° F (37° C)
Axillary	97.6° F (36.5° C)	96.6° to 98.6° F (35.9° to 37.0° C)

Delegation Guidelines

Body Temperature

The nurse may ask you to take temperatures. If so, you need this information from the nurse and the care plan:

- What site to use—oral, rectal, axillary, or tympanic membrane
- What thermometer to use—glass, electronic, or other type
- How long to leave a glass thermometer in place
- When to take temperatures
- Which persons are at risk for elevated temperatures
- What observations to report and record

Safety Alert

Body Temperature

Thermometers are inserted into the mouth, rectum, and axilla. Each area has many microbes. The area may contain blood. Therefore each person has his or her own glass thermometer. Follow Standard Precautions and the Bloodborne Pathogen Standard when taking temperatures.

Rectal temperatures are dangerous for persons with heart disease. The thermometer can stimulate the vagus nerve in the rectum. This nerve also affects the heart. Stimulation of the vagus nerve slows the heart rate. The heart rate can slow to dangerous levels in some persons.

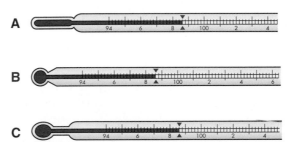

Fig. 7-1 Types of glass thermometers. **A,** The long or slender tip. **B,** The stubby tip (rectal thermometer). **C,** The pear-shaped tip.

Glass Thermometers

The glass thermometer is a hollow glass tube (Fig. 7-1). The tube is filled with a substance—mercury or a mercury-free mixture. When heated, the substance expands and rises in the tube. When cooled, the substance contracts and moves down the tube.

Long- or slender-tip thermometers are used for oral and axillary temperatures. So are thermometers with stubby and pear-shaped tips. Rectal thermometers have stubby tips that are color-coded in red.

Glass thermometers are reusable. However, the following are problems:

- They take a long time to register.
- They break easily. Broken rectal thermometers can injure the rectum and colon.
- The person may bite down and break an oral thermometer. Cuts in the mouth are risks. Swallowed mercury can cause mercury poisoning.

Safety Alert

Glass Thermometers

If a mercury–glass thermometer breaks, tell the nurse at once. Mercury is a hazardous substance. Do not touch the mercury. Do not let the person do so. The center must follow special procedures for handling all hazardous materials. See Chapter 4.

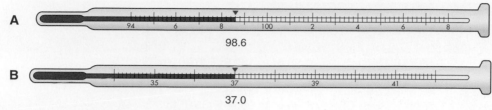

Fig. 7-2 A, Fahrenheit thermometer. The temperature measurement is 98.6° F. **B,** Centigrade thermometer. The temperature measurement is 37.0° C.

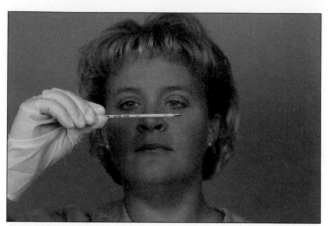

Fig. 7-3 The thermometer is held at the stem. It is read at eye level.

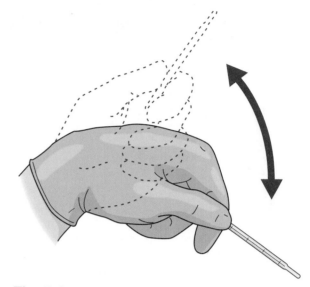

Fig. 7-4 The wrist is snapped to shake down the thermometer.

Reading a Glass Thermometer. Fahrenheit thermometers have long and short lines. Every other long line is marked in an even degree from 94° to 108° F. The short lines mean 0.2 (two tenths) of a degree (Fig. 7-2, *A*).

On a centigrade thermometer, each long line means 1 degree. Degrees range from 34° to 42° C. Each short line means 0.1 (one tenth) of a degree (Fig. 7-2, *B*).

To read a glass thermometer:

- Hold it at the stem (Fig. 7-3). Bring it to eye level.
- Turn it until you can see the numbers and the long and short lines.
- Turn it back and forth slowly until you see the silver or red line.
- Read the nearest degree (long line).
- Read the nearest tenth of a degree (short line)—an even number on a Fahrenheit thermometer.

Using a Glass Thermometer. Do the following to prevent infection, promote safety, and obtain an accurate measurement:

- Use only the person's thermometer.
- Use only a rectal thermometer for rectal temperatures.
- Rinse the thermometer under cold running water if it was soaking in a disinfectant. Dry it from the stem to the bulb end with tissues.

- Check the thermometer for breaks, cracks, and chips. Discard it following center policy if it is broken, cracked, or chipped.
- Shake down the thermometer so the substance moves down in the tube. Hold it at the stem. Stand away from walls, tables, or other hard surfaces. Flex and snap your wrist until the substance is below the lowest number on the thermometer (94° F or 34° C). See Figure 7-4.
- Clean and store the thermometer following center policy. Wipe it with tissues first to remove mucus, feces, or sweat. Do not use hot water. It causes the mercury or mercury-free mixture to expand so much that the thermometer could break. After cleaning, rinse the thermometer under cold running water. Then store it in a container with disinfectant solution.
- Use plastic covers following center policy (Fig. 7-5). To take a temperature, insert the thermometer into a cover. Remove the cover to read the thermometer. Discard the cover after use.
- Practice medical asepsis.
- Follow Standard Precautions and the Bloodborne Pathogen Standard.

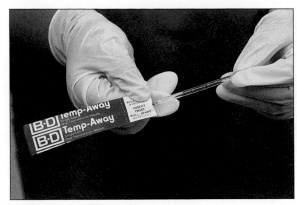

Fig. 7-5 The thermometer is inserted into a plastic cover.

🌀 Taking Temperatures.   Glass thermometers are used for oral, rectal, and axillary temperatures. Special measures are needed for each site:

• *The oral site*—The glass thermometer remains in place 2 to 3 minutes or as required by center policy.
• *The rectal site*—Lubricate the rectal thermometer for easy insertion and to prevent tissue injury. Hold it in place so it is not lost into the rectum or broken. A glass thermometer remains in the rectum for 2 minutes or as required by center policy. Privacy is important. The buttocks and anus are exposed. The procedure embarrasses many people.
• *The axillary site*—The axilla must be dry. Do not use this site right after bathing. Hold the glass thermometer in place for 5 to 10 minutes or as required by center policy.

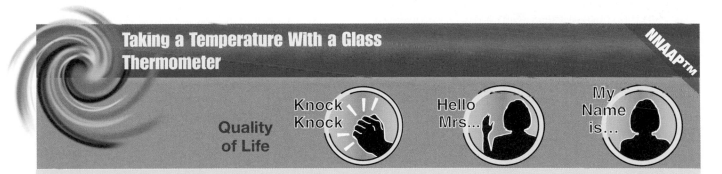

Taking a Temperature With a Glass Thermometer

NNAAP™

Quality of Life

Knock Knock

Hello Mrs...

My Name is...

Pre-Procedure

1 Follow *Delegation Guidelines: Body Temperature*, p. 119. *See Safety Alerts: Body Temperature; Glass Thermometers*, p. 119.
2 Explain the procedure to the person. For an oral temperature, ask the person not to eat, drink, smoke, or chew gum for at least 15 to 20 minutes or as required by center policy.
3 Collect the following:
    • Oral or rectal thermometer and holder
    • Tissues

• Plastic covers if used
• Gloves
• Toilet tissue (rectal temperature)
• Water-soluble lubricant (rectal temperature)
• Towel (axillary temperature)
4 Practice hand hygiene.
5 Identify the person. Check the ID bracelet against the assignment sheet. Call the person by name.
6 Provide for privacy.

Procedure

7 Put on the gloves.
8 Rinse the thermometer in cold water if it was soaking in a disinfectant. Dry it with tissues.
9 Check for breaks, cracks, or chips.
10 Shake down the thermometer below the lowest number.
11 Insert it into a plastic cover if used.
12 For an *oral temperature*:
    a Ask the person to moisten his or her lips.

b Place the bulb end of the thermometer under the tongue (Fig. 7-6, p. 123).
c Ask the person to close the lips around the thermometer to hold it in place.
d Ask the person not to talk. Remind the person not to bite down on the thermometer.
e Leave it in place for 2 to 3 minutes or as required by center policy.

Continued

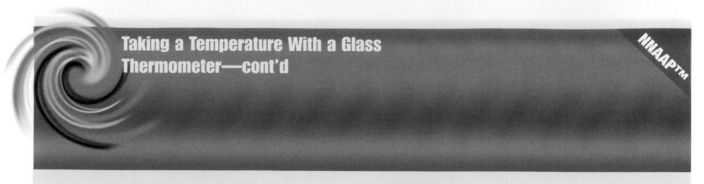

Procedure—cont'd

13 For a *rectal temperature:*
   a   Position the person in Sims' position (Chapter 16).
   b   Put a small amount of lubricant on a tissue. Lubricate the bulb end of the thermometer.
   c   Fold back top linens to expose the anal area.
   d   Raise the upper buttock to expose the anus (Fig. 7-7).
   e   Insert the thermometer 1 inch into the rectum. Do not force the thermometer. Remember, glass thermometers can break.
   f   Hold the thermometer in place for 2 minutes or as required by center policy. Do not let go of it while it is in the rectum.

14 For an *axillary temperature:*
   a   Help the person remove an arm from the gown. Do not expose the person.
   b   Dry the axilla with the towel.
   c   Place the bulb end of the thermometer in the center of the axilla.
   d   Ask the person to place the arm over the chest to hold the thermometer in place (Fig. 7-8). Hold it and the arm in place if he or she cannot help.
   e   Leave the thermometer in place for 5 to 10 minutes or as required by center policy.

15 Remove the thermometer.
16 Use tissues to remove the plastic cover. Wipe the thermometer with a tissue if no cover was used. Wipe from the stem to the bulb end.
17 For a *rectal temperature:*
   a   Place used toilet tissue on several thicknesses of clean toilet tissue.
   b   Place the thermometer on clean toilet tissue.
   c   Wipe the anal area to remove excess lubricant and any feces.
   d   Cover the person.
18 For an *axillary temperature:* Help the person put the gown back on.
19 Read the thermometer.
20 Record the person's name and temperature on your note pad or assignment sheet. Write *R* for a rectal temperature. Write *A* for an axillary temperature.
21 Shake down the thermometer.
22 Clean it according to center policy.
23 Discard tissue and the paper towel.
24 Remove the gloves. Decontaminate your hands.

Post-Procedure

25 Provide for comfort.
26 Place the signal light within reach.
27 Unscreen the person.
28 Complete a safety check of the room. (See inside of front book cover.)

29 Decontaminate your hands.
30 Report any abnormal temperature to the nurse. Record the temperature in the proper place. Note the temperature site when reporting and recording.

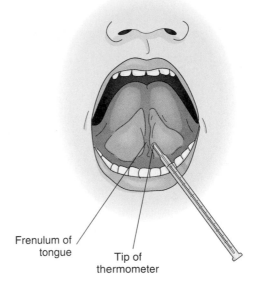

Fig. 7-6 The thermometer is placed at the base of the tongue.

Frenulum of tongue

Tip of thermometer

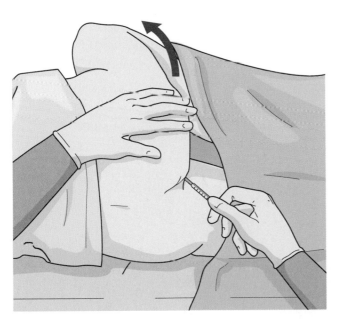

Fig. 7-7 The rectal temperature is taken with the person in Sims' position. The buttock is raised to expose the anus.

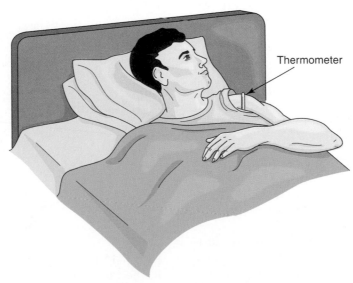

Thermometer

Fig. 7-8 The thermometer is held in place in the axilla by bringing the person's arm over the chest.

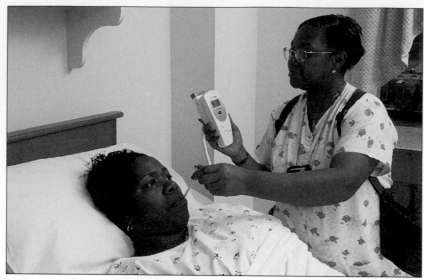

Fig. 7-9 The covered probe of the electronic thermometer is inserted under the tongue.

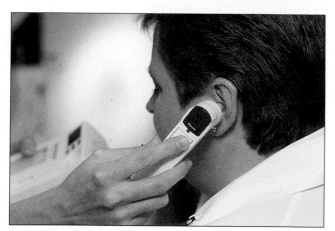

Fig. 7-10 Tympanic membrane thermometer.

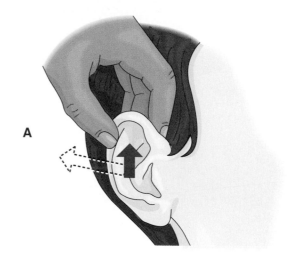

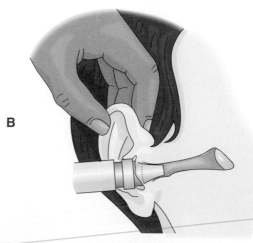

Fig. 7-11 Using a tympanic membrane thermometer. **A,** The ear is pulled up and back. **B,** The probe is inserted into the ear canal.

Electronic Thermometers

Electronic thermometers are battery-operated (Fig. 7-9). They measure temperature in a few seconds. The temperature is shown on the front of the device. The hand-held unit is kept in a battery charger when not in use.

Electronic thermometers have oral and rectal probes. A disposable cover (sheath) covers the probe. The probe cover is discarded after use. This helps prevent the spread of infection.

Tympanic Membrane Thermometers. Tympanic membrane thermometers measure temperature at the tympanic membrane in the ear (Fig. 7-10). The covered probe is gently inserted into the ear. The temperature is measured in 1 to 3 seconds.

Tympanic membrane thermometers are comfortable. They are not invasive like rectal thermometers. They are useful for confused persons because of their speed and comfort.

Taking a Temperature With an Electronic Thermometer

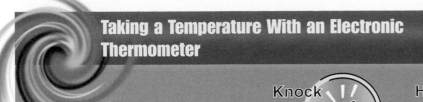

Quality of Life

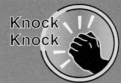
Knock Knock

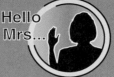
Hello Mrs...

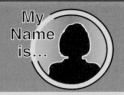
My Name is...

Pre-Procedure

1 Follow *Delegation Guidelines: Body Temperature,* p. 119. *See Safety Alert: Body Temperature,* p. 119.
2 Explain the procedure to the person. For an oral temperature, ask him or her not to eat, drink, smoke, or chew gum for at least 15 to 20 minutes.
3 Collect the following:
   • Thermometer—electronic or tympanic membrane
   • Probe (Blue for an oral or axillary temperature. Red for a rectal temperature.)
   • Probe covers
   • Toilet tissue (rectal temperature)
   • Water-soluble lubricant (rectal temperature)
   • Gloves
   • Towel (axillary temperature)
4 Plug the probe into the thermometer. (This is not done for a tympanic membrane thermometer.)
5 Practice hand hygiene.
6 Identify the person. Check the ID bracelet against the assignment sheet. Call the person by name.

Procedure

7 Provide for privacy.
8 Position the person for an oral, rectal, axillary, or tympanic membrane temperature.
9 Put on gloves if contact with blood, body fluids, secretions, or excretions is likely.
10 Insert the probe into a probe cover.
11 For an *oral temperature*:
   a Ask the person to open the mouth and raise the tongue.
   b Place the covered probe at the base of the tongue.
   c Ask the person to lower the tongue and close the mouth.
12 For a *rectal temperature*:
   a Place some lubricant on toilet tissue.
   b Lubricate the end of the covered probe.
   c Expose the anal area.
   d Raise the upper buttock.
   e Insert the probe ½ inch into the rectum.
   f Hold the probe in place.
13 For an *axillary temperature*:
   a Help the person remove an arm from the gown. Do not expose the person.
   b Dry the axilla with the towel.
   c Place the covered probe in the center of the axilla.
   d Place the person's arm over the chest.
   e Hold the probe in place.
14 For a *tympanic membrane temperature*:
   a Ask the person to turn his or her head so the ear is in front of you.
   b Pull up and back on the ear to straighten the ear canal (Fig. 7-11).
   c Insert the covered probe gently.
15 Start the thermometer.
16 Hold the probe in place until you hear a tone or see a flashing or steady light.
17 Read the temperature on the display.
18 Remove the probe. Press the eject button to discard the cover.
19 Record the person's name and temperature on your note pad or assignment sheet. Note the temperature site.
20 Return the probe to the holder.
21 Provide for comfort. Help the person put the gown back on (axillary temperature). For a rectal temperature:
   a Wipe the anal area with toilet tissue to remove lubricant.
   b Cover the person.
   c Discard used toilet tissue.
   d Remove the gloves. Decontaminate your hands.

Continued

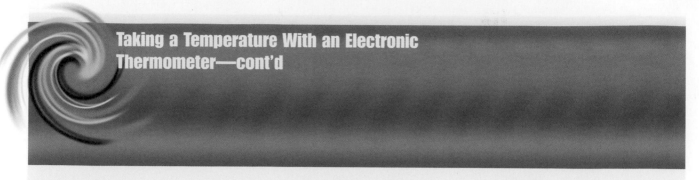

Taking a Temperature With an Electronic Thermometer—cont'd

Post-Procedure

22 Place the signal light within reach.
23 Unscreen the person.
24 Complete a safety check of the room. (See inside of front book cover.)
25 Return the thermometer to the charging unit.

26 Decontaminate your hands.
27 Report any abnormal temperature. Record the temperature in the proper place. Note the temperature site when reporting and recording.

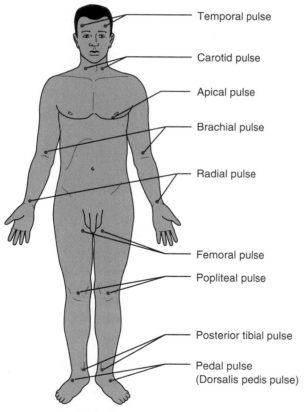

— Temporal pulse

— Carotid pulse

— Apical pulse

— Brachial pulse

— Radial pulse

— Femoral pulse

— Popliteal pulse

— Posterior tibial pulse

— Pedal pulse (Dorsalis pedis pulse)

Fig. 7-12 The pulse sites.

Pulse

The **pulse** is the beat of the heart felt at an artery as a wave of blood passes through the artery. A pulse is felt every time the heart beats.

The temporal, carotid, brachial, radial, femoral, popliteal, posterior tibial, and dorsalis pedis (pedal) pulses are on both sides of the body (Fig. 7-12). The radial site is used most often. It is easy to reach and find. You can take a radial pulse without disturbing or exposing the person. The apical pulse is over the heart. It is taken with a stethoscope.

Using a Stethoscope. A *stethoscope* is an instrument used to listen to the sounds produced by the heart, lungs, and other body organs (Fig. 7-13). Follow these rules when using a stethoscope:

- Wipe the earpieces and diaphragm with antiseptic wipes before and after use.
- Warm the diaphragm in your hand (Fig. 7-14).
- Place the earpiece tips in your ears. The bend of the tips points forward. Earpieces should fit snugly to block out noises. They should not cause pain or ear discomfort.
- Place the diaphragm over the artery. Hold it in place as in Figure 7-15.
- Prevent noise. Do not let anything touch the tubing. Ask the person to be silent.

Safety Alert

Stethoscopes

Stethoscopes are in contact with many persons and staff. Therefore you must prevent infection. Wipe the earpieces and diaphragm with antiseptic wipes before and after use.

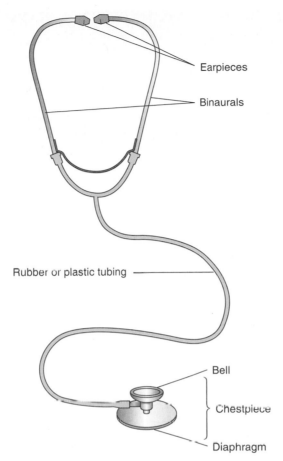

Earpieces

Binaurals

Rubber or plastic tubing

Bell

Chestpiece

Diaphragm

Fig. 7-13 Parts of a stethoscope.

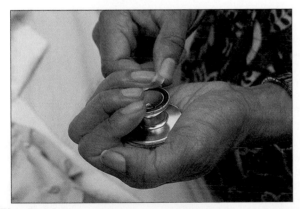

Fig. 7-14 The diaphragm of the stethoscope is warmed in the palm of the hand.

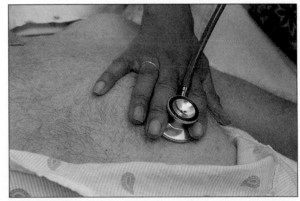

Fig. 7-15 The stethoscope is held in place with the fingertips of the index and middle fingers.

Pulse Rate. The **pulse rate** is the number of heartbeats or pulses felt in 1 minute. The pulse rate is affected by many factors—age, fever, exercise, fear, anger, anxiety, excitement, heat, position, pain, circulatory system problems (Box 7-1, p. 128), and diseases and injuries to other body systems. Some drugs increase the pulse rate. Other drugs slow the pulse.

The adult pulse rate is between 60 and 100 beats per minute. A rate of less than 60 or more than 100 is considered abnormal. Report abnormal rates to the nurse at once.

Text continued on p. 130

BOX 7-1   The Circulatory System

Structure and Function

The circulatory system is made up of the blood, heart, and blood vessels. The heart pumps blood through the blood vessels. The circulatory system has many functions:

- Blood carries food, oxygen, and other substances to the cells.
- Blood removes waste products from cells.
- Blood and blood vessels help regulate body temperature. Blood vessels in the skin dilate to cool the body. They constrict to retain heat.
- The system produces and carries cells that defend against disease-causing microbes.

The Blood

The blood consists of blood cells and *plasma.* Plasma is mostly water. It carries blood cells to other body cells. Plasma also carries substances that cells need to function. This includes food (proteins, fats, and carbohydrates), hormones, and chemicals.

Red blood cells (RBCs) are called *erythrocytes.* They give the blood its red color because of a substance in the cell called *hemoglobin.* The hemoglobin in *RBCs* picks up oxygen in the lungs, giving the blood a bright-red color. As blood circulates through the body, oxygen is given to the cells. Cells release carbon dioxide (a waste product). It is picked up by the hemoglobin. RBCs saturated with carbon dioxide make the blood look dark red. RBCs live for 3 or 4 months. Bone marrow produces new RBCs.

White blood cells (WBCs) are called *leukocytes.* They have no color. They protect the body against infection. At the first sign of infection, WBCs rush to the infection site. WBCs increase in number when there is an infection. WBCs are produced by the bone marrow. They live about 9 days.

Platelets (thrombocytes) are needed for blood clotting. They are produced by the bone marrow. A platelet lives about 4 days.

The Heart

The heart is a muscle. It pumps blood through the blood vessels to the tissues and cells. The heart lies in the middle to lower part of the chest cavity toward the left side (Fig. 7-16).

The heart has four chambers (Fig. 7-17, p. 130). Upper chambers receive blood and are called the *atria.* The *right atrium* receives blood from body tissues. The *left atrium* receives blood from the lungs. Lower chambers are called the *ventricles.* Ventricles pump blood. The *right ventricle* pumps blood to the lungs for oxygen. The *left ventricle* pumps blood to all parts of the body.

Heart action has two phases. *Diastole* is the resting phase. Heart chambers fill with blood. *Systole* is the working phase. The heart contracts. Blood is pumped through the blood vessels when the heart contracts.

The Blood Vessels

Blood flows to body tissues and cells through the blood vessels. *Arteries* carry blood away from the heart. Arterial blood is rich in oxygen. The *aorta* is the largest artery. It receives blood directly from the left ventricle. The aorta branches into other arteries that carry blood to all parts of the body (see Fig. 7-17). *Veins* return blood to the heart.

Changes With Aging

The heart muscle weakens. It pumps blood with less force. Problems may not occur at rest. Activity, exercise, excitement, and illness increase the body's need for oxygen and nutrients. A damaged or weak heart cannot meet these needs.

Arteries narrow and are less elastic. Less blood flows through them. Poor circulation occurs in many body parts. A weak heart must work harder to pump blood through narrowed vessels.

Common Disorders

Cardiovascular disorders are the leading causes of death in the United States. Problems occur in the heart or blood vessels.

Hypertension

With hypertension *(high blood pressure),* the resting blood pressure is too high. The systolic pressure is 140 mm Hg or higher. Or the diastolic pressure is 90 mm Hg or higher. Narrowed blood vessels are a common cause. Kidney disorders, head injuries, and adrenal gland tumors are other causes.

Signs and symptoms develop over time. Headache, blurred vision, dizziness, and nose bleeds occur. Hypertension can lead to stroke, heart attack, heart failure, kidney failure, and blindness.

Certain drugs can lower blood pressure. A healthy diet, a healthy weight, and regular exercise are needed. No smoking is allowed. Alcohol and caffeine are limited. Managing stress and sleeping well also lower blood pressure.

Coronary Artery Disease

The coronary arteries are in the heart. In coronary artery disease (CAD), the coronary arteries narrow. Therefore the heart muscle gets less blood. The most common cause is atherosclerosis (Fig. 7-18, p. 130). Fatty material collects on the arterial walls. The narrowed arteries block blood flow. Blockage may be total or partial. Permanent damage occurs in the part of the heart receiving its blood supply from the blocked artery.

BOX 7-1   The Circulatory System—cont'd

Men, older persons, people with a family history of CAD, and African-Americans are at risk. Treatment involves reducing risk factors that can be controlled—being overweight, smoking, lack of exercise, high blood cholesterol, hypertension, diabetes, and stress. The major complications of CAD are angina pectoris and myocardial infarction (heart attack):

- *Angina pectoris.* Angina *(pain)* pectoris *(chest)* means chest pain. The chest pain is from reduced blood flow to a part of the heart muscle (myocardium). Commonly called *angina,* it occurs when the heart needs more oxygen. Exertion, a heavy meal, stress, and excitement increase the heart's need for oxygen. In CAD, narrowed vessels prevent increased blood flow. Chest pain is described as a tightness or pressure. Some complain of discomfort in the chest. Pain in the jaw, neck, and down one or both arms is common. The person may be pale, feel faint, and perspire. Difficulty breathing is common. The person stops activity to rest. Rest often relieves symptoms in 3 to 15 minutes. Besides rest, a *nitroglycerin* tablet is taken when an angina attack occurs. It is placed under the tongue. There it dissolves and is rapidly absorbed into the bloodstream. Tablets are kept with the person at all times. The person takes a tablet and then tells the nurse. Angina pectoris often leads to heart attack. Chest pain that is not relieved by rest and nitroglycerin may signal a heart attack. The person needs emergency care.
- *Myocardial infarction (MI, heart attack). Myocardial* refers to the heart muscle. *Infarction* means tissue death. With MI, part of the heart muscle dies. This is from lack of blood flow to the heart muscle. Blood flow to the heart muscle is suddenly blocked. A thrombus (blood clot) blocks blood flow through an artery with atherosclerosis. The area of damage may

be small or large. Sudden cardiac death *(cardiac arrest)* can occur (Chapter 5). Signs and symptoms of MI include sudden, severe chest pain usually on the left side; indigestion; difficulty breathing; nausea; pallor; perspiration; and cold, clammy skin. The person is fearful, apprehensive, and has a feeling of doom. MI is an emergency. Efforts are made to relieve pain and prevent life-threatening problems.

Heart Failure

Heart failure or congestive heart failure (CHF) occurs when the heart cannot pump blood normally. Blood backs up. Tissue congestion occurs.

With left-sided failure, blood backs up into the lungs. The person has difficulty breathing, increased sputum, cough, and gurgling sounds in the lungs. Also, the rest of the body does not get enough blood. Poor blood flow to the brain causes confusion, dizziness, and fainting. The kidneys produce less urine. The skin is pale. Blood pressure falls.

With right-sided failure, blood backs up into the venous system. Feet and ankles swell. Neck veins bulge. Liver congestion affects liver function. The abdomen becomes congested with fluid. The right side of the heart pumps less blood to the lungs. Blood flow from the lungs to the left side of the heart is not normal. The left side has less blood to pump to the body. Organs receive less blood. The signs and symptoms described for left-sided failure occur.

Drugs strengthen the heart. They also reduce the amount of fluid in the body. A sodium-controlled diet is ordered. Oxygen is given. Semi-Fowler's or Fowler's position is preferred for breathing. Bedrest, intake and output, daily weight, elastic stockings, and range-of-motion exercises are part of the person's care plan.

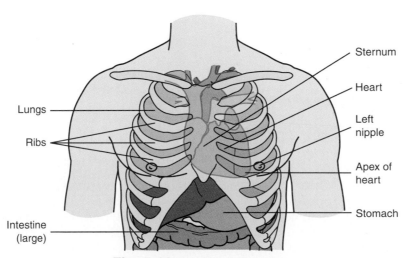

Fig. 7-16 Location of the heart.

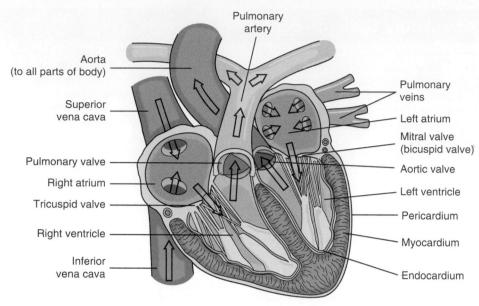

Fig. 7-17 Structures of the heart.

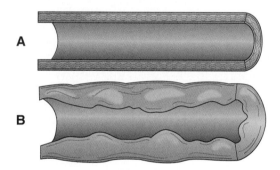

Fig. 7-18 A, Normal artery. **B,** Fatty deposits collect on the walls of arteries in atherosclerosis.

Delegation Guidelines

Taking Pulses

Before taking a pulse, you need this information from the nurse and the care plan:

- What pulse to take—radial or apical (p. 132)
- When to take the pulse
- What other vital signs to measure
- How long to count the pulse—30 seconds or 1 minute
- If the nurse has concerns about certain residents
- What observations to report and record:
  —The pulse site.
  —The pulse rate: report a pulse rate less than 60 or more than 100 beats per minute at once
  —If the pulse is regular or irregular
  —The pulse force: strong, full, bounding, weak, thready, or feeble

Rhythm and Force of the Pulse. The rhythm of the pulse should be regular. That is, pulses are felt in a pattern. The same time interval occurs between beats. An irregular pulse occurs when the beats are not evenly spaced or beats are skipped (Fig. 7-19).

Force relates to pulse strength. A forceful pulse is easy to feel. It is described as *strong, full,* or *bounding.* Hard-to-feel pulses are described as *weak, thready,* or *feeble.*

Safety Alert

Taking Pulses

Do not use your thumb to take a pulse. The thumb has a pulse. You could mistake the pulse in your thumb for the person's pulse. Reporting the wrong pulse rate can harm the person.

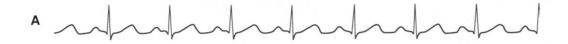

A

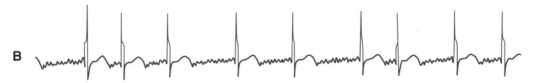

B

Fig. 7-19 A, The electrocardiogram shows a regular pulse. The beats occur at regular intervals. **B,** These beats occur at irregular intervals.

Taking a Radial Pulse.   The radial pulse is used for routine vital signs. Place the first 2 or 3 fingers of one hand against the radial artery. The radial artery is on the thumb side of the wrist (Fig. 7-20). Count the pulse for 30 seconds. Then multiply the number by 2. This gives the number of beats per minute. If the pulse is irregular, count it for 1 minute.

In some centers, all radial pulses are taken for 1 minute. Follow center policy.

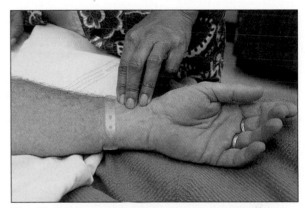

Fig. 7-20 The middle 3 fingers are used to take the radial pulse.

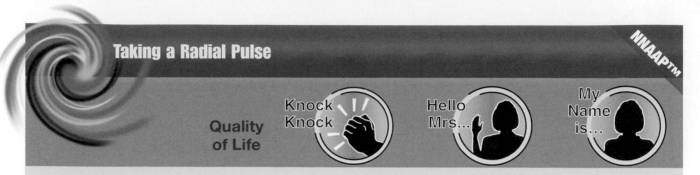

Taking a Radial Pulse

NNAAP™

Quality of Life

Knock Knock

Hello Mrs...

My Name is...

Pre-Procedure

1 Follow *Delegation Guidelines: Taking Pulses*, p. 130. See *Safety Alert: Taking Pulses*, p. 130.
2 Practice hand hygiene.
3 Identify the person. Check the ID bracelet against the assignment sheet. Call the person by name.
4 Explain the procedure to the person.
5 Provide for privacy.

Procedure

6 Have the person sit or lie down.
7 Locate the radial pulse. Use your first 2 or 3 middle fingers (see Fig. 7-20).
8 Note if the pulse is strong or weak, and regular or irregular.
9 Count the pulse for 30 seconds. Multiply the number of beats by 2. Or count the pulse for 1 minute as directed by the nurse or if required by center policy. (NNAAP™ skills evaluation requires counting the pulse for 1 minute.)
10 Count the pulse for 1 minute if it is irregular.
11 Record the person's name and pulse on your note pad or assignment sheet. Note the strength of the pulse. Note if it was regular or irregular.

Post-Procedure

12 Provide for comfort.
13 Place the signal light within reach.
14 Unscreen the person.
15 Complete a safety check of the room. (See inside of front book cover.)
16 Decontaminate your hands.
17 Report and record the pulse rate and your observations.

Taking an Apical Pulse.   The apical pulse is taken with a stethoscope. Apical pulses are taken on persons who have heart disease, who have irregular heart rhythms, or who take drugs that affect the heart. The apical pulse is on the left side of the chest slightly below the nipple (Fig. 7-21).

Count the apical pulse for 1 minute. The heartbeat normally sounds like a *lub-dub*. Count each *lub-dub* as 1 beat. Do not count the *lub* as 1 beat and the *dub* as another.

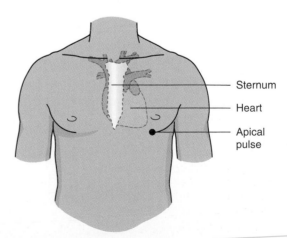

Sternum

Heart

Apical pulse

Fig. 7-21 The apical pulse is located 2 to 3 inches to the left of the sternum (breastbone) and below the left nipple.

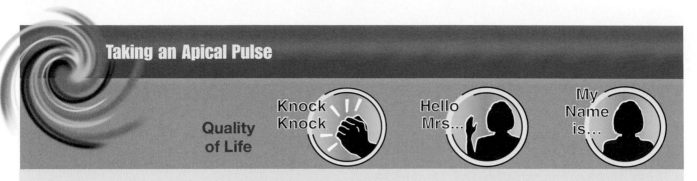

Taking an Apical Pulse

Quality of Life

Knock Knock

Hello Mrs...

My Name is...

Pre-Procedure

1 Follow *Delegation Guidelines: Taking Pulses*, p. 130. See *Safety Alert: Stethoscopes*, p. 130.
2 Collect a stethoscope and antiseptic wipes.
3 Practice hand hygiene.
4 Identify the person. Check the ID bracelet against the assignment sheet. Call the person by name.
5 Explain the procedure to the person.
6 Provide for privacy.

Procedure

7 Clean the earpieces and diaphragm with the wipes.
8 Have the person sit or lie down.
9 Expose the nipple area of the left chest. Do not expose a woman's breasts.
10 Warm the diaphragm in your palm.
11 Place the earpieces in your ears.
12 Find the apical pulse. Place the diaphragm 2 to 3 inches to the left of the breastbone and below the left nipple (see Fig. 7-21).
13 Count the pulse for 1 minute. Note if it is regular or irregular.
14 Cover the person. Remove the earpieces.
15 Record the person's name and pulse on your note pad or assignment sheet. Note if the pulse was regular or irregular.

Post-Procedure

16 Provide for comfort.
17 Place the signal light within reach.
18 Unscreen the person.
19 Complete a safety check of the room. (See inside of front book cover.)
20 Clean the earpieces and diaphragm with the wipes.
21 Return the stethoscope to its proper place.
22 Decontaminate your hands.
23 Report and record your observations. Record the pulse rate with *Ap* for apical pulse.

Respirations

Respiration means breathing air into (inhalation) and out of (exhalation) the lungs. Each respiration involves 1 inhalation and 1 exhalation. The chest rises during inhalation. It falls during exhalation. Respirations are normally quiet, effortless, and regular. Both sides of the chest rise and fall equally.

The healthy adult has 12 to 20 respirations per minute. The respiratory rate is affected by the factors that affect temperature and pulse. Heart and respiratory diseases (Box 7-2, p. 134) usually increase the respiratory rate.

People tend to change breathing patterns when they know their respirations are being counted. Therefore the person should not know that you are counting them. Respirations are counted right after taking a pulse. Keep your fingers or stethoscope over the pulse site. (The person assumes you are taking the pulse.) To count respirations, watch the chest rise and fall. Count them for 30 seconds. Multiply the number by 2 for the number of respirations in 1 minute. If an abnormal pattern is noted, count the respirations for 1 minute.

BOX 7-2   The Respiratory System

Structure and Function

Oxygen is needed to live. Every cell needs oxygen. The respiratory system (Fig. 7-22) brings oxygen into the lungs and removes carbon dioxide. *Respiration* is the process of supplying the cells with oxygen and removing carbon dioxide from them. Respiration involves *inhalation* (breathing in) and *exhalation* (breathing out). The terms *inspiration* (breathing in) and *expiration* (breathing out) are also used.

Air enters the body through the *nose*. Then air passes into the *pharynx* (throat). It is a tube-shaped passageway for air and food. Air passes from the pharynx into the *larynx* (voice box) and then into the *trachea* (the windpipe).

The trachea divides at its lower end into the *right bronchus* and *left bronchus*. Each bronchus enters a lung. Upon entering the lungs, the bronchi divide many times into smaller branches. The smaller branches are called *bronchioles.* Eventually the bronchioles subdivide. They end up in tiny one-celled air sacs called *alveoli*.

Alveoli are supplied by *capillaries.* Oxygen (O_2) and carbon dioxide (CO_2) are exchanged between the alveoli and capillaries. Blood in the capillaries picks up oxygen from the alveoli. Then the blood is returned to the left side of the heart and pumped to the rest of the body. Alveoli pick up carbon dioxide from the capillaries for exhalation.

Changes With Aging

Respiratory muscles weaken. Lung tissue becomes less elastic. Difficulty breathing may occur with activity. The person may lack strength to cough and clear the airway of secretions. Respiratory infections and diseases may develop. These can threaten the older person's life.

Turning, repositioning, and deep breathing help prevent respiratory complications from bed rest. Breathing usually is easier in semi-Fowler's position. The person should be as active as possible.

Common Disorders

Respiratory disorders interfere with bringing oxygen into the lungs and removing carbon dioxide from the body. They threaten life.

Chronic Obstructive Pulmonary Disease

Three disorders are grouped under chronic obstructive pulmonary disease (COPD). They obstruct air flow and interfere with the exchange of O_2 and CO_2 in the lungs:

- *Chronic bronchitis.* Chronic bronchitis is an inflammation *(itis)* of the bronchi *(bronch).* Smoking is the major cause. *Smoker's cough* in the morning is often the first symptom. At first the cough is dry. Over time, the person coughs up mucus. Mucus may contain pus. The cough becomes more frequent. The person has difficulty breathing and tires easily. Mucus and inflamed breathing passages *obstruct* airflow into the lungs. The body cannot get normal amounts of oxygen.

- *Emphysema.* The alveoli enlarge and become less elastic. They do not expand and shrink normally with breathing in and out. Some air is trapped in the alveoli when exhaling. Over time, more alveoli are involved and more air is trapped. The person develops a barrel chest (Fig. 7-23). Smoking is the most common cause. The person has shortness of breath and a cough. Sputum may contain pus. Breathing is easier when the person sits upright and slightly forward. The person must stop smoking. Respiratory therapy, breathing exercises, oxygen, and drug therapy are ordered.

- *Asthma.* The airway narrows. Difficulty breathing results. Allergies and emotional stress are common causes. Sudden attacks *(asthma attacks)* can occur. There is shortness of breath, wheezing, coughing, rapid pulse, sweating, and cyanosis (bluish color). Asthma is treated with drugs.

Pneumonia

Pneumonia is an inflammation and infection of lung tissue. Bacteria, viruses, aspiration, and immobility are causes. The person is very ill. Fever, chills, painful cough, chest pain on breathing, and a rapid pulse occur. Cyanosis may be present. Sputum is thick and green, yellowish, or rust colored. The color depends on the cause.

Drugs are ordered for infection and pain. Fluid intake is increased because of fever and to thin secretions. Thin secretions are easier to cough up. IV fluids and oxygen may be needed. Semi-Fowler's position eases breathing. Standard Precautions are followed. Transmission-Based Precautions are used depending on the cause.

Tuberculosis

Tuberculosis (TB) is a bacterial infection in the lungs. TB is spread by airborne droplets with coughing, sneezing, speaking, and singing (Chapter 3). People who have close, frequent contact with an infected person are at risk. So are people with human immunodeficiency virus (HIV) infection.

An active infection may not occur for many years. Chest x-ray and TB testing can detect the disease. Signs and symptoms are tiredness, loss of appetite, weight loss, fever, and night sweats. Cough and sputum production increase over time. Chest pain occurs.

Drugs for TB are given. The mouth and nose are covered with tissues when coughing or sneezing. Tissues are flushed down the toilet. Or they are placed in a biohazard bag. Standard Precautions and Airborne Precautions are practiced.

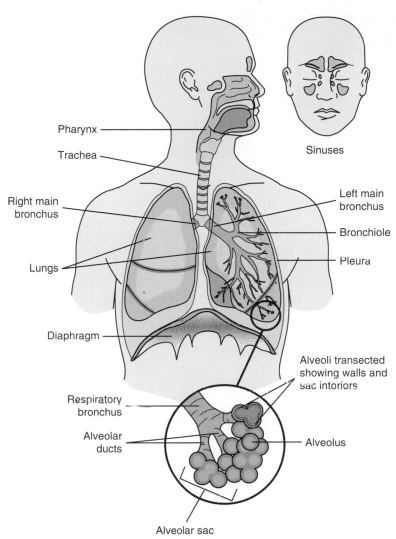

Fig. 7-22 The respiratory system.

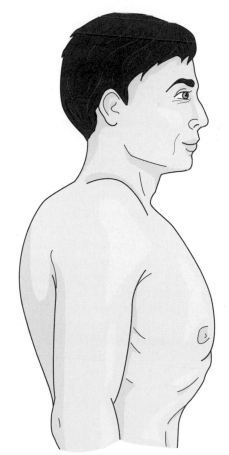

Fig. 7-23 Barrel chest with emphysema.

Delegation Guidelines

Counting Respirations

Before counting respirations, you need this information from the nurse and the care plan:

- How long to count respirations—30 seconds or 1 minute
- When to count respirations
- What other vital signs to measure
- What observations to report and record:
  —The respiratory rate
  —Equality and depth of respirations
  —If the respirations were regular or irregular
  —If the person has pain or difficulty in breathing
  —Any respiratory noises
  —Any abnormal respiratory patterns

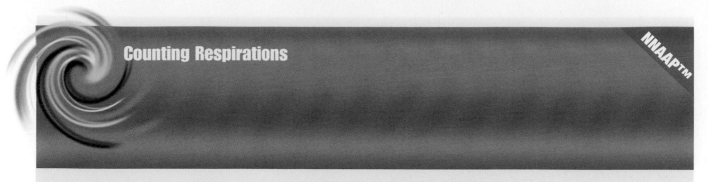

Counting Respirations

Procedure

1 Follow *Delegation Guidelines: Counting Respirations*, p. 135.
2 Keep your fingers or the stethoscope over the pulse site.
3 Do not tell the person you are counting respirations.
4 Begin counting when the chest rises. Count each rise and fall of the chest as 1 respiration.
5 Note the following:
   • If respirations are regular
   • If both sides of the chest rise equally
   • The depth of respirations
   • If the person has any pain or difficulty breathing
6 Count respirations for 30 seconds. Multiply the number by 2. (The NNAAP™ skills evaluation requires counting respirations for 1 minute.)
7 Count respirations for 1 minute if they are abnormal or irregular.
8 Record the person's name, respiratory rate, and other observations on your note pad or assignment sheet.

Post-Procedure

9   Provide for comfort.
10 Place the signal light within reach.
11 Complete a safety check of the room. (See inside of front book cover.)
12 Decontaminate your hands.
13 Report and record your observations.

Blood Pressure

Blood pressure is the amount of force exerted against the walls of an artery by the blood. The period of heart muscle contraction is called *systole*. The heart is pumping blood. The period of heart muscle relaxation is called *diastole*. The heart is at rest.

Systolic and diastolic pressures are measured. The **systolic pressure** represents the amount of force needed to pump blood out of the heart into the arterial circulation. It is the higher pressure. The **diastolic pressure** reflects the pressure in the arteries when the heart is at rest. It is the lower pressure.

Blood pressure is measured in millimeters (mm) of mercury (Hg). The systolic pressure is recorded over the diastolic pressure. A systolic pressure of 120 mm Hg and a diastolic pressure of 80 mm Hg are written as 120/80 mm Hg.

Normal and Abnormal Blood Pressures. Blood pressure can change from minute to minute. It can vary easily. Guidelines for normal blood pressure are as follows:

• *Systolic pressure*—less than 120 mm Hg
• *Diastolic pressure*—less than 80 mm Hg

Treatment is indicated for systolic pressures that remain above *(hyper)* 140 mm Hg and diastolic pressures that remain above 90 mm Hg. This condition is known as **hypertension.** Report any systolic pressure above 120 mm Hg or a diastolic pressure above 80 mm Hg. Likewise, systolic pressures below *(hypo)* 90 mm Hg and diastolic pressures below 60 mm Hg are reported. This is called **hypotension.** Some people normally have low blood pressures. However, hypotension may signal a life-threatening problem.

In older persons, arteries narrow and lose elasticity. The heart has to work harder to pump blood through the vessels. Therefore both the systolic and diastolic pressures are higher in older persons. A blood pressure of 160/90 mm Hg is normal for many older persons.

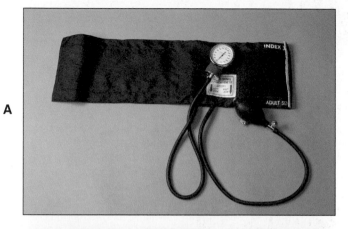

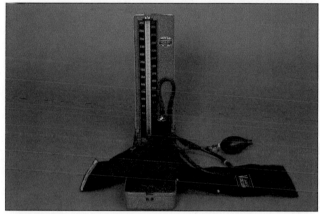

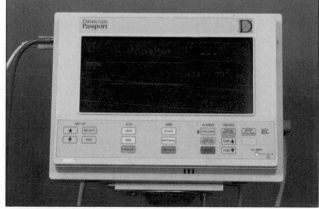

Fig. 7-24 Blood pressure equipment. **A,** Aneroid manometer and cuff. **B,** Mercury manometer and cuff. **C,** Electronic sphygmomanometer.

Equipment.   A stethoscope and a sphygmomanometer are used to measure blood pressure. The **sphygmomanometer** has a cuff and a measuring device. There are three types of sphygmomanometers:

- The *aneroid* type has a round dial and a needle that points to the numbers (Fig. 7-24, A).
- The *mercury* type is more accurate than the aneroid type. It has a column of mercury within a calibrated tube (Fig. 7-24, B).

- The *electronic* type shows the systolic and diastolic blood pressures on the front of the device (Fig. 7-24, C). It also shows the pulse rate. Follow the manufacturer's instructions.

The blood pressure cuff is wrapped around the upper arm. Tubing connects the cuff to the manometer. Another tube connects the cuff to a small hand-held bulb. A valve on the bulb is turned so the cuff inflates as the bulb is squeezed. The inflated cuff causes pressure over the brachial artery. The valve is turned the other way for cuff deflation. Blood pressure is measured as the cuff is deflated.

Sounds are produced as blood flows through the arteries. The stethoscope is used to listen to the sounds in the brachial artery as the cuff is deflated. Stethoscopes are not used with electronic manometers.

Safety Alert

Equipment
Mercury is a hazardous substance. Handle mercury manometers carefully. If one breaks, call for the nurse at once. Do not touch the mercury. Do not let the person touch it. The center must follow special procedures for handling all hazardous substances. See Chapter 4.

Measuring Blood Pressure.   Blood pressure is normally measured in the brachial artery. Box 7-3 on p. 138 lists the guidelines for measuring blood pressure.

Delegation Guidelines

Measuring Blood Pressure
Before measuring blood pressure, you need this information from the nurse and the care plan:
- When to measure blood pressure
- If the person has an arm with an IV infusion, a cast, or a dialysis access site
- If the person had breast surgery, what side was the surgery done on
- If the person needs to be lying down, sitting, or standing
- What size cuff to use—regular, pediatric, or extra-large
- What observations to report and record

BOX 7-3 Guidelines for Measuring Blood Pressure

- Do not take blood pressure on an arm with an IV infusion, a cast, or a dialysis access site. If a person had breast surgery, do not take blood pressure on that side. Avoid taking blood pressure on an injured arm.
- Let the person rest for 10 to 20 minutes before measuring blood pressure.
- Measure blood pressure with the person sitting or lying. Sometimes the doctor orders blood pressure measured in the standing position.
- Apply the cuff to the bare upper arm. Clothing can affect the measurement.
- Make sure the cuff is snug. Loose cuffs can cause inaccurate readings.
- Use a larger cuff if the person is obese or has a large arm. Use a smaller cuff if the person has very small arms. Ask the nurse what size to use.
- Place the diaphragm of the stethoscope firmly over the brachial artery. The entire diaphragm must have contact with the skin.
- Make sure the room is quiet. Talking, TV, radio, and sounds from the hallway can affect an accurate measurement.
- Have the sphygmomanometer where you can clearly see it.
- Measure the systolic and diastolic pressures. Expect to hear the first blood pressure sound at the point where you felt the radial or brachial pulse. The first sound is the systolic pressure. The point where the sound disappears is the diastolic pressure.
- Take the blood pressure again if you are not sure of an accurate measurement. Wait 30 to 60 seconds before repeating the measurement.
- Tell the nurse at once if you cannot hear the blood pressure.

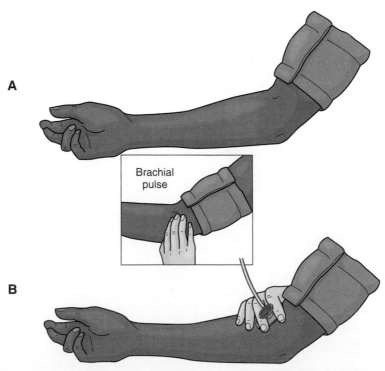

Brachial pulse

Fig. 7-25 Measuring blood pressure. **A,** The cuff is over the brachial artery. **B,** The diaphragm of the stethoscope is over the brachial artery.

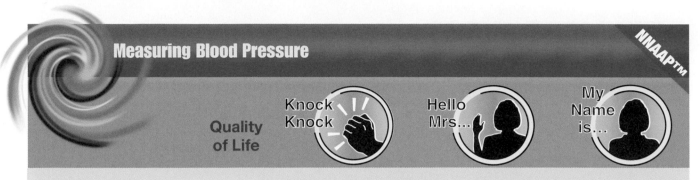

Measuring Blood Pressure

Quality of Life
- Knock Knock
- Hello Mrs...
- My Name is...

Pre-Procedure

1 Follow *Delegation Guidelines: Measuring Blood Pressure*, p. 137. See *Safety Alerts: Stethoscopes*, p. 126; *Equipment*, p. 137.
2 Collect the following:
   - Sphygmomanometer
   - Stethoscope
   - Antiseptic wipes
3 Practice hand hygiene.
4 Identify the person. Check the ID bracelet against the assignment sheet. Call the person by name.
5 Explain the procedure to the person.
6 Provide for privacy.

Procedure

7 Wipe the stethoscope earpieces and diaphragm with the wipes.
8 Have the person sit or lie down.
9 Position the person's arm level with the heart. The palm is up.
10 Stand no more than 3 feet away from the manometer. A mercury model is vertical, on a flat surface, and at eye level. The aneroid type is directly in front of you.
11 Expose the upper arm.
12 Squeeze the cuff to expel any remaining air. Close the valve on the bulb.
13 Find the brachial artery at the inner aspect of the elbow.
14 Place the arrow on the cuff over the brachial artery (Fig. 7-25, *A*). Wrap the cuff around the upper arm at least 1 inch above the elbow. It is even and snug.
15 *Method 1:*
   a Place the stethoscope earpieces in your ears.
   b Find the radial or brachial artery.
   c Inflate the cuff until you can no longer feel the pulse. Note this point.
   d Inflate the cuff 30 mm Hg beyond the point where you last felt the pulse.
   Method 2:
   a Find the radial or brachial artery.
   b Inflate the cuff until you can no longer feel the pulse. Note this point.
   c Inflate the cuff 30 mm Hg beyond the point where you last felt the pulse.
   d Deflate the cuff slowly. Note the point when you feel the pulse.
   e Wait 30 seconds.
   f Place the stethoscope earpieces in your ears.
   g Inflate the cuff 30 mm Hg beyond the point where you felt the pulse return.
16 Place the diaphragm over the brachial artery (Fig. 7-25, *B*). Do not place it under the cuff.
17 Deflate the cuff at an even rate of 2 to 4 millimeters per second. Turn the valve counterclockwise to deflate the cuff.
18 Note the point where you hear the first sound. This is the systolic reading. It is near the point where the radial pulse disappeared.
19 Continue to deflate the cuff. Note the point where the sound disappears. This is the diastolic reading.
20 Deflate the cuff completely. Remove it from the person's arm. Remove the stethoscope.
21 Record the person's name and blood pressure on your note pad or assignment sheet.
22 Return the cuff to the case or wall holder.

Post-Procedure

23 Provide for comfort.
24 Place the signal light within reach.
25 Unscreen the person.
26 Complete a safety check of the room. (See inside of front book cover.)
27 Clean the earpieces and diaphragm with the wipes.
28 Return the equipment to its proper place.
29 Decontaminate your hands.
30 Report any abnormal blood pressure to the nurse.

MEASURING HEIGHT AND WEIGHT

Height and weight are measured on admission to the center. Some residents are weighed daily, weekly, or monthly to monitor weight loss or gain. Weigh the person at the same time of day. Before breakfast is the best time. Food and fluids add weight.

Standing, chair, and lift scales are used. Chair and lift scales are used for persons who cannot stand. Balance the scale at zero before weighing the person. For balance scales, move the weights to zero. A digital scale should read at zero.

Delegation Guidelines

Measuring Height and Weight

Before measuring height and weight, you need this information from the nurse and the care plan:
- When to measure height and weight
- What scale to use

Safety Alert

Measuring Height and Weight

Follow the manufacturer's instructions when using chair or lift scales. Also follow the center's procedures. Practice safety measures to prevent falls.

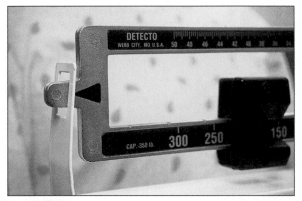

Fig. 7-26 The weight is read when the balance pointer is in the middle.

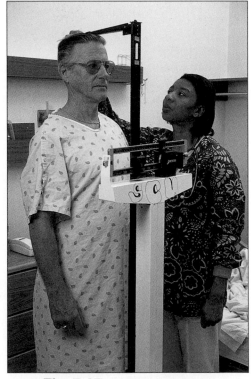

Fig. 7-27 Height is measured.

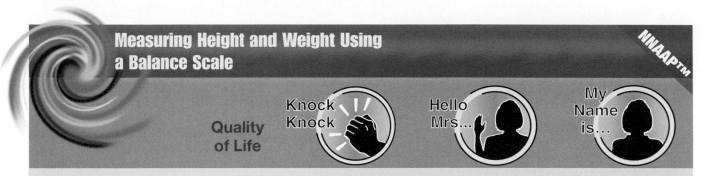

Measuring Height and Weight Using a Balance Scale

NNAAP™

Quality of Life

Knock Knock

Hello Mrs...

My Name is...

Pre-Procedure

1   Follow *Delegation Guidelines: Measuring Height and Weight.* See *Safety Alert: Measuring Height and Weight.*
2   Explain the procedure to the person.
3   Ask the person to void.
4   Practice hand hygiene.
5   Bring the scale and paper towels to the person's room.
6   Decontaminate your hands.
7   Identify the person. Check the ID bracelet against the assignment sheet. Call the person by name.
8   Provide for privacy.

Procedure

9   Place the paper towels on the scale platform.
10   Raise the height rod.
11   Move the weights to zero (0). The pointer is in the middle.
12   Have the person remove the robe and footwear. Assist as needed.
13   Help the person onto the scale.
14   Move the weights until the balance pointer is in the middle (Fig. 7-26).
15   Record the weight on your note pad or assignment sheet.
16   Ask the person to stand very straight.
17   Lower the height rod until it rests on the person's head (Fig. 7-27).
18   Record the height on your note pad or assignment sheet.
19   Help the person put on a robe and nonskid footwear if he or she will be up. Or help the person back to bed.

Post-Procedure

20   Provide for comfort.
21   Place the signal light within reach.
22   Raise or lower bed rails. Follow the care plan.
23   Unscreen the person.
24   Discard the paper towels.
25   Complete a safety check of the room. (See inside of front book cover.)
26   Return the scale to its proper place.
27   Decontaminate your hands.
28   Report and record the measurements.

INTAKE AND OUTPUT

The doctor or nurse may order intake and output (I&O) measurements. I&O records are kept. They are used to evaluate fluid balance and kidney function. They also are kept when the person has special fluid orders (Chapter 14).

All fluids taken by mouth are measured and recorded—water, milk, coffee, tea, juices, soups, and soft drinks. So are foods that melt at room temperature—ice cream, sherbet, custard, pudding, gelatin, and Popsicles. The nurse measures and records IV fluids and tube feedings. Output includes urine, vomitus, diarrhea, and wound drainage.

Intake and output are measured in milliliters (ml). Know these amounts:

* 1 ounce equals 30 ml
* A pint is about 500 ml
* A quart is about 1000 ml

You need to know the serving sizes of the bowls, dishes, cups, pitchers, glasses, and other containers. The information may be on the I&O record (Fig. 7-28, p. 142).

OSF ™
DEUS MEUS ET OMNIA
ST. JOSEPH MEDICAL CENTER
Bloomington, Illinois

FLUID BALANCE CHART

Water Glass	250ml
Styrofoam Cup	180ml
Cup (coffee)	250ml
Milk Carton	240ml
Pop (1 can)	360ml
Broth-Soup	175ml
Juice Carton	120ml
Juice Glass	120ml
Jello	120ml

Ice Cream	120ml
Ice Chips	1/2 amt. of ml's in cup
Pitcher (Yellow)	1000ml

DATE   6/15

TIME	INTAKE ORAL	Parenteral	Amt. ml Absbd.	OUTPUT URINE Method Collected	URINE Amt. (ml)	OTHER Method Collected	OTHER Amt. (ml)	CONT. IRRIGATION In	CONT. IRRIGATION Out
2400-0100		ml from previous shift		V	150				
0100-0200						Vom.	150		
0200-0300									
0300-0400									
0400-0500									
0500-0600	125			V	200				
0600-0700									
0700-0800									
	125	8 - hour Sub-total		8-hr T	350	8-hr T	150		
0800-0900	400	ml from previous shift		V	250				
0900-1000	100								
1000-1100									
1100-1200									
1200-1300	400			V	250				
1300-1400									
1400-1500	200								
1500-1600									
	1100	8 - hour Sub-total		8-hr T	500	8-hr T			
1600-1700		ml from previous shift		V	270				
1700-1800	350								
1800-1900	50								
1900-2000	200								
2000-2100				V	400				
2100-2200									
2200-2300									
2300-2400									
	600	8 - hour Sub-total		8-hr T	670	8-hr T			
	1825	24 - hour Sub-total		24-hr T	1520	24-hr T	750		

Source Key:

URINE	
V	- Voided
C	- Catheter
INC	- Incontinent
U.C.	- Ureteral Catheter

Source Key:

OTHER	
G.I.T.	- Gastric Intestinal Tube
T.T.	- T. Tube
Vom.	- Vomitus
Liq S.	- Liquid Stool
H.V.	- Hemovac

310' Marie Mills

Form No. MF36722 (Rev. 5/97) *MFI*

Fig. 7-28 An intake and output record. (Modified from OSF St. Joseph Medical Center, Bloomington, Ill.)

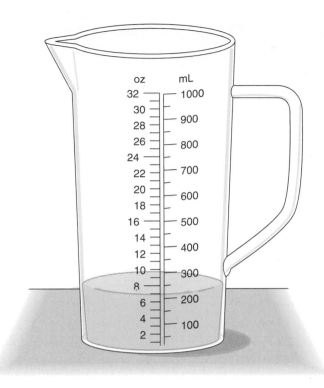

Fig. 7-29 A graduate marked in ounces and milliliters.

A measuring container for fluid is called a *graduate.* It is used to measure leftover fluids, urine, vomitus, and drainage from suction. Like a measuring cup, the graduate is marked in ounces and in milliliters (Fig. 7-29). Plastic urinals and kidney basins often have amounts marked.

An I&O record is kept at the bedside. When intake or output is measured, the amount is recorded in the correct column (see Fig. 7-28). Amounts are totaled at the end of the shift. The totals are recorded in the person's chart. They also are shared during the end-of-shift report.

The urinal, commode, bedpan, or specimen pan is used for voiding. Remind the person not to void in the toilet. Also remind the person not to put toilet tissue into the receptacle.

Delegation Guidelines
Intake and Output
When measuring I&O, you need this information from the nurse and the care plan:
- Does the person have a special fluid order—encourage fluids, restrict fluids, or NPO (See Chapter 14.)
- When to report measurements—hourly or end-of-shift
- What the person uses for voiding—urinal, bedpan, commode, or specimen pan (See Chapter 13.)
- Does the person have a catheter (See Chapter 13.)

Safety Alert
Intake and Output
Urine may contain microbes or blood. Microbes can grow in urinals, commodes, bedpans, specimen pans, and drainage systems. Follow Standard Precautions and the Bloodborne Pathogen Standard when handling such equipment. Thoroughly clean the item after it is used.

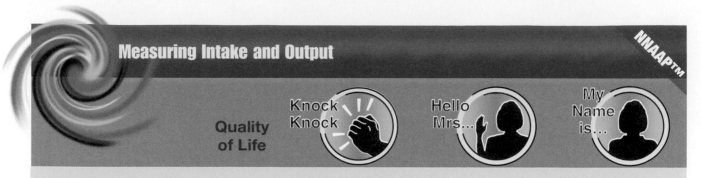

Measuring Intake and Output

Quality of Life

Knock Knock

Hello Mrs...

My Name is...

Pre-Procedure

1 Follow *Delegation Guidelines: Intake and Output*, p. 143. See *Safety Alert: Intake and Output*.
2 Explain the procedure to the person.
3 Practice hand hygiene.

4 Collect the following:
   • Intake and output (I&O) record
   • Graduates
   • Gloves

Procedure

5 Put on gloves.
6 Measure intake as follows:
   a Pour liquid remaining in a container into the graduate.
   b Measure the amount at eye level. Keep the container level.
   c Check the serving amount on the I&O record.
   d Subtract the remaining amount from the full serving amount. Record the amount.
   e Pour the fluid in the graduate back in the container.
   f Repeat steps 6a through 6e for each liquid.
   g Add the amounts from each liquid together.
   h Record the time and amount on the I&O record.

7 Measure output as follows:
   a Pour the fluid into the graduate used to measure output.
   b Measure the amount at eye level. Keep the container level.
8 Dispose of fluid in the toilet. Avoid splashes.
9 Clean and rinse the graduates. Dispose of rinse into the toilet. Return the graduates to their proper place.
10 Clean the bedpan, urinal, kidney basin, or other drainage container. Discard the rinse into the toilet. Return the item to its proper place.
11 Remove the gloves. Decontaminate your hands.
12 Record the amount on the I&O record.

Post-Procedure

13 Report and record your observations.

PAIN

Pain means to ache, hurt, or be sore. Pain is a warning from the body. It means there is tissue damage.

Pain is personal. It differs for each person. What *hurts* to one person may *ache* to another. What one person calls *sore*, another may call *aching*. If a person complains of pain, the person *has* pain. You must believe the person.

There are different types of pain:

• *Acute pain* is felt suddenly from injury, disease, trauma, or surgery. There is tissue damage. Acute pain lasts a short time, usually less than 6 months. It lessens with healing.

• *Chronic pain* lasts longer than 6 months. Pain is constant or occurs off and on. There is no longer tissue damage. Chronic pain remains long after healing. Arthritis and cancer are common causes.
• *Radiating pain* is felt at the site of tissue damage and in nearby areas. Pain from a heart attack is often felt in the left chest, left jaw, left shoulder, and left arm. Gallbladder disease can cause pain in the right upper abdomen, the back, and right shoulder (Fig. 7-30).
• *Phantom pain* is felt in a body part that is no longer there. A person with an amputated leg may still sense leg pain.

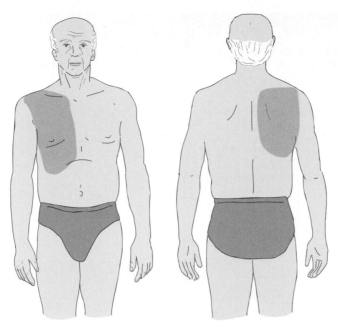

Fig. 7-30 Gallbladder pain radiates to the right upper abdomen, the back, and the right shoulder.

PAIN: Ask person to rate pain on scale of 1-10										
No pain									Worst pain imaginable	
0	1	2	3	4	5	6	7	8	9	10

Fig. 7-31 Pain rating scale. (Modified from deWit SC: *Fundamental concepts and skills for nursing,* Philadelphia, 2001, Saunders.)

Signs and Symptoms

You cannot see, hear, feel, or smell a person's pain. You must rely on what the person tells you. Promptly report any information you collect about pain. Use the person's exact words when reporting and recording. The nurse needs the following information:

- *Location.* Where is the pain? Ask the person to point to the area of pain. Pain can radiate. Ask the person if the pain is anywhere else and to point to those areas.
- *Onset and duration.* When did the pain start? How long has it lasted?
- *Intensity.* Does the person complain of mild, moderate, or severe pain? Ask the person to rate the pain on a scale of 1 to 10, with 10 as the most severe (Fig. 7-31).

- *Description.* Ask the person to describe the pain.
- *Factors causing pain.* These are called *precipitating* factors. To *precipitate* means to cause. Such factors include moving or turning in bed, coughing or deep breathing, and exercise. Ask what the person was doing before the pain started and when it started.
- *Vital signs.* Measure the person's pulse, respirations, and blood pressure. Increases in these vital signs often occur with acute pain. Vital signs may be normal with chronic pain.
- *Other signs and symptoms.* Does the person have other symptoms—dizziness, nausea, vomiting, weakness, numbness or tingling, or others? Box 7-4 on p. 146 lists the signs and symptoms that often occur with pain.

BOX 7-4 Signs and Symptoms of Pain

Body Responses

- Increased pulse, respirations, and blood pressure
- Nausea
- Pale skin (pallor)
- Sweating (diaphoresis)
- Vomiting

Behaviors

- Changes in speech: slow or rapid; loud or quiet
- Crying
- Gasping
- Grimacing
- Groaning
- Grunting
- Holding the affected body part (splinting)
- Irritability
- Maintaining one position; refusing to move
- Moaning
- Quietness
- Restlessness
- Rubbing
- Screaming

Review Questions

Circle the BEST answer.

1   Which statement is *false?*
   a   The vital signs are temperature, pulse, respirations, and blood pressure.
   b   Vital signs detect changes in body function.
   c   Vital signs change only during illness.
   d   Sleep, exercise, drugs, emotions, and noise affect vital signs.

2   Which should you report at once?
   a   An oral temperature of 98.4° F
   b   A rectal temperature of 101.6° F
   c   An axillary temperature of 97.6° F
   d   An oral temperature of 99.0° F

3   A rectal temperature is taken when the person
   a   Is confused
   b   Has heart disease
   c   Has a nasogastric tube
   d   Has diarrhea

Review Questions

4 Which gives the *least* accurate measurement of body temperature?
  a Oral site
  b Rectal site
  c Axillary site
  d Tympanic site

5 Which is usually used to take a pulse?
  a The radial pulse
  b The carotid pulse
  c The apical pulse
  d The brachial pulse

6 Which is reported to the nurse at once?
  a A pulse of 120 beats per minute
  b A pulse of 98 beats per minute
  c A pulse of 80 beats per minute
  d A pulse of 64 beats per minute

7 The following describe normal respirations *except*
  a There are 12 to 20 per minute
  b They are quiet and effortless
  c They are regular with both sides of the chest rising and falling equally
  d The person breathes through the mouth

8 Respirations are usually counted
  a After taking the temperature
  b After taking the pulse
  c Before taking the pulse
  d After taking the blood pressure

9 Which blood pressure is normal for an adult?
  a 88/54 mm Hg
  b 210/100 mm Hg
  c 116/76 mm Hg
  d 152/90 mm Hg

10 When taking a blood pressure, you should do the following *except*
  a Take the blood pressure in the arm with an IV infusion
  b Apply the cuff to a bare upper arm
  c Turn off the TV and radio
  d Locate the brachial artery

11 Which is the systolic blood pressure?
  a The point where the pulse is no longer felt
  b The point where the first sound is heard
  c The point where the last sound is heard
  d The point 30 mm Hg above where the pulse was felt

12 For an accurate weight measurement, the person
  a Wears footwear
  b Wears a robe
  c Urinates first
  d Chooses what scale to use

13 Which is *not* measured as output?
  a Urine
  b Vomitus
  c Perspiration
  d Wound drainage

14 Which is *not* measured for intake?
  a Coffee
  b Melted cheese
  c Ice cream
  d Jell-O

15 A person has pain in the left chest, the left jaw, and the left shoulder and arm. This is
  a Acute pain
  b Chronic pain
  c Radiating pain
  d Phantom pain

16 Mr. Smith complains of pain. You should do the following *except*
  a Ask him to point to where the pain is felt
  b Ask him to rate the pain on a scale of 1 to 10
  c Ask him to describe the pain
  d Ask to look at the pain

Answers to these questions are on p. 389.

CHAPTER 8

Care of the Resident's Environment

Objectives

- Define the key terms listed in this chapter
- Explain how to keep the resident's unit clean and safe
- Describe how to control temperature, odors, noise, and lighting
- Describe how to use furniture and equipment in the person's unit
- Describe open, closed, occupied, and surgical beds
- Explain the purpose of plastic and cotton drawsheets
- Handle linens following the rules of medical asepsis
- Perform the procedures described in this chapter

Key Terms

Fowler's position A semi-sitting position; the head of the bed is raised 45 to 90 degrees

full visual privacy Having the means to be completely free from public view while in bed

reverse Trendelenburg's position The head of the bed is raised, and the foot of the bed is lowered

semi-Fowler's position The head of the bed is raised 30 degrees; or the head of the bed is raised 30 degrees and the knee portion is raised 15 degrees

Trendelenburg's position The head of the bed is lowered, and the foot of the bed is raised

---

Resident rooms are designed for comfort, safety, and privacy. They need to be as homelike as possible.

THE RESIDENT'S UNIT

The resident's unit is the space, furniture, and equipment provided by the center. This area is considered private. It is treated like the person's home.

The person's unit must be clean, neat, safe, and comfortable. Follow the rules in Box 8-1.

Temperature and Ventilation

Most healthy people are comfortable when the temperature is 68° F to 74° F. Older and ill persons may need higher temperatures. OBRA requires that nursing centers maintain a temperature range of 71° F to 81° F.

Ventilation systems provide fresh air and move room air. Drafts occur as air moves. Older persons and ill persons are sensitive to drafts and cool temperatures. You need to:

- Make sure they wear the correct clothing.
- Provide enough blankets for warmth.
- Offer lap blankets to people in chairs or wheelchairs. Lap blankets cover the legs.
- Move them from drafty areas.

Odors

Draining wounds, vomitus, bowel movements, and urine cause odors. And they embarrass the person. Body, breath, and smoke odors offend others. To control odors, promptly do the following:

- Empty and clean bedpans, urinals, commodes, and kidney (emesis) basins.
- Change soiled linens and clothing.
- Follow center policy for soiled linens and clothing.
- Check incontinent persons often (Chapter 13).
- Clean persons who are wet or soiled from urine, feces, vomitus, or wound drainage.
- Dispose of incontinence and ostomy products promptly (Chapter 13).
- Keep laundry containers closed.
- Provide good hygiene (Chapter 11).

If you smoke, follow the center's policy. Practice hand hygiene after handling smoking materials and before giving care. Give careful attention to your uniforms, hair, and breath because of clinging smoke odors.

BOX 8-1   Maintaining the Person's Unit

- Make sure the person can reach the overbed table and the bedside stand.
- Arrange personal items as the person prefers. Make sure they are easily reached.
- Keep the signal light within the person's reach at all times.
- Make sure the person can reach the phone, TV, and light controls.
- Provide the person with enough tissues and toilet paper.
- Adjust lighting, temperature, and ventilation for the person's comfort.
- Handle equipment carefully to prevent noise.

- Explain the causes of strange noises.
- Empty wastebaskets as often as needed. They are emptied at least once a day.
- Respect the person's belongings. An item may not be important or valuable to you. Yet it has great meaning for the person. Even a scrap of paper can have great meaning to the person.
- Do not throw away any items belonging to the person.
- Do not move furniture or the person's belongings. Persons with poor vision rely on memory or feel for the location of items.
- Straighten bed linens as often as needed.

Noise

Clanging equipment, the clatter of dishes and trays, and loud voices are annoying. So are TVs, radios, phones, signal lights, intercoms, and noise from equipment needing repair or oil.

Residents may find sounds dangerous, frightening, or irritating. They may become upset, anxious, and uncomfortable. To decrease noise:

- Control your voice
- Handle equipment carefully
- Keep equipment working properly
- Answer phones, signal lights, and intercoms promptly

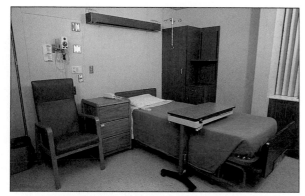

Fig. 8-1 Furniture in a typical unit.

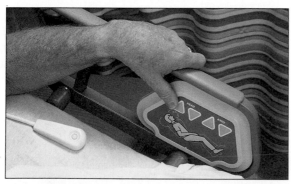

Fig. 8-2 Controls for an electric bed.

Lighting

Good lighting is needed for safety and comfort. Glares, shadows, and dull lighting can cause falls, headaches, and eyestrain. A bright room is cheerful. Dim light is relaxing and restful.

Adjust lighting, shades, and drapes to meet the person's needs. Adjust the overbed light for soft, medium, and bright lighting. Keep light controls within the person's reach. This protects the right to personal choice.

Room Furniture and Equipment

Rooms are furnished and equipped to meet basic needs (Fig 8-1). The right to privacy is also considered.

Rooms must be as homelike as possible. Residents can bring some furniture and personal items from home. This promotes their dignity and self-esteem.

The Bed. Beds have electrical or manual controls. Beds are raised to give care. This reduces bending and reaching. The lowest position lets the person get out of bed with ease.

Electric bed controls are on a side panel, bed rail, or the foot board (Fig. 8-2). Residents need to use the controls safely. They are warned not to raise the bed to the high position and not to adjust the bed to harmful positions. They are told of position limits or restrictions.

Manual beds have cranks at the foot of the bed (Fig. 8-3). The cranks are pulled up for use. They are kept down at all other times. Cranks in the *up* position are safety hazards. People can bump into them.

There are five basic bed positions:

- The *flat* position.
- **Fowler's position** is a semi-sitting position. The head of the bed is raised 45 to 90 degrees (Fig. 8-4).
- In **semi-Fowler's position,** the head of the bed is raised 30 degrees (Fig. 8-5). Some centers define this position as when the head of the bed is raised 30 degrees and the knee portion is raised 15 degrees. To give safe care, know the definition your center uses.
- In **Trendelenburg's position,** the head of the bed is lowered and the foot of the bed is raised (Fig. 8-6). A doctor orders the position. Blocks are placed under the legs at the foot of the bed. Or the bedframe is tilted.
- In **reverse Trendelenburg's position,** the head of the bed is raised and the foot of the bed is lowered (Fig. 8-7). Blocks are put under the legs at the head of the bed. Or the bed frame is tilted. This position requires a doctor's order.

Safety Alert

The Bed

Use bed rails as the nurse and care plan direct. Lock bed wheels at all times except when moving the bed. They must be locked to:

- Give bedside care
- Transfer a person to and from the bed. The person can be injured if the bed moves.

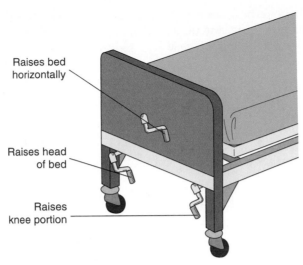

Raises bed
horizontally

Raises head
of bed

Raises
knee portion

Fig. 8-3 Manually operated bed.

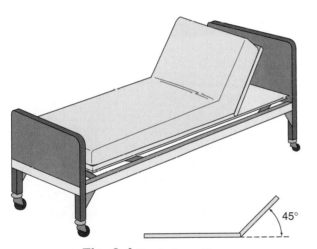

45°

Fig. 8-4 Fowler's position.

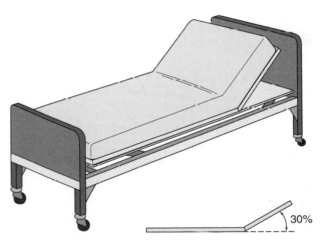

30%

Fig. 8-5 Semi-Fowler's position.

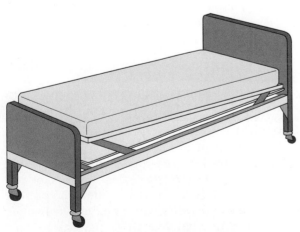

Fig. 8-6 Trendelenburg's position.

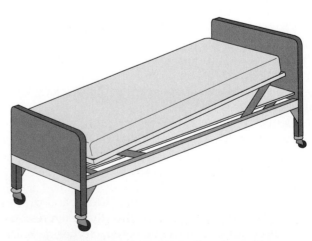

Fig. 8-7 Reverse Trendelenburg's position.

The Overbed Table. The overbed table (see Fig. 8-1) is used for meals, writing, reading, and other activities. It is placed over the bed by sliding the base under the bed. The table is raised or lowered for the person in bed or in a chair.

The overbed table is a work area for the nursing team. Only clean and sterile items are placed on the table. Never place bedpans, urinals, or soiled linen on an overbed table. Clean the table after using it for a work surface.

The Bedside Stand. The bedside stand has a top and a lower cabinet with a shelf (Fig. 8-8). The drawer is used for money, eyeglasses, books, and other items.

The top shelf is used for the wash basin. The wash basin can hold personal care items—soap, powder, lotion, deodorant, towels, washcloth, and a bath blanket. An emesis or kidney basin (shaped like a kidney) holds oral hygiene items. The kidney basin is stored on the top shelf or in the drawer. The bedpan and cover, urinal, and toilet paper are on the lower shelf.

The top of the stand is often used for tissues and the phone. The person may put a radio, flowers, gifts, cards, and other items there.

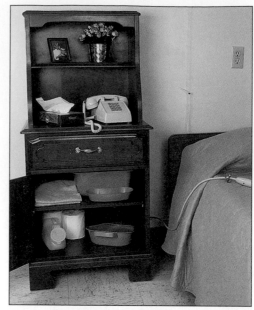

Fig. 8-8 The bedside stand.

Chairs. The person has at least 1 chair (Fig. 8-9). It must be comfortable and sturdy. It must not move or tip during transfers. The person should be able to get in and out of it with ease.

Privacy Curtains. The person has the right to full visual privacy. **Full visual privacy** is having the means to be completely free from public view while in bed. The privacy curtain is a means to full visual privacy. Always pull it completely around the bed when giving care. Privacy curtains prevent others from seeing the person. They do not block sound or conversations.

The Bathroom. A toilet, sink, call system, and mirror are standard equipment. Some bathrooms have showers. For safety, grab bars are by the toilet. The person uses them for support when lowering to or raising from the toilet. Some centers have raised toilet seats. The higher toilets make wheelchair transfers easier. They also are helpful for persons with joint problems.

The bathroom has towel racks, toilet paper, soap, a paper towel dispenser, and wastebasket. They are placed within easy reach of the person.

Closet and Drawer Space. Closet and drawer space are provided. OBRA requires that each resident have closet space with shelves and a clothes rack. The person must have free access to the closet and its contents. Items in the closet and drawers are the person's private property.

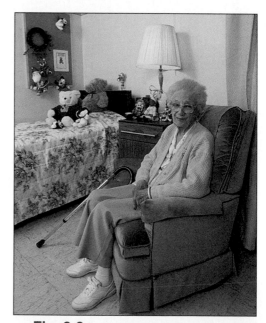

Fig. 8-9 Resident's chair from home.

Safety Alert

Closet and Drawer Space

Some residents hoard items. Straws, napkins, and salt and pepper packets are examples. The nurse may ask you to inspect a closet, drawers, or personal property. If so, the person must be present. Also have a co-worker with you. Your co-worker is a witness to what you are doing. This protects you if the person claims that something was stolen or damaged.

Other Equipment.   Many centers provide a TV, radio, and clock for comfort and relaxation. Many rooms have phones. Residents may bring furniture and items from home.

BEDMAKING

A clean, dry, and wrinkle-free bed increases comfort. It also helps prevent skin breakdown and pressure ulcers (Chapter 15).

A complete linen change is done on the person's bath day. This is done after the bath or shower when the person is up for the day. Follow the rules for bedmaking in Box 8-2.

BOX 8-2   Rules for Bedmaking

- Use good body mechanics at all times.
- Follow the rules of medical asepsis.
- Follow Standard Precautions and the Bloodborne Pathogen Standard.
- Practice hand hygiene before handling clean linen.
- Practice hand hygiene after handling dirty linen.
- Bring enough linen to the person's room.
- Bring only the linens that you will need. Extra linens cannot be used for another person.
- Do not use torn linen.
- Never shake linens. Shaking linens spreads microbes.
- Extra linen in a person's room is considered contaminated. Do not use it for other people. Put it with the dirty laundry.
- Hold linens away from your uniform. Dirty and clean linen must not touch your uniform.

- Check linens for dentures, eyeglasses, hearing aids, sharp objects, and other items.
- Never put dirty linens on the floor or on clean linens. Follow center policy for dirty linen.
- Keep bottom linens tucked in and wrinkle-free.
- Cover a plastic drawsheet with a cotton drawsheet. A plastic drawsheet must not touch the person's body.
- Straighten and tighten loose sheets, blankets, and bedspreads as needed.
- Make as much of one side of the bed as possible before going to the other side. This saves time and energy.
- Change wet, damp, and soiled linens right away.

Beds are made in these ways:

- A *closed bed* is not in use until bedtime. Top linens are not folded back. The bed is ready for a new resident (Fig. 8-10).
- An *open bed* is in use. Top linens are folded back so the person can get into bed. To open a closed bed, fold back the top linens (Fig. 8-11).

- An *occupied bed* is made with the person in it (Fig. 8-12).
- A *surgical bed* is made to transfer a person from a stretcher to the bed (Fig. 8-13). The bed is made for persons who arrive at the center by ambulance.

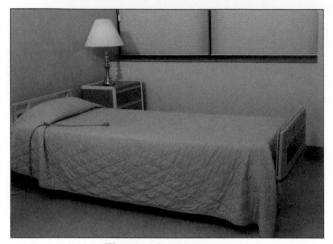

Fig. 8-10 Closed bed.

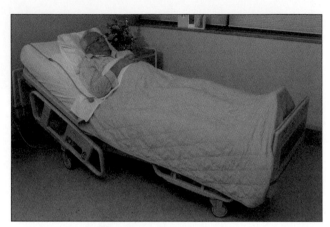

Fig. 8-12 Occupied bed.

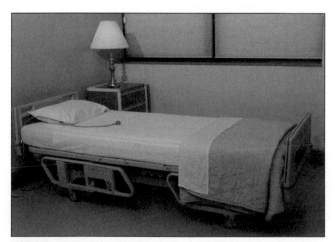

Fig. 8-11 Open bed. Top linens are folded to the foot of the bed.

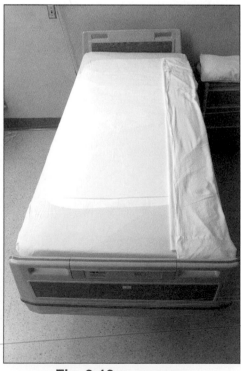

Fig. 8-13 Surgical bed.

Linens

Collect linens in the order you will use them:

- Mattress pad (if needed)
- Bottom sheet (flat or fitted)
- Plastic drawsheet, waterproof drawsheet, or waterproof pad (optional)
- Cotton drawsheet (if needed)
- Top sheet (if needed)
- Blanket
- Bedspread
- Pillowcase(s)
- Bath towel(s)
- Hand towel
- Washcloth
- Bath blanket

Use one arm to hold the linens. Use your other hand to pick them up. The item you will use first is at the bottom of your stack. (You picked up the mattress pad first. It is at the bottom. The bath blanket is on top.) You need the mattress pad first. To get it on top, place your arm over the bath blanket. Then turn the stack over onto the arm on the bath blanket (Fig. 8-14). The arm that held the linens is now free. Place the clean linens on a clean surface.

A 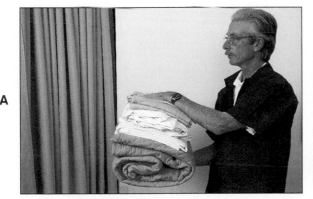 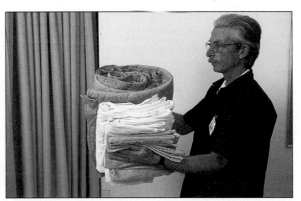 B

Fig. 8-14 Collecting linens. **A,** The arm is placed over the top of the stack of linens. **B,** The stack of linens is turned over onto the arm. Note that linens are held away from the body.

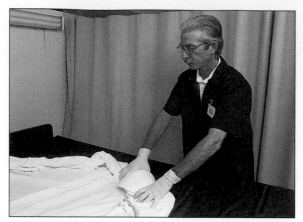

Fig. 8-15 Roll linens away from you when removing them from the bed.

Remove dirty linen one piece one at a time. Roll each piece away from you. The side that touched the person is inside the roll and away from you (Fig. 8-15).

Some linens are reused for the open bed—mattress pad, plastic drawsheet, blanket, and bedspread are reused for the same person. They are not reused if soiled, wet, or wrinkled. *Wet, damp, or soiled linens are changed right away.*

A *cotton drawsheet* is a small sheet placed over the middle of the bottom sheet. It helps keep the mattress and bottom linens clean and dry. A *plastic drawsheet* is waterproof. It is placed between the bottom sheet and cotton drawsheet. It protects the mattress and bottom linens from dampness and soiling. In some centers, it is called a *waterproof drawsheet*.

The cotton drawsheet protects the person from contact with the plastic and absorbs moisture. However, discomfort and skin breakdown may occur. Plastic retains heat. Plastic drawsheets are hard to keep tight and wrinkle-free. Many centers use waterproof pads instead of drawsheets.

Cotton drawsheets are often used without plastic drawsheets. Plastic-covered mattresses cause some persons to perspire heavily. This increases discomfort. A cotton drawsheet reduces heat retention and absorbs moisture. Cotton drawsheets are often used as lift or turning sheets (Chapter 16). When used for this purpose, do not tuck them in at the sides.

The bedmaking procedures that follow include plastic and cotton drawsheets. This is so you learn how to use them. Ask the nurse about their use.

The Closed Bed

A closed bed is made if the person will be out of bed most of the day or after a person is discharged. If the bed is made for a new resident, the bed frame and mattress are cleaned and disinfected before making the bed. A complete linen change is done on the person's bath day.

The Open Bed

To open a closed bed, fold back the top linens. Open beds are made for persons who:

- Arrive at the center by wheelchair
- Are out of bed for a short time

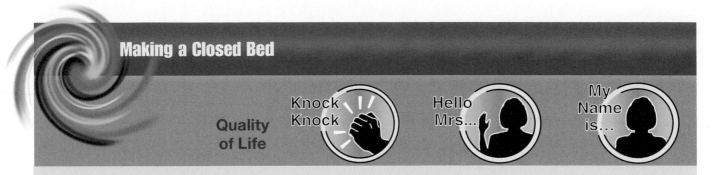

Making a Closed Bed

Quality of Life — Knock Knock — Hello Mrs... — My Name is...

Pre-Procedure

1 Follow *Delegation Guidelines: Making Beds*. See *Safety Alert: Making Beds*.
2 Practice hand hygiene.
3 Collect clean linen:
  - Mattress pad (if needed)
  - Bottom sheet (flat sheet or fitted sheet)
  - Plastic drawsheet or waterproof pad (if needed)
  - Cotton drawsheet (if needed)
  - Top sheet
  - Blanket
  - Bedspread
  - Two pillowcases
  - Bath towel(s)
  - Hand towel
  - Washcloth
  - Bath blanket
  - Gloves
  - Laundry bag
4 Place linen on a clean surface.
5 Raise the bed for body mechanics.

Procedure

6 Put on the gloves.
7 Remove linen. Roll each piece away from you. Place each piece in a laundry bag.
8 Clean the bed frame and mattress if this is part of your job.
9 Remove and discard the gloves. Decontaminate your hands.
10 Move the mattress to the head of the bed.
11 Put the mattress pad on the mattress. It is even with the top of the mattress.
12 Place the bottom sheet on the mattress pad (Fig. 8-16, p. 158):
  a Unfold it lengthwise.
  b Place the center crease in the middle of the bed.
  c Position the lower edge even with the bottom of the mattress.
  d Place the large hem at the top and the small hem at the bottom.
  e Face hem-stitching downward, away from the person.
13 Open the sheet. Fanfold it to the other side of the bed (Fig. 8-17, p. 158).
14 Tuck the top of the sheet under the mattress. The sheet is tight and smooth.
15 Make a mitered corner if using a flat sheet (Fig. 8-18, p. 158).
16 Place the plastic drawsheet on the bed. It is about 14 inches from the top of the mattress. Or put the waterproof pad on the bed.

17 Open the plastic drawsheet. Fanfold it to the other side of the bed.
18 Place a cotton drawsheet over the plastic drawsheet. It covers the entire plastic drawsheet (Fig. 8-19, p. 159).
19 Open the cotton drawsheet. Fanfold it to the other side of the bed.
20 Tuck both drawsheets under the mattress. Or tuck each in separately.
21 Go to the other side of the bed.
22 Miter the top corner of the flat bottom sheet.
23 Pull the bottom sheet tight so there are no wrinkles. Tuck in the sheet.
24 Pull the drawsheets tight so there are no wrinkles. Tuck both in together or separately (Fig. 8-20, p. 159).
25 Go to the other side of the bed.
26 Put the top sheet on the bed:
  a Unfold it lengthwise.
  b Place the center crease in the middle.
  c Place the large hem even with the top of the mattress.
  d Open the sheet. Fanfold it to the other side.
  e Face hem-stitching outward, away from the person.
  f Do not tuck the bottom in yet.
  g Never tuck top linens in on the sides.
27 Place the blanket on the bed:
  a Unfold it so the center crease is in the middle.
  b Put the upper hem about 6 to 8 inches from the top of the mattress.

Continued

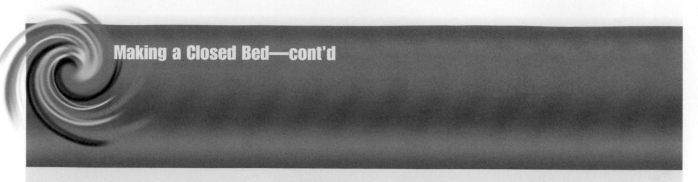

Making a Closed Bed—cont'd

Procedure—cont'd

c　Open the blanket. Fanfold it to the other side.

d　If steps 33 and 34 are not done, turn the top sheet down over the blanket. Hem-stitching is down, away from the person.

28　Place the bedspread on the bed:

a　Unfold it so the center crease is in the middle.

b　Place the upper hem even with the top of the mattress.

c　Open and fanfold the spread to the other side.

d　Make sure the spread facing the door is even. It covers all top linens.

29　Tuck in top linens together at the foot of the bed. They should be smooth and tight. Make a mitered corner.

30　Go to the other side.

31　Straighten all top linen. Work from the head of the bed to the foot.

32　Tuck in the top linens together at the foot of the bed. Make a mitered corner.

33　Turn the top hem of the spread under the blanket to make a cuff (Fig. 8-21).

34　Turn the top sheet down over the spread. Hem-stitching is down. (Steps 33 and 34 are not done in some centers. The spread covers the pillow. If so, tuck the spread under the pillow.)

35　Put the pillowcase on the pillow as in Figure 8-22 or Figure 8-23, p. 162. Fold extra material under the pillow at the seam end of the pillow-case.

36　Place the pillow on the bed. The open end of the pillowcase is away from the door. The seam is toward the head of the bed.

Post-Procedure

37　Attach the signal light to the bed.

38　Lower the bed to its lowest position. Lock the bed wheels.

39　Put towels, washcloth, and bath blanket in the bedside stand.

40　Complete a safety check of the room. (See inside of front book cover.)

41　Follow center policy for dirty linen.

42　Decontaminate your hands.

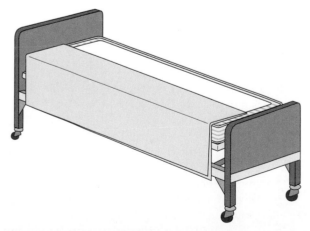

Fig. 8-16 The bottom sheet is on the bed with the center crease in the middle. The lower edge of the sheet is even with the bottom of the mattress.

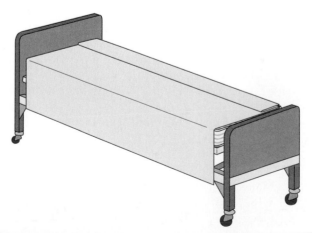

Fig. 8-17 The bottom sheet is fanfolded to the other side of the bed.

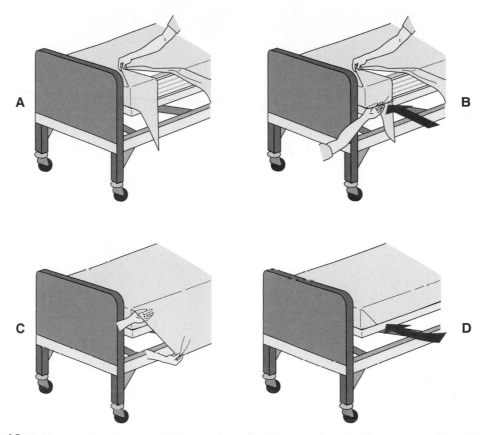

Fig. 8-18 Making a mitered corner. **A,** The bottom sheet is tucked under the mattress. The side of the sheet is raised onto the mattress. **B,** The remaining portion of the sheet is tucked under the mattress. **C,** The raised portion of the sheet is brought off the mattress. **D,** The entire side of the sheet is tucked under the mattress.

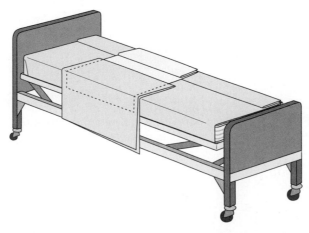

Fig. 8-19 A cotton drawsheet is over the plastic drawsheet. The cotton drawsheet completely covers the plastic drawsheet.

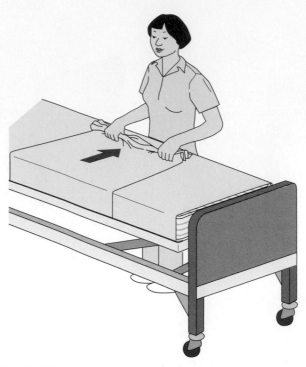

Fig. 8-20 The drawsheet is pulled tight to remove wrinkles.

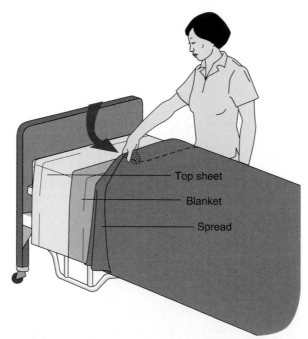

Top sheet

Blanket

Spread

Fig. 8-21 The top hem of the bedspread is turned under the top hem of the blanket to make a cuff.

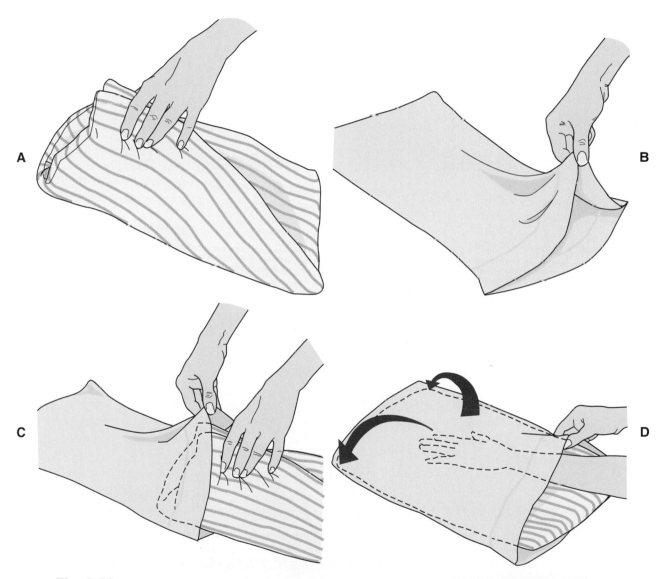

Fig. 8-22 Putting a pillowcase on a pillow. **A,** Open the pillowcase so it is flat on the bed. Grasp the corners of the pillow at the seam end and form a "V" with the pillow. **B,** The pillowcase is flat on the bed. The pillowcase is opened with the free hand. **C,** The "V" end of the pillow is guided into the pillowcase. **D,** The "V" end of the pillow falls into the corners of the pillowcase.

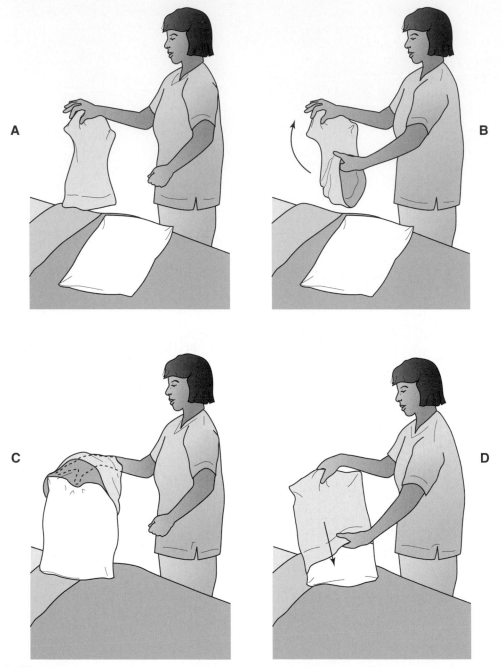

Fig. 8-23 Putting a pillowcase on the pillow. **A,** Grasp the closed end of the pillowcase. **B,** Using your other hand, gather up the pillowcase. The pillowcase should cover your hand holding the closed end. **C,** Grasp the pillow with the hand covered by the pillowcase. **D,** Pull the pillowcase down over the pillow with your other hand.

The Occupied Bed

An occupied bed is made when a person stays in bed. When making an occupied bed, keep the person in good alignment. You must know about restrictions or limits in the person's movement or position.

Explain each procedure step to the person before it is done. This is important even if the person cannot respond to you or is in a coma.

Making an Occupied Bed

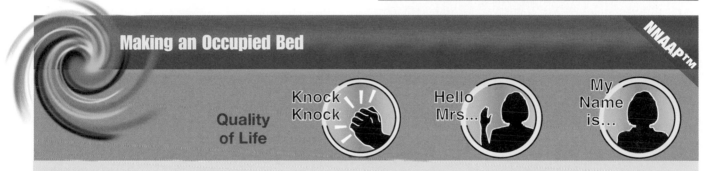

Quality of Life — Knock Knock — Hello Mrs... — My Name is... — NNAAP™

Pre-Procedure

1 Follow *Delegation Guidelines: Making Beds*. See *Safety Alerts: Making Beds; The Occupied Bed.*
2 Explain the procedure to the person.
3 Practice hand hygiene.
4 Collect the following:
   • Gloves
   • Laundry bag
   • Clean linen (see procedure: *Making a Closed Bed*, p. 157)
5 Place linen on a clean surface.
6 Identify the person. Check the ID bracelet against the assignment sheet. Call the person by name.
7 Provide for privacy.
8 Remove the signal light.
9 Raise the bed for body mechanics. Bed rails are up if used.
10 Lower the head of the bed. It is as flat as possible.

Procedure

11 Lower the bed rail near you.
12 Put on gloves.
13 Loosen top linens at the foot of the bed.
14 Remove the bedspread and then the blanket (Fig. 8-24, p. 165). Place each over the chair.
15 Cover the person with a bath blanket. It provides warmth and privacy:
   a Unfold a bath blanket over the top sheet.
   b Ask the person to hold onto the bath blanket. If he or she cannot, tuck the top part under the person's shoulders.
   c Grasp the top sheet under the bath blanket at the shoulders. Bring the sheet down to the foot of the bed. Remove the sheet from under the blanket (Fig. 8-25, p. 165).
16 Move the mattress to the head of the bed.
17 Position the person on the side of the bed away from you. Adjust the pillow for comfort.
18 Loosen bottom linens from the head to the foot of the bed.
19 Fanfold bottom linens one at a time toward the person. Start with the cotton drawsheet (Fig. 8-26, p. 166). If reusing the mattress pad, do not fanfold it.
20 Place a clean mattress pad on the bed. Unfold it lengthwise. The center crease is in the middle. Fanfold the top part toward the person. If reusing the mattress pad, straighten and smooth any wrinkles.
21 Place the bottom sheet on the mattress pad. Hem-stitching is away from the person. Unfold the sheet so the crease is in the middle. The small hem is even with the bottom of the mattress. Fanfold the top part toward the person.

Continued

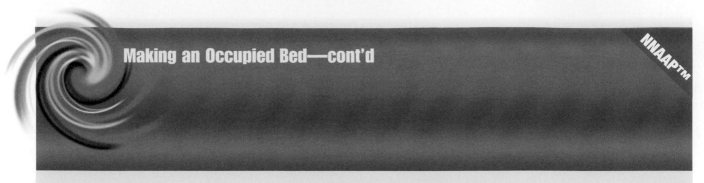

Making an Occupied Bed—cont'd

Procedure—cont'd

22 Make a mitered corner at the head of the bed. Tuck the sheet under the mattress from the head to the foot.

23 Pull the plastic drawsheet toward you over the bottom sheet. Tuck excess material under the mattress. Do the following for a clean plastic drawsheet (Fig. 8-27, p. 166):
   a Place the plastic drawsheet on the bed. It is about 14 inches from the mattress top.
   b Fanfold the top part toward the person.
   c Tuck in the excess fabric.

24 Place the cotton drawsheet over the plastic drawsheet. It covers the entire plastic drawsheet. Fanfold the top part toward the person. Tuck in excess fabric.

25 Raise the bed rail if used. Go to the other side, and lower the bed rail.

26 Explain to the person that he or she will roll over a bump. Assure the person that he or she will not fall.

27 Help the person turn to the other side. Adjust the pillow for comfort.

28 Loosen bottom linens. Remove one piece at a time. Place each piece in the laundry bag.

29 Remove and discard the gloves. Decontaminate your hands.

30 Straighten and smooth the mattress pad.

31 Pull the clean bottom sheet toward you. Make a mitered corner at the top. Tuck the sheet under the mattress from the head to the foot of the bed.

32 Pull the drawsheets tightly toward you. Tuck both under together or separately.

33 Position the person supine in the center of the bed. Adjust the pillow for comfort.

34 Put the top sheet on the bed. Unfold it lengthwise. The crease is in the middle. The large hem is even with the top of the mattress. Hemstitching is on the outside.

35 Ask the person to hold onto the top sheet so you can remove the bath blanket. Or tuck the top sheet under the person's shoulders. Remove the bath blanket.

36 Place the blanket on the bed. Unfold it so the crease is in the middle and it covers the person. The upper hem is 6 to 8 inches from the top of the mattress.

37 Place the bedspread on the bed. Unfold it so the center crease is in the middle and it covers the person. The top hem is even with the mattress top.

38 Turn the top hem of the spread under the blanket to make a cuff.

39 Bring the top sheet down over the spread to form a cuff.

40 Go to the foot of the bed.

41 Make a toe pleat. Make a 2-inch pleat across the foot of the bed. The pleat is about 6 to 8 inches from the foot of the bed.

42 Lift the mattress corner with one arm. Tuck all top linens under the mattress together. Make a mitered corner.

43 Raise the bed rail if used. Go to the other side, and lower the bed rail if used.

44 Straighten and smooth top linens.

45 Tuck the top linens under the bottom of the mattress. Make a mitered corner.

46 Change the pillowcase(s).

Post-Procedure

47 Place the signal light within reach.

48 Raise or lower bed rails. Follow the care plan.

49 Raise the head of the bed to a level appropriate for the person. Provide for comfort.

50 Lower the bed to its lowest position. Lock the bed wheels.

51 Put towels, washcloth, and bath blanket in the bedside stand.

52 Unscreen the person.

53 Complete a safety check of the room. (See inside of front book cover.)

54 Follow center policy for dirty linen.

55 Decontaminate your hands.

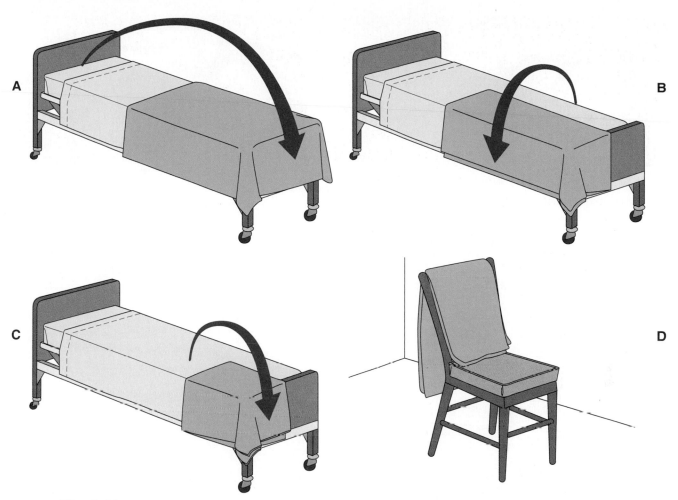

Fig. 8-24 Folding linen for reuse. **A,** The top edge of the blanket is folded down to the bottom edge. **B,** The blanket is folded from the far side of the bed to the near side. **C**, The top edge of the blanket is folded down to the bottom edge again. **D,** The folded blanket is placed over the back of a straight chair.

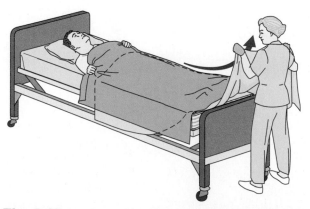

Fig. 8-25 The person holds onto the bath blanket. The top sheet is removed from under the bath blanket.

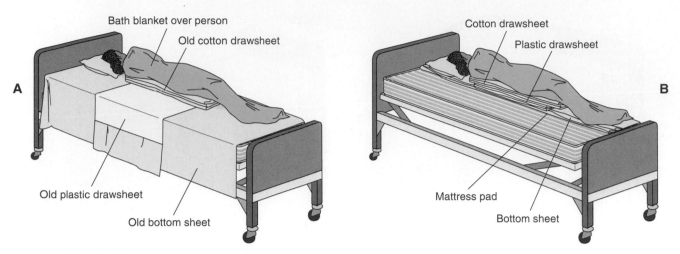

Fig. 8-26 Occupied bed. **A,** The cotton drawsheet is fanfolded and tucked under the person. **B,** All bottom linens are tucked under the person.

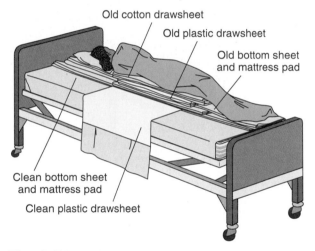

Fig. 8-27 A clean bottom sheet and plastic drawsheet are on the bed with both fanfolded and tucked under the person.

The Surgical Bed

Surgical beds are made for persons who arrive at the center by ambulance. They also are used for persons who are taken by stretcher to treatment or therapy areas. Surgical beds are made when portable tubs are used. To make a surgical bed:

- Do not tuck the top linens under the mattress.
- Fold all top linens at the foot of the bed back onto the bed. The fold is even with the bottom edge of the mattress (Fig. 8-28, A).
- Fanfold linen lengthwise to the side of the bed farthest from the door (Fig. 8-28, B).
- Leave the bed in its highest position.
- Leave both bed rails down.

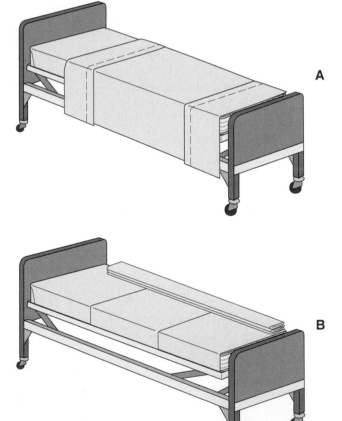

Fig. 8-28 Surgical bed. **A,** The bottom of the top linens is folded back onto the bed. The fold is even with the bottom edge of the mattress. **B,** Top linens are fanfolded lengthwise to the opposite side of the bed.

Review Questions

Circle the **BEST** answer.

1. Nursing center residents need a temperature range between
   a 60° F and 66° F   c 71° F and 81° F
   b 68° F and 74° F   d 80° F and 86° F

2. Which does *not* protect a person from drafts?
   a Wearing enough clothing
   b Being covered with enough blankets
   c Being moved out of a drafty area
   d Sitting by the air conditioner

3. To prevent odors, you need to do the following *except*
   a Check incontinent persons often
   b Dispose of incontinence and ostomy products at the end of your shift
   c Keep laundry containers closed
   d Clean persons who are wet or soiled

4. Beds are raised horizontally to
   a Prevent bending and reaching when giving care
   b Let the person get in and out of bed with ease
   c Raise the head of the bed
   d Lock the bed in position

5. The head of the bed is raised 30 degrees. This is called
   a Fowler's position
   b Semi-Fowler's position
   c Trendelenburg's position
   d Reverse Trendelenburg's position

6. The bedpan is stored
   a In the closet
   b In the bedside stand
   c On the overbed table
   d Under the bed

7. To maintain a person's unit, you can do the following *except*
   a Save items that do not look important
   b Provide enough tissues and toilet paper
   c Place personal items as you choose
   d Straighten bed linens as needed

8. Which requires a linen change?
   a The resident will have visitors
   b Wet linen
   c Wrinkled linen
   d Crumbs in the bed

9. When handling linens,
   a Put dirty linens on the floor
   b Hold linens away from your body and uniform
   c Shake linens to remove crumbs
   d Take extra linen to another person's room

10. A person is out of the room most of the day. What type of bed should you make?
    a A closed bed   c An occupied bed
    b An open bed   d A surgical bed

11. A complete linen change is done when
    a The bottom linens are wet or soiled
    b The bed is made for a new person
    c The person will transfer from a stretcher to the bed
    d Linens are loose or wrinkled

12. You are using a plastic drawsheet. Which is *true*?
    a A cotton drawsheet must completely cover the plastic drawsheet.
    b Waterproof bed protectors are needed.
    c The person's consent is needed.
    d The plastic is in contact with the person's skin.

Circle **T** if the statement is true or **F** if the statement is false.

13. **T F**   Soft, dim lighting is relaxing.
14. **T F**   The privacy curtain prevents others from hearing conversations.
15. **T F**   The overbed table and bedside stand should be within the person's reach.
16. **T F**   You should explain the cause of strange noises.
17. **T F**   Residents must be able to reach items in their closets.

Answers to these questions are on p. 389.

CHAPTER 9

Observing, Reporting, and Recording

Objectives

- Define the key terms listed in this chapter
- Explain the difference between objective and subjective data
- Identify the observations that you need to report to the nurse
- List the basic rules for recording
- Explain the purpose, parts, and information found in the medical record
- Describe the legal and ethical aspects of medical records
- Explain how computers are used in health care
- Explain how to protect the right to privacy when using computers
- Use the 24-hour clock, medical terminology, and abbreviations

Key Terms

objective data Information that is seen, heard, felt, or smelled; signs
observation Using the senses of sight, hearing, touch, and smell to collect information
recording The written account of care and observations; charting
reporting The oral account of care and observations

signs Objective data
subjective data Things a person tells you about that you cannot observe through your senses; symptoms
symptoms Subjective data

You make many observations when caring for residents. The nurse needs this information to plan and evaluate the person's care. You communicate information to the nurse through reporting and recording.

OBSERVING

Observation is using the senses of sight, hearing, touch, and smell to collect information:

- You *see* how the person lies, sits, or walks. You see flushed or pale skin. You see red and swollen body areas.
- You *listen* to the person breathe, talk, and cough. You use a stethoscope to listen to the heartbeat and to measure blood pressure.
- Through *touch*, you feel if the skin is hot or cold, or moist or dry. You use touch to take the person's pulse.
- *Smell* is used to detect body, wound, and breath odors. You also smell odors from urine and bowel movements.

Objective data (**signs**) are seen, heard, felt, or smelled. You can feel a pulse. You can see urine. You cannot feel or see the person's pain, fear, or nausea. **Subjective data** (**symptoms**) are things a person tells you about that you cannot observe through your senses.

Box 9-1 on p. 170 lists the basic observations you need to make and report to the nurse. Make notes of your observations. Use them when reporting and recording observations. Carry a note pad and pen in your pocket to note observations as you make them.

REPORTING AND RECORDING

The health team communicates by reporting and recording. Both are accounts of what was done for and observed about the person. **Reporting** is the oral account of care and observations. **Recording** (*charting*) is the written account of care and observations.

Reporting

You report care and observations to the nurse. Follow these rules:

- Be prompt, thorough, and accurate.
- Give the person's name and room and bed number.
- Give the time your observations were made or the care was given.
- Report only what you observed or did yourself.
- Give reports as often as the person's condition requires. Or give them as often as the nurse asks you to.
- Report any changes from normal or changes in the person's condition. Report these changes at once.
- Use your written notes to give a specific, concise, and clear report (Fig. 9-1, p. 171).

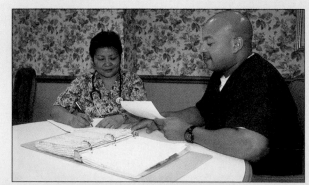

Fig. 9-1 The nursing assistant uses notes when reporting to the nurse.

BOX 9-1   Basic Observations

Ability to Respond

- Is the person easy or hard to arouse?
- Can the person give his or her name, the time, and location when asked?
- Does the person identify others correctly?
- Does the person answer questions correctly?
- Does the person speak clearly?
- Are instructions followed correctly?
- Is the person calm, restless, or excited?
- Is the person conversing, quiet, or talking a lot?

Movement

- Can the person squeeze your fingers with each hand?
- Can the person move arms and legs?
- Are the person's movements shaky or jerky?
- Does the person complain of stiff or painful joints?

Pain or Discomfort

- Where is the pain? (Ask the person to point to the pain.)
- Does the pain go anywhere else?
- When did the pain begin?
- What was the person doing when the pain began?
- How long does the pain last?
- How does the person describe the pain?
  - —Sharp
  - —Severe
  - —Knifelike
  - —Dull
  - —Burning
  - —Aching
  - —Comes and goes
  - —Depends on position
- How severe is the pain? Ask the person to rate the pain on a scale of 1 to 10 (Chapter 7).
- Was medication given?
- Did medication help relieve the pain? Is pain still present?
- Is the person able to sleep and rest?
- What is the position of comfort?

Skin

- Is the skin pale or flushed?
- Is the skin cool, warm, or hot?
- Is the skin moist or dry?
- What color are the lips and nails?
- Is the skin intact? Are there broken areas? If so, where?
- Are sores or reddened areas present? If yes, where?
- Are bruises present? Where are they?
- Does the person complain of itching? If yes, where?

Eyes, Ears, Nose, and Mouth

- Is there drainage from the eyes? What color is the drainage?
- Are the eyelids closed?
- Are the eyes reddened?
- Does the person complain of spots, flashes, or blurring?
- Is the person sensitive to bright lights?
- Is there drainage from the ears? What color is the drainage?
- Can the person hear? Is repeating necessary? Are questions answered appropriately?
- Is there drainage from the nose? What color is the drainage?
- Can the person breathe through the nose?
- Is there breath odor?
- Does the person complain of a bad taste in the mouth?
- Does the person complain of painful gums or teeth?

Respirations

- Do both sides of the person's chest rise and fall with respirations?
- Is breathing noisy?
- Does the person complain of difficulty breathing?
- What is the amount and color of sputum?
- What is the frequency of the person's cough? Is it dry or productive?

Bowels and Bladder

- Is the abdomen firm or soft?
- Does the person complain of gas?
- What are the amount, color, and consistency of bowel movements?
- What is the frequency of bowel movements?
- Can the person control bowel movements?
- Does the person have pain or difficulty urinating?
- What is the amount of urine?
- What is the color of urine?
- Is urine clear? Are there particles in the urine?
- Does urine have a foul smell?
- Can the person control the passage of urine?
- What is the frequency of urination?

Appetite

- Does the person like the diet?
- How much of the meal is eaten?
- What are the person's food preferences?
- Can the person chew food?
- How much liquid was taken?
- What are the person's liquid preferences?
- How often does the person drink liquids?
- Can the person swallow food and fluids?
- Does the person complain of nausea?
- What is the amount and color of material vomited?
- Does the person have hiccups?
- Is the person belching?
- Does the person cough when swallowing?

Activities of Daily Living

- Can the person perform personal care without help?
  - —Bathing?
  - —Brushing teeth?
  - —Combing and brushing hair?
  - —Shaving?
- Which does the person use: toilet, commode, bedpan, or urinal?
- Does the person feed himself or herself?
- Can the person walk?
- What amount and kind of help is needed?

BOX 9-2	**Rules for Recording**

- Always use ink. Use the ink color required by the center.
- Include the date and the time for every recording. Use conventional time (AM or PM) or 24-hour clock time according to center policy (p. 172).
- Make sure writing is readable and neat.
- Use only center-approved abbreviations (p. 177).
- Use correct spelling, grammar, and punctuation.
- Never erase errors or use correction fluid. Cross out the incorrect part, and write "error" or "mistaken entry" over it. Sign your initials to the error or mistaken entry. Then rewrite the part. Follow center policy for correcting errors.
- Sign all entries with your name and title as required by center policy.
- Do not skip lines. Draw a line through the blank space of a partially completed line or to the end of a page. This prevents others from recording in a space with your signature.
- Make sure each form is stamped with the person's name and other identifying information.

- Record only what you observed and did yourself.
- Never chart a procedure or treatment until after it is completed.
- Be accurate, concise, and factual. Do not record judgments or interpretations.
- Record in a logical and sequential manner.
- Be descriptive. Avoid terms with more than one meaning.
- Use the person's exact words whenever possible. Use quotation marks to show that the statement is a direct quote.
- Chart any changes from normal or changes in the person's condition. Also chart that you informed the nurse (include the nurse's name), what you told the nurse, and the time you made the report.
- Do not omit information.
- Record safety measures such as placing the signal light within reach or reminding someone not to get out of bed. This helps protect you if the person falls.

End-of-Shift Report.   The nurse gives a report at the end of the shift. This is called the *end-of-shift report*. It is given to the nursing team of the oncoming shift. Information is shared about the care given and the care to be given. Information about the person's condition is included.

Some centers have all nursing team members hear the end-of-shift report as they come on duty. Others have nursing assistants perform routine tasks while nurses hear the report. After report, nurses share important information with the nursing assistants.

Recording

Recording is done on the person's medical record. The *medical record (chart)* is a written account of a person's condition and response to treatment and care. The record is permanent and a legal document. It can be used as evidence in a court of law of the person's problems, treatment, and care.

Centers have policies about medical records and who can access them. Policies address who records, when to record, abbreviations, correcting errors, ink color, and signing entries.

Professional staff involved in a person's care can look at the chart. If you have access, you must keep the information confidential. This is an ethical and legal responsibility. If you are not involved in the person's care, you have no right to review that person's chart. To do so is an invasion of privacy.

The record has many forms. They are organized into sections for easy use. Each page is stamped with the person's name, room number, and other identifying information. This helps prevent errors and improper placement of records.

When recording on the person's chart, you must communicate clearly and thoroughly. Follow the rules in Box 9-2. The charting sample in Figure 9-2 on p. 172 shows how the rules apply. Anyone who reads your charting should know:

- What you observed
- What you did
- The person's response

Recording Time.   The 24-hour clock (military time or international time) has four digits (Fig. 9-3, p. 172). The first two digits are for the hour: 0100 = 1:00 AM; 1300 = 1:00 PM. The last two digits are for minutes: 0110 = 1:10 AM. The AM and PM abbreviations are not used.

As Figure 9-3 shows, the hour is the same for morning times, but AM is not used. For PM times, add 12 to the clock time. If it is 2:00 PM, add 12 and 2 for 1400. For 8:35 PM, add 12 and 835 for 2035.

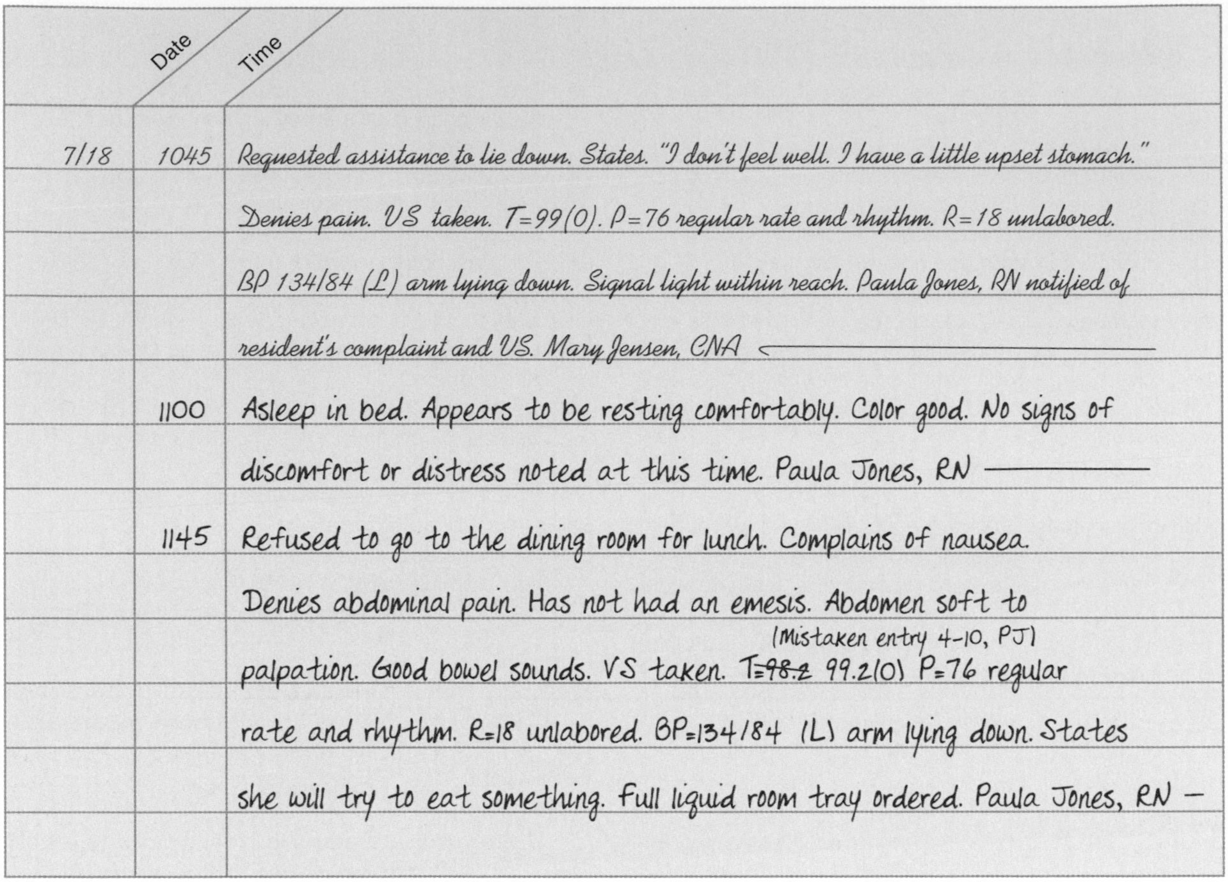

	Date	Time	
7/18	1045		Requested assistance to lie down. States. "I don't feel well. I have a little upset stomach."
			Denies pain. VS taken. T=99 (O). P=76 regular rate and rhythm. R=18 unlabored.
			BP 134/84 (L) arm lying down. Signal light within reach. Paula Jones, RN notified of
			resident's complaint and VS. Mary Jensen, CNA
	1100		Asleep in bed. Appears to be resting comfortably. Color good. No signs of
			discomfort or distress noted at this time. Paula Jones, RN
	1145		Refused to go to the dining room for lunch. Complains of nausea.
			Denies abdominal pain. Has not had an emesis. Abdomen soft to
			palpation. Good bowel sounds. VS taken. T=~~98.2~~ 99.2(O) P=76 regular (Mistaken entry 4-10, PJ)
			rate and rhythm. R=18 unlabored. BP=134/84 (L) arm lying down. States
			she will try to eat something. Full liquid room tray ordered. Paula Jones, RN —

Fig. 9-2 Charting sample.

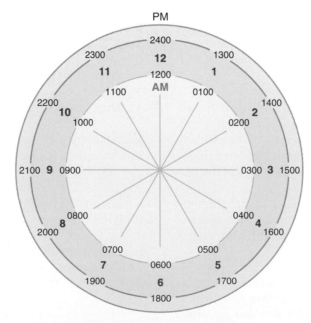

Fig. 9-3 The 24-hour clock.

Date	Time	Weight	T	P	R	BP				Signatures
10/19	0700	126	98.4	72	20	142/84				Mary Smith CNA
10/26	0715	125	98.6	72	18	140/84				Jane Doe LPN
11/2	0715	126	98.6	70	18	144/82				Mary Smith CNA

Fig. 9-4 Vital signs and daily weight flow sheet. (Modified from Evangelical Lutheran Good Samaritan Society, Sioux Falls, S.D.)

Medical Record Forms.   The following parts of the medical record relate to your work:

- *Admission sheet*—is completed when the person is admitted to the center. It has identifying information about the person. Use it to fill out forms that require the same information.
- *Progress notes*—are written accounts of observations, the care given, and the person's response (see Fig. 9-2).

- *Flow sheets*—are used to record frequent measurements or observations. Flow sheets are used for vital signs and daily weight (Fig. 9-4). The activities-of-daily-living flow sheet is used to record the person's everyday activities (Chapter 2). They also are used for recording intake and output (Chapter 7).

Using Computers. Computer systems collect, send, record, and store information. It is retrieved when needed. Centers can store charts and care plans on computers. Entering information on a computer is easier and faster than charting.

Computers are easy to use. They contain vast amounts of information. Therefore the right to privacy must be protected. Only certain staff members use the computer. Each has a code (password) to access computer files. If allowed access, you will learn how to use the center's system. You must follow the center's policy. Also follow the rules in Box 9-3 and the ethical and legal rules about privacy, confidentiality, and defamation (Chapter 1).

MEDICAL TERMINOLOGY AND ABBREVIATIONS

Medical terminology and abbreviations are used when reporting and recording. Like all words, medical terms are made up of parts or word elements. They are combined to form medical terms. A term is translated by separating the word into its elements. Word elements are prefixes, roots, and suffixes (Box 9-4). Most are from Greek or Latin.

BOX 9-3   Using the Center's Computer

- Do not tell anyone your password. If someone has your password, he or she can access the computer under your name. It will be hard to prove that someone else made the entries.
- Change your password often.
- Do not use another person's password.
- Follow the rules for recording (see Box 9-2).
- Enter information carefully. Double-check your entries.
- Prevent others from seeing what is on the screen. Do not leave the computer unattended.
- Log off after making an entry.
- Position equipment so the screen cannot be seen in the hallway.
- Do not leave printouts where others can read them or pick them up.
- Destroy or shred computer printouts according to center policy.
- Send e-mail and messages only to those needing the information.
- Do not use e-mail for information or messages that require immediate reporting. Give the report in person. (The person may not read e-mail in a timely manner.)

- Do not use e-mail or messages to report confidential information. This includes addresses, phone numbers, and Social Security numbers. The computer system may not be secure.
- Do not use the center's computer to:
  —Send personal e-mail or messages
  —Send or receive e-mail or messages that are offensive, illegal, or sexual
  —Send or receive e-mail or messages for illegal activities, jokes, politics, gambling (including football and other pools), chain letters, advertising, or other non-work activities
  —Post information, opinions, or comments on Internet message boards
  —Take part in Internet discussion groups
  —Upload, download, or transmit materials containing a copyright, trademark, or patent
- Remember that any communication may be read or heard by someone other than the intended person.
- Remember that deleted communications can be retrieved by authorized personnel.
- Remember that the center has the right to monitor your computer use. This includes Internet use.
- Do not open another person's e-mail or messages.

Prefixes, Roots, and Suffixes

A *prefix* is a word element placed before a root. It changes the meaning of the word. The prefix *olig* (scant, small amount) is placed before the word *uria* (urine) to make *oliguria*. It means a scant amount of urine. Prefixes are always combined with other word elements. They are never used alone.

The *root* contains the word's basic meaning. It is combined with another root, with prefixes, and with suffixes. A vowel (an *o* or an *i*) is added between two roots or between a root and a suffix. The vowel makes pronunciation easier.

A *suffix* is placed after a root. It changes the meaning of a word. Suffixes are not used alone. When translating medical terms, begin with the suffix. For example, *nephritis* means inflammation of the kidney. It was formed by combining *nephro* (kidney) and *itis* (inflammation).

Medical terms are formed by combining word elements. Prefixes always come before roots. Suffixes always come after roots. A root can be combined with prefixes, roots, or suffixes. Combining a prefix, root, and suffix is another way to form medical terms. *Endocarditis* has the prefix *endo* (inner), the root *card* (heart), and the suffix *itis* (inflammation). *Endocarditis* means inflammation of the inner part of the heart.

BOX 9-4	Medical Terminology		
Prefix	**Meaning**	**Prefix**	**Meaning**
a-, an-	without, not, lack of	leuk-	white
ab-	away from	macro-	large
ad-	to, toward, near	mal-	bad, illness, disease
ante-	before, forward, in front of	meg-	large
anti-	against	micro-	small
auto-	self	mono-	one, single
bi-	double, two, twice	neo-	new
brady-	slow	non-	not
circum-	around	olig-	small, scant
contra-	against, opposite	para-	beside, beyond, after
de-	down, from	per-	by, through
dia-	across, through, apart	peri-	around
dis-	apart, free from	poly-	many, much
dys-	bad, difficult, abnormal	post-	after, behind
ecto-	outer, outside	pre-	before, in front of, prior to
en-	in, into, within	pro-	before, in front of
endo-	inner, inside	re-	again, backward
epi-	over, on, upon	retro-	backward, behind
eryth-	red	semi-	half
eu-	normal, good, well, healthy	sub-	under, beneath
ex-	out, out of, from, away from	super-	above, over, excess
hemi-	half	supra-	above, over
hyper-	excessive, too much, high	tachy-	fast, rapid
hypo-	under, decreased, less than normal	trans-	across
in-	in, into, within, not	uni-	one
infra-	within		
inter-	between		
intro-, intra-	into, within		

Continued

BOX 9-4 Medical Terminology—cont'd

Root (combining vowel)	Meaning	Root (combining vowel)	Meaning
		necro	death
abdomin (o)	abdomen	nephr (o)	kidney
aden (o)	gland	neur (o)	nerve
adren (o)	adrenal gland	ocul (o)	eye
angi (o)	vessel	oophor (o)	ovary
arterio	artery	ophthalm (o)	eye
arthr (o)	joint	orth (o)	straight, normal, correct
broncho	bronchus, bronchi	oste (o)	bone
card, cardi (o)	heart	ot (o)	ear
cephal (o)	head	ped (o)	child, foot
chole, chol(o)	bile	pharyng (o)	pharynx
chondr (o)	cartilage	phleb (o)	vein
colo	colon, large intestine	pnea	breathing, respiration
cost (o)	rib	**Root (combining vowel)**	**Meaning**
crani (o)	skull	pneum (o)	lung, air, gas
cyan (o)	blue	proct (o)	rectum
cyst (o)	bladder, cyst	psych (o)	mind
cyt (o)	cell	pulmo	lung
dent (o)	tooth	py (o)	pus
derma	skin	rect (o)	rectum
duoden (o)	duodenum	rhin (o)	nose
encephal (o)	brain	salping (o)	eustachian tube, uterine tube
enter (o)	intestines		
fibr (o)	fiber, fibrous	splen (o)	spleen
gastr (o)	stomach	sten (o)	narrow, constriction
gloss (o)	tongue	stern (o)	sternum
gluc (o)	sweetness, glucose	stomat (o)	mouth
glyc (o)	sugar	therm (o)	heat
gyn, gyne, gyneco	woman	thoraco	chest
hem, hema, hemo, hemat (o)	blood	thromb (o)	clot, thrombus
		thyr (o)	thyroid
hepat (o)	liver	toxic (o)	poison, poisonous
hydr (o)	water	toxo	poison
hyster (o)	uterus	trache (o)	trachea
ile (o), ili (o)	ileum	urethr (o)	urethra
laparo	abdomen, loin, or flank	urin (o)	urine
laryng (o)	larynx	uro	urine, urinary tract, urination
lith (o)	stone		
mamm (o)	breast, mammary gland	uter (o)	uterus
mast (o)	mammary gland, breast	vas (o)	blood vessel, vas deferens
meno	menstruation		
my (o)	muscle	ven (o)	vein
myel (o)	spinal cord, bone marrow	vertebr (o)	spine, vertebrae

BOX 9-4	Medical Terminology—cont'd		
Suffix	**Meaning**	**Suffix**	**Meaning**
-algia	pain	-oma	tumor
-asis	condition, usually abnormal	-osis	condition
-cele	hernia, herniation, pouching	-pathy	disease
-centesis	puncture and aspiration of	-penia	lack, deficiency
-cyte	cell	-phagia	to eat or consume; swallowing
-ectasis	dilation, stretching	-phasia	speaking
-ectomy	excision, removal of	-phobia	an exaggerated fear
-emia	blood condition	-plasty	surgical repair or reshaping
-genesis	development, production, creation	-plegia	paralysis
		-ptosis	falling, sagging, dropping, down
-genic	producing, causing	-rrhage, -rrhagia	excessive flow
-gram	record	-rrhaphy	stitching, suturing
-graph	a diagram, a recording instrument	-rrhea	profuse flow, discharge
		-scope	examination instrument
-graphy	making a recording	-scopy	examination using a scope
-iasis	condition of	-stasis	maintenance, maintaining a constant level
-ism	a condition		
-itis	inflammation	-stomy, -ostomy	creation of an opening
-logy	the study of	-tomy, -otomy	incision, cutting into
-lysis	destruction of, decomposition	-uria	condition of the urine
-megaly	enlargement		
-meter	measuring instrument		
-metry	measurement		

Directional Terms

Certain terms describe the position of one body part in relation to another. These terms give the direction of the body part when a person is standing and facing forward (Fig. 9-5):

- *Anterior (ventral)*—at or toward the front of the body or body part
- *Distal*—the part farthest from the center or from the point of attachment
- *Lateral*—at the side of the body or body part
- *Medial*—at or near the middle or midline of the body or body part
- *Posterior (dorsal)*—at or toward the back of the body or body part
- *Proximal*—the part nearest to the center or to the point of origin

Abbreviations

Abbreviations are shortened forms of words or phrases. They save time and space when recording. Each center has a list of accepted abbreviations. Obtain the list when you are hired. Use only those accepted by the center. If you are unsure if an abbreviation is acceptable, write the term out in full. This ensures accurate communication.

Common abbreviations are on the inside of the back book cover for easy use.

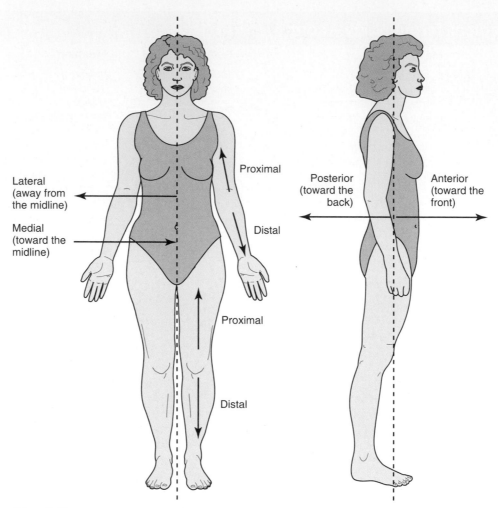

Fig. 9-5 Directional terms describe the position of one body part in relation to another.

Review Questions

Circle the **BEST** answer.

1 Which is a symptom?
   a Redness   c Pain
   b Vomiting   d Pulse rate of 78

2 Which is a sign?
   a Nausea   c Dizziness
   b Headache   d Dry skin

3 When recording, you do the following *except*
   a Use ink
   b Include the date and time
   c Erase errors
   d Sign all entries with your name and title

4 These statements are about recording. Which is *false?*
   a Use the person's exact words when possible.
   b Record only what you did and observed.
   c Sign your initials to a mistaken entry.
   d Chart a procedure before completing it.

5 In the evening the clock shows 9:26. In 24-hour clock time this is
   a 9:26 PM   c 0926
   b 926   d 2126

6 These statements are about medical records. Which is *false?*
   a The record is used to communicate information about the person.
   b The record is a written account of the person's illness and response to treatment.
   c The record can be used as evidence of the care given.
   d Anyone working in the center can read the medical record.

7 A person is weighed daily. The measurement is recorded on the
   a Admission sheet
   b Graphic sheet
   c Flow sheet
   d Progress notes

8 These statements are about using computers. Which is *false?*
   a Computers are used to collect, send, record, and store information.
   b The person's privacy must be protected.
   c You should e-mail confidential information.
   d Employees each have different passwords.

9 Which is *not* a word element used in medical terms?
   a Prefix
   b Suffix
   c Root
   d Abbreviation

10 *Distal* means
   a The part nearest to the center or point of origin
   b Relating to or located at or near the middle or the midline of the body or body part
   c The part farthest from the center or point of attachment
   d Relating to or located at the side of the body or body part

Answers to these questions are on p. 389.

CHAPTER 10

The Dying Person

Objectives

- Define the key terms listed in this chapter
- Explain how religion, culture, and age affect attitudes about death
- Describe the five stages of dying
- Explain how to meet the needs of the dying person and family
- Explain how people can legally express their end-of-life wishes
- Identify the signs of approaching death and the signs of death
- Perform the procedure described in this chapter

postmortem After (*post*) death (*mortem*)
rigor mortis The stiffness or rigidity (*rigor*) of skeletal muscles that occurs after death (*mortis*)

terminal illness An illness or injury for which there is no reasonable expectation of recovery

---

Some deaths are sudden; others are expected. Many illnesses and diseases have no cure. After some injuries, the body cannot function. The disease or injury ends in death. An illness or injury for which there is no reasonable expectation of recovery is a **terminal illness.** A common terminal illness, cancer is the second leading cause of death in the United States (Box 10-1, p. 182).

Some people need hospice care (Chapter 1). Hospice care focuses on physical, emotional, social, and spiritual needs. Cure and life-saving measures are not concerns. Pain relief and comfort are stressed. The goal is to improve the dying person's quality of life.

You will help meet the dying person's needs. Therefore you must understand the dying process. Then you can approach the dying person with caring, kindness, and respect.

ATTITUDES ABOUT DEATH

Many people fear death. Some look forward to and accept death. Attitudes often change as a person grows older and with changing circumstances.

Culture and Religion

Death practices and attitudes differ among cultures (see *Caring About Culture: Death Rites*). In some cultures, the family cares for the dying person at home. Some families prepare the body for burial.

Religion affects attitudes about death. Some believe the afterlife is free of suffering and hardship. They also believe in reunion with loved ones. Many believe sins and misdeeds are punished in the afterlife. Others believe there is no afterlife. To them, death is the end of life.

Some religions believe that the body keeps its physical form after death. Others believe that only the spirit or soul is present in the afterlife. *Reincarnation* is the belief that the spirit or soul is reborn in another human body or in another form of life.

Many people strengthen their religious beliefs when dying. Religion also provides comfort for the dying person and the family.

Age

Children ages 3 to 5 years know when family members or pets die. They notice dead birds or bugs. To them, death is temporary. They think death is punishment for being bad.

Children between the ages of 5 and 7 years know death is final. Death happens to other people but not to them. Death can be avoided. Children relate death to punishment and body mutilation. It also involves witches, ghosts, goblins, and monsters. These ideas come from fairy tales, cartoons, movies, video games, and TV.

Adults fear pain and suffering, dying alone, and the invasion of privacy. They also fear loneliness and separation from loved ones. They worry about the care and

Caring About Culture
Death Rites

In *Vietnam*, quality of life is more important than length of life because of beliefs in reincarnation. Less suffering in the next life is expected. Therefore dying persons are helped to recall past good deeds and to achieve a fitting mental state. Death at home is preferred over death in the hospital. Upon death, the body is washed and wrapped in clean, white sheets. In some areas a coin or jewels (a wealthy family) and rice (a poor family) are put in the dead person's mouth. This is from the belief that they will help the soul go through the encounters with gods and devils and the soul will be born rich in the next life. Relatives sew small pillows to place under the body's neck, feet, and wrists. The body is placed in a coffin for in-ground burial.

The *Chinese* have an aversion to anything concerning death. Autopsy and disposal of the body are not prescribed by religion. Donating body parts is encouraged. The eldest son makes all arrangements. The body is buried in a coffin. After 7 years, the body is exhumed and cremated. The urn is reburied in the tomb. White or yellow and black clothing is worn for mourning.

In *India*, Hindu persons are often accepting of God's will. The person's desire to be clearheaded as death nears must be assessed in planning medical treatment. A time and place for prayer are essential for the family and the person. Prayer helps them deal with anxiety and conflict. The Hindu priest reads from Holy Sanskrit books. Some priests tie strings (meaning a blessing) around the neck or wrist. After death, the son pours water into the mouth of the deceased. Blood transfusions, organ transplants, and autopsies are allowed. Cremation is preferred. Reincarnation is a Hindu belief.

From D'Avanzo CE, Geissler EM: *Pocket guide to cultural health assessment*, ed 3, St Louis, 2003, Mosby.

BOX 10-1 Cancer

Cells reproduce for tissue growth and repair. Cells divide in an orderly way. Sometimes cell division and growth are out of control. A mass or clump of cells develops. This new growth of abnormal cells is called a *tumor:*

- *Benign tumors* grow slowly and within a local area. They do not spread to other body parts. They usually do not cause death.
- A *malignant tumor (cancer)* grows fast. It invades other tissues.

Metastasis is the spread of cancer to other body parts (Fig. 10-1). Cancer cells break off the tumor and travel to other body parts. New tumors grow in other body parts. This occurs if the cancer is not treated and controlled.

The most common cancer sites are the skin, lungs, colon, rectum, breast, prostate, uterus, and urinary tract. Cancer occurs in all ages. Exact causes are unknown. The National Cancer Institute cites these risk factors:

- Tobacco—smoking tobacco, chewing tobacco and snuff, and secondhand smoke.
- Exposure to radiation—sun, sunlamps, tanning booths, x-ray procedures.
- Alcohol.
- Diet—high-fat diet, being seriously overweight.
- Chemicals and other substances—metals, pesticides, asbestos, and others.
- Hormone replacement therapy (HRT).
- Diethylstilbestrol—a synthetic form of estrogen used between the early 1940s and 1971. It was given during pregnancy to prevent certain problems.
- Close relatives with certain types of cancer—melanoma and cancers of the breast, ovary, prostate, and colon.

If detected early, cancer can be treated and controlled. According to the National Cancer Institute, some signs and symptoms of cancer are:

- Thickening or lump in the breast or any other part of the body
- Obvious change in a wart or mole
- A sore that does not heal
- Nagging cough or hoarseness
- Changes in bowel or bladder habits
- Indigestion or difficulty swallowing
- Unexplained changes in weight
- Unusual bleeding or discharge

Treatment depends on the type of tumor, its site and size, and if it has spread. One or more of the following treatments are commonly used:

- *Surgery* removes tumors. It is done to cure or control cancer. It also relieves pain from advanced cancer. Some surgeries are very disfiguring. Self-esteem and body image are affected.
- *Radiation therapy (radiotherapy)* kills cells. X-ray beams are aimed at the tumor. Cancer cells and normal cells receive radiation. Both are destroyed. Burns, skin breakdown, and hair loss can occur at the treatment site. Discomfort, nausea and vomiting, diarrhea, and loss of appetite (anorexia) are other side effects.
- *Chemotherapy* involves drugs that kill cells. Normal cells and cancer cells are affected. Side effects include gastrointestinal irritation, poor appetite, nausea, vomiting, and diarrhea. *Stomatitis*, an inflammation (*itis*) of the mouth (*stomat*), and hair loss (*alopecia*) may occur. Blood cell production decreases. Bleeding and infection are risks. The person may feel weak and tired.

Persons with cancer have physical, psychological, social, and spiritual needs. Many need pain relief or control. Anger, fear, and depression are common. Some surgeries are disfiguring. The person may feel unwhole, unattractive, or unclean. The person and family need support.

---

support of those left behind. Adults often resent death because it affects plans, hopes, dreams, and ambitions.

Older persons usually have fewer fears. They know death will occur. Some welcome death as freedom from pain, suffering, and disability. Death also means reunion with those who have died. Like younger adults, they often fear dying alone.

THE STAGES OF DYING

Dr. Elisabeth Kübler-Ross described five stages of dying:

- *Denial* is the first stage. Persons refuse to believe they are dying. "No, not me" is a common response. The person believes a mistake was made.
- *Anger* is stage two. The person thinks "Why me?" There is anger, rage, and envy of those with life and health. Family, friends, and the health team are often targets of anger.
- *Bargaining* is the third stage. Anger has passed. The person now says "Yes, me, but. . . . "Promises are made in exchange for more time. Bargaining is usually private and on a spiritual level.
- *Depression* is the fourth stage. The person thinks "Yes, me," and is very sad. The person mourns things that were lost and the future loss of life.
- *Acceptance* is the last stage. The person is calm and at peace. The person has said what needs to be said. Unfinished business is completed.

PSYCHOLOGICAL, SOCIAL, AND SPIRITUAL NEEDS

Dying people may want family and friends present. They may want to talk about their fears and worries. Some want to be alone. Often they need to talk at night. Things are quiet, distractions are few, and there is more time to think. You need to listen and use touch:

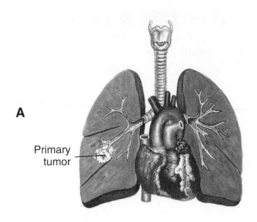
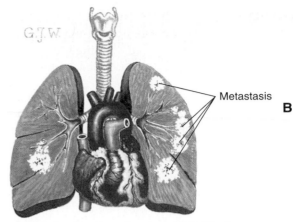

Fig. 10-1 A, Tumor in the lung. **B,** Tumor has metastasized to the other lung. (Modified from Belcher AE: *Cancer nursing,* St Louis, 1992, Mosby.)

- *Listening.* Let the person express feelings and emotions in his or her own way. Do not worry about saying the wrong thing or finding comforting words. You do not need to say anything. Being there for the person is what counts.
- *Touch.* Touch shows caring and concern when words cannot. Sometimes the person does not want to talk but needs you nearby.

Some people want to see a spiritual leader or to take part in religious practices. Provide privacy during prayer and spiritual moments. The person may have religious objects nearby (medals, pictures, statues, or religious writings). Handle these valuables with care and respect.

PHYSICAL NEEDS

Comfort is promoted. The person is allowed to die in peace and with dignity.

- *Vision.* Vision blurs and gradually fails. The person turns toward light. A dark room may frighten the person. The eyes may be half-open. Secretions may collect in the corners of the eyes. Because of failing vision, explain what you are doing to the person or in the room. The room should be well lit. However, avoid bright lights and glares. Good eye care is needed (Chapter 11).
- *Hearing.* Hearing is one of the last functions lost. Many people hear until the moment of death. Even unconscious persons may hear. Always assume that the person can hear. Speak in a normal voice. Give reassurance and explanations about care. Offer words of comfort. Avoid topics that could upset the person.
- *Speech.* Speech becomes difficult. It may be hard to understand the person. Sometimes the person cannot speak. Anticipate his or her needs. Ask "yes" or "no" questions. Do not ask questions with long answers. Despite speech problems, you must talk to the person.
- *Mouth.* Routine mouth care is given if the person can eat and drink. Frequent oral care is given as death nears and when taking oral fluids is difficult. Oral hygiene is needed if mucus collects in the mouth and the person cannot swallow.
- *Nose.* Crusting and irritation of the nostrils can occur. Nasal secretions, an oxygen cannula, and a nasogastric (NG) tube (Chapter 14) are common causes. Carefully clean the nose. Apply lubricant as directed by the nurse and the care plan.
- *Circulation.* Circulation fails and body temperature rises as death nears. The skin is cool, pale, and mottled (blotchy). Perspiration increases. Skin care, bathing, and preventing pressure ulcers are necessary. Linens and gowns are changed whenever needed. Despite cool skin, only light bed coverings are needed. Blankets may make the person feel too warm and cause restlessness.
- *Elimination.* Urinary and fecal incontinence may occur. Use incontinence products and give perineal care as needed. Constipation and urinary retention are common. Enemas and catheters may be needed (Chapter 13).
- *Comfort and positioning.* Skin care, personal and oral hygiene, back massages, and good alignment promote comfort. The nurse gives pain-relief drugs ordered by the doctor. Frequent position changes and supportive devices also promote comfort. Turn the person slowly and gently. Semi-Fowler's position is usually best for breathing problems.
- *The person's room.* The person's room should be pleasant, well lit, and well ventilated. Some equipment is upsetting to look at (suction machines, drainage containers). If possible, keep such items out of the person's sight. Mementos, pictures, cards, flowers, and religious items provide comfort. The person and family arrange these items to reflect the person's choices. This helps meet love, belonging, and self-esteem needs.

THE FAMILY

This is a hard time for the family. You may not find comforting words. Show your feelings by being available, courteous, and considerate. Use touch to show your concern.

You must respect the right to privacy. The person and family need time together. However, you cannot neglect care because the family is present. Most centers let family members help give care. Or you can suggest that they take a break for a beverage or meal.

The family may be very tired, sad, and tearful. Watching a loved one die is very painful. So is dealing with the eventual loss of that person. The family needs support, understanding, courtesy, and respect.

LEGAL ISSUES

Some people make end-of-life wishes known. Living wills and durable power of attorney are common advance directives (Chapter 6). *"Do Not Resuscitate"* (DNR) orders also are common. The orders mean that the person will not be resuscitated. The doctor writes the orders after consulting with the person and family.

SIGNS OF DEATH

There are signs that death is near. They may occur rapidly or slowly:

- Movement, muscle tone, and sensation are lost. This usually starts in the feet and legs. It eventually spreads to other body parts. When mouth muscles relax, the jaw drops. The mouth may stay open. The facial expression is often peaceful.
- Peristalsis and other gastrointestinal functions slow. Abdominal distention, fecal incontinence, fecal impaction, nausea, and vomiting are common.
- Body temperature rises. The person feels cool or cold, looks pale, and perspires heavily.
- Circulation fails. The pulse is fast, weak, and irregular. Blood pressure starts to fall.
- The respiratory system fails. Slow respirations or rapid and shallow respirations are observed. Mucus collects in the airway. This causes the *death rattle* that is heard.
- Pain decreases as the person loses consciousness. Some people are conscious until the moment of death.

The signs of death include no pulse, respirations, or blood pressure. Pupils are fixed and dilated. A doctor determines that death has occurred and pronounces the person dead.

CARE OF THE BODY AFTER DEATH

Care of the body after *(post)* death *(mortem)* is called **postmortem** care. The nurse may ask you to assist with this care. The care begins when the doctor pronounces the person dead.

Postmortem care is done to maintain good body appearance. Discoloration and skin damage are prevented. Valuables and personal items are gathered for the family. The right to privacy and the right to be treated with dignity and respect apply after death.

Rigor mortis is the stiffness or rigidity *(rigor)* of skeletal muscles that occurs after death *(mortis)*. It occurs within 2 to 4 hours after death. The body is positioned in normal alignment before rigor mortis sets in. The family may want to see the body. The body should appear in a comfortable and natural position for this viewing.

In some centers the body is prepared only for viewing. The funeral director completes postmortem care.

Postmortem care may involve repositioning the body. Moving the body can cause remaining air in the lungs, stomach, and intestines to be expelled. When air is expelled, sounds are produced. Do not let these sounds alarm or frighten you. They are normal and expected.

Delegation Guidelines

Care of the Body After Death

When assisting with postmortem care, you need this information from the nurse:

- If dentures will be inserted or placed in a denture container
- If tubes will be removed or left in place
- If the family wants to view the body
- Special center policies and procedures

Safety Alert

Care of the Body After Death

Standard Precautions and the Bloodborne Pathogen Standard are followed. You may have contact with infected blood, body fluids, secretions, or excretions.

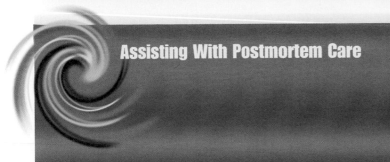

Pre-Procedure

1 Follow *Delegation Guidelines: Care of the Body After Death.* See *Safety Alert: Care of the Body After Death.*
2 Practice hand hygiene.
3 Collect the following:
   • Postmortem kit (shroud or body bag, gown, ID tags, gauze squares, safety pins)
   • Bed protectors
   • Wash basin
   • Bath towels and washcloths
   • Denture cup
   • Tape
   • Dressings
   • Gloves
   • Cotton balls
   • Gown
   • Valuables envelope
4 Provide for privacy.
5 Raise the bed for body mechanics.
6 Make sure the bed is flat.

Procedure

7 Put on the gloves.
8 Position the body supine. Arms and legs are straight. A pillow is under the head and shoulders.
9 Close the eyes. Gently pull the eyelids over the eyes. Apply moist cotton balls gently over the eyelids if the eyes will not stay closed.
10 Insert dentures if it is center policy. If not, put them in a labeled denture cup.
11 Close the mouth. If necessary, put a rolled towel under the chin to keep the mouth closed.
12 Follow center policy for jewelry. Remove all jewelry, except for wedding rings (if center policy). List the removed jewelry. Place the jewelry and list in a valuables envelope.
13 Place a cotton ball over the rings. Tape them in place.
14 Remove drainage containers. Leave tubes and catheters in place if there will be an autopsy. Ask the nurse about removing tubes.
15 Bathe soiled areas with plain water. Dry thoroughly.
16 Place a bed protector under the buttocks.
17 Remove soiled dressings. Replace them with clean ones.
18 Put a clean gown on the body. Position the body as in step 8.
19 Brush and comb the hair if necessary.
20 Cover the body to the shoulders with a sheet if the family will view the body.
21 Gather the person's belongings. Put them in a bag labeled with the person's name.
22 Remove supplies, equipment, and linens. Straighten the room. Provide soft lighting.
23 Remove the gloves. Decontaminate your hands.
24 Let the family view the body. Provide for privacy. Return to the room after they leave.
25 Decontaminate your hands. Put on gloves.
26 Fill out the ID tags. Tie one to the ankle or to the right big toe.
27 Place the body in the body bag, or cover it with a sheet. Or apply the shroud (Fig. 10-2, p. 186):
   a Bring the top down over the head.
   b Fold the bottom up over the feet.
   c Fold the sides over the body.
   d Pin or tape the shroud in place.
28 Attach the second ID tag to the shroud, sheet, or body bag.
29 Leave the denture cup with the body.
30 Pull the privacy curtain around the bed. Or close the door.

Post-Procedure

31 Remove the gloves. Decontaminate your hands.
32 Strip the unit after the body has been removed. Wear gloves for this step.
33 Remove the gloves. Decontaminate your hands.
34 Report the following to the nurse:
   • The time the body was taken by the funeral director
   • What was done with jewelry and personal items
   • What was done with dentures

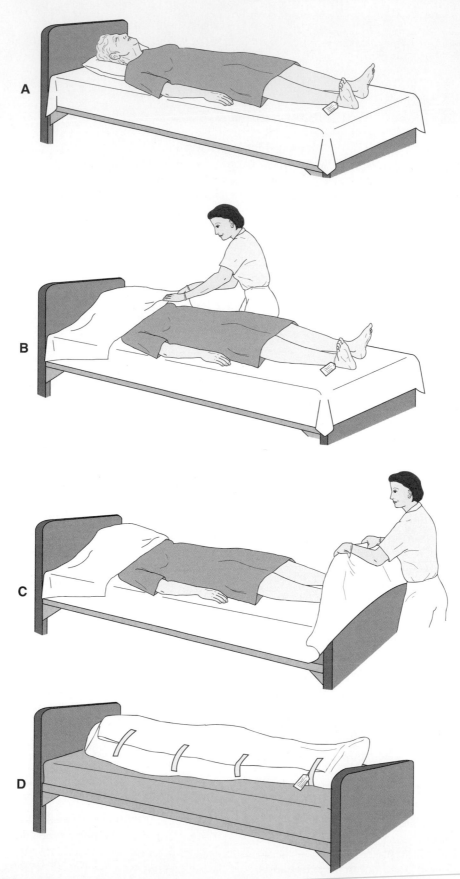

Fig. 10-2 Applying a shroud. **A,** Place the body on the shroud. **B,** Bring the top of the shroud down over the head. **C,** Fold the bottom up over the feet. **D,** Fold the sides over the body. Tape or pin the sides together. Attach the ID tag.

Review Questions

Circle the **BEST** answer.

1 Reincarnation is the belief that
  a There is no afterlife
  b The spirit or soul is reborn into another human body or another form of life
  c The body keeps its physical form in the afterlife
  d Only the spirit or soul is present in the afterlife

2 Children between the ages of 5 and 7 view death as
  a Temporary
  b Final
  c Adults do
  d Going to sleep

3 Adults and older persons usually fear
  a Dying alone
  b Reincarnation
  c The five stages of dying
  d Advance directives

4 A dying person tries to gain more time during the stage of
  a Anger
  b Bargaining
  c Depression
  d Acceptance

5 When caring for a dying person, you should
  a Use touch and listen
  b Do most of the talking
  c Keep the room darkened
  d Speak in a loud voice

6 As death nears, the last sense lost is
  a Sight
  b Taste
  c Smell
  d Hearing

7 The dying person's care includes the following *except*
  a Eye care
  b Mouth care
  c Exercise
  d Position changes

8 A "Do Not Resuscitate" order was written. This means that
  a CPR will not be done
  b The person has a living will
  c Life-prolonging measures will be carried out
  d The person is kept alive as long as possible

9 The signs of death are
  a Convulsions and incontinence
  b No pulse, respirations, or blood pressure
  c Loss of consciousness and convulsions
  d The eyes stay open, no muscle movements, and the body is rigid

10 Postmortem care is done
  a After rigor mortis sets in
  b After the doctor pronounces the person dead
  c When the funeral director arrives for the body
  d After the family has viewed the body

Answers to these questions are on p. 389.

CHAPTER 11

Oral Hygiene and Bathing

Objectives

- Define the key terms listed in this chapter
- Describe the care given before and after breakfast, after lunch, and in the evening
- Explain the importance of oral hygiene and bathing
- Identify safety measures for tub baths and showers
- Explain the purposes of a back massage
- Explain the purposes of perineal care
- Perform the procedures described in this chapter

oral hygiene Mouth care

perineal care Cleaning the genital and anal areas; pericare

Intact skin prevents microbes from entering the body and causing an infection. Likewise, mucous membranes of the mouth, genital area, and anus must be clean and intact. Good hygiene also prevents body and breath odors. It is relaxing and increases circulation.

Culture and personal choice affect hygiene. (See *Caring About Culture: Personal Hygiene*). The person's preferences are part of the care plan.

DAILY CARE

Most people have hygiene routines and habits. For example, teeth are brushed and face and hands washed on awakening. These and other hygiene measures are often done before and after meals and at bedtime. Certain measures are needed:

- Before breakfast. This is called *early morning care* or AM *care.*
- After breakfast. This is called *morning care.*
- During the afternoon. This is called *afternoon care.*
- Before bedtime. This is called *evening care* or PM *care.*

Care measures at such times include:

- Assisting with elimination
- Cleaning incontinent persons
- Changing wet or soiled linens
- Assisting with hygiene (Face and hand washing and oral hygiene are done before breakfast, in the afternoon, and at bedtime. Morning care includes oral hygiene, bathing, and perineal care.)
- Assisting with dressing and hair care
- Helping residents change into sleepwear (evening care)
- Providing back massages (morning care and evening care)
- Making beds and straightening units

ORAL HYGIENE

Oral hygiene (mouth care) keeps the mouth and teeth clean. It prevents mouth odors and infections, increases comfort, and makes food taste better. Oral hygiene also reduces the risk for *dental caries (cavities)* and *periodontal disease (gum disease).*

Illness, disease, and some drugs often cause a bad taste in the mouth. They may cause a whitish coating in the mouth and on the tongue. Others cause redness

Caring About Culture

Personal Hygiene

Personal hygiene is very important to *East Indian Hindus.* Their religion requires at least one bath a day. Some believe it is harmful to bathe after a meal. Another Hindu belief is that a cold bath prevents blood disease. Some believe that eye injuries can occur if a bath is too hot. Hot water can be added to cold water. However, cold water is not added to hot water. After bathing, the body is carefully dried with a towel.

From Giger JN, Davidhizar RE: *Transcultural nursing: assessment and intervention,* ed 4, St Louis, 2004, Mosby.

Delegation Guidelines

Oral Hygiene

To assist with oral hygiene, you need this information from the nurse and the care plan:
- The type of oral hygiene to give (pp. 190-194)
- What cleaning agent and equipment to use
- If lubricant is applied to the lips (if so, what lubricant to use)
- How often to give oral hygiene
- How much help the person needs
- What observations to report and record:
  —Dry, cracked, swollen, or blistered lips
  —Mouth or breath odor
  —Redness, swelling, irritation, sores or white patches in the mouth or on the tongue
  —Bleeding, swelling, or redness of the gums
  —Loose teeth
  —Rough, sharp, or chipped areas on dentures

and swelling of the mouth and tongue. Dry mouth is common from oxygen, smoking, decreased fluid intake, and anxiety. Some drugs cause dry mouth.

Oral hygiene is given on awakening, after meals, and at bedtime. Many people practice oral hygiene before meals. Some persons need mouth care every 2 hours or more often. Always follow the care plan. Use a toothbrush with soft bristles.

Safety Alert

Oral Hygiene

Follow Standard Precautions and the Bloodborne Pathogen Standard when giving oral hygiene. You have contact with the person's mucous membranes. Gums may bleed during mouth care. Also, the mouth has many microbes. Pathogens spread through sexual contact may be in the mouths of some persons.

Brushing Teeth

Many people perform oral hygiene themselves. Others need help gathering and setting up equipment. You may have to brush the teeth of persons who are very weak, cannot use or move their arms, or are too confused to brush their teeth.

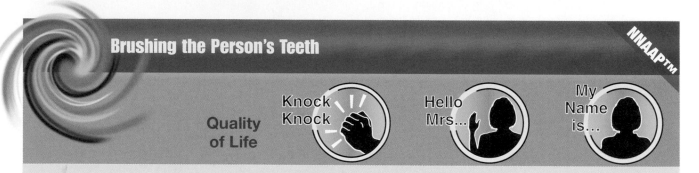

Brushing the Person's Teeth

NNAAP™

Quality of Life

Knock Knock · Hello Mrs... · My Name is...

Pre-Procedure

1   Follow *Delegation Guidelines: Oral Hygiene*, p. 189. See *Safety Alert: Oral Hygiene*.
2   Explain the procedure to the person.
3   Practice hand hygiene.
4   Collect the following:
   • Toothbrush
   • Toothpaste
   • Mouthwash (or solution on the care plan)
   • Water glass with cool water
   • Straw
   • Kidney basin
   • Hand towel
   • Paper towels
   • Gloves
5   Place the paper towels on the overbed table. Arrange items on top of them.
6   Identify the person. Check the ID bracelet against the assignment sheet. Call the person by name.
7   Provide for privacy.
8   Raise the bed for body mechanics. Bed rails are up if used.

Procedure

9   Lower the bed rail near you if up.
10   Assist the person to a sitting position or to a side-lying position near you.
11   Place the towel over the person's chest.
12   Adjust the overbed table so you can reach it with ease.
13   Decontaminate your hands. Put on the gloves.
14   Apply toothpaste to the toothbrush.
15   Hold the toothbrush over the kidney basin. Pour some water over the brush.
16   Brush the teeth gently (Fig. 11-1).
17   Brush the tongue gently.
18   Let the person rinse the mouth with water. Hold the kidney basin under the person's chin. Repeat this step as needed.
19   Let the person use mouthwash or other solution. Hold the kidney basin under the chin.
20   Wipe the person's mouth. Remove the towel.
21   Remove and discard the gloves. Decontaminate your hands.

Post-Procedure

22   Provide for comfort.
23   Place the signal light within reach.
24   Lower the bed to its lowest position.
25   Raise or lower bed rails. Follow the care plan.
26   Clean and return equipment to its proper place. Wear gloves.
27   Wipe off the overbed table with the paper towels. Discard the paper towels.
28   Remove the gloves. Decontaminate your hands.
29   Adjust the overbed table for the person.
30   Unscreen the person.
31   Complete a safety check of the room. (See inside of front book cover.)
32   Follow center policy for dirty linen.
33   Decontaminate your hands.
34   Report and record your observations.

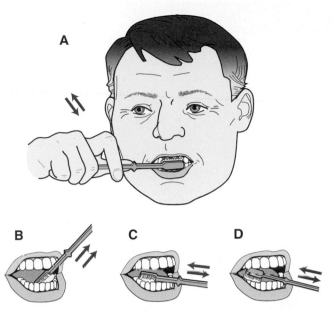

Fig. 11-1 Brushing teeth. **A,** The brush is at a 45-degree angle to the gums. Teeth are brushed with short strokes. **B,** The brush is at a 45-degree angle against the inside of the front teeth. Teeth are brushed from the gum to the crown of the tooth with short strokes. **C,** The brush is held horizontally against the inner surfaces of the teeth. The teeth are brushed back and forth. **D,** The brush is positioned on the biting surfaces of the teeth. The teeth are brushed back and forth.

Mouth Care for the Unconscious Person

Unconscious persons cannot eat or drink. They may breathe with their mouths open. Many receive oxygen. These factors cause mouth dryness and crusting on the tongue and mucous membranes. Oral hygiene keeps the mouth clean and moist. It also helps prevents infection.

The care plan tells you what cleaning agent to use. Use sponge swabs to apply the cleaning agent. After cleaning, apply lubricant to the lips. It prevents cracking of the lips.

Unconscious persons usually cannot swallow. Protect them from choking and aspiration. Aspiration can cause pneumonia and death. To prevent aspiration, position the person on one side with the head turned well to the side (Fig. 11-2). In this position, excess fluid runs out of the mouth. Use only a small amount of fluid.

Keep the person's mouth open with a padded tongue blade (see Fig. 11-2). Do not use your fingers. The person can bite down on them. The bite breaks the skin and creates a portal of entry for microbes. Infection is a risk.

Always assume that unconscious persons can hear. Explain what you are doing step-by-step. Also tell the person when you are done and when you are leaving the room.

Give mouth care at least every 2 hours. Follow the nurse's directions and the care plan.

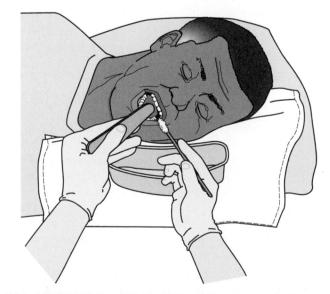

Fig. 11-2 The head of the unconscious person is turned well to the side to prevent aspiration. A padded tongue blade is used to keep the mouth open while cleaning the mouth with swabs.

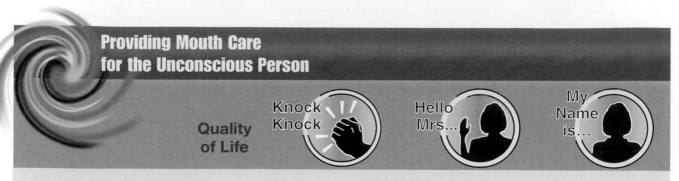

**Providing Mouth Care
for the Unconscious Person**

Quality
of Life

Knock
Knock

Hello
Mrs...

My
Name
is...

Pre-Procedure

1 Follow *Delegation Guidelines: Oral Hygiene*, p. 189.
   See *Safety Alert: Oral Hygiene*, p. 190.
2 Practice hand hygiene.
3 Collect the following:
   • Cleaning agent (check the care plan)
   • Sponge swabs
   • Padded tongue blade
   • Water glass with cool water
   • Hand towel
   • Kidney basin
   • Lip lubricant
   • Paper towels
   • Gloves
4 Place the paper towels on the overbed table. Arrange items on top of them.
5 Identify the person. Check the ID bracelet against the assignment sheet. Call the person by name.
6 Explain the procedure to the person.
7 Provide for privacy.
8 Raise the bed for body mechanics. Bed rails are up if used.

Procedure

9   Lower the bed rail near you if up.
10 Decontaminate your hands. Put on the gloves.
11 Position the person in a side-lying position near you. Turn his or her head well to the side.
12 Place the towel under the person's face.
13 Place the kidney basin under the chin.
14 Adjust the overbed table so you can reach it with ease.
15 Separate the upper and lower teeth. Use the padded tongue blade. Be gentle. Never use force. If you have problems, ask the nurse for help.
16 Clean the mouth using sponge swabs moistened with the cleaning agent (see Fig. 11-2):
    a Clean the chewing and inner surfaces of the teeth.
    b Clean the outer surfaces of the teeth.
    c Swab the roof of the mouth, inside of the cheeks, and the lips.
    d Swab the tongue.
    e Moisten a clean swab with water. Swab the mouth to rinse.
    f Place used swabs in the kidney basin.
17 Apply lubricant to the lips.
18 Wipe the person's mouth. Remove the towel.
19 Remove and discard the gloves. Decontaminate your hands.
20 Explain that the procedure is done. Explain that you will reposition him or her.
21 Reposition the person. Provide for comfort.
22 Raise or lower bed rails. Follow the care plan.

Post-Procedure

23 Place the signal light within reach.
24 Lower the bed to its lowest position.
25 Clean and return equipment to its proper place. Discard disposable items. (Wear gloves.)
26 Wipe off the overbed table with paper towels. Discard the paper towels.
27 Remove the gloves. Decontaminate your hands.
28 Unscreen the person.
29 Complete a safety check of the room. (See inside of front book cover.)
30 Tell the person that you are leaving the room.
31 Follow center policy for dirty linen.
32 Decontaminate your hands.
33 Report and record observations.

Denture Care

Dentures are cleaned as often as natural teeth. Dentures are slippery when wet. They easily break or chip if dropped onto a hard surface (floors, sinks). Hold them firmly. During cleaning, firmly hold them over a basin of water lined with a towel. This protects them from the hard sink.

Use a cleaning agent. Follow the manufacturer's instructions for cleaner use and water temperature. Dentures lose their shape (warp) in hot water. If not worn, store clean dentures in a container with cool water or a denture soaking solution. Otherwise they can dry out and warp.

Dentures are usually removed at bedtime. Some people do not wear their dentures. Others wear dentures for eating and remove them after meals. Remind them not to wrap dentures in tissues or napkins. Otherwise, they are easily discarded.

Safety Alert

Denture Care

Dentures are costly. Handle them very carefully. Label the denture cup with the person's name and room number. Report lost or damaged dentures to the nurse at once.

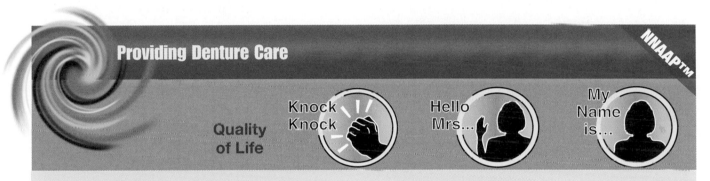

Providing Denture Care

Pre-Procedure

1   Follow *Delegation Guidelines: Oral Hygiene*, p. 189. See *Safety Alerts: Oral Hygiene: Denture Care*, p. 190.
2   Explain the procedure to the person.
3   Practice hand hygiene.
4   Collect the following:
    • Denture brush or soft-bristled toothbrush
    • Denture cup labeled with the person's name and room number
    • Cleaning agent
    • Water glass with cool water
    • Straw
    • Mouthwash (or other noted solution)
    • Kidney basin
    • Two hand towels
    • Gauze squares
    • Gloves
5   Identify the person. Check the ID bracelet against the assignment sheet. Call the person by name.
6   Provide for privacy.

Procedure

7   Lower the bed rail near you if used.
8   Place a towel over the person's chest.
9   Decontaminate your hands. Put on the gloves.
10 Ask the person to remove the dentures. Carefully place them in the kidney basin.
11 Remove the dentures if the person cannot do so. Use gauze squares to get a good grip on the slippery dentures:
    a   Grasp the upper denture with your thumb and index finger (Fig. 11-3, p. 194). Move it up and down slightly to break the seal. Remove the denture. Place it in the kidney basin.
    b   Grasp and remove the lower denture with your thumb and index finger. Turn it slightly, and lift it out of the mouth. Place it in the kidney basin.
12 Follow the care plan for raising bed rails.
13 Take the kidney basin, denture cup, brush, and cleaning agent to the sink.
14 Line the sink with a towel. Fill the sink with water until it is half full.
15 Rinse each denture under warm running water. (Some states require cool water.) Rinse out the denture cup.
16 Return dentures to the denture cup.
17 Apply the cleaning agent to the brush.

Continued

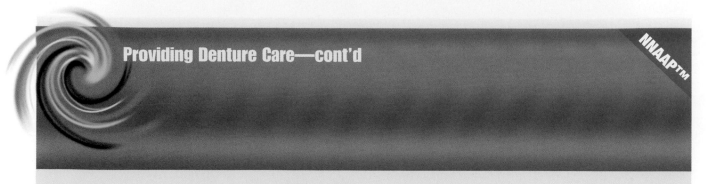

Providing Denture Care—cont'd

Procedure—cont'd

18 Brush the dentures as in Figure 11-4.
19 Rinse dentures under running water. Use warm or cool water as directed by the cleaning agent manufacturer. (Some states require cool water.)
20 Rinse the denture cup. Place dentures in the denture cup. Cover the dentures with cool water.
21 Clean the kidney basin.
22 Take the denture cup and kidney basin to the bedside table.
23 Lower the bed rail if up.
24 Position the person for oral hygiene.
25 Let the person use mouthwash (or noted solution). Hold the kidney basin under the chin.
26 Ask the person to insert the dentures. Insert them if the person cannot:

a Hold the upper denture firmly with your thumb and index finger. Raise the upper lip with the other hand. Insert the denture. Gently press on the denture with your index fingers to make sure it is in place.
b Hold the lower denture with your thumb and index finger. Pull the lower lip down slightly. Insert the denture. Gently press down on it to make sure it is in place.

27 Place the denture cup in the top drawer of the bedside stand if the dentures are not worn. The dentures must be in water or in a denture soaking solution.
28 Wipe the person's mouth. Remove the towel.
29 Remove the gloves. Decontaminate your hands.

Post-Procedure

30 Assist with hand washing.
31 Provide for comfort.
32 Place the signal light within reach.
33 Raise or lower bed rails. Follow the care plan.
34 Unscreen the person.
35 Clean and return equipment to its proper place. Discard disposable items. (Wear gloves.)

36 Complete a safety check of the room. (See inside of front book cover.)
37 Follow center policy for dirty linen.
38 Decontaminate your hands.
39 Report and record your observations.

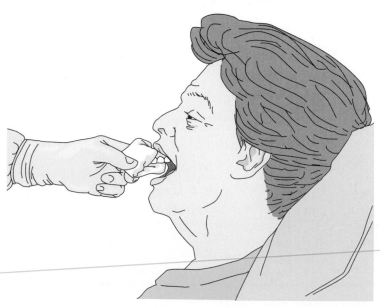

Fig. 11-3 Remove the upper denture by grasping it with the thumb and index finger of one hand. Use a piece of gauze to grasp the slippery denture.

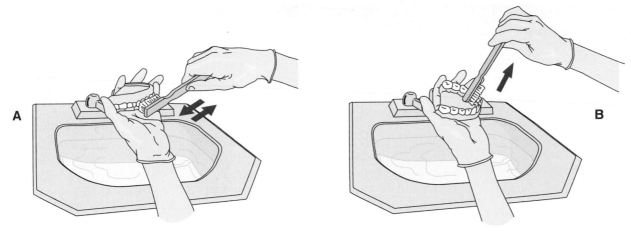

Fig. 11-4 Cleaning dentures. **A,** Outer surfaces of the upper denture are brushed with back-and-forth motions. Note that the denture is held over the sink, which is filled halfway with water and lined with a towel. **B,** Position the brush vertically to clean the inner surfaces of the denture. Use upward strokes

BATHING

Bathing cleans the skin and the genital and anal areas. Bathing is refreshing and relaxing. Circulation is stimulated and body parts exercised. Observations are made, and you have time to talk to the person. The rules for bathing are in Box 11-1.

Complete or partial bed baths, tub baths, or showers are given. The method depends on the person's condition, self-care abilities, and personal choice. In nursing centers, bathing usually is done after breakfast or the evening meal. The person's choice of bath time is respected.

Dry skin occurs with aging. Soap also dries the skin. Dry skin is easily damaged. Therefore older persons usually need a complete bath or shower 2 times a week. Partial baths are taken the other days. Some bathe daily but not with soap. Thorough rinsing is needed when using soap. Lotions and oils help keep the skin soft.

BOX 11-1 | Rules for Bathing

- Follow the care plan for bathing method and skin care products.
- Allow personal choice whenever possible.
- Follow Standard Precautions and the Bloodborne Pathogen Standard.
- Collect needed items before starting the procedure.
- Provide for privacy. Screen the person. Close doors, shades, blinds, or drapes.
- Assist the person with elimination. Bathing stimulates the need to urinate. Comfort and relaxation increase if urination needs are met.
- Cover the person for warmth and privacy.
- Reduce drafts. Close doors and windows.
- Protect the person from falling.
- Use good body mechanics at all times.
- Know what water temperature to use. See *Delegation Guidelines: Bathing,* p. 196.
- Keep bar soap in the soap dish between latherings. This prevents soapy water.
- Wash from the cleanest to the dirtiest areas.
- Encourage the person to help as much as is safely possible.
- Rinse the skin thoroughly. You must remove all soap.
- Pat the skin dry to avoid irritating or breaking the skin. Do not rub the skin.
- Dry under the breasts, between skin folds, in the perineal area, and between the toes.
- Bathe the skin whenever feces or urine is present. This prevents skin breakdown and odors.

Delegation Guidelines

Bathing

To assist with bathing, you need this information from the nurse and the care plan:

- What bath to give—complete bed bath, partial bath, tub bath, or shower
- How much help the person needs
- The person's activity or position limits
- What water temperature to use (Bath water cools fast. Therefore water temperature for a complete bed bath is usually between 110° and 115° F [43.3° and 46.1° C] for adults.)
- What skin care products to use and what the person prefers
- What observations to report and record:
  —The color of the skin, lips, nail beds, and sclera (whites of the eyes)
  —The location and description of rashes
  —Dry skin
  —Bruises or open skin areas
  —Pale or reddened areas, particularly over bony parts
  —Drainage or bleeding from wounds or body openings
  —Swelling of the feet and legs
  —Corns or calluses on the feet
  —Skin temperature
  —Complaints of pain or discomfort

Safety Alert

Bathing

Hot water can burn delicate and fragile skin. Measure water temperature according to center policy. If unsure if the water is too hot, ask the nurse to check it.

Protect the person from falls. Practice the measures presented in Chapter 4.

Use caution when applying powder. Do not use powders near persons with respiratory disorders. Inhaling powder can irritate the airway and lungs. Before applying powder, check with the nurse and the care plan. To safely apply powder:

- Do not shake or sprinkle powder onto the person.
- Turn away from the person.
- Sprinkle a small amount of powder onto your hands or a cloth.
- Apply the powder in a thin layer.

Beds are made after baths. After making the bed, lower the bed to its lowest position. Then lock the wheels. For an occupied bed, raise or lower bed rails according to the care plan.

Contact with blood, body fluids, secretions, and excretions is likely. Follow Standard Precautions and the Bloodborne Pathogen Standard.

The Complete Bed Bath

The *complete bed bath* involves washing the person's body in bed. Some people are embarrassed to have others see their bodies. Some fear exposure. Explain how the bed bath is given. Also explain how you cover the body for privacy.

Text continued on p. 202

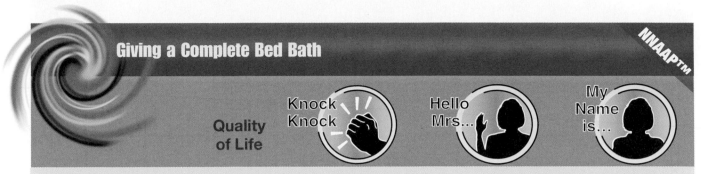

Giving a Complete Bed Bath

Pre-Procedure

1 Follow *Delegation Guidelines: Bathing*. See *Safety Alert: Bathing*.
2 Practice hand hygiene.
3 Identify the person. Check the ID bracelet against the assignment sheet. Call the person by name.
4 Explain the procedure to the person.
5 Offer the bedpan or urinal (Chapter 13). Provide for privacy.
6 Collect clean linen for a closed bed (see procedure: *Making an Occupied Bed*, p. 163). Place linen on a clean surface.
7 Collect the following:
- Wash basin
- Soap
- Bath thermometer
- Orange stick or nail file
- Washcloth
- Two bath towels and two hand towels
- Bath blanket
- Clothing, gown, or pajamas
- Items for oral hygiene
- Lotion
- Powder
- Deodorant or antiperspirant
- Brush and comb
- Other grooming items if requested
- Paper towels
- Gloves
8 Arrange items on the overbed table. Adjust the height as needed.
9 Close doors and windows to prevent drafts.
10 Provide for privacy.
11 Raise the bed for body mechanics. Bed rails are up if used.

Procedure

12 Remove the signal light. Lower the bed rail near you if up.
13 Decontaminate your hands. Put on gloves.
14 Provide oral hygiene.
15 Cover the person with a bath blanket. Remove top linens (see procedure: *Making an Occupied Bed*, p. 163).
16 Lower the head of the bed. It is as flat as possible. The person has at least one pillow.
17 Cover the overbed table with paper towels.
18 Raise the bed rail near you if bed rails are used. Both bed rails must be up.
19 Fill the wash basin ⅔ full with water. Water temperature is usually 110° to 115° F (43.3° to 46.1° C) for adults. Measure water temperature. Use a bath thermometer. Or test the water by dipping your elbow or inner wrist into the basin.
20 Place the basin on the overbed table.
21 Lower the bed rail if up.
22 Place a hand towel over the person's chest.
23 Make a mitt with the washcloth (Fig. 11-5, p. 199). Use a mitt for the entire bath.
24 Wash around the person's eyes with water. Do not use soap. Gently wipe from the inner to the outer aspect of the eyelid with a corner of the mitt (Fig. 11-6, p. 199). Clean the far eye first. Repeat this step for the near eye. Use a clean part of the washcloth for each stroke.
25 Ask the person if you should use soap to wash the face.
26 Wash the face, ears, and neck. Rinse and pat dry with the towel on the chest.
27 Help the person move to the side of the bed near you.
28 Remove the gown. Do not expose the person.
29 Place a bath towel lengthwise under the far arm.
30 Support the arm with your palm under the person's elbow. His or her forearm rests on your forearm.
31 Wash the arm, shoulder, and underarm. Use long, firm strokes (Fig. 11-7, p. 199). Rinse and pat dry.
32 Place the basin on the towel. Put the person's hand into the water (Fig. 11-8, p. 200). Wash it well. Clean under fingernails with an orange stick or nail file.
33 Remove the basin. Dry the hand well. Cover the arm with the bath blanket.
34 Repeat steps 29 through 33 for the near arm.

Continued

Procedure—cont'd

35 Place a bath towel over the chest crosswise. Hold the towel in place. Pull the bath blanket from under the towel to the waist.

36 Lift the towel slightly, and wash the chest (Fig. 11-9, p. 200). Do not expose the person. Rinse and pat dry, especially under breasts.

37 Move the towel lengthwise over the chest and abdomen. Do not expose the person. Pull the bath blanket down to the pubic area.

38 Lift the towel slightly, and wash the abdomen (Fig. 11-10, p. 200). Rinse and pat dry.

39 Pull the bath blanket up to the shoulders, covering both arms. Remove the towel.

40 Change soapy or cool water. Measure bath water temperature as in step 19. If bed rails are used, raise the bed rail near you before leaving the bedside. Lower it when you return.

41 Uncover the far leg. Do not expose the genital area. Place a towel lengthwise under the foot and leg.

42 Bend the knee, and support the leg with your arm. Wash it with long, firm strokes. Rinse and pat dry.

43 Place the basin on the towel near the foot.

44 Lift the leg slightly. Slide the basin under the foot.

45 Place the foot in the basin (Fig. 11-11, p. 201). Use an orange stick or nail file to clean under toenails if necessary. If the person cannot bend the knees:
  a Wash the foot. Carefully separate the toes. Rinse and pat dry.
  b Clean under the toenails with an orange stick or nail file if necessary.

46 Remove the basin. Dry the leg and foot. Cover the leg with the bath blanket. Remove the towel.

47 Repeat steps 41 through 46 for the near leg.

48 Change the water. Measure water temperature as in step 19. If bed rails are used, raise the bed rail near you before leaving the bedside. Lower it when you return.

49 Turn the person onto the side away from you.

50 Uncover the back and buttocks. Do not expose the person. Place a towel lengthwise on the bed along the back.

51 Wash the back. Work from the back of the neck to the lower end of the buttocks. Use long, firm, continuous strokes (Fig. 11-12, p. 201). Rinse and dry well.

52 Turn the person onto his or her back.

53 Change the water for perineal care. Measure water temperature as in step 19. (Some states also require changing gloves and hand hygiene at this time.) If bed rails are used, raise the bed rail near you before leaving the bedside. Lower it when you return.

54 Let the person wash the genital area. Adjust the overbed table so he or she can reach the wash basin, soap, and towels with ease. Place the signal light within reach. Ask the person to signal when finished. Make sure the person understands what to do.

55 Remove the gloves. Decontaminate your hands.

56 Answer the signal light promptly. Provide perineal care if the person cannot do so (p. 209). (Decontaminate your hands and wear gloves for perineal care.)

57 Give a back massage (p. 207).

58 Apply deodorant or antiperspirant. Apply lotion and powder as requested. See *Safety Alert: Bathing.*

59 Put clean garments on the person.

60 Comb and brush the hair (Chapter 12).

61 Make the bed. Attach the signal light.

Post-Procedure

62 Provide for comfort.

63 Lower the bed to its lowest position.

64 Raise or lower bed rails. Follow the care plan.

65 Put on gloves.

66 Empty and clean the wash basin. Return it and other supplies to their proper place.

67 Wipe off the overbed table with the paper towels. Discard the paper towels.

68 Unscreen the person.

69 Complete a safety check of the room. (See inside of front book cover.)

70 Follow center policy for dirty linen.

71 Remove the gloves. Decontaminate your hands.

72 Report and record your observations.

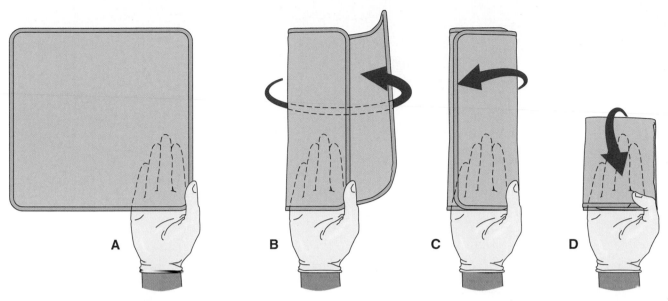

Fig. 11-5 Making a mitted washcloth. **A,** Grasp the near side of the washcloth with your thumb. **B,** Bring the washcloth around and behind your hand. **C,** Fold the side of the washcloth over your palm as you grasp it with your thumb. **D,** Fold the top of the washcloth down and tuck it under next to your palm.

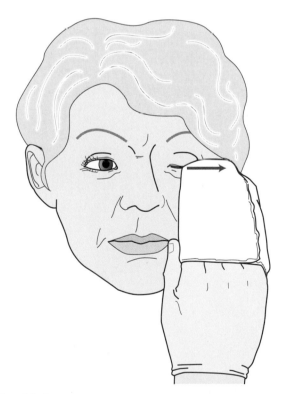

Fig. 11-6 Wash the person's eyelids with a mitted washcloth. Wipe from the inner to the outer aspect of the eye.

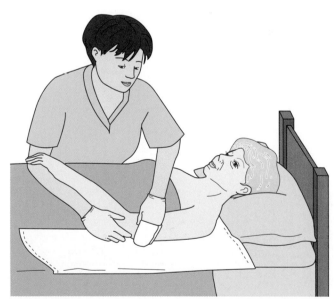

Fig. 11-7 Wash the person's arm with firm, long strokes using a mitted washcloth.

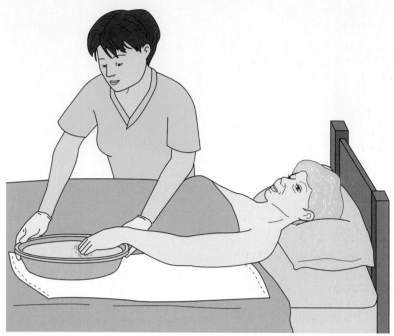

Fig. 11-8 The person's hands are washed by placing the wash basin on the bed.

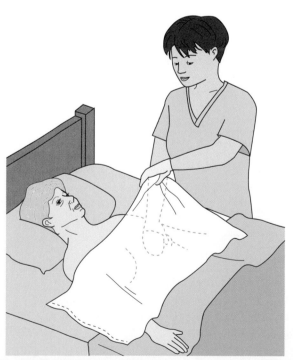

Fig. 11-9 The person's breasts are not exposed during the bath. A bath towel is placed horizontally over the chest area. The towel is lifted slightly to reach under to wash the breasts and chest.

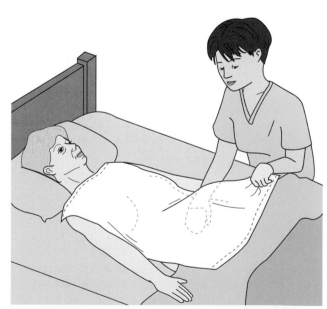

Fig. 11-10 The bath towel is turned so that it is vertical to cover the breasts and abdomen. The towel is lifted slightly to bathe the abdomen. The bath blanket covers the pubic area.

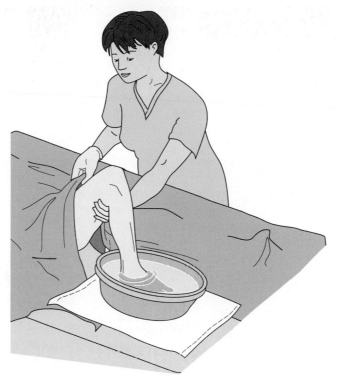

Fig. 11-11 The foot is washed by placing it in the wash basin on the bed.

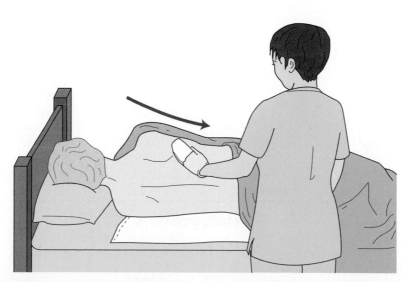

Fig. 11-12 The back is washed with long, firm, continuous strokes. Note that the person is in a side-lying position. A towel is placed lengthwise on the bed to protect the linens from water.

The Partial Bath

The *partial bath* involves bathing the face, hands, axillae (underarms), back, buttocks, and perineal area. Odors or discomfort occurs if these areas are not clean. Some persons bathe themselves in bed or at the sink. You assist as needed. Most need help washing the back. You give partial baths to persons who cannot bathe themselves.

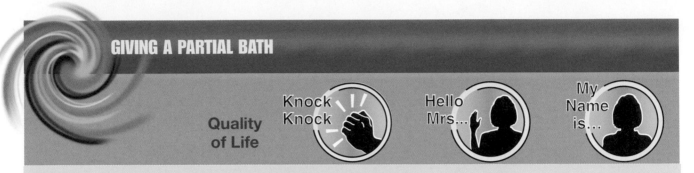

GIVING A PARTIAL BATH

Quality of Life — Knock Knock — Hello Mrs... — My Name is...

Pre-Procedure

1 Follow *Delegation Guidelines: Bathing*. See *Safety Alert: Bathing*.

2 Follow steps 2 through 10 in procedure: *Giving a Complete Bed Bath*, p. 197.

Procedure

3 Make sure the bed is in the lowest position.
4 Assist with oral hygiene. (Wear gloves.)
5 Remove top linen. Cover the person with a bath blanket.
6 Cover the overbed table with paper towels.
7 Fill the wash basin (⅔) full with water. Water temperature is 110° to 115° F (43.3° to 46.1° C) for adults or as directed by the nurse. Measure water temperature with the bath thermometer. Or test bath water by dipping your elbow or inner wrist into the basin.
8 Place the basin on the overbed table.
9 Position the person in Fowler's position. Or assist him or her to sit at the bedside.
10 Adjust the overbed table so the person can reach the basin and supplies.
11 Help the person undress.
12 Ask the person to wash easy-to-reach body parts (Fig. 11-13). Explain that you will wash the back and areas the person cannot reach.
13 Place the signal light within reach. Ask him or her to signal for help or when done bathing.

14 Leave the room after decontaminating your hands.
15 Return when the signal light is on. Knock before entering. Decontaminate your hands.
16 Change the bath water. Measure bath water temperature as in step 7.
17 Raise the bed for body mechanics. The far bed rail is up if used.
18 Ask what was washed. Put on gloves. Wash and dry areas the person could not reach.
19 Remove the gloves. Decontaminate your hands.
20 Give a back massage.
21 Apply lotion, powder, and deodorant or antiperspirant as requested.
22 Help the person put on clean garments.
23 Assist with hair care and other grooming needs.
24 Assist the person to a chair. (Lower the bed if the person transfers to a chair.) Otherwise, turn the person onto the side away from you.
25 Make the bed.
26 Lower the bed to its lowest position.

Post-Procedure

27 Provide for comfort.
28 Place the signal light within reach.
29 Raise or lower bed rails. Follow the care plan.
30 Put on gloves.
31 Empty and clean the basin. Return the basin and supplies to their proper place.
32 Wipe off the overbed table with the paper towels. Discard the paper towels.

33 Unscreen the person.
34 Complete a safety check of the room. (See inside of front book cover.)
35 Follow center policy for dirty linen.
36 Remove the gloves. Decontaminate your hands.
37 Report and record your observations.

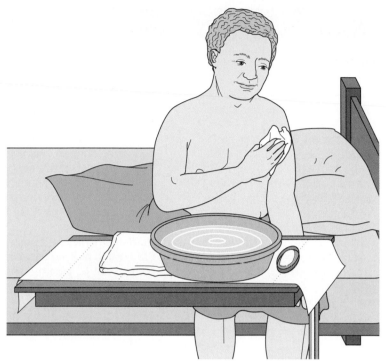

Fig. 11-13 The person is bathing himself while sitting on the side of the bed.

Tub Baths and Showers

Many residents take tub baths or showers. Falls, chilling, and burns from hot water are risks. Safety is important (Box 11-2, p. 204). The measures in Box 11-1 also apply.

Tub Baths.   A tub bath can cause a person to feel faint, weak, or tired. These are greater risks for persons who were on bed rest. A bath lasts no longer than 20 minutes.

Some centers have portable tubs. The sides are lowered to transfer the person from bed to the tub. The sides are raised after the transfer. Then the person is transported to the tub room.

Whirlpool tubs have special lifts. The person is transported to the tub room in a special wheelchair or stretcher. The chair or stretcher and person are lifted into the tub (Fig. 11-14). The tub has a whirlpool action that cleanses. You wash the upper body. Carefully wash under breasts, between skin folds, and in the perineal area. Dry the person after the bath.

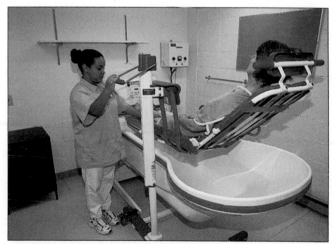

Fig. 11-14 The stretcher and person are lowered into the tub.

BOX 11-2   Safety Measures for Tub Baths and Showers

- Know what water temperature to use. See *Delegation Guidelines: Tub Baths and Showers.*
- Clean the tub or shower before and after use.
- Dry the tub or shower room floor.
- Check hand rails, grab bars, hydraulic lifts, and other safety aids. They must be in working order.
- Place a bath mat in the tub or on the shower floor. This is not needed if there are nonskid strips or a nonskid surface.
- Cover the person for warmth and privacy. This includes during transport to and from the shower room or tub room.
- Place needed items within the person's reach.
- Place the signal light within the person's reach.
- Show the person how to use the signal light in the shower or tub room.
- Have the person use grab bars when getting in and out of the tub. The person must not use towel bars for support.
- Turn cold water on first, then hot water. Turn hot water off first, then cold water.
- Adjust water temperature and pressure to prevent chilling or burns. Do this before the person gets into the shower. If a shower chair is used, position it first.
- Direct water away from the person while adjusting water temperature and pressure.
- Fill the tub before the person gets into it.
- Measure water temperature. For showers and tub baths, use the digital display. Or you can use a bath thermometer for a tub bath.
- Keep the water spray directed toward the person during the shower. This helps keep him or her warm.
- Keep bar soap in the soap dish between latherings. This prevents soapy water. It reduces the risk of slipping and falls in showers and tubs.
- Avoid using bath oils. They make tub and shower surfaces slippery.
- Do not leave weak or unsteady persons unattended.
- Stay within hearing distance if the person can be left alone. Wait outside the shower curtain or door. You will be nearby if the person calls for you or has an accident.
- Drain the tub before the person gets out of the tub. Cover him or her to protect from exposure and chilling.

Showers.   Some residents use shower chairs (Fig. 11-15). Water drains through an opening in the seat. The chair is used to transport the person to and from the shower. The wheels are locked during the shower to prevent the chair from moving.

Some people can stand in the shower. Have them use the grab bars for support during the shower. Like tubs, showers have nonskid surfaces. If not, a bath mat is used. Never let weak or unsteady persons stand in the shower. They need to use a shower chair.

Protect the person's privacy. The person has the right not to have his or her body seen by others. Properly screen and cover the person. Also, close doors and the shower curtain.

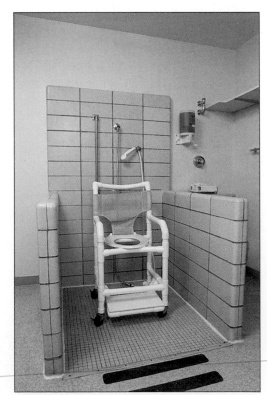

Fig. 11-15 Shower chair in a shower stall.

Delegation Guidelines

Tub Baths and Showers

For a tub bath or shower, you need this information from the nurse and the care plan:

- If the person takes a tub bath or shower
- What water temperature to use (usually 105° F; 40.5° C)
- If any special equipment is needed
- How much help the person needs
- If the person bathes unattended
- What observations to report and record (p. 196)

Safety Alert

Tub Baths and Showers

Some persons are very weak or large. Two staff members are needed to safely assist them with tub baths and showers.

You may use portable tubs, whirlpool equipment, and shower chairs. Always follow the manufacturer's instructions. Also, protect the person from falls, chilling, and burns. Follow the safety measures in Chapter 4. Remember to measure water temperature.

Prevent infection. Clean and disinfect tubs and showers before and after use.

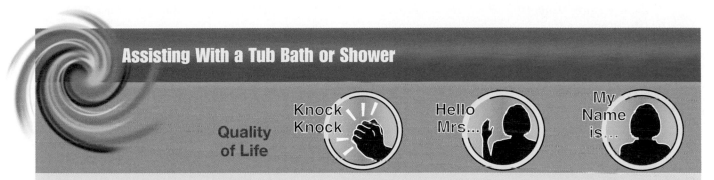

Assisting With a Tub Bath or Shower

Pre-Procedure

1 Follow *Delegation Guidelines: Tub Baths and Showers.* See *Safety Alert: Tub Baths and Showers.*
2 Reserve the bathtub or shower.
3 Practice hand hygiene.
4 Identify the person. Check the ID bracelet against the assignment sheet. Call the person by name.
5 Explain the procedure to the person.
6 Collect the following:
- Washcloth and two bath towels
- Soap
- Bath thermometer (for a tub bath)
- Clothing, gown, or pajamas
- Grooming items as requested
- Robe and nonskid footwear
- Rubber bath mat if needed
- Disposable bath mat
- Gloves
- Wheelchair or shower chair

Procedure

7 Place items in the tub or shower room. Use the space provided or a chair.
8 Clean and disinfect the tub or shower.
9 Place a rubber bath mat in the tub or on the shower floor. Do not block the drain.
10 Place the disposable bath mat on the floor in front of the tub or shower.
11 Put the *Occupied* sign on the door.
12 Return to the person's room. Decontaminate your hands.
13 Provide for privacy.
14 Help the person sit on the side of the bed.
15 Help the person put on a robe and nonskid footwear.
16 Assist or transport the person to the tub or shower room.
17 Have the person sit on the chair. Provide for privacy.
18 *For a tub bath:* Fill the tub halfway with warm water (105° F; 40.5° C). Measure water temperature with the bath thermometer. Or check the digital display (Fig. 11-16).
19 *For a shower:* Turn on the shower. Adjust water temperature and pressure.
20 Help the person undress and remove footwear.
21 Help the person into the tub or shower. Position the shower chair, and lock the wheels.
22 Assist with washing if necessary. Wear gloves.

Continued

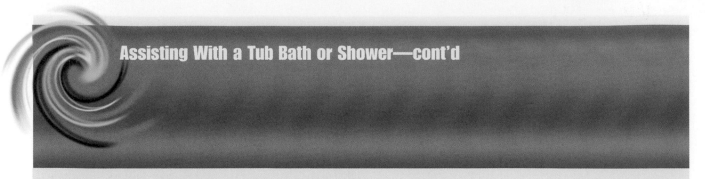

Assisting With a Tub Bath or Shower—cont'd

Procedure—cont'd

23 Ask the person to use the signal light when done or when help is needed. Remind the person that a tub bath lasts no longer than 20 minutes.

24 Place a towel across the chair.

25 Leave the room if the person can bathe unattended. If not, stay in the room or remain nearby. Remove the gloves and decontaminate your hands if you will leave the room.

26 Check the person every 5 minutes.

27 Return when the signal light is on. Knock before entering. Decontaminate your hands.

28 Turn off the shower, or drain the tub. Cover the person while the tub drains.

29 Help the person out of the tub or shower and onto the chair.

30 Help the person dry off. Pat gently. Dry under breasts, between skin folds, in the perineal area, and between the toes.

31 Assist with lotion and other grooming items as needed.

32 Help the person dress and put on footwear.

33 Help the person return to the room. Provide for privacy.

34 Assist the person to a chair or into bed.

35 Provide a back massage.

36 Assist with hair care and other grooming needs.

Post-Procedure

37 Make the bed. Provide for comfort.

38 Raise or lower bed rails. Follow the care plan.

39 Place the signal light within reach.

40 Unscreen the person.

41 Complete a safety check of the room. (See inside of front book cover.)

42 Clean and disinfect the tub or shower. Remove soiled linen. Wear gloves for this step.

43 Discard disposable items. Put the *Unoccupied* sign on the door. Return supplies to their proper place.

44 Follow center policy for dirty linen.

45 Decontaminate your hands.

46 Report and record your observations.

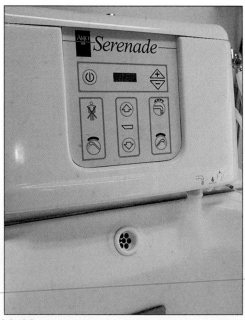

Fig. 11-16 The digital display shows water temperature.

THE BACK MASSAGE

The back massage (back rub) relaxes muscles and stimulates circulation. Back massages last 3 to 5 minutes. Observe the skin before the massage. Look for breaks in the skin, bruises, reddened areas, and other signs of skin breakdown.

Lotion reduces friction during the massage. Warm lotion before applying it. Place the bottle in the warm bath water, hold the bottle under warm water, or rub some lotion between your hands.

The prone position is best for a massage. The side-lying position is often used for older and disabled persons. Use firm strokes. Always keep your hands in contact with the person's skin. After the massage, apply some lotion to the elbows, knees, and heels. This keeps the skin soft. These bony areas are at risk for skin breakdown.

Delegation Guidelines

Back Massage

To give a back massage, you need this information from the nurse and the care plan:

- Can the person have a back massage (see *Safety Alert: Back Massage*)
- How to position the person
- Does the person have position limits
- When should the person receive a back massage
- Does the person need frequent back massages for comfort and to relax
- What observations to report and record:
  - Bruising
  - Reddened areas
  - Signs of skin breakdown

Safety Alert

Back Massage

Back massages are dangerous for persons with certain heart diseases, back injuries, back surgeries, skin diseases, and some lung disorders. Check with the nurse and care plan before giving back massages to persons with these conditions.

Do not massage bony areas that are reddened. Reddened areas signal skin breakdown and pressure ulcers. Massage can lead to further tissue damage.

Wear gloves if the person's skin is not intact. Always follow Standard Precautions and the Bloodborne Pathogen Standard.

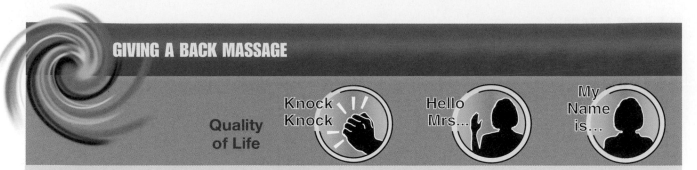

GIVING A BACK MASSAGE

Quality
of Life

Knock
Knock

Hello
Mrs...

My
Name
is...

Pre-Procedure

1 Follow *Delegation Guidelines: Back Massage*, p. 207. See *Safety Alert: Back Massage*, p. 207.
2 Practice hand hygiene.
3 Identify the person. Check the ID bracelet against the assignment sheet. Call the person by name.
4 Explain the procedure to the person.

5 Collect the following:
   • Bath blanket
   • Bath towel
   • Lotion
6 Provide for privacy.
7 Raise the bed for body mechanics. Bed rails are up if used.

Procedure

8 Lower the bed rail near you if up.
9 Position the person in the prone or side-lying position. The back is toward you.
10 Expose the back, shoulders, upper arms, and buttocks. Cover the rest of the body with the bath blanket.
11 Lay the towel on the bed along the back.
12 Warm the lotion.
13 Apply lotion to the lower back area.
14 Stroke up from the buttocks to the shoulders. Then stroke down over the upper arms. Stroke up the upper arms, across the shoulders, and down the back to the buttocks (Fig. 11-17). Use firm strokes. Keep your hands in contact with the person's skin.

15 Repeat step 14 for at least 3 minutes.
16 Knead by grasping skin between your thumb and fingers (Fig. 11-18). Knead half of the back. Start at the buttocks and move up to the shoulder. Then knead down from the shoulder to the buttocks. Repeat on the other half of the back.
17 Apply lotion to bony areas. Use circular motions with the tips of your index and middle fingers. (Do not massage reddened bony areas.)
18 Use fast movements to stimulate. Use slow movements to relax the person.
19 Stroke with long, firm movements to end the massage. Tell the person you are finishing.
20 Cover the person. Remove the towel and bath blanket.

Post-Procedure

21 Provide for comfort.
22 Lower the bed to its lowest position.
23 Raise or lower bed rails. Follow the care plan.
24 Place the signal light within reach.
25 Return lotion to its proper place.
26 Unscreen the person.

27 Complete a safety check of the room. (See inside of front book cover.)
28 Follow center policy for dirty linen.
29 Decontaminate your hands.
30 Report and record your observations.

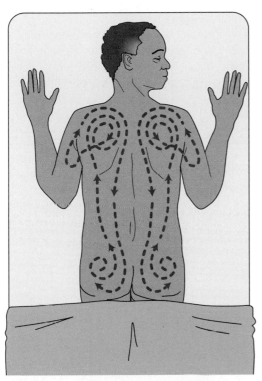

Fig. 11-17 The person lies in the prone position for a back massage. Stroke upward from the buttocks to the shoulders, down over the upper arms, back up the upper arms, across the shoulders, and down the back to the buttocks.

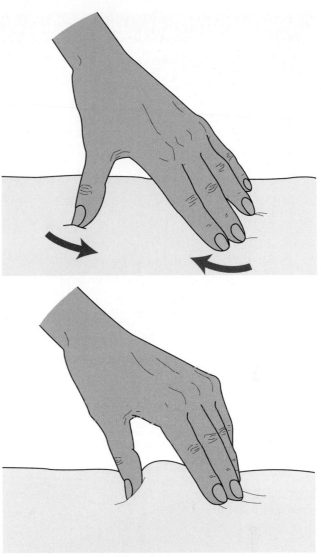

Fig. 11-18 Kneading is done by picking up tissue between the thumb and fingers.

PERINEAL CARE

Perineal care *(pericare)* involves cleaning the genital and anal areas. It prevents infection and odors, and it promotes comfort. Perineal care is done daily during the bath. It also is done whenever the area is soiled with urine or feces.

The person does perineal care if able. Otherwise, it is given by nursing staff. The procedure embarrasses many people and nursing staff, especially when it involves the other sex. *Perineum* and *perineal* are not common terms. Most people understand *privates, private parts, crotch, genitals,* or the *area between your legs.*

Use terms the person understands. The term must also be in good taste professionally.

Work from the cleanest area to the dirtiest. This is commonly called cleaning from "front to back." The urethral area (the front) is the cleanest. The anal area (the back) is the dirtiest. Therefore clean from the urethra to the anal area.

The perineal area is delicate and easily injured. Use warm water, not hot. Use washcloths, towelettes, cotton balls, or swabs according to center policy. Rinse thoroughly. Pat dry after rinsing. This reduces moisture and promotes comfort.

Delegation Guidelines

Perineal Care

Before giving perineal care, you need this information from the nurse and the care plan:

- When perineal care needs to be done
- What terms the person understands—perineum, privates, private parts, crotch, genitals, area between the legs, and so on
- How much help the person needs
- What water temperature to use—usually 105° to 109° F (40.5° to 42.7° C)
- Any position restrictions or limits
- What observations to report and record:
  —Odors
  —Redness, swelling, discharge, or irritation
  —Complaints of pain, burning, or other discomfort
  —Signs of urinary or fecal incontinence (Chapter 13)

Safety Alert

Perineal Care

Hot water can burn delicate perineal tissues. To prevent burns, measure water temperature according to center policy. If the water seems too hot, ask the nurse to check it.

Protect yourself and the person from infection. Contact with blood, body fluids, secretions, and excretions is likely during perineal care. Follow Standard Precautions and the Bloodborne Pathogen Standard.

NOTE: Persons who are incontinent need perineal care. You must protect the person and dry garments from the wet incontinence product. After cleaning and drying the perineal area, remove the wet incontinence products, garments, and linen. Then apply clean, dry ones. (See Chapter 13.)

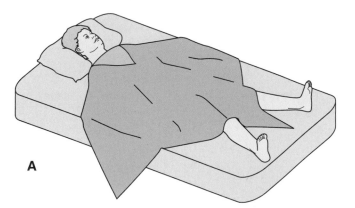
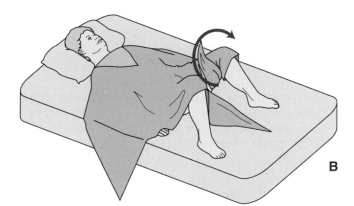

Fig. 11-19 Draping for perineal care. **A,** Position the bath blanket like a diamond: one corner is at the neck, there is a corner at each side, and one corner is between the person's legs. **B,** Wrap the blanket around the leg by bringing the corner around under the leg and over the top. Tuck the corner under the hip.

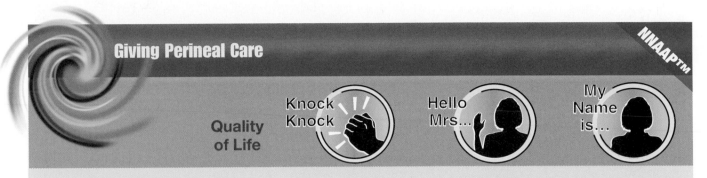

Giving Perineal Care

Pre-Procedure

1. Follow *Delegation Guidelines: Perineal Care.* See *Safety Alert: Perineal Care.*
2. Explain the procedure to the person.
3. Practice hand hygiene.
4. Collect the following:
   - Soap
   - At least 4 washcloths
   - Bath towel
   - Bath blanket
   - Bath thermometer
   - Wash basin
   - Waterproof pad
   - Gloves
   - Paper towels
5. Cover the overbed table with paper towels. Arrange items on top of them.
6. Identify the person. Check the ID bracelet against the assignment sheet. Call the person by name.
7. Provide for privacy.
8. Raise the bed for body mechanics. Bed rails are up if used.

Procedure

9. Lower the bed rail near you if up.
10. Cover the person with a bath blanket. Move top linens to the foot of the bed.
11. Position the person supine.
12. Drape the person as in Figure 11-19.
13. Raise the bed rail if used.
14. Fill the wash basin ⅔ full with water. Water temperature is about 105° to 109° F (40.5° to 42.7° C). Measure water temperature according to center policy.
15. Place the basin on the overbed table.
16. Lower the bed rail if up.
17. Decontaminate your hands. Put on the gloves.
18. Help the person flex the knees and spread the legs. Or help the person spread the legs as much as possible with the knees straight.
19. Place a waterproof pad under the buttocks.
20. Fold the corner of the bath blanket between the legs onto the abdomen.
21. Wet the washcloths. Squeeze out excess water before using them.
22. Apply soap to a washcloth.
23. *For female perineal care:*
    a. Separate the labia. Clean downward from front to back with one stroke (Fig. 11-20, p. 212).
    b. Repeat steps 22 and 23a until the area is clean. Use a clean part of the washcloth for each stroke. Use more than one washcloth if needed.
    c. Rinse the perineum with a clean washcloth. Separate the labia. Stroke downward from front to back. Repeat as necessary. Use a clean part of the washcloth for each stroke. Use more than one washcloth if needed.
    d. Pat the area dry with the towel.
24. *For male perineal care:*
    a. Retract the foreskin if the person is uncircumcised (Fig. 11-21, p. 213).
    b. Grasp the penis.
    c. Clean the tip. Use a circular motion. Start at the meatus of the urethra, and work outward (Fig. 11-22, p. 213). Repeat as needed. Use a clean part of the washcloth each time.
    d. Rinse the area with another washcloth.
    e. Return the foreskin to its natural position.
    f. Clean the shaft of the penis. Use firm downward strokes. Rinse the area.
    g. Help the person flex his knees and spread his legs. Or help him spread his legs as much as possible with his knees straight.
    h. Clean the scrotum. Rinse well. Observe for redness and irritation in the skin folds.
    i. Pat dry the penis and scrotum.
25. Fold the blanket back between the legs.
26. Help the person lower the legs and turn onto the side away from you.
27. Apply soap to a washcloth.

Continued

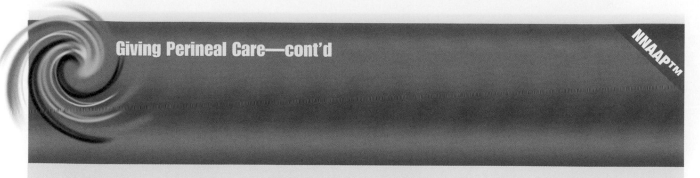

Giving Perineal Care—cont'd

Procedure—cont'd

28 Clean the rectal area with one stroke. For a female, clean from the vagina to the anus (Fig. 11-23).

29 Repeat steps 27 and 28 until the area is clean. Use a clean part of the washcloth for each stroke. Use more than one washcloth if needed.

30 Rinse the rectal area with a washcloth. For a female, stroke from the vagina to the anus.

Repeat as necessary. Use a clean part of the washcloth for each stroke. Use more than one washcloth if needed.

31 Pat the area dry with the towel.

32 Remove the waterproof pad.

33 Remove and discard the gloves. Decontaminate your hands.

Post-Procedure

34 Provide for comfort.

35 Cover the person. Remove the bath blanket.

36 Lower the bed to its lowest position.

37 Raise or lower bed rails. Follow the care plan.

38 Place the signal light within reach.

39 Empty and clean the wash basin. Wear gloves.

40 Return the basin and supplies to their proper place.

41 Wipe off the overbed table with the paper towels. Discard the paper towels.

42 Remove the gloves. Decontaminate your hands.

43 Unscreen the person.

44 Complete a safety check of the room. (See inside of front book cover.)

45 Follow center policy for dirty linen.

46 Decontaminate your hands.

47 Report and record your observations.

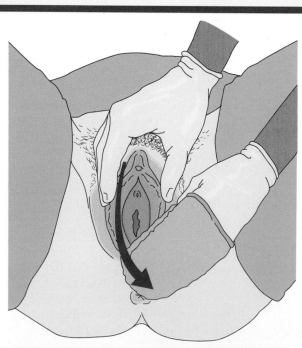

Fig. 11-20 Separate the labia with one hand. Use a mitted washcloth to cleanse between the labia with downward strokes.

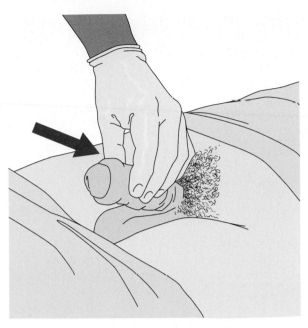

Fig. 11-21 The foreskin of the uncircumcised male is pulled back for perineal care. It is returned to the normal position immediately after cleaning.

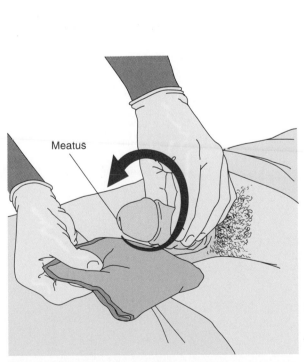

Fig. 11-22 The penis is cleaned with circular motions starting at the meatus of the urethra.

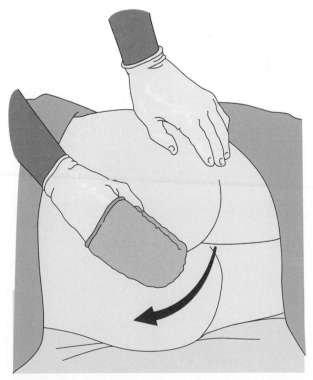

Fig. 11-23 The rectal area is cleaned by wiping from the vagina to the anus. The side-lying position allows the anal area to be cleaned more thoroughly.

Review Questions

Circle **T** if the statement is true or **F** if the statement is false.

1   **T F**   After lunch Mr. Lee wants a back massage. You can give a back massage then.

2   **T F**   Mrs. Bell's toothbrush has hard bristles. They are good for oral hygiene.

3   **T F**   Unconscious persons are supine for mouth care.

4   **T F**   Your fingers keep an unconscious person's mouth open for oral hygiene.

5   **T F**   Mrs. Bell has a lower denture. It is washed over a counter.

6   **T F**   A tub bath lasts 30 minutes.

7   **T F**   You can give permission for showers, but not tub baths.

8   **T F**   Weak persons are left alone in the shower if they are sitting.

9   **T F**   A back massage relaxes muscles and stimulates circulation.

10   **T F**   Perineal care helps prevent infection.

11   **T F**   Foreskin is returned to its normal position immediately after cleaning.

Circle the **BEST** answer.

12   You brush Mrs. Bell's teeth and note the following. Which is *not* reported to the nurse?
  a   Bleeding, swelling, or redness of the gums
  b   Irritations, sores, or white patches in the mouth or on the tongue
  c   Lips that are dry, cracked, swollen, or blistered
  d   Food between the teeth.

13   Which action is *wrong* when bathing Mrs. Bell?
  a   Covering her for warmth and privacy.
  b   Rinsing her skin thoroughly to remove all soap.
  c   Washing from the dirtiest to cleanest area.
  d   Patting her skin dry.

14   What is a safe water temperature for a complete bed bath?
  a   95° F
  b   100° F
  c   110° F
  d   120° F

15   You are going to give a back massage. Which is *false?*
  a   It should last 3 to 5 minutes.
  b   Lotion is warmed before being applied.
  c   Your hands are always in contact with the skin.
  d   The side-lying position is best.

Answers to these questions are on p. 389.

CHAPTER 12

Grooming

Objectives

- Define the key terms listed in this chapter
- Explain the importance of hair care, shaving, and nail and foot care
- Describe the safety measures for shaving a person
- Describe the rules for changing gowns and clothing
- Perform the procedures described in this chapter

alopecia Hair loss
dandruff Excessive amount of dry, white flakes from the scalp

hirsutism Excessive body hair in women and children

Hair care, shaving, nail and foot care, and clean clothes promote comfort and well-being. They also promote quality of life. Hair and nails are discussed in Box 12-1.

HAIR CARE

Many nursing centers have beauty and barber shops where residents can have hair shampooed, cut, and styled. Men also can have mustaches and beards groomed. You assist with daily hair care.

The care plan reflects the person's culture, personal choice, skin and scalp condition, health history, and self-care ability. These terms are common in care plans:

- **Alopecia** means hair loss. Hair loss may be complete or partial. Male pattern baldness occurs with aging and is the result of heredity. Hair also thins in some women with aging. Cancer treatments often cause alopecia in males and females.
- **Hirsutism** is excessive body hair in women and children. It results from heredity and abnormal amounts of male hormones.
- **Dandruff** is the excessive amount of dry, white flakes from the scalp. Itching often occurs. Sometimes eyebrows and ear canals are involved.

Brushing and Combing Hair

Brushing and combing hair are part of early morning care, morning care, and afternoon care. They also are done whenever needed. Encourage residents to do their own hair care. Assist as needed. The person chooses how to brush, comb, and style hair.

Long hair easily mats and tangles. Daily brushing and combing prevent the problem. So does braiding. Do not braid hair without the person's consent. *Never cut matted or tangled hair.*

When brushing and combing hair, start at the scalp. Then brush or comb to the hair ends. To brush or comb through matted or tangled hair or cut hair for any other reason.

- Take a small section of hair near the ends.
- Comb or brush through to the hair ends.
- Working up to the scalp, add small sections of hair.
- Comb or brush through each longer section to the hair ends.
- Brush or comb from the scalp to the hair ends.

Special measures are needed for curly, coarse, and dry hair. Use a wide-toothed comb for curly hair. Start at the neckline. Working upward, lift and fluff hair outward. Continue to the forehead. To make combing easier, wet hair or apply a conditioner or petroleum jelly as directed. The person's hair care practices and hair care products used are part of the care plan. Also, the person can guide you when giving hair care. See *Caring About Culture: Braiding Hair.*

Caring About Culture

Braiding Hair

Styling hair in small braids is a common practice of some cultural groups. The braids are left intact for shampooing. To undo these braids, the nurse obtains the person's consent.

Delegation Guidelines

Brushing and Combing Hair

To brush and comb hair, you need this information from the nurse and care plan:
- How much help the person needs
- What to do if hair is matted and tangled
- What measures are needed for curly, coarse, or dry hair
- What hair care products to use
- The person's preferences and routine hair care measures
- What observations to report and record:
  —Scalp sores
  —Flaking
  —Presence of lice
  —Patches of hair loss
  —Very dry or very oily hair

Safety Alert

Brushing and Combing Hair

Sharp brush bristles can injure the scalp. So can a comb with sharp or broken teeth. Tell the nurse if you have concerns about the person's brush or comb.

BOX 12-1 The Hair and Nails

Structure and Function

The entire body, except the palms of the hands and soles of the feet, is covered with hair. Hair in the nose and ears and around the eyes protects these organs from dust, insects, and other objects.

Oil glands secrete an oily substance into the space near the hair shaft. Oil travels to the skin surface, helping to keep the hair and skin soft and shiny.

Nails protect the tips of fingers and toes. Nails help fingers pick up and handle small items.

Changes With Aging

White or gray hair is common. Some men lose a lot of hair. Hair thins on men and women. Hair is drier from decreases in scalp oils. Nails become thick and tough.

Common Disorders

- *Pediculosis (lice)* is the infestation with lice. (Infestation means being in or on a host.) Lice are parasites. Lice bites cause severe itching in the affected area.
- *Pediculosis capitis* is the infestation of the scalp *(capitis)* with lice.
- *Pediculosis pubis* is the infestation of the pubic *(pubis)* hair with lice. Head and pubic lice attach their eggs to hair shafts.
- *Pediculosis corporis* is the infestation of the body *(corporis)* with lice. Lice eggs attach to clothing and furniture. Lice easily spread to others through clothing, furniture, bed linen, and sexual contact. They also are spread by sharing combs and brushes. Medicated shampoos, lotions, and creams are used to treat lice. Thorough bathing is needed. So is washing clothing and linen in hot water. Report signs of lice to the nurse at once.

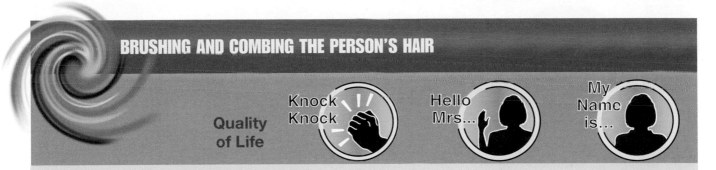

BRUSHING AND COMBING THE PERSON'S HAIR

Quality of Life — Knock Knock — Hello Mrs... — My Name is...

Pre-Procedure

1 Follow *Delegation Guidelines: Brushing and Combing Hair.* See *Safety Alert: Brushing and Combing Hair.*
2 Practice hand hygiene.
3 Identify the person. Check the ID bracelet against the assignment sheet. Call the person by name.
4 Explain the procedure to the person. Ask the person how to style hair.
5 Collect the following:
 - Comb and brush
 - Bath towel
 - Hair care items as requested
6 Arrange items on the bedside stand.
7 Provide for privacy.

Procedure

8 Lower the bed rail if used.
9 Help the person to the chair. The person puts on a robe and nonskid footwear when up. (If the person is in bed, raise the bed for body mechanics. Bed rails are up if used. Lower the near bed rail. Assist the person to semi-Fowler's position if allowed.)
10 Place a towel across the shoulders or across the pillow.
11 Ask the person to remove eyeglasses. Put them in the eyeglass case: Put the case inside the bedside stand.
12 Part hair into 2 sections (Fig. 12-1, A, p. 218). Divide one side into 2 sections (Fig. 12-1, B, p. 218). Use the comb for this step.
13 Brush the hair. Start at the scalp, and brush toward the hair ends (Fig. 12-2, p. 218).
14 Use the comb to divide the other side into sections. Brush the hair as in step 13.
15 Style the hair as the person prefers.
16 Remove the towel.
17 Let the person put on the eyeglasses.

Continued

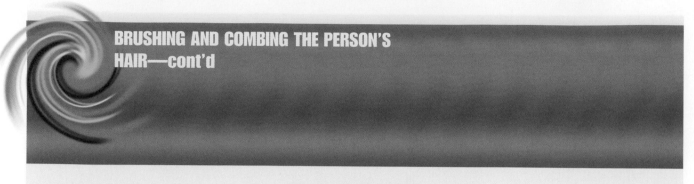

BRUSHING AND COMBING THE PERSON'S HAIR—cont'd

Post-Procedure

18 Provide for comfort.
19 Lower the bed to its lowest position.
20 Raise or lower bed rails. Follow the care plan.
21 Place the signal light within reach.
22 Unscreen the person.
23 Clean and return items to their proper place.
24 Complete a safety check of the room. (See inside of front book cover.)
25 Follow center policy for dirty linen.
26 Decontaminate your hands.

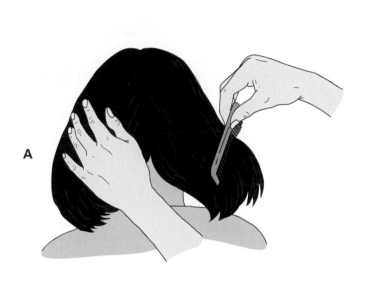

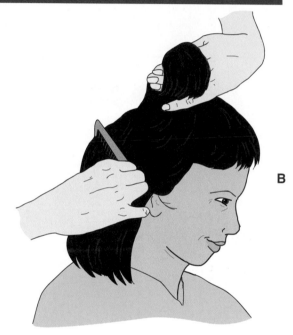

Fig. 12-1 Parting hair. **A,** Part hair down the middle. Divide it into two main sections. **B,** Then part the main section into two smaller sections.

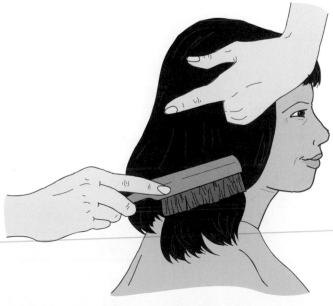

Fig. 12-2 Brush hair by starting at the scalp. Brush down to the hair ends.

Shampooing

Shampooing is usually done weekly on the person's bath or shower day. If a woman's hair is done in the beauty shop, do not shampoo her hair. She wears a shower cap during the tub bath or shower.

After shampooing, dry and style hair as quickly as possible. Women may want hair curled or rolled up before drying. Check with the nurse before doing so.

The shampoo method depends on the person's condition, safety, and personal choice:

* *Shampoo during the shower or tub bath.* A hand-held nozzle is used. A spray of water is directed to the hair.
* *Shampoo at the sink.* The person sits facing away from the sink. A folded towel is placed over the sink edge to protect the neck. The person's head is tilted back over the edge of the sink. A water pitcher or hand-held nozzle is used to wet and rinse the hair.
* *Shampoo on a stretcher.* The stretcher is in front of the sink. A towel is placed under the neck. The head is tilted over the edge of the sink (Fig. 12-3, p. 220). A water pitcher or hand-held nozzle is used to wet and rinse the hair. Remember to lock the stretcher wheels, use the safety straps, and raise the far side rail.
* *Shampoo in bed.* The person's head and shoulders are moved to the edge of the bed if possible. A shampoo tray is placed under the head to protect the linens and mattress from water. The tray also drains water into a basin placed on a chair by the bed (Fig. 12-4, p. 220). Use a water pitcher to wet and rinse the hair.

Delegation Guidelines

Shampooing

Before shampooing hair, you need this information from the nurse and the care plan:

* When to shampoo the person's hair
* What method to use
* What shampoo and conditioner to use
* The person's position restrictions or limits
* What water temperature to use—usually 105° F (40.5° C)
* If hair is curled or rolled up before drying
* What observations to report and record:
  —Scalp sores
  —Hair falling out in patches
  —The presence of lice
  —How the person tolerated the procedure

Safety Alert

Shampooing

When shampooing during the tub bath or shower, the person tips his or her head back to keep shampoo and water out of the eyes. Support the back of the head with one hand as you shampoo with the other. Some older people cannot tip their heads back. They lean forward and hold a washcloth over the eyes. Support the forehead with one hand as you shampoo with the other. Make sure the person can breathe easily.

Many older people have limited range of motion in their necks. They cannot tolerate shampooing at the sink or on a stretcher.

You must keep shampoo out of the eyes. The person holds a hand towel or washcloth over the eyes. Do not let shampoo get near the eyes. When rinsing, cup your hand at the person's forehead. This keeps soapy water from running down the person's forehead and into the eyes.

If a medicated shampoo or conditioner is used, return it to the nurse. Never leave it at the bedside unless instructed to do so.

Follow Standard Precautions if the person has scalp lesions. Also follow the Bloodborne Pathogen Standard.

Text continued on p. 222

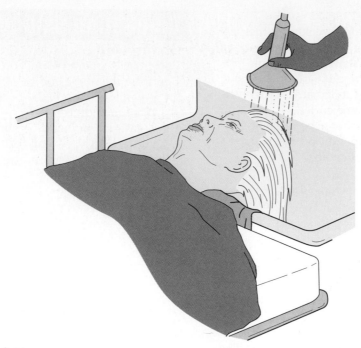

Fig. 12-3 Shampooing while the person is on a stretcher. The stretcher is in front of the sink.

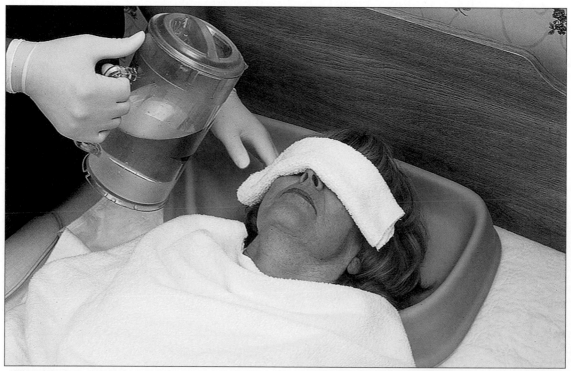

Fig. 12-4 A shampoo tray is used to shampoo a person in bed. The tray is directed to the side of the bed so water drains into a collecting basin.

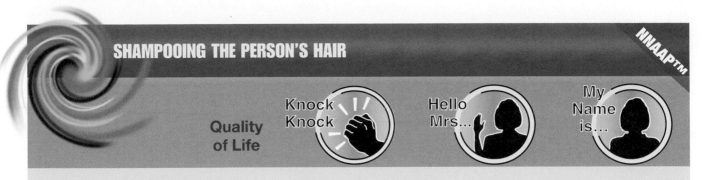

SHAMPOOING THE PERSON'S HAIR

Pre-Procedure

1 Follow *Delegation Guidelines: Shampooing*, p. 219. See *Safety Alert: Shampooing*, p. 219.
2 Explain the procedure to the person.
3 Practice hand hygiene.
4 Collect the following:
   - Two bath towels
   - Hand towel or washcloth
   - Shampoo
   - Hair conditioner (if requested)
   - Bath thermometer
   - Pitcher or nozzle (if needed)
   - Shampoo tray (if needed)
   - Basin or pan (if needed)
   - Waterproof pad (if needed)
   - Gloves (if needed)
   - Comb and brush
   - Hair dryer
5 Arrange items nearby.
6 Identify the person. Check the ID bracelet against the assignment sheet. Call the person by name.
7 Provide for privacy.
8 Raise the bed for body mechanics for a shampoo in bed. The far bed rail is up if bed rails are used.

Procedure

9 Position the person for the method you will use. Place the waterproof pad and shampoo tray under the head and shoulders if needed.
10 Place a bath towel across the shoulders or across the pillow.
11 Brush and comb the hair to remove snarls and tangles.
12 Raise the bed rail if used.
13 Obtain water. Water temperature should be about 105° F (40.5° C). Test temperature according to center policy.
14 Lower the bed rail (if used).
15 Put on gloves (if needed).
16 Ask the person to hold a dampened hand towel or washcloth over the eyes. It should not cover the nose and mouth. (A damp towel or washcloth is easier to hold. It will not slip.)
17 Use the pitcher or nozzle to wet the hair.
18 Apply a small amount of shampoo.
19 Work up a lather with both hands. Start at the hairline. Work toward the back of the head.
20 Massage the scalp with your fingertips. Do not scratch the scalp.
21 Rinse the hair.
22 Repeat steps 18 through 21.
23 Apply conditioner. Follow directions on the container.
24 Squeeze water from the person's hair.
25 Cover hair with a bath towel.
26 Dry the person's face with a towel.
27 Help the person raise the head if appropriate. For the person in bed, raise the head of the bed.
28 Rub the hair and scalp with the towel. Use the second towel if the first is wet.
29 Comb the hair to remove snarls and tangles.
30 Dry and style hair as quickly as possible.

Post-Procedure

31 Remove and discard the gloves (if used). Decontaminate your hands.
32 Provide for comfort.
33 Lower the bed to its lowest position.
34 Raise or lower bed rails. Follow the care plan.
35 Place the signal light within reach.
36 Unscreen the person.
37 Clean and return equipment to its proper place. Discard disposable items.
38 Complete a safety check of the room. (See inside of front book cover.)
39 Follow center policy for dirty linen.
40 Decontaminate your hands.

SHAVING

Many men shave for comfort and mental well-being. Many women shave their legs and underarms. Women with coarse facial hair may shave. Or they may use other hair removal methods. See Box 12-2 for shaving rules.

Blade and electric shavers are used. Clean electric shavers after each use. Safety razors (blade razors) can cause nicks or cuts. They are not used for persons:

- With dementia. They may resist care and move suddenly.
- Who take drugs that prevent or slow down blood clotting. Bleeding occurs easily. A nick or cut can cause serious bleeding.

Soften the beard and skin before using a safety razor. Apply a warm washcloth or towel to the face for a few minutes. Then lather the face with soap and water or a shaving cream. Women's legs and underarms are shaved after bathing when the skin is soft.

Beards and mustaches need daily care. Food can collect in hair. So can mouth and nose drainage. Daily washing and combing are needed. Ask the person how to groom his beard or mustache. *Never trim or shave a beard or mustache without the person's consent.*

Delegation Guidelines

Shaving

To shave a person, you need this information from the nurse and care plan:

- What shaver to use—electric or safety razor
- When to shave the person

Safety Alert

Shaving

Safety razors are very sharp. Protect the person and yourself from nicks or cuts. Prevent contact with blood.

You will rinse the razor often during the shaving procedure. Then you will wipe the razor with tissues or paper towels. To protect yourself from cuts, place the tissues or paper towels on the overbed table. Do not hold them in your hand.

Follow Standard Precautions and the Bloodborne Pathogen Standard. Discard used razor blades and disposable shavers in the sharps container.

BOX 12-2   Rules for Shaving

- Use electric shavers for persons taking drugs that prevent blood clotting (anticoagulant drugs). Never use safety razors.
- Protect bed linens. Place a towel under the part being shaved. Or place a towel across the shoulders to protect clothing.
- Soften the skin before shaving.
- Encourage the person to do as much as safely possible.
- Hold the skin taut as needed.
- Shave in the direction of hair growth when shaving the face and underarms.
- Shave up from the ankles when shaving legs. This is against hair growth.
- Do not cut, nick, or irritate the skin.
- Rinse the body part thoroughly.
- Apply direct pressure to nicks or cuts.
- Report nicks, cuts, or irritation to the nurse at once.

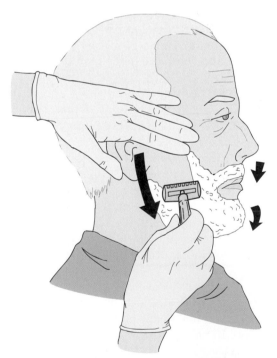

Fig. 12-5 Shave in the direction of hair growth. Use longer strokes on the larger areas of the face. Use short strokes around the chin and lips.

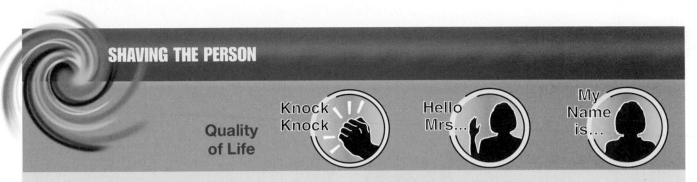

SHAVING THE PERSON

Quality of Life — Knock Knock — Hello Mrs... — My Name is...

Pre-Procedure

1 Follow *Delegation Guidelines: Shaving.* See *Safety Alert: Shaving.*
2 Explain the procedure to the person.
3 Practice hand hygiene.
4 Collect the following:
   - Wash basin
   - Bath towel
   - Hand towel
   - Washcloth
   - Safety razor
   - Mirror
   - Shaving cream, soap, or lotion
   - Shaving brush
   - After-shave lotion (men only)
   - Tissues or paper towels
   - Paper towels
   - Gloves
5 Arrange paper towels and supplies on the overbed table.
6 Identify the person. Check the ID bracelet against the assignment sheet. Call the person by name.
7 Provide for privacy.
8 Raise the bed for body mechanics. Bed rails are up if used.

Procedure

9 Fill the basin with warm water.
10 Place the basin on the overbed table.
11 Lower the bed rail near you if up.
12 Assist the person to semi-Fowler's position if allowed or to the supine position.
13 Adjust lighting to clearly see the person's face.
14 Place the bath towel over the chest.
15 Adjust the overbed table for easy reach.
16 Tighten the razor blade to the shaver.
17 Wash the person's face. Do not dry.
18 Wet the washcloth or towel. Wring it out.
19 Apply the washcloth or towel to the face for a few minutes.
20 Put on gloves.
21 Apply shaving cream with your hands. Or use a shaving brush to apply lather.
22 Hold the skin taut with one hand.
23 Shave in the direction of hair growth. Use short strokes around the chin and lips (Fig. 12-5).
24 Rinse the razor often. Wipe it with tissues or paper towels.
25 Apply direct pressure to any bleeding areas.
26 Wash off any remaining shaving cream or soap. Dry with a towel.
27 Apply after-shave lotion if requested.
28 Remove the towel and gloves. Decontaminate your hands.
29 Move the overbed table to the side of the bed.

Post-Procedure

30 Provide for comfort.
31 Place the signal light within reach.
32 Lower the bed to its lowest position.
33 Raise or lower bed rails. Follow the care plan.
34 Clean and return equipment and supplies to their proper place. Discard disposable items. Wear gloves.
35 Wipe off the overbed table with the paper towels. Discard the paper towels.
36 Remove the gloves. Decontaminate your hands.
37 Position the overbed table for the person.
38 Unscreen the person.
39 Complete a safety check of the room. (See inside of front book cover.)
40 Follow center policy for dirty linen.
41 Decontaminate your hands.
42 Report nicks, cuts, or bleeding to the nurse. Also report and record other observations.

NAIL AND FOOT CARE

Nail and foot care prevent infection, injury, and odors. Hangnails, ingrown nails (nails that grow in at the side), and nails torn away from the skin cause skin breaks. Long or broken nails can scratch skin or snag clothing. Dirty feet, socks, or stockings harbor microbes and cause odors. Nails are easier to trim and clean after soaking or bathing. Use nail clippers to cut fingernails. *Never use scissors.* Use extreme caution to prevent damage to nearby tissues.

Some centers do not let nursing assistants cut or trim toenails. Follow center policy.

Delegation Guidelines

Nail and Foot Care

To give nail and foot care, you need this information from the nurse and the care plan:

- What water temperature to use
- How long to soak fingernails (usually 5 to 10 minutes)
- How long to soak the feet (usually 15 to 20 minutes)
- What observations to report and record:
  —Reddened, irritated, or calloused areas
  —Breaks in the skin
  —Corns on top of and between toes
  —Very thick nails
  —Loose nails

Safety Alert

Nail and Foot Care

You do not cut or trim toenails if a person:

- Has diabetes
- Has poor circulation to the legs and feet
- Takes drugs that affect blood clotting
- Has very thick nails or ingrown toenails

The RN or podiatrist (foot [pod] doctor) cuts toenails and provides foot care for these persons.

Check between the toes for cracks and sores. These areas often are overlooked. If left untreated, a serious infection could occur.

The feet are easily burned. Persons with decreased sensation or circulatory problems may not feel hot temperatures.

Breaks in the skin and bleeding can occur. Follow Standard Precautions and the Bloodborne Pathogen Standard.

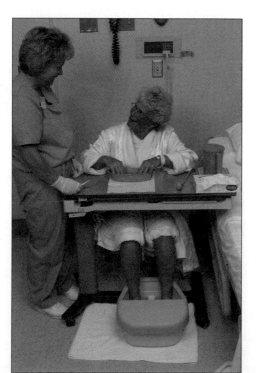

Fig. 12-6 Nail and foot care. The feet soak in a whirlpool foot bath, and the fingers soak in a kidney basin.

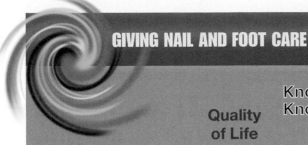

Quality
of Life

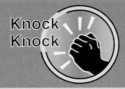

Knock
Knock

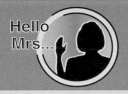

Hello
Mrs...

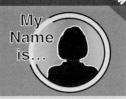

My
Name
is...

Pre-Procedure

1 Follow *Delegation Guidelines: Nail and Foot Care.* See *Safety Alert: Nail and Foot Care.*
2 Explain the procedure to the person.
3 Practice hand hygiene.
4 Collect the following:
   - Wash basin or whirlpool foot bath
   - Soap
   - Bath thermometer
   - Bath towel
   - Hand towel
   - Washcloth
   - Kidney basin
   - Nail clippers
   - Orange stick
   - Emery board or nail file
   - Lotion for hands; lotion or petroleum jelly for feet.
   - Paper towels
   - Disposable bath mat
   - Gloves
5 Arrange paper towels and other items on the overbed table.
6 Identify the person. Check the ID bracelet against the assignment sheet. Call the person by name.
7 Provide for privacy.
8 Assist the person to the bedside chair. Place the signal light within reach.

Procedure

9 Place the bath mat under the feet.
10 Fill the wash basin or whirlpool foot bath ⅔ full with water. The nurse tells you what water temperature to use. (Measure water temperature with a bath thermometer. Or test it by dipping your elbow or inner wrist into the basin.)
11 Place the basin or foot bath on the bath mat.
12 Help the person put the feet into the basin or foot bath.
13 Adjust the overbed table in front of the person.
14 Fill the kidney basin ⅔ full with water. See step 10 for water temperature.
15 Place the kidney basin on the overbed table.
16 Place the person's fingers into the basin. Position the arms for comfort (Fig. 12-6).
17 Let the fingers soak for 5 to 10 minutes. Let the feet soak for 15 to 20 minutes. Rewarm water as needed.
18 Decontaminate your hands. Put on gloves.
19 Clean under the fingernails with the orange stick. Use a towel to wipe the orange stick after each nail.
20 Remove the kidney basin. Dry the hands and between the fingers thoroughly.
21 Clip fingernails straight across with the nail clippers (Fig. 12-7, p. 226).
22 Shape nails with an emery board or nail file.
23 Push cuticles back with the orange stick or a washcloth (Fig. 12-8, p. 226).
24 Apply lotion to the hands. Warm lotion before applying it.
25 Move the overbed table to the side.
26 Wash the feet with soap and a washcloth. Wash between the toes.
27 Remove the feet from the basin or foot bath. Dry thoroughly, especially between the toes.
28 Apply lotion or petroleum jelly to the tops and soles of the feet. Do not apply between the toes. Warm lotion before applying it.
29 Remove and discard the gloves. Decontaminate your hands.
30 Help the person put on socks and nonskid footwear.

Post-Procedure

31 Provide for comfort.
32 Place the signal light within reach.
33 Raise or lower bed rails. Follow the care plan.
34 Clean and return equipment and supplies to their proper place. Discard disposable items. Wear gloves for this step.
35 Remove the gloves. Decontaminate your hands.
36 Unscreen the person.
37 Complete a safety check of the room. (See inside of front book cover.)
38 Follow center policy for dirty linen.
39 Decontaminate your hands.
40 Report and record your observations.

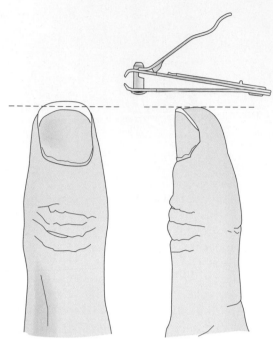

Fig. 12-7 Clip fingernails straight across. Use a nail clipper.

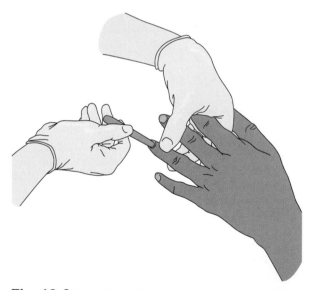

Fig. 12-8 Push the cuticle back with an orange stick.

CHANGING CLOTHING AND GOWNS

Some residents wear regular clothes. They dress in the morning and change into sleepwear for bed. Incontinent persons may change more often. Other residents wear hospital gowns (p. 232).

Some persons need help changing clothing and gowns. Follow these rules:

- Provide for privacy. Do not expose the person.
- Encourage the person to do as much as possible.
- Let the person choose what to wear. Make sure the right undergarments are chosen.
- Remove clothing from the strong or "good" side first.
- Put clothing on the weak side first.
- Support the arm or leg when removing or putting on a garment.

Text continued on p. 232

Delegation Guidelines

Changing Clothing
Before changing clothing, you need this information from the nurse and the care plan:
- How much help the person needs
- The person's strong side and weak side
- If the person needs to wear certain garments
- What observations to report and record:
  —How much help was given
  —How the person tolerated the procedure
  —Any complaints by the person

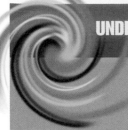

UNDRESSING THE PERSON

Quality of Life

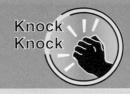 Knock Knock

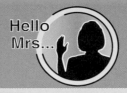 Hello Mrs...

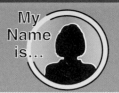 My Name is...

Pre-Procedure

1 Follow *Delegation Guidelines: Changing Clothing.*
2 Explain the procedure to the person.
3 Practice hand hygiene.
4 Get a bath blanket and clothing requested by the person.
5 Identify the person. Check the ID bracelet against the assignment sheet. Call the person by name.
6 Provide for privacy.
7 Raise the bed for body mechanics. Bed rails are up if used.
8 Lower the bed rail on the person's weak side.
9 Position him or her supine.
10 Cover the person with the bath blanket. Fanfold linens to the foot of the bed.

Procedure

11 Remove garments that open in the back:
  a Raise the head and shoulders. Or turn him or her onto the side away from you.
  b Undo buttons, zippers, ties, or snaps.
  c Bring the sides of the garment to the sides of the person (Fig. 12-9, p. 228). If he or she is in a side-lying position, tuck the far side under the person. Fold the near side onto the chest (Fig. 12-10, p. 228).
  d Position the person supine.
  e Slide the garment off the shoulder on the strong side. Remove it from the arm (Fig. 12-11, p. 228).
  f Repeat step 11e for the weak side.
12 Remove garments that open in the front:
  a Undo buttons, zippers, ties, or snaps.
  b Slide the garment off the shoulder and arm on the strong side.
  c Raise the head and shoulders. Bring the garment over to the weak side (Fig. 12-12, p. 228). Lower the head and shoulders.
  d Remove the garment from the weak side.
  e If you cannot raise the head and shoulders:
    (1) Turn the person toward you. Tuck the removed part under the person.
    (2) Turn him or her onto the side away from you.
    (3) Pull the side of the garment out from under the person. Make sure he or she will not lie on it when supine.
    (4) Return the person to the supine position.
    (5) Remove the garment from the weak side.
13 Remove pullover garments:
  a Undo buttons, zippers, ties, or snaps.

  b Remove the garment from the strong side.
  c Raise the head and shoulders. Or turn the person onto the side away from you. Bring the garment up to the person's neck (Fig. 12-13, p. 228).
  d Remove the garment from the weak side.
  e Bring the garment over the person's head.
  f Position him or her in the supine position.
14 Remove pants or slacks:
  a Remove footwear.
  b Position the person supine.
  c Undo buttons, zippers, ties, snaps, or buckles.
  d Remove the belt.
  e Ask the person to lift the buttocks off the bed. Slide the pants down over the hips and buttocks (Fig. 12-14, p. 229). Have the person lower the hips and buttocks.
  f If the person cannot raise the hips off the bed:
    (1) Turn the person toward you.
    (2) Slide the pants off the hip and buttock on the strong side (Fig. 12-15, p. 229).
    (3) Turn the person away from you.
    (4) Slide the pants off the hip and buttock on the weak side (Fig. 12-16, p. 229).
  g Slide the pants down the legs and over the feet.
15 Dress the person. See procedure: *Dressing the Person*, p. 230.
16 Help the person get out of bed if he or she is to be up. If the person will stay in bed:
  a Cover the person, and remove the bath blanket.
  b Provide for comfort.
  c Lower the bed to its lowest position.
  d Raise or lower bed rails. Follow the care plan.

Post-Procedure

17 Place the signal light within the person's reach.
18 Unscreen the person.
19 Complete a safety check of the room. (See inside of front book cover.)
20 Follow center policy for soiled clothing.
21 Decontaminate your hands.
22 Report and record your observations.

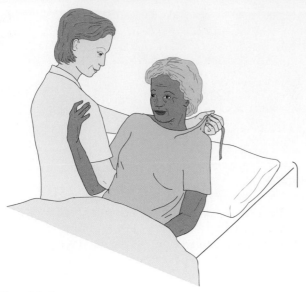

Fig. 12-9 The sides of the garment are brought from the back to the sides of the person.

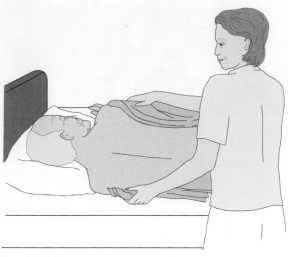

Fig. 12-10 A garment that opens in back is removed from the person in the side-lying position. The far side of the garment is tucked under the person. The near side is folded onto the person's chest.

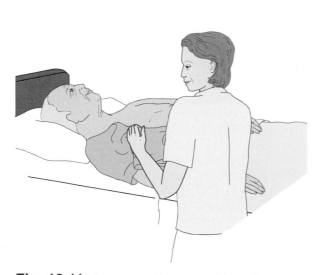

Fig. 12-11 The garment is removed from the strong side first.

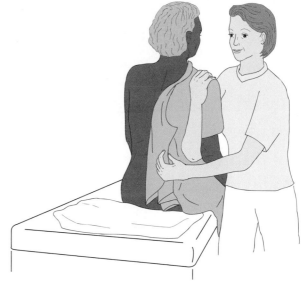

Fig. 12-12 A front-opening garment is removed with the person's head and shoulders raised. The garment is removed from the strong side first. Then it is brought around the back to the weak side.

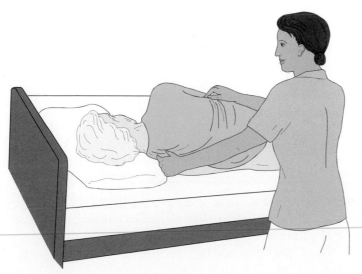

Fig. 12-13 A pullover garment is removed from the strong side first. Then the garment is brought up to the person's neck so that it can be removed from the weak side.

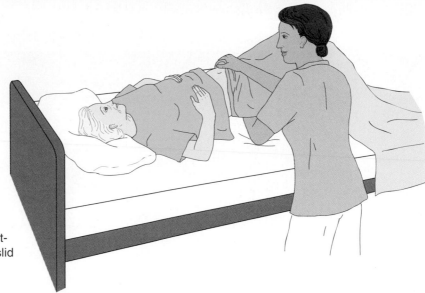

Fig. 12-14 The person lifts the hips and buttocks for removing the pants. The pants are slid down over the hips and buttocks.

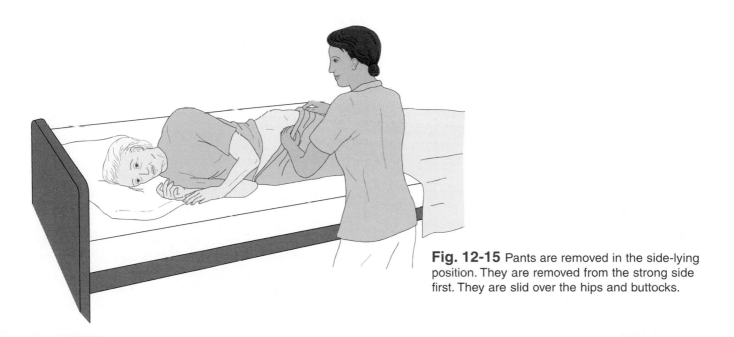
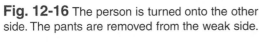

Fig. 12-15 Pants are removed in the side-lying position. They are removed from the strong side first. They are slid over the hips and buttocks.

Fig. 12-16 The person is turned onto the other side. The pants are removed from the weak side.

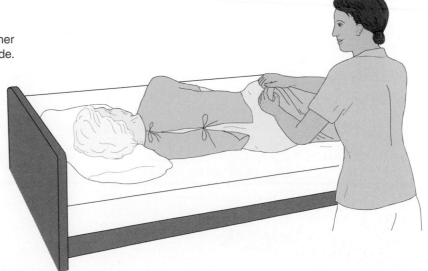

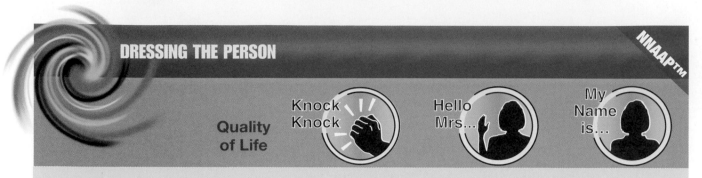

DRESSING THE PERSON

Quality of Life • Knock Knock • Hello Mrs... • My Name is...

Pre-Procedure

1 Follow *Delegation Guidelines: Changing Clothing,* p. 226.
2 Explain the procedure to the person.
3 Practice hand hygiene.
4 Get a bath blanket and clothing requested by the person.
5 Identify the person. Check the ID bracelet against the assignment sheet. Call the person by name.
6 Provide for privacy.
7 Raise the bed for body mechanics. Bed rails are up if used.
8 Lower the bed rail (if up) on the person's strong side.
9 Undress the person. (See procedure: *Undressing the Person*, p. 227).
10 Position the person supine.

Procedure

11 Cover the person with the bath blanket. Fanfold linens to the foot of the bed.
12 Put on garments that open in the back:
   a Slide the garment onto the arm and shoulder of the weak side.
   b Slide the garment onto the arm and shoulder of the strong side.
   c Raise the person's head and shoulders.
   d Bring the sides to the back.
   e If the person is in a side-lying position:
      (1) Turn the person toward you.
      (2) Bring one side of the garment to the person's back (Fig. 12-17, A).
      (3) Turn the person away from you.
      (4) Bring the other side to the person's back (Fig. 12-17, B).
   f Fasten buttons, snaps, ties, or zippers.
   g Position the person supine.
13 Put on garments that open in the front:
   a Slide the garment onto the arm and shoulder on the weak side.
   b Raise the head and shoulders. Bring the side of the garment around to the back. Lower the person down. Slide the garment onto the arm and shoulder of the strong arm.
   c If the person cannot raise the head and shoulders:
      (1) Turn the person toward you.
      (2) Tuck the garment under him or her.

   (3) Turn the person away from you.
   (4) Pull the garment out from under him or her.
   (5) Turn the person back to the supine position.
   (6) Slide the garment over the arm and shoulder of the strong arm.
   d Fasten buttons, snaps, ties, or zippers.
14 Put on pullover garments:
   a Position the person supine.
   b Bring the neck of the garment over the head.
   c Slide the arm and shoulder of the garment onto the weak side.
   d Raise the person's head and shoulders.
   e Bring the garment down.
   f Slide the arm and shoulder of the garment onto the strong side.
   g If the person cannot assume a semi-sitting position:
      (1) Turn the person toward you.
      (2) Tuck the garment under the person.
      (3) Turn the person away from you.
      (4) Pull the garment out from under him or her.
      (5) Position the person supine.
      (6) Slide the arm and shoulder of the garment onto the strong side.
   h Fasten buttons, snaps, ties, or zippers.

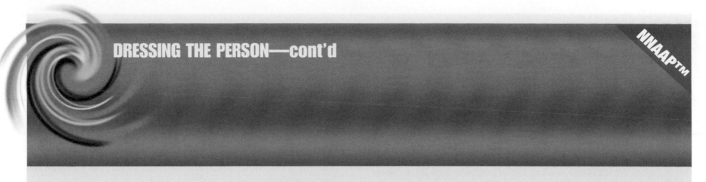

DRESSING THE PERSON—cont'd

NNAAP™

Procedure—cont'd

15 Put on pants or slacks:
- a Slide the pants over the feet and up the legs.
- b Ask the person to raise the hips and buttocks off the bed.
- c Bring the pants up over the buttocks and hips.
- d Ask the person to lower the hips and buttocks.
- e If the person cannot raise the hips and buttocks:
  - (1) Turn person onto the strong side.
  - (2) Pull the pants over the buttock and hip on the weak side.
  - (3) Turn the person onto the weak side.
  - (4) Pull the pants over the buttock and hip on the strong side.
  - (5) Position the person supine.
- f Fasten buttons, ties, snaps, zipper, and the belt buckle.

16 Put socks and footwear on the person.

17 Help the person get out of bed. If the person will stay in bed:
- a Cover the person, and remove the bath blanket.
- b Provide for comfort.
- c Lower the bed to its lowest position.
- d Raise or lower bed rails. Follow the care plan.

Post-Procedure

18 Place the signal light within reach.
19 Unscreen the person.
20 Complete a safety check of the room. (See inside of front book cover.)
21 Follow center policy for soiled clothing.
22 Decontaminate your hands.
23 Report and record your observations.

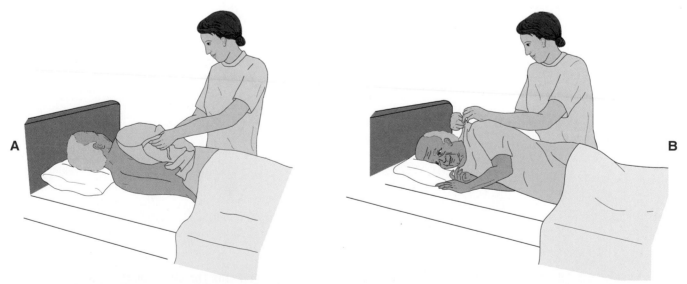

A   B

Fig. 12-17 Dressing a person. **A,** The side-lying position can be used to put on garments that open in the back. Turn the person toward you after the garment is put on the arms. The side of the garment is brought to the person's back. **B,** Then turn the person away from you. The other side of the garment is brought to the back and fastened.

Changing Gowns

Some residents wear hospital gowns. Gowns are usually worn for IV therapy. Some centers have special gowns for IV therapy. They open along the entire sleeve and close with ties, snaps, or Velcro. Sometimes standard hospital gowns are used.

Delegation Guidelines

Changing Gowns

Before changing a gown, you need this information from the nurse and the care plan:

- Which arm has the IV
- If the person has an IV pump (see *Safety Alert: Changing Gowns*)

Safety Alert

Changing Gowns

IV pumps control the rate of infusion. If the person has an IV pump and a standard gown, do not use the following procedure. The arm with the IV is not put through the sleeve.

After changing the gown, ask the nurse to check the IV flow rate.

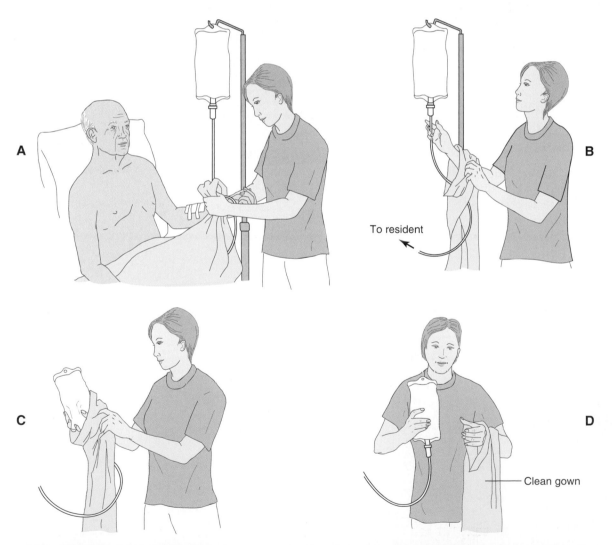

To resident

Clean gown

Fig. 12-18 Changing a gown. **A,** The gown is removed from the good arm. The sleeve on the arm with the IV is gathered up, slipped over the IV site and tubing, and removed from the arm and hand. **B,** The gathered sleeve is slipped along the IV tubing to the bag. **C,** The IV bag is removed from the pole and passed through the sleeve. **D,** The gathered sleeve of the clean gown is slipped over the IV bag at the shoulder part of the gown.

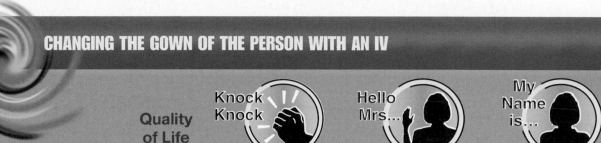

CHANGING THE GOWN OF THE PERSON WITH AN IV

Quality of Life

Knock Knock

Hello Mrs...

My Name is...

Pre-Procedure

1 Follow *Delegation Guidelines: Changing Gowns.* See *Safety Alert: Changing Gowns.*
2 Explain the procedure to the person.
3 Practice hand hygiene.
4 Get a clean gown and a bath blanket.
5 Identify the person. Check the ID bracelet against the assignment sheet. Call the person by name.
6 Provide for privacy.
7 Raise the bed for body mechanics. Bed rails are up if used.

Procedure

8 Lower the bed rail near you (if up).
9 Cover the person with a bath blanket. Fanfold linens to the foot of the bed.
10 Untie the gown. Free parts that the person is lying on.
11 Remove the gown from the arm with no IV.
12 Gather up the sleeve of the arm with the IV. Slide it over the IV site and tubing. Remove the arm and hand from the sleeve (Fig. 12-18, A).
13 Keep the sleeve gathered. Slide your arm along the tubing to the bag (Fig. 12-18, B).
14 Remove the bag from the pole. Slide the bag and tubing through the sleeve (Fig. 12-18, C). Do not pull on the tubing. Keep the bag above the person.
15 Hang the IV bag on the pole.
16 Gather the sleeve of the clean gown that will go on the arm with the IV infusion.
17 Remove the bag from the pole. Slip the sleeve over the bag at the shoulder part of the gown (Fig. 12-18, D). Hang the bag.
18 Slide the gathered sleeve over the tubing, hand, arm, and IV site. Then slide it onto the shoulder.
19 Put the other side of the gown on the person. Fasten the gown.
20 Cover the person. Remove the bath blanket.

Post-Procedure

21 Provide for comfort.
22 Place the signal light within reach.
23 Lower the bed to its lowest position.
24 Raise or lower bed rails. Follow the care plan.
25 Unscreen the person.
26 Complete a safety check of the room. (See inside of front book cover.)
27 Follow center policy for dirty linen.
28 Decontaminate your hands.
29 Ask the nurse to check the flow rate.

Review Questions

Circle the **BEST** answer.

1   Mr. Lee has alopecia. This is
   a Excessive body hair
   b Dry, white flakes from the scalp
   c An infestation of lice
   d Hair loss

2   Which prevents hair from matting and tangling?
   a Bed rest
   b Daily brushing and combing
   c Daily shampooing
   d Cutting hair

3   Mrs. Clark's hair is not matted or tangled. When brushing the hair, start at
   a The forehead
   b The hair ends
   c The scalp
   d The back of the neck

4   Mr. Lee wants his hair washed. You should
   a Wash his hair during his shower
   b Wash his hair at the sink
   c Shampoo him in bed
   d Follow the care plan

5   When shaving Mr. Lee, do the following *except*
   a Practice Standard Precautions
   b Follow the Bloodborne Pathogen Standard
   c Shave in the direction of hair growth
   d Shave when the skin is dry

6   Mr. Lee is nicked during shaving. Your first action is to
   a Wash your hands
   b Apply direct pressure
   c Tell the nurse
   d Use an electric razor

7   Fingernails are cut with
   a Toenail clippers
   b Scissors
   c A nail file
   d Nail clippers

8   Fingernails are trimmed
   a Before soaking
   b After soaking
   c Before trimming toenails
   d After trimming toenails

Circle **T** if the statement is true or **F** if the statement is false.

9   **T F** Mr. Lee has a mustache and beard. You think he would be more comfortable without facial hair. You can shave his beard and mustache.
10 **T F** Clothing is removed from the strong side first.
11 **T F** The person chooses what to wear.
12 **T F** You can cut matted hair.

Answers to these questions are on p. 389.

CHAPTER 13

Elimination

Objectives

- Define the key terms listed in this chapter
- Describe the structures and functions of the urinary and gastrointestinal systems
- Explain how aging affects the urinary and gastrointestinal systems
- Describe the common disorders of the urinary and gastrointestinal systems
- Describe the measures that promote elimination
- List the observations to make about urine and bowel movements
- Describe urinary incontinence and the care required
- Explain how to care for persons with catheters
- Describe the methods for bladder and bowel training
- Explain how to collect urine and stool specimens
- Describe the purpose, solutions, and methods of enema administration
- Describe how to care for a person with an ostomy
- Perform the procedures described in this chapter

Key Terms

catheter A tube used to drain or inject fluid through a body opening

colostomy A surgically created opening *(stomy)* between the colon *(colo)* and abdominal wall

constipation The passage of a hard, dry stool

defecation The process of excreting feces from the rectum through the anus; a bowel movement

diarrhea The frequent passage of liquid stools

dysuria Painful or difficult *(dys)* urination *(uria)*

enema The introduction of fluid into the rectum and lower colon

fecal impaction The prolonged retention and buildup of feces in the rectum

fecal incontinence The inability to control the passage of feces and gas through the anus

feces The semisolid mass of waste products in the colon that are expelled through the anus

flatulence The excessive formation of gas in the stomach and intestines

flatus Gas or air passed through the anus

hematuria Blood *(hemat)* in the urine *(uria)*

ileostomy A surgically created opening *(stomy)* between the ileum (small intestine; *ileo*) and the abdominal wall

nocturia Frequent urination *(uria)* at night *(noct)*

oliguria Scant amount *(olig)* of urine *(uria)*; less than 500 ml in 24 hours

ostomy A surgically created opening

polyuria Abnormally large amounts *(poly)* of urine *(uria)*

stoma An opening; see *colostomy* and *ileostomy*

stool Excreted feces

urinary frequency Voiding at frequent intervals

urinary incontinence The loss of bladder control

urinary urgency The need to void at once

urination The process of emptying urine from the bladder; voiding

voiding Urination

Eliminating waste is a physical need. The urinary system removes waste products from the blood. It also maintains the body's water balance. The gastrointestinal system removes solid wastes from the body.

URINARY ELIMINATION

The healthy adult produces about 1500 ml (milliliters) (3 pints) of urine a day. Many factors affect urine production. Age and disease affect the amount of urine produced (Box 13-1). So do the amount and kinds of fluid ingested, dietary salt, body temperature, perspiration, and drugs. Some substances increase urine production—coffee, tea, alcohol, and some drugs. A diet high in salt causes the body to retain water. When water is retained, less urine is produced.

Urination (**voiding**) mean the process of emptying urine from the bladder. The amount of fluid intake, habits, and available toilet facilities affect frequency. So do activity, work, and illness. People usually void at bedtime, after getting up, and before meals. Some people void every 2 to 3 hours. The need to void at night disturbs sleep.

Some persons need help getting to the bathroom. Others use bedpans, urinals, or commodes. To promote urination, follow the measures in Box 13-2 and the person's care plan.

Observations

Normal urine is pale yellow, straw-colored, or amber. It is clear with no particles. A faint odor is normal. Observe urine for color, clarity, odor, amount, and particles.

Ask the nurse to observe urine that looks or smells abnormal. Report the following problems:

- **Dysuria**—painful or difficult *(dys)* urination *(uria)*
- **Hematuria**—blood *(hemat)* in the urine *(uria)*
- **Nocturia**—frequent urination *(uria)* at night *(noct)*
- **Oliguria**—scant amount *(olig)* of urine *(uria)*, less than 500 ml in 24 hours
- **Polyuria**—abnormally large amounts *(poly)* of urine *(uria)*
- **Urinary frequency**—voiding at frequent intervals
- **Urinary urgency**—the need to void at once

BOX 13-1 **The Urinary System**

Body Structure and Function

The two kidneys (Fig. 13-1, p. 238) lie in the upper abdomen against the muscles of the back on each side of the spine. Blood passes through the two kidneys. Urine is formed in the kidneys.

Urine consists of wastes and excess fluids filtered out of the blood. Urine flows through the two ureters to the urinary bladder. Urine is stored in the bladder. The urethra connects the bladder to the outside of the body. Urine passes from the body through the urethra.

Changes With Aging

Kidney function decreases. The kidneys shrink (atrophy). Blood flow to the kidneys is reduced. Waste removal is less efficient. Urine is more concentrated.

Bladder muscles weaken. Bladder size decreases. It holds less urine. Urinary frequency or urgency may occur. Many older persons have to urinate during the night. Urinary incontinence (inability to control the passage of urine from the bladder) may occur (p. 245).

In men, the prostate gland enlarges. This puts pressure on the urethra. Difficulty urinating or frequent urination occurs.

Urinary tract infections are risks. Persons with incontinence may need bladder training programs. Sometimes catheters are needed.

Common Disorders

- *Urinary retention*—is when the person does not empty the bladder completely. Urine is left in the bladder after voiding. The person feels like the bladder is full but voids in small amounts. Dribbling may occur. Nervous system and prostate disorders are common causes.
- *Urinary tract infections (UTIs)*—are common. Microbes can enter the system through the urethra. Catheters (p. 246), urological exams, intercourse, poor perineal hygiene, and poor fluid intake are common causes.

Women are at high risk. Microbes can easily enter the short female urethra. Prostate gland secretions help protect men from UTIs. An enlarged prostate increases the risk of a UTI in older men. Incomplete bladder emptying, perineal soiling from fecal incontinence, and poor nutrition increase the risk of UTI in older men and women.
  - —*Cystitis* is a bladder *(cyst)* infection *(itis)*. It is caused by bacteria. Urinary frequency, urgency, pain or burning on urination, blood or pus in the urine, foul-smelling urine, and fever may occur. Antibiotics are ordered. Fluids are encouraged—usually 2000 ml per day. If untreated, cystitis can lead to pyelonephritis.
  - —*Pyelonephritis* is inflammation *(itis)* of the kidney *(nephr)* pelvis *(pyelo)*. Infection is the most common cause. Cloudy urine may contain pus, mucus, and blood. Chills, fever, back pain, and nausea and vomiting occur. So do the signs and symptoms of cystitis. Treatment involves antibiotics and fluids.
- *Renal calculi*—are kidney *(renal)* stones *(calculi)*. Bedrest, immobility, and poor fluid intake are risk factors. Stones vary in size. The person has severe, cramping pain in the back and side just below the ribs and pain in the abdomen, thigh, and urethra. Nausea, vomiting, fever, and chills are common. Painful, frequent, and urgent urination may occur. So can blood in the urine. Drugs are given for pain relief. The person needs to drink about 2000 to 3000 ml of fluid a day. Increased fluids help stones pass through the urine. All urine is strained. Surgical removal of the stone may be necessary. Some dietary changes can prevent stones.
- *Renal failure*—is when the kidneys do not function or are severely impaired. Waste products are not removed from the blood. The body retains fluid. Heart failure and hypertension easily result. Renal failure may be acute or chronic. The person is very ill.

BOX 13-2 **Nursing Measures to Promote Elimination**

- Provide fluids as the nurse and care plan direct.
- Follow the person's elimination routines and habits. Check with the nurse and the care plan.
- Help the person to the bathroom when the request is made. Or provide the commode, bedpan, or urinal. The need to void or have a bowel movement may be urgent.
- Help the person assume a normal position for voiding if possible. Women sit or squat. Men stand.
- Warm the bedpan or urinal.
- Cover the person for warmth and privacy.
- Provide for privacy. Ask visitors to leave the room. Close room and bathroom doors, pull privacy curtains, and pull window drapes, shades, or blinds. Leave the room if the person can be alone.
- Tell the person that running water, flushing the toilet, or playing music can mask elimination sounds. Voiding or having a bowel movement with others close by embarrasses some people.
- Stay nearby if the person is weak or unsteady.
- Place the signal light and toilet tissue within reach.
- Allow enough time for voiding or bowel movements. Do not rush the person.
- Promote relaxation. Some people like to read.
- Run water in a sink if the person cannot start a urine stream. Or place the person's fingers in warm water.
- Provide perineal care and skin care as needed.
- Assist with hand washing after elimination. Provide a wash basin, soap, washcloth, and towel.
- Dispose of urine and feces promptly. This reduces odors and prevents the spread of microbes.
- Assist the person to the bathroom or offer the bedpan, urinal, or commode at regular times. Some people are embarrassed or are too weak to ask for help.

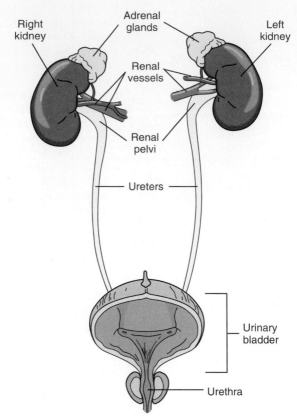

Fig. 13-1 The urinary system.

Bedpans

Bedpans are used by persons who cannot be out of bed. Women use bedpans for voiding and bowel movements. Men use them for bowel movements.

A *fracture pan* has a thin rim. It is only about ½-inch deep at one end (Fig. 13-2). The smaller end is placed under the buttocks (Fig. 13-3). Fracture pans are used:

- By persons with casts
- By persons in traction
- By persons with limited back motion
- After spinal cord injury or surgery
- After a hip fracture
- After hip replacement surgery
- By persons with osteoporosis (Chapter 4)
- By persons with painful joints

Text continued on p. 242

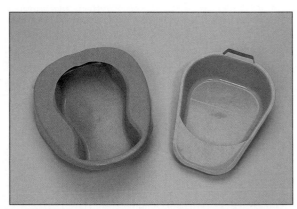

Fig. 13-2 Standard bedpan *(left)* and the fracture pan *(right)*.

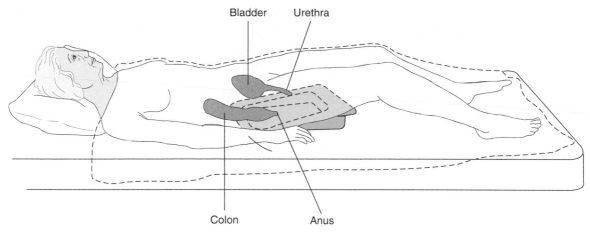

Bladder   Urethra

Colon   Anus

Fig. 13-3 A person positioned on a fracture pan. The smaller end is under the buttocks.

Delegation Guidelines

Bedpans

Before assisting with a bedpan, you need this information from the nurse and care plan:

- What bedpan to use—standard bedpan or fracture pan
- Position or activity limits
- If the nurse needs to observe the results before you dispose of the contents
- What observations to report and record:
  —Urine color, clarity, and odor
  —Amount
  —Presence of particles
  —Complaints of urgency, burning, dysuria, or other problems
  —For bowel movements, see p. 256

Safety Alert

Bedpans

Urine and bowel movements may contain blood and microbes. Microbes can live and grow in dirty bedpans. Follow Standard Precautions and the Bloodborne Pathogen Standard when handling bedpans and their contents. Thoroughly clean and disinfect bedpans after use.

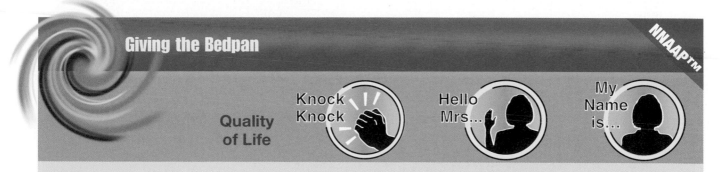

Giving the Bedpan

NNAAP™

Quality of Life

Knock Knock

Hello Mrs...

My Name is...

Pre-Procedure

1 Follow *Delegation Guidelines: Bedpans*. See *Safety Alert: Bedpans*.
2 Provide for privacy.
3 Practice hand hygiene.
4 Put on gloves.
5 Collect the following:

- Bedpan
- Bedpan cover
- Toilet tissue

6 Arrange equipment on the chair or bed.
7 Explain the procedure to the person.

Continued

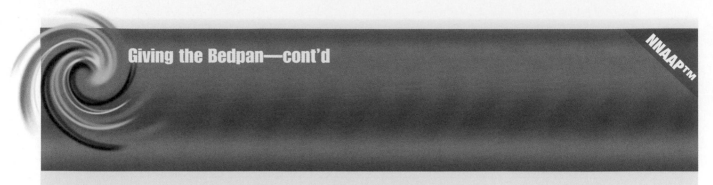

Procedure

8   Warm and dry the bedpan if necessary.

9   Lower the bed rail near you if up.

10   Position the person supine. Raise the head of the bed slightly.

11   Fold the top linens and gown out of the way. Keep the lower body covered.

12   Ask the person to flex the knees and raise the buttocks by pushing against the mattress with his or her feet.

13   Slide your hand under the lower back. Help raise the buttocks.

14   Slide the bedpan under the person (Fig. 13-4).

15   If the person cannot assist in getting on the bedpan:

   a   Turn the person onto the side away from you.

   b   Place the bedpan firmly against the buttocks (Fig. 13-5, *A*).

   c   Push the bedpan down and toward the person (Fig. 13-5, *B*).

   d   Hold the bedpan securely. Turn the person onto the back.

   e   Make sure the bedpan is centered under the person.

16   Cover the person.

17   Raise the head of the bed so the person is in a sitting position.

18   Make sure the person is correctly positioned on the bedpan (Fig. 13-6, p. 242).

19   Raise the bed rail if used.

20   Place the toilet tissue and signal light within reach.

21   Ask the person to signal when done or when help is needed.

22   Remove the gloves. Decontaminate your hands.

23   Leave the room, and close the door.

24   Return when the person signals. Or check the person every 5 minutes. Knock before entering.

25   Decontaminate your hands. Put on gloves.

26   Raise the bed for body mechanics. Lower the bed rail (if used) and the head of the bed.

27   Ask the person to raise the buttocks. Remove the bedpan. Or hold the bedpan and turn him or her onto the side away from you.

28   Clean the genital area if the person cannot do so. Clean from front (urethra) to back (anus) with toilet tissue. Use fresh tissue for each wipe. Provide perineal care if needed.

29   Cover the bedpan. Take it to the bathroom. Lower the bed, and raise the bed rail (if used) before leaving the bedside.

30   Note the color, amount, and character of urine or feces.

31   Empty the bedpan contents into the toilet and flush. Rinse the bedpan. Pour the rinse into the toilet and flush. Clean the bedpan with a disinfectant.

32   Remove soiled gloves. Practice hand hygiene, and put on clean gloves.

33   Return the bedpan and clean cover to the bedside stand.

34   Help the person with hand washing.

35   Remove the gloves. Decontaminate your hands.

Post-Procedure

36   Provide for comfort.

37   Place the signal light within reach.

38   Raise or lower bed rails. Follow the care plan.

39   Unscreen the person.

40   Complete a safety check of the room. (See inside of front book cover.)

41   Follow center policy for soiled linen.

42   Decontaminate your hands.

43   Report and record your observations.

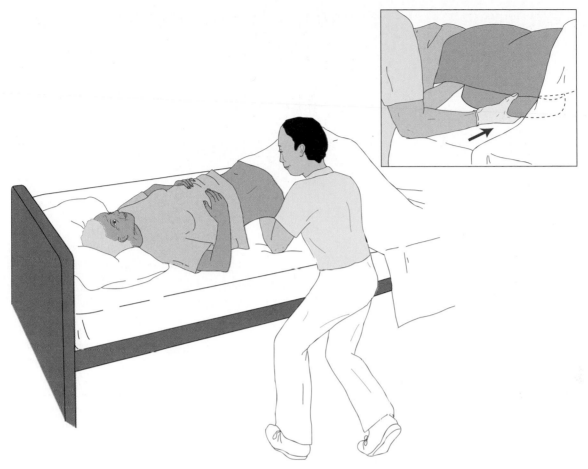

Fig. 13-4 The person raises the buttocks off the bed with help. The bedpan is slid under the person.

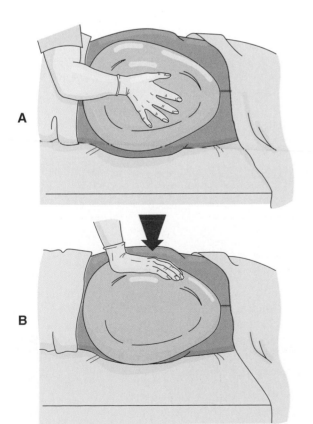

A

B

Fig. 13-5 Giving a bedpan. **A,** Position the person on one side. Place the bedpan firmly against the buttocks. **B,** Push downward on the bedpan and toward the person.

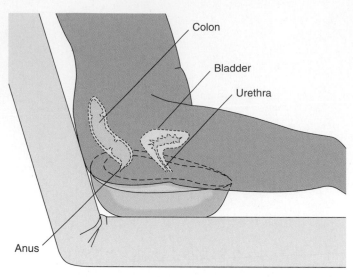

Fig. 13-6 The person is positioned on the bedpan so the urethra and anus are directly over the opening.

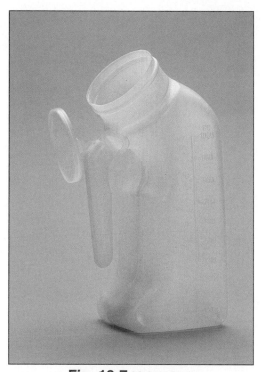

Fig. 13-7 Male urinal.

Urinals

Men use urinals to void (Fig. 13-7). Plastic urinals have caps and hook-type handles. The urinal hooks to the bed rail within the man's reach. He stands to use the urinal if possible. Or he sits on the side of the bed or lies in bed to use it. Some men need support when standing. You may have to place and hold the urinal for some men.

Remind men to hang urinals on bed rails and to signal after using them. Remind them not to place urinals on overbed tables and bedside stands. These surfaces must not be contaminated with urine. Some centers do not use bed rails. Follow center policy for where to place urinals.

Urinals

Before assisting with urinals, you need this information from the nurse and care plan:

- How the urinal is used—standing, sitting, or lying in bed
- If help is needed with placing or holding the urinal
- If the man needs support to stand (if yes, how many staff members are needed)
- If the nurse needs to observe the urine before you dispose of it
- What observations to report and record (see *Delegation Guidelines: Bedpans,* p. 239)

Urinals

Follow Standard Precautions and the Bloodborne Pathogen Standard when handling urinals and their contents. Empty them promptly to prevent odors and the spread of microbes. A filled urinal spills easily, causing safety hazards. Also, it is an unpleasant site and a source of odor. Urinals are cleaned and disinfected like bedpans.

Giving the Urinal

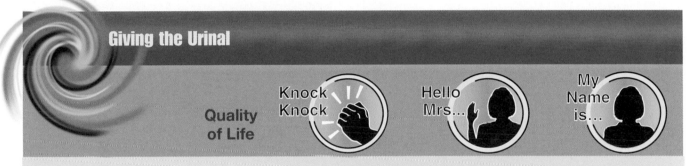

Quality of Life — Knock Knock — Hello Mrs... — My Name is...

Pre-Procedure

1. Follow *Delegation Guidelines: Urinals.* See *Safety Alert: Urinals.*
2. Provide for privacy.
3. Determine if the man will stand, sit, or lie in bed.
4. Practice hand hygiene.
5. Put on gloves.

Procedure

6. Give him the urinal if he is in bed. Remind him to tilt the bottom down to prevent spills.
7. If he is going to stand:
   a. Help him sit on the side of the bed.
   b. Put nonskid footwear on him.
   c. Help him stand. Provide support if he is unsteady.
   d. Give him the urinal.
8. Position the urinal if necessary. Position his penis in the urinal if he cannot do so.
9. Provide for privacy.
10. Place the signal light within reach. Ask him to signal when done or when he needs help.
11. Remove the gloves. Decontaminate your hands.
12. Leave the room, and close the door.
13. Return when he signals for you. Or check on the person every 5 minutes. Knock before entering.
14. Decontaminate your hands. Put on gloves.
15. Close the cap on the urinal. Take it to the bathroom.
16. Note the color, amount, and character of the urine.
17. Empty the urinal contents into the toilet and flush. Rinse it with cold water. Pour the rinse into the toilet and flush. Rinse the urinal with cold water. Clean the urinal with a disinfectant.
18. Return the urinal to its proper place.
19. Remove soiled gloves. Practice hand hygiene, and put on clean gloves.
20. Assist with hand washing.
21. Remove the gloves. Decontaminate your hands.

Post-Procedure

22. Provide for comfort.
23. Place the signal light within reach.
24. Raise or lower bed rails. Follow the care plan.
25. Unscreen him.
26. Complete a safety check of the room. (See inside of front book cover.)
27. Follow center policy for soiled linen.
28. Decontaminate your hands.
29. Report and record your observations.

Commodes

A commode is a chair or wheelchair with an opening for a bedpan or container (Fig. 13-8). It allows a normal position for elimination. Some commodes are wheeled into bathrooms and placed over toilets. The container is removed if the commode is used with the toilet. Wheels are locked after the commode is positioned over the toilet.

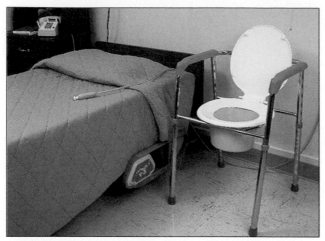

Fig. 13-8 The commode has a toilet seat with a container. The container slides out from under the seat for emptying.

Delegation Guidelines

Commodes

You need this information from the nurse and care plan when assisting with commodes:

- Is the commode used at the bedside or over the toilet
- How much help the person needs
- If the person can be left alone
- Does the nurse need to observe urine or bowel movements
- What observations to report and record (See *Delegation Guidelines: Bedpans*, p. 239)

Safety Alert

Commodes

To use a commode, the person is transferred to or from bed or a chair or wheelchair. Practice safe transfer procedures (Chapter 16). Use the transfer belt.

Urine and feces may contain blood and microbes. Follow Standard Precautions and the Bloodborne Pathogen Standard. Thoroughly clean and disinfect the commode container after use.

Helping the Person to the Commode

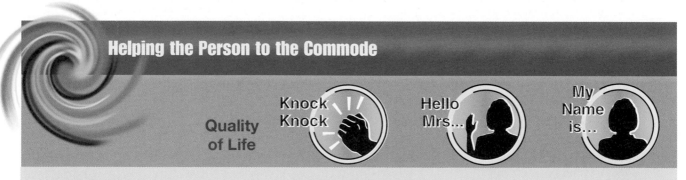

Quality of Life   Knock Knock   Hello Mrs...   My Name is...

Pre-Procedure

1. Follow *Delegation Guidelines: Commodes*. See *Safety Alert: Commodes*.
2. Explain the procedure to the person.
3. Provide for privacy.
4. Practice hand hygiene.
5. Put on gloves.
6. Collect the following:
   - Commode
   - Toilet tissue
   - Bath blanket
   - Transfer belt
7. Bring the commode next to the bed. Remove the chair seat and container lid.

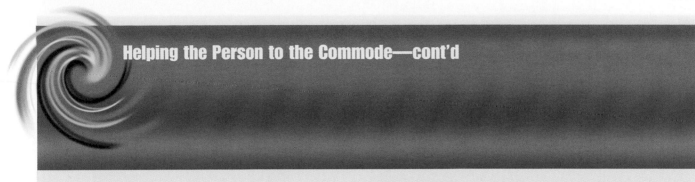

Helping the Person to the Commode—cont'd

Procedure

8 Help the person sit on the side of the bed.
9 Help him or her put on a robe and nonskid footwear.
10 Assist the person to the commode. Use the transfer belt.
11 Cover the person with a bath blanket for warmth.
12 Place the toilet tissue and signal light within reach.
13 Ask him or her to signal when done or when help is needed. (Stay with the person if necessary. Be respectful. Provide as much privacy as possible.)
14 Remove the gloves. Decontaminate your hands.
15 Leave the room. Close the door.
16 Return when the person signals. Or check on the person every 5 minutes. Knock before entering.
17 Decontaminate your hands. Put on the gloves.
18 Help the person clean the genital area as needed. Remove the gloves, and practice hand hygiene.

19 Help the person back to bed using the transfer belt. Remove the transfer belt, robe, and footwear. Raise the bed rail if used.
20 Put on clean gloves. Remove and cover the commode container. Clean the commode.
21 Take the container to the bathroom.
22 Check urine and feces for color, amount, and character.
23 Empty the container contents into the toilet and flush. Rinse the container. Pour the rinse into the toilet and flush. Clean and disinfect the container.
24 Return the container to the commode. Return other supplies to their proper place.
25 Return the commode to its proper place.
26 Remove soiled gloves. Practice hand hygiene, and put on clean gloves.
27 Assist with hand washing.
28 Remove the gloves. Decontaminate your hands.

Post-Procedure

29 Provide for comfort.
30 Place the signal light within reach.
31 Raise or lower bed rails. Follow the care plan.
32 Unscreen the person.
33 Complete a safety check of the room. (See inside of front book cover.)

34 Follow center policy for soiled linen.
35 Decontaminate your hands.
36 Report and record your observations.

Urinary Incontinence

Urinary incontinence is the loss of bladder control. It may be temporary or permanent. The basic types of incontinence are:

- *Stress incontinence*—Urine leaks during exercise and certain movements. Urine loss is small (less than 50 ml). Often called *dribbling,* it occurs with laughing, sneezing, coughing, lifting, or other activities.
- *Urge incontinence*—Urine is lost in response to a sudden, urgent need to void. The person cannot get to a toilet in time. Urinary frequency, urinary urgency, and night-time voidings are common.

- *Overflow incontinence*—Urine leaks when the bladder is too full. The person feels like the bladder is not empty. The person only dribbles or has a weak urine stream.
- *Functional incontinence*—The person has bladder control but cannot use the toilet in time. Immobility, restraints, unanswered signal lights, no signal light within reach, and not knowing where to find the bathroom are causes. So is difficulty removing clothing. Confusion and disorientation are other causes.
- *Reflex incontinence*—Urine is lost at predictable intervals. Urine is lost when the bladder is full. The person does not feel the need to void.

BOX 13-3   Nursing Measures for Persons With Urinary Incontinence

- Record the person's voidings. This includes incontinent times and successful use of the toilet, commode, bedpan, or urinal.
- Answer signal lights promptly. The need to void may be urgent.
- Promote normal urinary and bowel elimination (see Box 13-2).
- Encourage voiding at scheduled intervals.
- Follow the person's bladder training program (p. 252).
- Have the person wear easy-to-remove clothing. Incontinence can occur while trying to deal with buttons, zippers, and undergarments.
- Encourage the person to do pelvic muscle exercises as instructed by the nurse.
- Help prevent urinary tract infections:
  —Promote fluid intake as the nurse directs.
  —Have the person wear cotton underwear.
  —Keep the perineal area clean and dry.
- Decrease fluid intake before bedtime.
- Provide good skin care.
- Provide dry garments and linens.
- Observe for signs of skin breakdown.
- Use incontinence products as the nurse directs. Follow the manufacturer's instructions.
- Provide perineal care as needed (Chapter 11). Remember to:
  —Use a safe and comfortable water temperature.
  —Follow Standard Precautions and the Bloodborne Pathogen Standard.
  —Protect the person and dry garments and linen from the wet incontinence product.
  —Expose only the perineal area.
  —Wash, rinse, and dry the perineal area and buttocks.
  —Remove wet incontinence products, garments, and linen. Apply clean, dry ones.

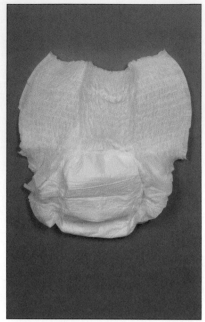

Fig. 13-9 Incontinence product.

Incontinence products help keep the person dry (Fig. 13-9). They have two layers and a waterproof back. Fluid passes through the first layer. It is absorbed by the second layer. The nurse selects products that best meet the person's needs.

Incontinence is beyond the person's control. It is not something the person chooses to do. The person needs frequent care. The person may wet again just after skin care and having wet garments and linens changed. Be patient. The person's needs are great. If you find yourself becoming short-tempered and impatient, talk to the nurse at once. The person has the right to be free from abuse, mistreatment, or neglect. Be kind, empathetic, understanding, and patient.

Catheters

A **catheter** is a tube used to drain or inject fluid through a body opening. Inserted through the urethra into the bladder, a urinary catheter drains urine. An *indwelling catheter* (*retention* or *Foley catheter*) is left in the bladder (Fig. 13-10). Tubing connects the catheter to the drainage bag. A doctor or nurse inserts the catheter (*catheterization*).

Some people are too weak or disabled to use the bedpan, urinal, commode, or toilet. For them, catheters can promote comfort and prevent incontinence. Catheters can protect wounds and pressure ulcers from contact with urine. They also allow hourly urinary output measurements. However, they are a last resort for incontinence. Catheters do not treat the cause of incontinence.

Persons with catheters are at high risk for infection. The measures in Box 13-4 promote comfort and safety.

Sometimes incontinence results from intestinal, rectal, and reproductive system surgeries. More than one type of incontinence can be present. This is called *mixed incontinence.*

Incontinence is embarrassing. Garments get wet, and odors develop. The person is uncomfortable. Skin irritation, infection, and pressure ulcers are risks. Falling is a risk when trying to get to the bathroom quickly. The person's pride, dignity, and self-esteem are affected. Loss of independence, social isolation, and depression are common.

Follow the nurse's instructions and the care plan. The care plan may include some of the measures in Box 13-3. *Good skin care and dry clothing and linens are essential.* The measures in Box 13-2 prevent incontinence in some people. Others need bladder training (p. 252). Sometimes catheters are ordered.

Text continued on p. 250

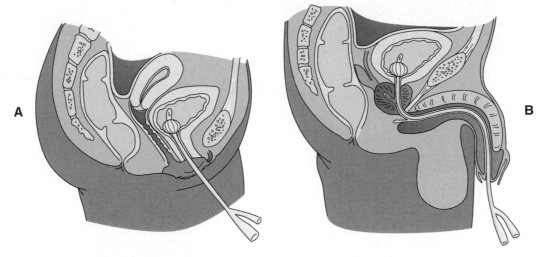

Fig. 13-10 Indwelling catheter. **A,** Indwelling catheter in the female bladder. The inflated balloon at the top prevents the catheter from slipping out through the urethra. **B,** Indwelling catheter with the balloon inflated in the male bladder.

BOX 13-4   Nursing Measures for Persons With Indwelling Catheters

- Follow the rules of medical asepsis.
- Follow Standard Precautions and the Bloodborne Pathogen Standard.
- Allow urine to flow freely through the catheter or tubing. Tubing should not have kinks. The person should not lie on the tubing.
- Keep the catheter connected to the drainage tubing. Follow the measures on p. 250 if the catheter and drainage tube are disconnected.
- Keep the drainage bag below the bladder. This prevents urine from flowing backward into the bladder.
- Attach the drainage bag to the bed frame, back of the chair, or lower part of an IV pole. *Never attach the drainage bag to the bed rail.* Otherwise it is higher than the bladder when the bed rail is raised.
- Do not let the drainage bag rest on the floor. This can contaminate the system.
- Coil the drainage tubing on the bed. Secure it to the bottom linen (Fig. 13-11, p. 249). Follow center policy. Use a clip, tape, safety pin with rubber band, or other device as directed by the nurse. Tubing must not loop below the drainage bag.
- Secure the catheter to the inner thigh (see Fig. 13-11). Or secure it to the man's abdomen. This prevents excess catheter movement and friction at the insertion site. Secure the catheter with tape or other devices as the nurse directs.
- Check for leaks. Check the site where the catheter connects to the drainage bag. Report any leaks to the nurse at once.
- Provide catheter care daily or twice a day (see procedure: *Giving Catheter Care,* p. 249). Some centers consider perineal care to be sufficient. Follow the care plan.
- Provide perineal care daily, after bowel movements, and when there is vaginal drainage. Follow the care plan.
- Empty the drainage bag at the end of the shift or as the nurse directs. Measure and record the amount of urine (see procedure: *Emptying a Urinary Drainage Bag,* p. 251). Report increases or decreases in the amount of urine.
- Use a separate measuring container for each person. This prevents the spread of microbes from one person to another.
- Do not the let the drain on the drainage bag touch any surface.
- Report complaints to the nurse at once—pain, burning, the need to void, or irritation. Also report the color, clarity, and odor of urine and the presence of particles.
- Encourage fluid intake as directed by the nurse and care plan.

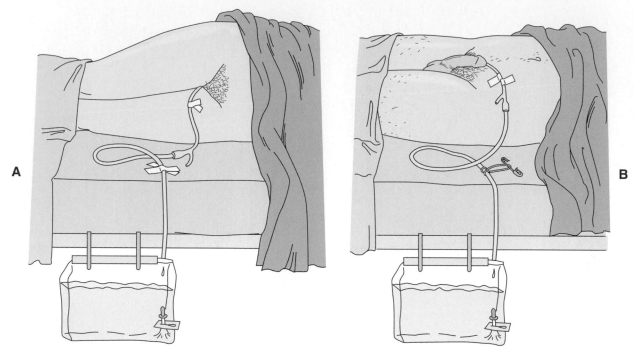

Fig. 13-11 Securing catheters. **A,** The drainage tube is coiled on the bed and secured to the bottom linens. The catheter is taped to the inner thigh. Enough slack is left on the catheter to prevent friction at the urethra. **B,** The catheter is secured to the man's abdomen.

Delegation Guidelines

Catheters

Before giving catheter care, you need this information from the nurse and the care plan:

- When to give catheter care—daily, twice a day, after bowel movements, or when vaginal discharge is present
- Where to secure the catheter—thigh or abdomen
- How to secure drainage tubing—clip, tape, safety pin and rubber band, or other device
- What observations to report and record:
  —Complaints of pain, burning, irritation, or the need to void
  —Crusting, abnormal drainage, or secretions
  —The color, clarity, and odor of urine
  —Particles in the urine
  —Drainage system leaks

Safety Alert

Catheters

Urine may contain microbes and blood. Follow Standard Precautions and the Bloodborne Pathogen Standard.

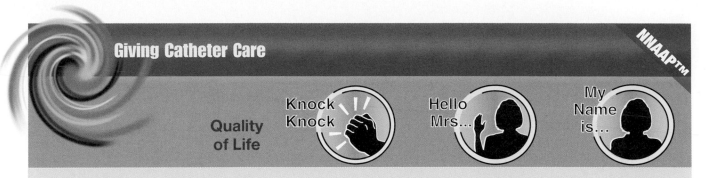

Giving Catheter Care

Quality of Life
- Knock Knock
- Hello Mrs...
- My Name is...

Pre-Procedure

1 Follow *Delegation Guidelines: Catheters.* See *Safety Alert: Catheters.*
2 Explain the procedure to the person.
3 Practice hand hygiene.
4 Collect the following:
- Items for perineal care (Chapter 11)
- Gloves
- Bed protector
- Bath blanket

5 Identify the person. Check the ID bracelet against the assignment sheet. Call the person by name.
6 Provide for privacy.
7 Raise the bed for body mechanics. Bed rails are up if used.

Procedure

8 Lower the bed rail near you if up.
9 Decontaminate your hands. Put on the gloves.
10 Cover the person with a bath blanket. Fanfold top linens to the foot of the bed.
11 Drape the person for perineal care (Chapter 11).
12 Fold back the bath blanket to expose the genital area.
13 Place the bed protector under the buttocks. Ask the person to flex the knees and raise the buttocks off the bed.
14 Give perineal care (Chapter 11).
15 Apply soap to a clean, wet washcloth.
16 Separate the labia (female). In an uncircumcised male, retract the foreskin (Fig. 13-12, p. 250). Check for crusts, abnormal drainage, or secretions.
17 Hold the catheter near the meatus.

18 Clean the catheter from the meatus down the catheter about 4 inches (Fig. 13-13, p. 250). Clean downward, away from the meatus, with 1 stroke. Do not tug or pull on the catheter. Repeat as needed with a clean area of the washcloth. Use a clean washcloth if needed.
19 Rinse the catheter with a clean washcloth. Rinse from the meatus down the catheter about 4 inches. Rinse downward, away from the meatus, with 1 stroke. Do not tug or pull on the catheter. Repeat as needed with a clean area of the washcloth. Use a clean washcloth if needed.
20 Secure the catheter. Coil and secure tubing (see Fig. 13-11).
21 Remove the bed protector.
22 Cover the person. Remove the bath blanket.
23 Remove the gloves. Decontaminate your hands.

Post-Procedure

24 Provide for comfort.
25 Place the signal light within reach.
26 Raise or lower bed rails. Follow the care plan.
27 Lower the bed to its lowest position.
28 Clean and return equipment to its proper place. Discard disposable items. (Wear gloves for this step.)
29 Remove the gloves. Decontaminate your hands.

30 Unscreen the person.
31 Complete a safety check of the room. (See inside of front book cover.)
32 Follow center policy for soiled linen.
33 Decontaminate your hands.
34 Report and record your observations.

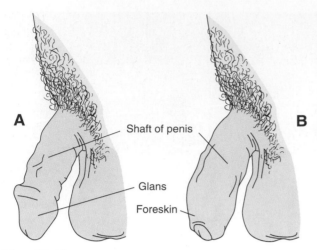

Fig. 13-12 A, Circumcised male. **B,** Uncircumcised male.

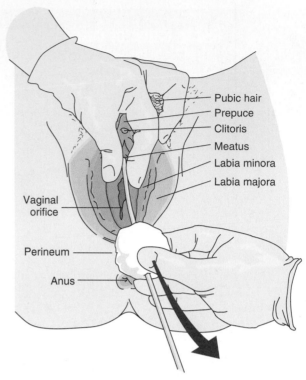

Fig. 13-13 The catheter is cleaned starting at the meatus. About 4 inches of the catheter is cleaned.

Drainage Systems. A closed drainage system is used for indwelling catheters. Nothing can enter the system from the catheter to the drainage bag. The urinary system is sterile. Infection can occur if microbes enter the drainage system. The microbes travel up the tubing or catheter into the bladder and kidneys. A urinary tract infection can threaten health and life.

The drainage system has tubing and a drainage bag. Tubing attaches at one end to the catheter. At the other end, it attaches to the drainage bag.

The bag hangs from the bed frame, chair, or wheelchair. It must not touch the floor. The bag is always kept lower than the person's bladder (see Fig. 13-11). Microbes can grow in urine. If the drainage bag is higher than the bladder, urine can flow back into the bladder. An infection can occur. Therefore do not hang the drainage bag on a bed rail. When the bed rail is raised, the bag is higher than bladder level. When the person walks, the bag is held lower than the bladder.

Sometimes drainage systems are disconnected accidentally. If that happens, tell the nurse at once. Do not touch the ends of the catheter or tubing. Do the following:

- Practice hand hygiene. Put on gloves.
- Wipe the end of the tube with an antiseptic wipe.
- Wipe the end of the catheter with another antiseptic wipe.
- Do not put the ends down. Do not touch the ends after you clean them.
- Connect the tubing to the catheter.
- Discard the wipes into a biohazard bag.
- Remove the gloves. Practice hand hygiene.

Delegation Guidelines

Drainage Systems

Before emptying a urinary drainage bag, you need this information from the nurse and the care plan:
- When to empty the drainage bag
- If you should clean or discard the drainage bag
- What observations to report and record:
  —The amount of urine measured
  —The color, clarity, and odor of urine
  —Particles in the urine
  —Complaints of pain, burning, irritation, or the need to urinate
  —Drainage system leaks

Safety Alert

Drainage Systems

Urine may contain microbes and blood. Follow Standard Precautions and the Bloodborne Pathogen Standard.

Some drainage bags are secured to a leg. Called "leg bags," they hold less than 1000 ml of urine (p. 252). Most drainage bags hold at least 2000 ml of urine. Therefore leg bags fill faster than drainage bags. Check leg bags often. Empty and measure urine when the bag is half full.

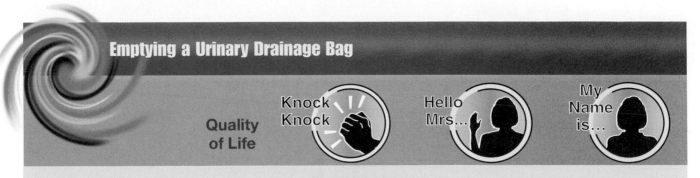

Emptying a Urinary Drainage Bag

Quality of Life

Knock Knock

Hello Mrs...

My Name is...

Pre-Procedure

1 Follow *Delegation Guidelines: Drainage Systems.* See *Safety Alert: Drainage Systems.*
2 Collect equipment:
   • Graduate (measuring container)
   • Gloves
   • Paper towels
3 Practice hand hygiene.
4 Explain the procedure to the person.
5 Identify the person. Check the ID bracelet against the assignment sheet. Call the person by name.
6 Provide for privacy.

Procedure

7 Put on the gloves.
8 Place a paper towel on the floor. Place the graduate on top of it.
9 Position the graduate under the collection bag.
10 Open the clamp on the drain.
11 Let all urine drain into the graduate. Do not let the drain touch the graduate (Fig. 13-14).
12 Close and position the clamp (see Fig. 13-11).
13 Measure urine.
14 Remove and discard the paper towel.
15 Rinse the graduate. Return it to its proper place.
16 Remove the gloves. Practice hand hygiene.
17 Record the time and amount on the intake and output (I&O) record (Chapter 7).

Post-Procedure

18 Unscreen the person.
19 Complete a safety check of the room. (See inside of front book cover.)
20 Report and record the amount and other observations.

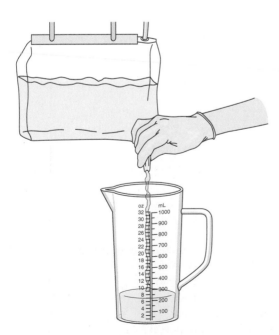

Fig. 13-14 The clamp on the drainage bag is opened. The drain is directed into the graduate. The drain must not touch the inside of the graduate.

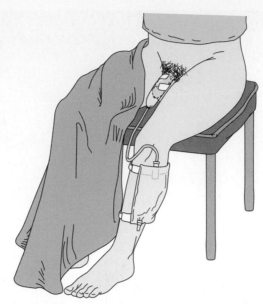

Fig. 13-15 Condom catheter attached to a leg bag.

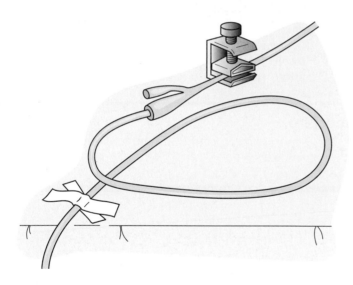

Fig. 13-16 The clamped catheter prevents urine from draining out of the bladder. The clamp is applied directly to the catheter—not to the drainage tubing.

Condom Catheters. Condom catheters are often used for incontinent men. They also are called *external catheters*, *Texas catheters*, and *urinary sheaths*. A condom catheter is a soft sheath that slides over the penis. Tubing connects the condom catheter and drainage bag. Many men prefer leg bags (Fig. 13-15).

Bladder Training

Bladder training programs help some persons with urinary incontinence. Some persons need bladder training after indwelling catheter removal. Control of urination is the goal. Bladder control promotes comfort and quality of life. It also increases self-esteem.

There are two basic methods for bladder training:

- The person uses the toilet, commode, bedpan, or urinal at certain times. The person is given 15 or 20 minutes to start voiding. Measures to promote urination are practiced.
- The person has a catheter. The catheter is clamped to prevent urine flow from the bladder (Fig. 13-16). It is usually clamped for 1 hour at first. Over time, it is clamped for 3 to 4 hours. Urine drains when the catheter is unclamped. When the catheter is removed, voiding is encouraged every 3 to 4 hours or as directed by the nurse and the care plan.

Urine Specimens

Urine specimens are collected for urine tests. Doctors use test results to make a diagnosis or evaluate treatment. Follow the rules in Box 13-5.

BOX 13-5 Rules for Collecting Specimens

- Follow the rules of medical asepsis.
- Follow Standard Precautions and the Bloodborne Pathogen Standard.
- Use a clean container for each specimen.
- Use the correct container.
- Label the container accurately.
- Do not touch the inside of the container or lid.
- Collect the specimen at the correct time.

- Ask the person not to have a bowel movement when collecting a urine specimen. The specimen must not contain feces.
- Ask the person to put toilet tissue in the toilet or wastebasket. Urine and stool specimens must not contain tissue.
- Place the specimen container in a plastic bag.
- Take the specimen and requisition slip to the storage area.

Delegation Guidelines

Urine Specimens

Before collecting a urine specimen, you need this information from the nurse:

- The type of specimen needed
- What time to collect the specimen
- What special measures are needed
- What observations to report and record:
  - —Problems obtaining the specimen
  - —Color, clarity, and odor of urine
  - —Particles in the urine
  - —Complaints of pain, burning, urgency, dysuria, or other problems

Safety Alert

Urine Specimens

Microbes can grow in urine. Urine also may contain blood. Follow Standard Precautions and the Bloodborne Pathogen Standard.

Random Urine Specimen. The random urine specimen is collected for a urinalysis. No special measures are needed. It is collected at any time. Many people can collect the specimen themselves. Weak and very ill persons need help.

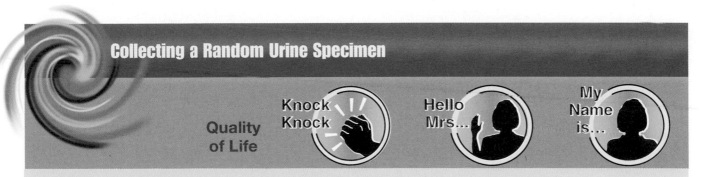

Collecting a Random Urine Specimen

Quality of Life

Knock Knock

Hello Mrs...

My Name is...

Pre-Procedure

1 Follow *Delegation Guidelines: Urine Specimens.* See *Safety Alert: Urine Specimens.*
2 Explain the procedure to the person.
3 Practice hand hygiene.
4 Collect the following:
   - Voiding receptacle—bedpan and cover, urinal, or specimen pan
   - Specimen container and lid
   - Label

   - Gloves
   - Plastic bag
5 Label the container. Put the container and lid in the bathroom.
6 Decontaminate your hands.
7 Identify the person. Check the ID bracelet against the requisition slip. Call the person by name.
8 Provide for privacy.

Continued

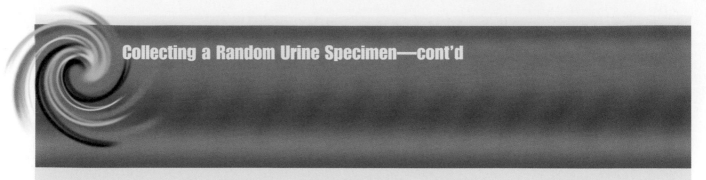

Collecting a Random Urine Specimen—cont'd

Procedure

9   Decontaminate your hands. Put on the gloves.
10 Ask the person to void into the receptacle. Remind him or her to put toilet tissue into the wastebasket or toilet. Toilet tissue is not put in the bedpan or specimen pan.
11 Take the receptacle to the bathroom.
12 Pour about 120 ml (4 oz) of urine into the specimen container. Dispose of excess urine.

13 Place the lid on the specimen container. Put the container in the plastic bag.
14 Clean and return the receptacle to its proper place.
15 Remove the gloves, and practice hand hygiene. Put on clean gloves.
16 Assist with hand washing.
17 Remove the gloves, and practice hand hygiene.

Post-Procedure

18 Provide for comfort.
19 Place the signal light within reach.
20 Raise or lower bed rails. Follow the care plan.
21 Unscreen the person.
22 Complete a safety check of the room. (See inside of front book cover.)

23 Decontaminate your hands.
24 Report and record your observations.
25 Take the specimen and the requisition slip to the storage area.

Midstream Specimen. The midstream specimen is also called a *clean-voided specimen* or a *clean-catch specimen.* The perineal area is cleaned before collecting the specimen. This reduces the number of microbes in the urethral area. The person starts to void into a receptacle. Then the person stops the stream of urine, and a sterile specimen container is positioned. The person voids into the container until the specimen is obtained.

Stopping the stream of urine is hard for many people. You may need to position and hold the specimen container in place after the person starts to void.

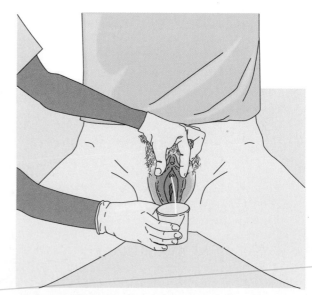

Fig. 13-17 The labia are separated to collect a midstream specimen.

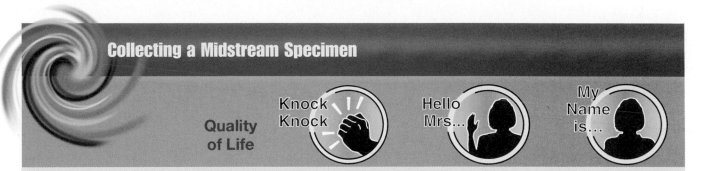

Collecting a Midstream Specimen

Pre-Procedure

1   Follow *Delegation Guidelines: Urine Specimens,* p. 253. See *Safety Alert: Urine Specimens,* p. 253.
2   Explain the procedure to the person.
3   Practice hand hygiene.
4   Collect the following:
   * Midstream specimen kit (with antiseptic solution)
   * Label
   * Disposable gloves
   * Sterile gloves (if not part of the kit)
   * Voiding receptacle—bedpan, urinal, or commode if needed
   * Plastic bag
   * Supplies for perineal care
5   Label the container. Decontaminate your hands.
6   Identify the person. Check the ID bracelet against the requisition slip. Call the person by name.
7   Provide for privacy.

Procedure

8   Provide perineal care. Remove the gloves, and decontaminate your hands.
9   Open the sterile kit.
10   Put on the sterile gloves.
11   Pour the antiseptic solution over the cotton balls.
12   Open the sterile specimen container. Do not touch the inside of the container or lid. Set the lid down so the inside is up.
13   *For a female*—clean the perineum with cotton balls:
   a   Spread the labia with your thumb and index finger. Use your non-dominant hand. (This hand is now contaminated. It must not touch anything sterile.)
   b   Clean down the urethral area from front to back. Use a clean cotton ball for each stroke.
   c   Keep the labia separated to collect the urine specimen (steps 16 and 17).
14   *For a male*—clean the penis with cotton balls:
   a   Hold the penis with your non-dominant hand.
   b   Clean the penis starting at the meatus. Use a cotton ball and clean in a circular motion. Start at the center and work outward.
   c   Keep holding the penis until the specimen is collected (steps 16 and 17).
15   Ask the person to void into the receptacle.
16   Pass the specimen container into the stream of urine. Keep the labia separated (Fig. 13-17).
17   Collect about 30 to 60 ml of urine (1 to 2 oz).
18   Remove the specimen container before the person stops voiding.
19   Release the labia or penis.
20   Let the person finish voiding into the receptacle.
21   Put the lid on the specimen container. Touch only the outside of the container or lid.
22   Wipe the outside of the container.
23   Place the container in a plastic bag.
24   Provide toilet tissue after the person is done voiding.
25   Take the receptacle to the bathroom.
26   Measure urine if intake and output is ordered. Include the amount in the specimen container.
27   Clean the receptacle and other items. Return equipment to its proper place.
28   Remove soiled gloves. Practice hand hygiene.
29   Put on clean gloves.
30   Assist with hand washing
31   Remove the gloves. Decontaminate your hands.

Post-Procedure

32   Follow steps 18-25 in procedure: *Collecting a Random Urine Specimen.*

BOX 13-6 The Gastrointestinal System

Body Structure and Function

Bowel elimination is the excretion of wastes from the gastrointestinal (GI) system (Fig. 13-18). Foods and fluids are normally taken in through the mouth. They are partially digested in the stomach. The partially digested foods and fluids are called *chyme*.

Chyme passes from the stomach into the small intestine. Further digestion and absorption of nutrients occur as the chyme passes through the small bowel. Then chyme enters the large intestine (large bowel or colon) where fluid is absorbed. Chyme becomes less fluid and more solid in consistency. **Feces** refers to the semisolid mass of waste products in the colon that are expelled through the anus.

Feces move through the intestines by peristalsis. *Peristalsis* is the alternating contraction and relaxation of intestinal muscles. The feces move through the large intestine to the rectum. Feces are stored in the rectum until excreted from the body. **Defecation** (bowel movement) is the process of excreting feces from the rectum through the anus. **Stool** refers to excreted feces.

Changes With Aging

Peristalsis decreases. The stomach and colon empty slower. Feces pass through the intestines at a slower rate. Flatulence and constipation are risks. Some older persons lose bowel control. Older persons are at risk for intestinal tumors and disorders.

Common Disorders

- **Constipation**—is the passage of a hard, dry stool. The person usually strains to have a bowel movement. Stools are large or marble-size. Large stools cause pain as they pass through the anus. Constipation occurs when feces move slowly through the bowel. This allows more time for water absorption. Common causes include a low-fiber diet, ignoring the urge to defecate, decreased fluid intake, inactivity, drugs, aging, and certain diseases. Dietary changes, fluids, and activity prevent or relieve constipation. So do drugs and enemas.
- **Fecal impaction**—is the prolonged retention and buildup of feces in the rectum. Feces are hard or putty-like. Fecal impaction results if constipation is not relieved. The person cannot defecate. More water is absorbed from already hard feces. Liquid feces pass around the hardened fecal mass in the rectum. The liquid feces seep from the anus. The person tries many times to have a bowel movement. Abdominal discomfort, nausea, cramping, and rectal pain are common. The doctor may order drugs and enemas to remove the impaction. Sometimes the nurse removes the fecal mass with a gloved finger. This is called *digital removal of an impaction*.
- **Diarrhea**—is the frequent passage of liquid stools. Feces move through the intestines rapidly. This reduces the time for fluid absorption. The need to defecate is urgent. Some people cannot get to a bathroom in time. Abdominal cramping, nausea, and vomiting may occur. Causes of diarrhea include infections, some drugs, irritating foods, and microbes in food and water. Good skin care is needed. Fluid lost through diarrhea is replaced. Microbes often cause diarrhea. Always practice Standard Precautions.
- **Fecal incontinence**—is the inability to control the passage of feces and gas through the anus. Causes include intestinal diseases and nervous system diseases and injuries. Fecal impaction, diarrhea, some drugs, and aging are other causes. Unanswered signal lights can result in fecal incontinence. Fecal incontinence affects the person emotionally. Frustration, embarrassment, anger, and humiliation are common. Good skin care is required. The person may need bowel training (p. 250).
- **Flatulence**—is the excessive formation of gas or air in the stomach and intestines. Gas and air passed through the anus is called **flatus.** Common causes of flatulence are gas-forming foods, bacterial action in the intestines, and constipation. If flatus is not expelled, the intestines distend. That is, they swell or enlarge from the pressure of the gases. Abdominal cramping or pain, shortness of breath, and a swollen abdomen occur. "Bloating" is a common complaint. Walking, moving in bed, and the left side-lying position often produce flatus. Doctors may order enemas, drugs, or rectal tubes to relieve flatulence.

BOWEL ELIMINATION

Some people have a bowel movement every day. Others have one every 2 to 3 days. Some people have 2 or 3 bowel movements a day. Many people defecate after breakfast. Others do so in the evening.

Stools are normally brown, soft, formed, moist, and shaped like the rectum. They have a normal odor caused by bacterial action in the intestines. Certain foods and drugs also cause odors. Age and disease can affect bowel elimination (Box 13-6).

Observations

Your observations are used for the nursing process. Carefully observe stools before disposing of them. Observe and report the following to the nurse: color, consistency, odor, shape, size, and frequency of defecation. Ask the nurse to observe abnormal stools.

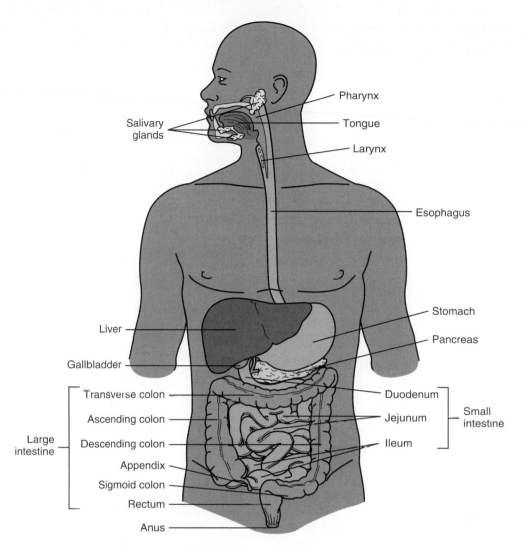

Fig. 13-18 The gastrointestinal system.

Factors Affecting Bowel Elimination

These factors affect stool frequency, consistency, color, and odor:

- *Privacy*—Lack of privacy can prevent defecation despite having the urge. Odors and sounds are embarrassing.
- *Habits*—Many people have a bowel movement after breakfast. Some drink a hot beverage, read, or take a walk. These activities are relaxing. Defecation is easier when a person is relaxed, not tense.
- *Diet*—A well-balanced diet and bulk are needed. High-fiber foods leave a residue for needed bulk. Fruits, vegetables, and whole grain cereals and breads are high in fiber. Gas-forming foods stimulate peristalsis, which aids defecation. They include onions, beans, cabbage, cauliflower, radishes, and cucumbers.

- *Fluids*—Feces contain water. Stool consistency depends on the amount of water absorbed in the colon. Feces harden and dry when large amounts of water are absorbed or when fluid intake is poor. Hard, dry feces move slowly through the colon. Constipation can occur. Drinking 6 to 8 glasses of water daily promotes normal bowel elimination. Warm fluids—coffee, tea, hot cider, and warm water—increase peristalsis.
- *Activity*—Exercise and activity maintain muscle tone and stimulate peristalsis.
- *Drugs*—Drugs can prevent constipation or control diarrhea. Other drugs have diarrhea or constipation as side effects.
- *Disability*—Some people cannot control bowel movements. They defecate whenever feces enter the rectum. A bowel training program is needed (p. 258).
- *Age*—Aging slows down the passage of feces through the intestines. This results in constipation. For some people, changes from aging cause fecal incontinence.

Comfort and Safety

The care plan includes measures to meet the person's elimination needs. It may involve diet, fluids, and exercise. Follow the measures in Box 13-2 to promote comfort and safety.

Bowel Training

Bowel training has two goals:

- To gain control of bowel movements.
- To develop a regular pattern of elimination. Fecal impaction, constipation, and fecal incontinence are prevented.

Meals, especially breakfast, stimulate the urge to defecate. The person's usual time of day for defecation is noted on the care plan. Toilet, commode, or bedpan use is offered at this time. Factors that promote elimination are part of the care plan and bowel training program.

The doctor may order a suppository to stimulate defecation. A *suppository* is a cone-shaped, solid drug that is inserted into a body opening. It melts at body temperature. A nurse inserts a rectal suppository into the rectum. A bowel movement occurs about 30 minutes later.

Enemas

An **enema** is the introduction of fluid into the rectum and lower colon. Doctors order enemas to remove feces and to relieve constipation, fecal impaction, or flatulence.

The doctor orders the type of enema and the enema solution. The solution depends on the enema's purpose:

- *Cleansing enemas*—clean the bowel of feces and flatus. They relieve constipation and fecal impaction. The doctor orders a soapsuds, tap-water, or saline solution. Usually 500 to 1000 ml of solution is given.

- *Small-volume enemas*—irritate and distend the rectum. This causes defecation. They are often ordered for constipation or when the bowel does not need complete cleansing. They contain about 120 ml of solution.
- *Oil-retention enemas*—relieve constipation and fecal impactions. The oil is retained for 30 to 60 minutes or longer (1 to 3 hours). Retaining oil softens feces and lubricates the rectum. This lets feces pass with ease. Most oil-retention enemas involve mineral, olive, or cottonseed oil.

Delegation Guidelines

Enemas

You may be asked to give a small-volume enema. Before doing so, you need this information from the nurse and the care plan:

- How to position the person—Sims' or the left side-lying position
- How long the person should try to retain the solution
- What to report and record

Safety Alert

Enemas

Enemas are usually safe procedures. Many people give themselves enemas at home. However, enemas are dangerous for older persons and those with certain heart and kidney diseases.

Contact with stools is likely when giving enemas. They may contain microbes and blood. Follow Standard Precautions and the Bloodborne Pathogen Standard.

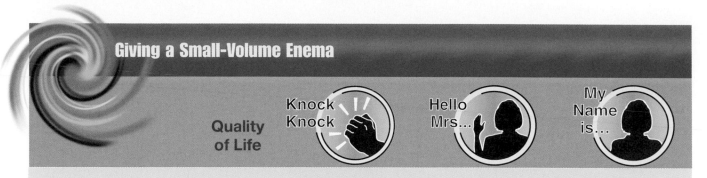

Giving a Small-Volume Enema

Quality of Life · Knock Knock · Hello Mrs... · My Name is...

Pre-Procedure

1   Follow *Delegation Guidelines: Enemas.* See *Safety Alert: Enemas.*
2   Explain the procedure to the person.
3   Practice hand hygiene.
4   Collect the following:
   - Small-volume enema
   - Bedpan or commode
   - Waterproof pad
   - Toilet tissue
   - Gloves
   - Robe and nonskid footwear
   - Bath blanket
5   Identify the person. Check the ID bracelet against the assignment sheet. Call the person by name.
6   Provide for privacy.
7   Raise the bed for body mechanics. Bed rails are up if used.

Procedure

8   Lower the bed rail near you if up.
9   Cover the person with a bath blanket. Fanfold top linens to the foot of the bed.
10 Position the person in Sims' or a left side-lying position.
11 Decontaminate your hands. Put on the gloves.
12 Place the waterproof pad under the buttocks.
13 Expose the anal area.
14 Position the bedpan near the person.
15 Remove the cap from the enema tip.
16 Separate the buttocks to see the anus.
17 Ask the person to take a deep breath through the mouth.
18 Insert the enema tip 2 inches into the rectum (Fig. 13-19, p. 260). Do this when the person is exhaling. Insert the tip gently. Stop if the person complains of pain, you feel resistance, or bleeding occurs.
19 Squeeze and roll the bottle gently. Release pressure on the bottle after you remove the tip from the rectum.
20 Put the bottle into the box, tip first.
21 Help the person onto the bedpan; raise the head of the bed. Raise or lower bed rails according to the care plan. Or assist the person to the bathroom or commode. The person wears a robe and nonskid footwear when up. The bed is in the lowest position.
22 Place the signal light and toilet tissue within reach. Remind the person not to flush the toilet.
23 Discard disposable items.
24 Remove the gloves. Decontaminate your hands.
25 Leave the room if the person can be left alone.
26 Return when the person signals. Or check on the person every 5 minutes. Knock before entering.
27 Decontaminate your hands. Lower the bed rail if up.
28 Put on gloves.
29 Observe enema results for amount, color, consistency, and odor.
30 Help the person with perineal care.
31 Remove the bed protector.
32 Empty, clean, and disinfect the bedpan or commode. Flush the toilet after the nurse observes the results.
33 Return equipment to its proper place.
34 Remove the gloves. Practice hand hygiene.
35 Assist with hand washing. Wear gloves.
36 Return top linens. Remove the bath blanket.

Post-Procedure

37 Provide for comfort.
38 Place the signal light within reach.
39 Lower the bed to its lowest position.
40 Raise or lower bed rails. Follow the care plan.
41 Unscreen the person.
42 Complete a safety check of the room. (See inside of front book cover.)
43 Follow center policy for soiled linen and used supplies.
44 Decontaminate your hands.
45 Report and record your observations.

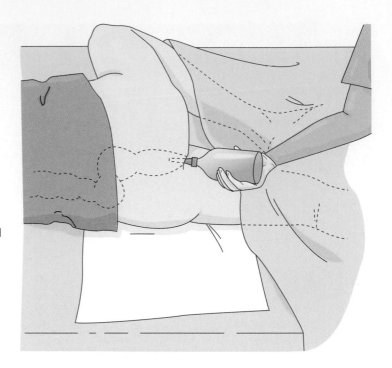

Fig. 13-19 The small-volume enema tip is inserted 2 inches into the rectum.

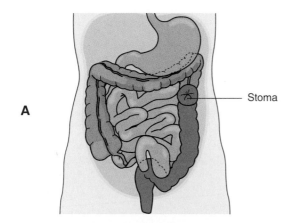

A

Stoma

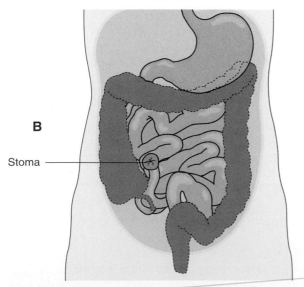

B

Stoma

Fig. 13-20 Ostomy sites. *Shading* shows the part of the bowel surgically removed. **A,** A colostomy in the descending colon. **B,** An ileostomy. The entire large intestine is removed.

The Person With an Ostomy

Cancer, bowel disease, and trauma (stab or bullet wounds) are common reasons for intestinal surgery. An ostomy is sometimes necessary. An **ostomy** is a surgically created opening. The opening is called a **stoma.** The person wears a pouch over the stoma to collect feces and flatus.

- A **colostomy** is a surgically created opening *(stomy)* between the colon *(colo)* and abdominal wall. Part of the colon is brought out onto the abdominal wall, and a stoma is made. Feces and flatus pass through the stoma, not the anus. With a permanent colostomy, the diseased part of the colon is removed. A temporary colostomy gives the diseased or injured bowel time to heal. After healing, surgery is done to reconnect the bowel. The colostomy site depends on the site of disease or injury (Fig. 13-20, *A*). Stool consistency depends on the colostomy site. Stools range from liquid to formed. The more colon remaining to absorb water, the more solid and formed the stool. If the colostomy is near the start of the colon, stools are liquid. A colostomy near the end of the colon results in formed stools.
- An **ileostomy** is a surgically created opening *(stomy)* between the ileum (small intestine *[ileo]*) and the abdominal wall. Part of the ileum is brought out onto the abdominal wall, and a stoma is made. The entire colon is removed (Fig. 13-20, *B*). Liquid feces drain constantly from an ileostomy. Water is not absorbed because the colon was removed. Feces in the small intestine contain digestive juices that are very irritating to the skin.

Ostomy Pouches.   Feces irritate the skin. The ostomy pouch must fit well. Good skin care is essential. Skin care prevents skin breakdown around the stoma. The skin is washed and dried. Then a skin barrier is applied around the stoma. It prevents feces from having contact with the skin. The skin barrier is part of the pouch or a separate device.

The pouch has an adhesive backing that is applied to the skin. Sometimes pouches are secured to ostomy belts (Fig. 13-21). Many pouches have a drain at the bottom that closes with clips, clamps, or wire closures. The drain is opened to empty the pouch. The pouch is emptied when feces are present. It is opened when it balloons or bulges with flatus. The drain is wiped with toilet tissue before it is closed. The pouch is changed every 3 to 7 days and when it leaks.

Odors are prevented by:

- Good hygiene
- Emptying the pouch
- Avoiding gas-forming foods
- Putting deodorants into the pouch (The nurse tells you what to use.)

The person can wear normal clothes. However, tight garments can prevent feces from entering the pouch. Also, bulging from feces and flatus can be seen with tight clothes.

Peristalsis increases after eating. Therefore stomas are usually quiet before breakfast. That is, expelling feces is less likely at this time. If the person showers or bathes with the pouch off, it is best done before breakfast. Showers and baths are delayed 1 or 2 hours after a new pouch is applied. This gives adhesive time to stick to the skin.

Do not flush pouches down the toilet. Follow center policy for disposing of them.

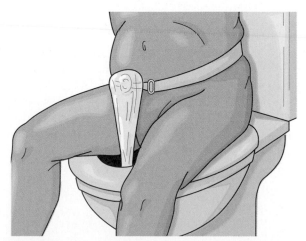

Fig. 13-21 The ostomy pouch is secured to an ostomy belt. The pouch is emptied by directing it into the toilet and unclamping the end.

Safety Alert

Ostomy Pouches
When handling ostomy pouches, contact with feces is likely. They may contain microbes or blood. Follow Standard Precautions and the Bloodborne Pathogen Standard.

Tell the nurse if you observe signs of skin breakdown.

Stool Specimens
When internal bleeding is suspected, feces are checked for blood. Stools also are studied for fat, microbes, worms, and other abnormal contents. The stool specimen must not be contaminated with urine. Some tests require a warm stool. The specimen is taken to the storage area where it is kept warm. When collecting stool specimens, follow the rules in Box 13-5.

Delegation Guidelines

Stool Specimens
Before collecting a stool specimen, you need this information from the nurse:
- What time to collect the specimen
- What special measures are needed
- What observations to report and record:
  —Problems obtaining the specimen
  —Color, amount, consistency, and odor of feces
  —Complaints of pain or discomfort

Safety Alert

Stool Specimens
Stools contain microbes. And they may contain blood. Follow Standard Precautions and the Bloodborne Pathogen Standard.

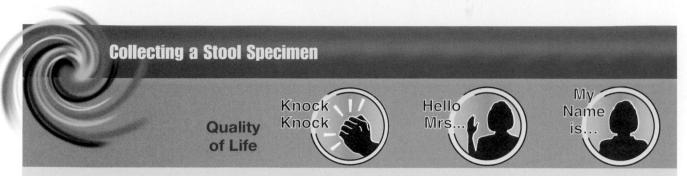

Collecting a Stool Specimen

Quality of Life

Knock Knock

Hello Mrs...

My Name is...

Pre-Procedure

1 Follow *Delegation Guidelines: Stool Specimens,* p. 261. See *Safety Alert: Stool Specimens,* p. 261.
2 Explain the procedure to the person.
3 Practice hand hygiene.
4 Collect the following:
   • Bedpan and cover or commode
   • Urinal for voiding
   • Specimen pan for the toilet or commode
   • Specimen container and lid
   • Tongue blade

   • Disposable bag
   • Gloves
   • Toilet tissue
   • Laboratory requisition slip
   • Plastic bag

5 Label the container. Decontaminate your hands.
6 Identify the person. Check the ID bracelet against the requisition slip. Call the person by name.
7 Provide for privacy.

Procedure

8 Decontaminate your hands. Put on gloves.
9 Ask the person to void. Provide the bedpan, commode, or urinal for voiding if the person does not use the bathroom. Empty and clean the device.
10 Put the specimen pan on the toilet if the person will use the bathroom. Place it at the back of the toilet.
11 Assist the person onto the bedpan or to the toilet or commode. The person wears a robe and nonskid footwear when up.
12 Ask the person not to put toilet tissue in the bedpan, commode, or specimen pan. Provide a bag for toilet tissue.
13 Place the signal light and toilet tissue within reach. Raise or lower bed rails. Follow the care plan.
14 Remove the gloves, and practice hand hygiene. Leave the room.
15 Return when the person signals. Or check on the person every 5 minutes. Knock before entering. Decontaminate your hands.

16 Lower the bed rail near you if up.
17 Put on the gloves. Provide perineal care if needed.
18 Use a tongue blade to take about 2 tablespoons of stool to the specimen container (Fig. 13-22). Take the sample from the middle of a formed stool. If required by center policy, take stool from 2 different places on the specimen.
19 Put the lid on the specimen container. Do not touch the inside of the lid or container. Place the container in the plastic bag.
20 Wrap the tongue blade in toilet tissue.
21 Discard the tongue blade into the bag.
22 Empty, clean, and disinfect equipment.
23 Remove the gloves. Decontaminate your hands.
24 Return equipment to its proper place.
25 Help the person with hand washing. Wear gloves.

Post-Procedure

26 Provide for comfort.
27 Place the signal light within reach.
28 Lower the bed to its lowest position.
29 Raise or lower bed rails. Follow the care plan.
30 Unscreen the person.
31 Complete a safety check of the room. (See inside of front book cover.)

32 Take the specimen and requisition slip to the storage area.
33 Decontaminate your hands.
34 Report and record your observations.

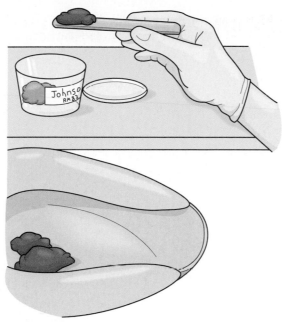

Fig. 13-22 A tongue blade is used to transfer a small amount of stool from the bedpan to the specimen container.

Review Questions

Circle the **BEST** answer.

1 Which is *false?*
    a Urine is normally clear and yellow or amber in color.
    b Urine normally has an ammonia odor.
    c Voiding usually occurs before going to bed and on rising.
    d A person normally voids about 1500 ml a day.

2 Which is *not* a rule for normal elimination?
    a Help the person assume a normal position for voiding.
    b Provide for privacy.
    c Help the person to the bathroom or commode. Or provide the bedpan or urinal as soon as requested.
    d Always stay with the person who is on a bedpan.

3 The best position for using a bedpan is
    a Fowler's position
    b The supine position
    c The prone position
    d The side-lying position

4 After using the urinal, the man should
    a Put it on the bedside stand
    b Use the signal light
    c Put it on the overbed table
    d Empty it

5 Urinary incontinence
    a Is always permanent
    b Requires good skin care
    c Is treated with a catheter
    d Requires bladder training

6 A person has an indwelling catheter. Which action is *not correct?*
    a Keep the drainage bag above the level of the bladder.
    b Keep drainage tubing free of kinks.
    c Coil the drainage tubing on the bed.
    d Secure the catheter according to center policy.

Review Questions

7 A person has a catheter. Which action is *not correct?*
   a Tape any leaks at the connection site.
   b Follow Standard Precautions and the Bloodborne Pathogen Standard.
   c Empty the drainage bag at the end of your shift.
   d Report complaints of pain, burning, the need to urinate, or irritation at once.

8 The goal of bladder training is to
   a Remove the catheter
   b Allow the person to walk to the bathroom
   c Gain control of urination
   d Void every 3 or 4 hours

9 You are going to collect a random urine specimen. You should do the following *except*
   a Label the container as requested
   b Use the correct container
   c Collect the specimen at the right time
   d Clean the perineum

10 Which is *false?*
    a A person must have a bowel movement every day.
    b Stools are normally brown, soft, and formed.
    c Diarrhea occurs when feces move rapidly through the bowels.
    d Constipation results when feces move slowly through the colon.

11 The prolonged retention and accumulation of feces in the rectum is called
    a Constipation
    b Fecal impaction
    c Diarrhea
    d Anal incontinence

12 Bowel training is aimed at
    a Gaining control of bowel movements and developing a regular elimination pattern
    b Ostomy control
    c Preventing fecal impaction, constipation, and anal incontinence
    d Preventing bleeding

13 Small-volume enemas
    a Are given in the Sims' or left side-lying position
    b Contain 500 to 1000 ml of solution
    c Are retained for 30 to 60 minutes
    d Soften feces

14 Which statement about ostomies is *false?*
    a Good skin care around the stoma is essential.
    b Deodorants can control odors.
    c The person wears a pouch.
    d Feces are always liquid.

15 A stool specimen must be kept warm. After collecting the specimen, you need to
    a Put in the oven
    b Take it to the storage area
    c Take it to the laboratory
    d Cover it with a towel

Answers to these questions are on p. 389.

CHAPTER 14

Nutrition

Objectives

- Define the key terms listed in this chapter
- Explain the purpose and use of the Food Guide Pyramid
- Describe factors that affect eating and nutrition
- Describe the special diets
- Identify the signs, symptoms, and precautions relating to regurgitation and aspiration
- Describe fluid requirements and the causes of dehydration
- Explain what to do when the person has special fluid orders
- Explain how to assist with enteral nutrition and IV therapy
- Perform the procedures described in this chapter

anorexia Loss of appetite

calorie The amount of energy produced when the body burns food

dysphagia Difficulty *(dys)* swallowing *(phagia)*

enteral nutrition Giving nutrients through the gastrointestinal tract *(enteral)*

gavage Tube feeding

intravenous (IV) therapy Giving fluids through a needle or catheter inserted into a vein; IV, IV therapy, and IV infusion

nutrient A substance that is ingested, digested, absorbed, and used by the body

nutrition The processes involved in the ingestion, digestion, absorption, and use of foods and fluids by the body

regurgitation The backward flow of food from the stomach into the mouth

---

Food and water are needed for life. They affect physical and mental well-being. Food and water are needed to help:

- Prevent infection
- Prevent acute and chronic diseases
- Prevent chronic illnesses from becoming worse
- Promote healing
- Decrease the risk for accidents and injuries

The digestive system is discussed in Box 14-1.

BASIC NUTRITION

Nutrition is the processes involved in the ingestion, digestion, absorption, and use of foods and fluids by the body. Foods and fluids contain nutrients. A **nutrient** is a substance that is ingested, digested, absorbed, and used by the body. Nutrients are grouped into fats, proteins, carbohydrates, vitamins, minerals, and water.

Fats, proteins, and carbohydrates give the body fuel for energy. The amount of energy provided by nutrients is measured in calories. A **calorie** is the amount of energy produced when the body burns food:

- 1 gram of fat—9 calories
- 1 gram of protein—4 calories
- 1 gram of carbohydrate—4 calories

Food Guide Pyramid

The *Food Guide Pyramid* promotes wise food choices (Fig. 14-2, p. 268). It suggests eating more foods at the bottom level (level 1) and lesser amounts at each level moving to the top (level 4). A low-fat diet is the goal. More bread, cereal, rice, and pasta (level 1) and more vegetables and fruits (level 2) are eaten. Food from the milk, yogurt, and cheese group are eaten in moderate amounts. So are foods from the meat, poultry, fish, beans, eggs, and nut group (level 3). Fats,

oils, and sweets (level 4) are used sparingly. See Box 14-2, p. 269 for serving sizes.

Foods from levels 1, 2, and 3 are needed daily. They contain the essential nutrients. No one food or food group contains every nutrient.

- *Breads, cereals, rice, and pasta group.* A person needs 6 to 11 servings a day. Foods come from grain (wheat, oats, rice, corn, and so on). They provide protein, carbohydrates, and some vitamins and minerals—thiamin, niacin, riboflavin, and iron.
- *Vegetable group.* A person needs 3 to 5 servings a day. Low in fat, vegetables provide fiber, vitamins A and C, carbohydrates, and minerals. A variety of vegetables are eaten—dark green and yellow vegetables, tomatoes, potatoes, and vegetable juices.
- *Fruit group.* A person needs 2 to 4 fruit servings daily. Fruits provide carbohydrates, vitamins A and C, potassium, and other minerals. Fresh fruits and juices are best. Frozen and canned fruits that are sweetened or syrupy juices are high in sugar and calories.
- *Milk, yogurt, and cheese group.* A person needs 2 to 3 servings daily. This group is high in protein, carbohydrates, fat, calcium, and riboflavin.
- *Meat, poultry, fish, dry beans, eggs, and nuts group.* A person needs 2 to 3 servings a day. This food group is high in fat and protein. Wise food choices lower fat intake and calories. Fish and shellfish are low in fat. Chicken and turkey have less fat than veal, beef, pork, and lamb. Veal has less fat than beef. Use lean cuts of beef and pork. Egg yolks have more fat than egg whites. Nuts and peanut butter have the most fat in this group. Peas and cooked dry beans are very low in fat.
- *Fats, oils, and sweets group.* Fats, oils, and sweets (foods with added sugar) are high in fat with few nutrients. Use them sparingly and as little as

Text continued on p. 269

BOX
14-1
Digestive System

Body Structure and Function

The digestive system breaks down food physically and chemically so it can be absorbed for use by the cells. This process is called *digestion*. The digestive system is also called the *gastrointestinal system (GI system)*. It consists of the *alimentary canal (GI tract)* and the accessory organs of digestion (Fig. 14-1, p. 268). The alimentary canal extends from the mouth to the anus. Its major parts are the mouth, pharynx, esophagus, stomach, small intestine, and large intestine. The accessory organs of digestion are the teeth, tongue, salivary glands, liver, gallbladder, and pancreas.

Digestion begins in the *mouth (oral cavity)*. The oral cavity receives food and prepares it for digestion. Using chewing motions, the *teeth* cut, chop, and grind food into smaller particles for digestion and swallowing. The *tongue* aids in chewing and swallowing. *Taste buds* on the tongue contain nerve endings. Taste buds sense sweet, sour, bitter, and salty tastes. *Salivary glands* in the mouth secrete *saliva*. Saliva moistens food particles for easier swallowing and begins the digestion of food. During swallowing, the tongue pushes food into the pharynx.

The *pharynx* (throat) is a muscular tube. Swallowing continues as the pharynx contracts. Contraction of the pharynx pushes food into the *esophagus*. The esophagus is a muscular tube about 10 inches long. It extends from the pharynx to the stomach. Involuntary muscle contractions called *peristalsis* move food down the esophagus into the stomach.

The *stomach* is a muscular, pouch-like sac in the upper left part of the abdominal cavity. Strong stomach muscles stir and churn food to break it up into even smaller particles. The stomach is lined with a mucous membrane containing glands that secrete *gastric juices*. Food is mixed and churned with the gastric juices to form a semi-liquid substance called *chyme*. Through peristalsis, the chyme is pushed from the stomach into the small intestine.

For structures and functions of the intestines, see Chapter 13.

Changes With Aging

Salivary glands produce less saliva. This can cause difficulty swallowing. Taste and smell dull. This decreases appetite.

Secretion of digestive juices decreases. As a result, fried and fatty foods are hard to digest. They may cause indigestion.

Loss of teeth and ill-fitting dentures cause chewing problems. This causes digestion problems. Hard-to-chew foods are avoided. Ground or chopped meat is easier to chew.

Peristalsis decreases. The stomach empties slower than when younger.

Fewer calories are needed. Energy and activity levels decline. More fluids are needed for chewing, swallowing, digestion, and kidney function. Foods are needed to prevent constipation and bone changes. High-protein foods are needed for tissue growth and repair. However, some older persons lack protein in their diets. High-protein foods (meat and fish) are costly.

Common Disorders

Diabetes, an endocrine disorder, affects nutrition. The body cannot produce or use insulin properly. Insulin is needed for sugar use. Insulin is secreted by the pancreas. Sugar builds up in the blood. Cells do not have enough sugar for energy. They cannot perform their functions. The three types of diabetes are:
- *Type 1*—occurs most often in children and young adults. The pancreas produces little or no insulin. Onset is rapid. There is increased thirst and urination, constant hunger, weight loss, blurred vision, and extreme fatigue.
- *Type 2*—occurs in adults. Persons over 40 years of age are at risk. Obesity and hypertension are risk factors. The pancreas secretes insulin. However, the body cannot use it well. Onset is slow. The person has fatigue, nausea, frequent urination, increased thirst, weight loss, and blurred vision. Infections are frequent. Wounds heal slowly.
- *Gestational diabetes*—develops during pregnancy. (Gestation comes from *gestare*. It means to *bear*.) It usually goes away after the baby is born. However, the woman is at risk for type 2 diabetes later in life.

Diabetes must be controlled. Otherwise complications occur. These include blindness, renal failure, nerve damage, hypertension, and circulatory disorders. Circulatory disorders can lead to stroke, heart attack, and slow wound healing. Foot and leg wounds are very serious. Infection and gangrene can occur. Sometimes amputation is needed.

Risk factors include a family history of the disease. For type 1, whites are at greater risk than non-whites. Type 2 is more common in older and overweight persons. These ethnic groups are at risk for type 2:
- African-Americans
- Native Americans
- Asian and Pacific Islander Americans
- Hispanics

Type 1 is treated with daily insulin therapy, healthy eating, and exercise. Type 2 is treated with healthy eating and exercise. Many persons with type 2 take oral drugs. Some need insulin. Overweight persons need to lose weight.

Both types require blood glucose monitoring. Good foot care is needed. Corns, blisters, and calluses can lead to an infection and amputation.

The person's blood sugar level can fall too low or go too high:
- *Hypoglycemia* means low *(hypo)* sugar *(glyc)* in the blood *(emia)*. Signs and symptoms include: hunger, weakness, trembling or shakiness, sweating, headache, dizziness, faintness, rapid pulse, low blood pressure, rapid and shallow respirations, confusion, changes in vision, cold and clammy skin, convulsions, and unconsciousness.
- *Hyperglycemia* means high *(hyper)* sugar *(glyc)* in the blood *(emia)*. Signs and symptoms include: weakness, drowsiness, thirst, hunger, frequent urination, leg cramps, flushed face, and sweet breath odor. Respirations are slow, deep, and labored; blood pressure is low; and the pulse is rapid and weak. Dry skin, blurred vision, headache, and nausea and vomiting are other symptoms. Convulsions and coma can occur.

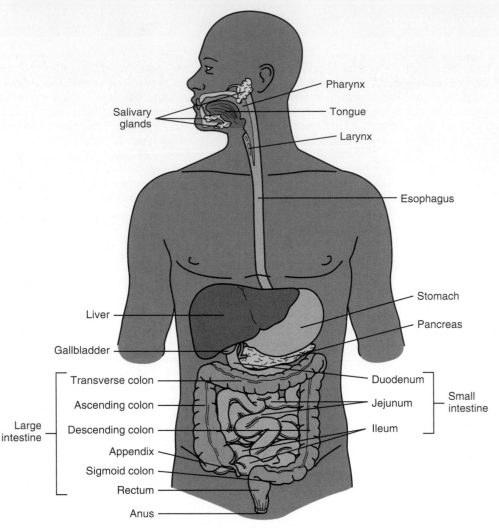

Fig. 14-1 The digestive system.

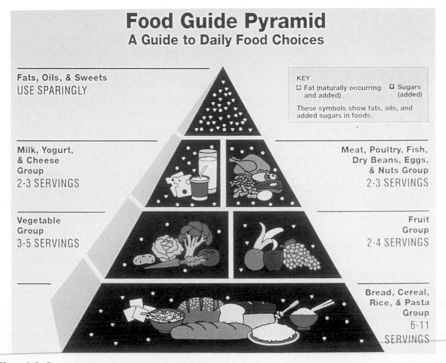

Fig. 14-2 Food Guide Pyramid. Courtesy U.S. Dept. of Agriculture, Washington, D.C.

BOX 14-2   Food Guide Pyramid Serving Sizes

Bread, Cereals, Rice, and Pasta Group (6 to 11 servings daily)

- 1 slice bread = 1 serving
- 1 ounce ready-to-eat cereal = 1 serving
- ½ cup cooked cereal, rice, or pasta = 1 serving

Vegetable Group (3 to 5 servings daily)

- 1 cup raw leafy vegetables = 1 serving
- ½ cup other cooked or chopped raw vegetables = 1 serving
- ¾ cup vegetable juice = 1 serving

Fruit Group (2 to 4 servings daily)

- 1 medium apple, orange, or banana = 1 serving
- ½ cup chopped, cooked, or canned fruit = 1 serving
- ¾ cup fruit juice = 1 serving

Milk, Cheese, and Yogurt Group (2 to 3 servings daily)

- 1 cup milk or yogurt = 1 serving
- ½ to 1 ounce cheese = 1 serving
- 2 ounces process cheese = 1 serving

Meat, Poultry, Fish, Dry Beans, Eggs, and Nuts Group (2 to 3 servings daily)

- 2 to 3 ounces cooked lean meat, poultry, or fish = 1 serving
- ½ cup cooked dry beans = 1 serving
- 1 egg = 1 serving
- 2 tablespoons peanut butter = 1 serving

Fats, Oils, and Sweets Group

- Use sparingly

---

possible. This group includes cooking oils, shortening, butter, margarine, salad dressing, soft drinks, sour cream, cream cheese, and frosting. All candy, most desserts, jelly and jam, syrup, and alcohol are included.

Nutrients

A well-balanced diet has food from levels 1, 2, and 3 of the Food Guide Pyramid. It ensures an adequate intake of essential nutrients:

- *Protein*—is the most important nutrient. It is needed for tissue growth and repair. Sources include meat, fish, poultry, eggs, milk and milk products, cereals, beans, peas, and nuts.
- *Carbohydrates*—provide energy and fiber for bowel elimination. They are found in fruits, vegetables, breads, cereals, and sugar. Fiber is not digested. It is needed for elimination (Chapter 13).
- *Fats*—provide energy. They add flavor to food and help the body use certain vitamins. Sources include meats, lard, butter, shortening, oils, milk, cheese, egg yolks, and nuts. Dietary fat not needed by the body is stored as body fat (adipose tissue).
- *Vitamins*—are needed for certain body functions. The lack of a vitamin results in signs and symptoms of an illness. The body stores vitamins A, D, E, and K. Vitamin C and the B complex vitamins are not stored. They must be ingested daily.
- *Minerals*—are needed for bone and tooth formation, nerve and muscle function, fluid balance, and other body processes. Calcium, phosphorus, iron, sodium, and potassium are common minerals.

FACTORS AFFECTING EATING AND NUTRITION

Many factors affect nutrition and eating habits. Some begin during infancy and continue throughout life. Others develop later.

- *Age*—Age affects nutrition. See Box 14-1.
- *Culture*—Culture influences food choices and food preparation. Frying, baking, smoking, and roasting food and eating raw food are cultural practices. So is the use of sauces and spices. (See *Caring About Culture: Food Practices*, p. 270.)
- *Religion*—Selecting, preparing, and eating food often involve religious practices. A person may follow all, some, or none of the dietary practices of his or her faith. You must respect the person's religious practices.
- *Appetite*—Appetite relates to the desire for food. When hungry, a person seeks food. He or she eats until the appetite is satisfied. However, loss of appetite (**anorexia**) can occur. Causes include illness, drugs, anxiety, pain, and depression. Unpleasant sights, thoughts, and smells are other causes.
- *Personal choice*—Food likes and dislikes are influenced by food served in the home. Body reactions affect food choices. People usually avoid foods that cause allergic reactions, nausea, vomiting, diarrhea, indigestion, or headaches.
- *Illness*—Appetite usually decreases during illness and recovery from injuries. However, nutritional needs are increased. The body must fight infection, heal tissue, and replace lost blood cells. Nutrients lost through vomiting and diarrhea are replaced. Some diseases and drugs cause a sore mouth. This makes eating painful.

Caring About Culture

Food Practices

Food practices vary among cultural groups. Rice and beans are protein sources in *Mexico*. In the *Philippines*, rice is preferred with every meal. A diet high in starch and fat is common in *Poland*. Potatoes, rye, and wheat are common. The diet in *China* is low in fat but high in sodium. The sodium content is from the use of soy sauce and dried and preserved foods.

Eating beef is common in the *United States*. Beef is not eaten in *India*. Organ meats are common in *England*.

From D'Avanzo CE, Geissler EM: *Pocket guide to cultural health assessment*, ed 3, St Louis, 2003, Mosby.

OBRA DIETARY REQUIREMENTS

OBRA has these requirements for food served in nursing centers:

- Each person's nutritional and dietary needs are met.
- The person's diet is well-balanced and nourishing. Food is well-seasoned and tastes good. It is not too salty nor too sweet.
- Food is appetizing. It smells good and is attractive.
- Hot food is served hot. Cold food is served cold. Food servers keep food at the correct temperature.
- Food is served promptly. Otherwise, hot food cools and cold food warms.
- Food is prepared to meet each person's needs. Some people need food cut, ground, or chopped. Others have special diets.
- Each person receives at least 3 meals a day. A bedtime snack is offered.
- The center provides any special eating equipment and utensils (Fig. 14-3). Called adaptive equipment, they allow the person to eat independently.

SPECIAL DIETS

Doctors may order special diets for a nutritional deficiency or a disease. They also order them to remove or decrease certain substances in the diet. The health team works together to meet the person's nutritional needs. See Box 14-3. *Regular diet, general diet,* and *house diet* mean no dietary limits or restrictions.

The Sodium-Controlled Diet

The average amount of sodium in the daily diet is 3000 to 5000 mg. The body needs no more than 1500 to 2400 mg. Healthy people excrete excess sodium in the urine. Heart, liver, and kidney diseases and certain drugs cause the body to retain extra sodium.

Sodium causes the body to retain water. If there is too much sodium, the body retains more water. Tissues swell with water. There is excess fluid in the blood vessels. The heart has to work harder. Sodium

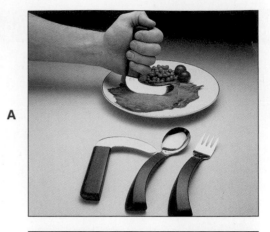

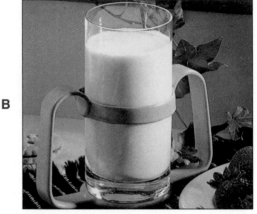

Fig. 14-3 Eating utensils for persons with special needs. **A,** Knives with rounded blades are rocked back and forth to cut food. The person does not need a fork in one hand and a knife in the other. The fork and spoon are curved. **B,** Glass or cup holder. Courtesy Sammons Preston: An AbilityOne Company, Bolingbrook, Ill.

control decreases the amount of sodium in the body. The body retains less water. Less water in the tissues and blood vessels reduces the heart's workload. The doctor orders the amount of sodium restriction.

Diabetes Meal Planning

Diabetes is a chronic disease from a lack of insulin (see Box 14-1). Diabetes is usually treated with insulin or other drugs, diet, and exercise. The dietitian and person develop a meal plan. Consistency is key. It involves:

- The person's food preferences—likes and dislikes, eating habits, meal times, culture, and life-style. It may be necessary to limit amounts of food or change how food is prepared.
- Calories needed. The same amounts of carbohydrates, protein, and fat are eaten each day.
- Meal and snack times are the same from day to day. Serve meals and snacks on time. The person eats at regular times to maintain a certain blood sugar level.

BOX 14-3   Special Diets

Diet	Foods Allowed
Clear liquid—foods liquid at body temperature and that leave small amounts of residue; non-irritating and non-gas forming	Water, tea, and coffee (without milk or cream); carbonated beverages; gelatin; clear fruit juices (apple, grape, cranberry); fat-free clear broth; hard candy, sugar, and Popsicles
Full liquid—foods liquid at room temperature or melt at body temperature	Foods on the clear liquid diet; custard; eggnog; strained soups; strained fruit and vegetable juices; milk and milk shakes; strained, cooked cereals; plain ice cream and sherbet; pudding; yogurt
Mechanical soft—semi-solid foods that are easily digested	All liquids; eggs (not fried); broiled, baked, or roasted meat, fish, or poultry that is chopped or shredded; mild cheeses (American, Swiss, cheddar, cream, cottage); strained fruit juices; refined bread (no crust) and crackers; cooked cereal; cooked or pureed vegetables; cooked or canned fruit without skin or seeds; pudding; plain cakes and soft cookies without fruit or nuts
High fiber—foods that increase the amount of residue and fiber in the colon to stimulate peristalsis	All fruits and vegetables; whole wheat bread; whole grain cereals; fried foods; whole grain rice; milk, cream, butter, and cheese; meats
High calorie—calorie intake is increased to about 3000 to 4000 a day; includes 3 full meals and between-meal snacks	Dietary increases in all foods; large portions of a regular diet with 3 between-meal snacks
Calorie controlled—provides adequate nutrients while controlling calories to promote weight loss and reduction of body fat	Foods low in fats and carbohydrates and lean meats; avoid butter, cream, rice, gravies, salad oils, noodles, cakes, pastries, carbonated and alcoholic beverages, candy, potato chips, and similar foods
High iron—foods that are high in iron	Liver and other organ meats; lean meats; egg yolks; shellfish; dried fruits; dried beans; green leafy vegetables; lima beans; peanut butter; enriched breads and cereals
Fat controlled (low cholesterol)—foods low in fat and foods prepared without adding fat	Skim milk or buttermilk; cottage cheese (no other cheeses allowed); gelatin; sherbet; fruit; lean meat, poultry, and fish (baked, broiled, roasted); fat-free broth; soups made with skim milk; margarine; rice, pasta, breads, and cereals; vegetables; potatoes
High protein—aids and promotes tissue healing	Meat, milk, eggs, cheese, fish, poultry; breads and cereals; green leafy vegetables
Sodium controlled—a certain amount of sodium is allowed	Fruits and vegetables and unsalted butter are allowed; adding salt at the table is not allowed; highly salted foods and foods high in sodium are not allowed; the use of salt during cooking may be restricted
Diabetes meal planning—the same amount of carbohydrates, protein, and fat are eaten at the same time each day	Determined by nutritional and energy requirements

Always check the tray to see what was eaten. Tell the nurse what the person did and did not eat. If all food was not eaten, a snack is needed. The nurse tells you what to give the person for a snack. It makes up for what was not eaten at the meal. The amount of insulin given also depends on daily food intake. Tell the nurse about changes in the person's eating habits.

The Dysphagia Diet

Dysphagia means difficulty *(dys)* swallowing *(phagia)*. In severe cases, food enters the airway. *Aspiration* is breathing fluid or an object into the lungs (Chapter 5 and p. 272).

The dysphagia diet involves changing food thickness to meet the person's needs. The health team chooses the right food thickness.

Safety Alert

The Dysphagia Diet

You may be asked to feed a person with dysphagia. To promote safety, you must:

- Know the signs and symptoms of dysphagia (Box 14-4).
- Position the person's head and neck correctly. Follow the care plan.
- Feed the person according to the care plan.
- Follow aspiration precautions (Box 14-5).
- Report changes in how the person eats.
- Report choking, coughing, or difficulty breathing during or after meals. Also report abnormal breathing or respiratory sounds. Report these observations at once.

FLUID BALANCE

Water is needed to live. Death can result from too much or too little water. Water is ingested through fluids and foods. Water is lost through urine, feces, and vomit. It is also lost through the skin (perspiration) and the lungs (expiration).

Fluid balance is needed for health. The amount of fluid taken in *(intake)* and the amount of fluid lost *(output)* must be equal. If fluid intake exceeds fluid output, body tissues swell with water. This is called *edema*. Edema is common in people with heart and kidney diseases. *Dehydration* is a decrease in the amount of water in body tissues. Fluid output exceeds intake. Common causes are poor fluid intake, vomiting, diarrhea, bleeding, excess sweating, and increased urine production.

Normal Fluid Requirements

An adult needs 1500 ml of water daily to survive. About 2000 to 2500 ml of fluid per day is needed for normal fluid balance. The water requirement increases with hot weather, exercise, fever, illness, and excess fluid losses.

Older persons may have a decreased sense of thirst. Their bodies need water, but they may not feel thirsty. Offer them water often. Follow special fluid orders.

BOX 14-4 Signs and Symptoms of Dysphagia

- The person avoids foods that need chewing.
- Food spills out of the person's mouth while eating.
- Food "pockets" or is "squirreled" in the person's cheeks.
- The person eats slowly, especially solid foods.
- The person complains that food will not go down or the food is stuck.
- The person frequently coughs or chokes before, during, or after swallowing.
- The person regurgitates food after eating (p. 279).
- The person spits out food suddenly and almost violently.
- Food comes up through the person's nose.
- The person is hoarse—especially after eating.
- After swallowing, the person makes gargling sounds while talking or breathing.
- There is excessive drooling of saliva.
- The person complains of frequent heartburn.
- The person's appetite is decreased.
- The person has unexplained weight loss.
- The person has recurrent pneumonia.

BOX 14-5 Aspiration Precautions

- Help the person with meals and snacks. Follow the care plan.
- Position the person in Fowler's position or upright in a chair for meals and snacks.
- Support the upper back, shoulders, and neck with a pillow. Follow the care plan.
- Observe for signs and symptoms of aspiration during meals and snacks.
- Check the person's mouth after each meal and snack for pocketing. Check inside the cheeks, under the tongue, and on the roof of the mouth. Remove any food present. Report your observations to the nurse.
- Position the person in a chair or in semi-Fowler's position after each meal or snack. The person maintains this position for at least 1 hour after eating. Follow the care plan.
- Provide mouth care after each meal or snack.

Special Orders

The doctor may order the amount of fluid a person can have during a 24-hour period. This is done to maintain fluid balance. Intake records are kept (Chapter 7). Found on the care plan, common orders are:

- *Encourage fluids*—The person drinks an increased amount of fluid. The order may be general or state the amount to ingest. Fluids are kept within the person's reach. They are served at the correct temperature. Fluids are offered often to persons who cannot feed themselves.
- *Restrict fluids*—Fluids are limited to a certain amount. They are offered in small amounts and in small containers. The water pitcher is removed from the room or kept out of sight. The person needs frequent oral hygiene to keep the mouth moist.
- *Nothing by mouth*—The person cannot eat or drink anything. *NPO* is the abbreviation for *non per os*. It means nothing *(non)* by *(per)* mouth *(os)*. NPO often is ordered before and after surgery, before some laboratory tests and diagnostic procedures, and to treat certain illnesses. The water pitcher and glass are removed. Frequent oral hygiene is needed, but the person must not swallow any fluid. The person is NPO 6 to 8 hours before surgery and before some laboratory tests and diagnostic procedures.

MEETING FOOD AND FLUIDS NEEDS

Weakness, illness, and confusion can affect appetite and eating. An uncomfortable position, the need for oral hygiene, the need to eliminate, and pain also affect appetite.

Preparing for Meals

You need to prepare residents for meals. They need to eliminate and have oral care. They need dentures, eyeglasses, and hearing aids in place. If incontinent, they need to be clean and dry. A comfortable position for eating is important.

The setting must be free of unpleasant sights, sounds, and odors. Remove unpleasant equipment from the room.

Delegation Guidelines

Preparing for Meals

To prepare a person for a meal, you need this information from the nurse and care plan:
- How much help the person needs
- Where the person will eat—dining area or room
- What the person uses for elimination—bathroom, commode, bedpan, urinal, or specimen pan
- The type of oral hygiene needed
- If the person wears dentures
- How to position the person—in bed or in a chair
- If the person wears eyeglasses or hearing aids
- How the person gets to the dining room—by self or with help
- If the person uses a wheelchair, walker, or cane

Safety Alert

Preparing for Meals

Before meals, the person needs to eliminate and have oral hygiene. Follow Standard Precautions and the Bloodborne Pathogen Standard. Also follow them when cleaning equipment and the room.

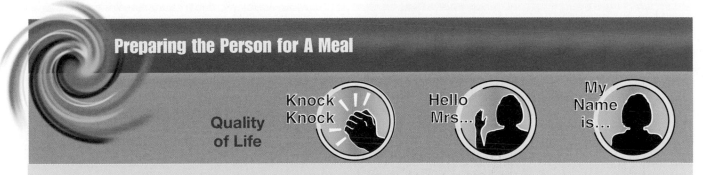

Preparing the Person for A Meal

Quality of Life — Knock Knock — Hello Mrs... — My Name is...

Pre-Procedure

1 Follow *Delegation Guidelines: Preparing for Meals.* See *Safety Alert: Preparing for Meals.*
2 Explain to the person that it is mealtime.
3 Practice hand hygiene.
4 Collect the following:
- Equipment for oral hygiene
- Bedpan, urinal, specimen pan, or commode and toilet tissue
- Wash basin
- Soap
- Washcloth
- Towel
- Gloves
5 Provide for privacy.

Continued

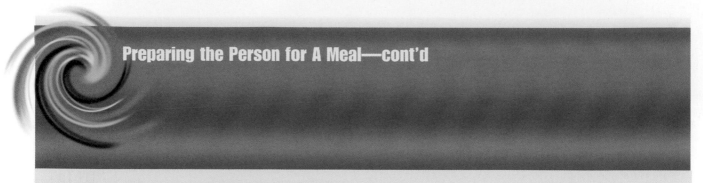

Preparing the Person for A Meal—cont'd

Procedure

6   Make sure eyeglasses and hearing aids are in place.

7   Assist with oral hygiene. Make sure dentures are in place. Decontaminate your hands and wear gloves.

8   Assist with elimination. Make sure the incontinent person is clean and dry. Wear gloves and practice hand hygiene.

9   Assist with hand washing. Wear gloves and decontaminate your hands.

10   Do the following if the person will eat in bed:
   a   Raise the head of the bed to a comfortable position.
   b   Clean the overbed table. Adjust it in front of the person.
   c   Place the signal light within reach.
   d   Unscreen the person.

11   Do the following if the person will sit in a chair:
   a   Position the person in a chair or wheelchair.
   b   Remove items from the overbed table. Clean the table.
   c   Adjust the overbed table in front of the person.
   d   Place the signal light within reach.
   e   Unscreen the person.

12   Complete a safety check of the room. (See inside of front book cover.)

13   Assist the person to the dining area. (This is for the person who eats in a dining area.)

Post-Procedure

14   Return to the room. Knock before entering.

15   Clean and return equipment to its proper place. Wear gloves for this step.

16   Straighten the room. Eliminate unpleasant noise, odors, or equipment.

17   Complete a safety check of the room. (See inside of front book cover.)

18   Remove the gloves. Decontaminate your hands.

Serving Meal Trays

Food is served in containers that keep foods at the correct temperature. Hot food is kept hot. Cold food is kept cold. Meal trays are served after residents are prepared for meals. You can serve trays promptly if residents are ready to eat. Prompt serving keeps food at the right temperature.

If food is not served within 15 minutes, recheck food temperature following center policy. If not at the right temperature, get other food. Some centers allow reheating in a microwave oven.

Delegation Guidelines

Serving Meal Trays

Before serving meal trays, you need this information from the nurse and care plan for each person:
- What adaptive equipment the person uses
- How much help is needed opening cartons, cutting food, buttering bread, and so on
- If I&O is measured

Safety Alert

Serving Meal Trays

Always check food temperature after reheating. Food that is too hot can burn the person.

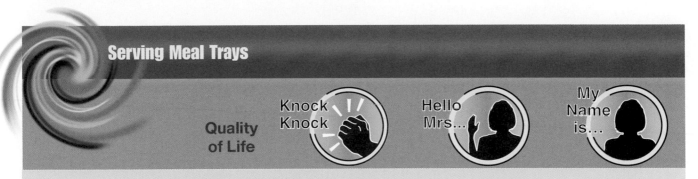

Serving Meal Trays

Quality of Life — Knock Knock — Hello Mrs... — My Name is...

Pre-Procedure

1   Follow *Delegation Guidelines: Serving Meal Trays.* See *Safety Alert: Serving Meal Trays.*

2   Practice hand hygiene.

Procedure

3   Make sure the tray is complete. Check items on the tray with the dietary card. Make sure adaptive equipment is included.

4   Identify the person. Check the ID bracelet against the dietary card. Call the person by name.

5   Place the tray within the person's reach. Adjust the overbed table as needed.

6   Remove food covers. Open cartons, cut meat, and butter bread as needed.

7   Place the napkin, clothes protector, adaptive equipment, and silverware within reach.

8   Measure and record intake if ordered (Chapter 7). Note the amount and type of foods eaten.

9   Check for and remove any food in the mouth (pocketing). Wear gloves. Decontaminate your hands after removing the gloves.

10 Remove the tray.

11 Clean spills. Change soiled linen.

12 Help the person return to bed if indicated.

Post-Procedure

13 Assist with oral hygiene and hand washing. Wear gloves.

14 Remove the gloves. Decontaminate your hands.

15 Provide for comfort.

16 Place the signal light within reach.

17 Raise or lower bed rails. Follow the care plan.

18 Complete a safety check of the room. (See inside of front book cover.)

19 Follow center policy for soiled linen.

20 Decontaminate your hands.

21 Report and record your observations.

Feeding the Person

Weakness, paralysis, casts, and other physical limits may make self-feeding impossible. These persons are fed.

Serve food and fluids in the order the person prefers. Offer fluids to help the person chew and swallow.

Spoons are used to feed the person. They are less likely to cause injury than forks. The spoon should be only one-third full. This portion is chewed and swallowed easily. Some people need smaller portions. Follow the care plan.

Persons who need to be fed are often angry, humiliated, and embarrassed. Some are also depressed, resentful, or refuse to eat. Let them do as much as possible. Some can manage "finger foods" (bread, cookies, crackers). If strong enough, they can hold milk or juice glasses (never hot drinks). Do not exceed activity limits ordered by the doctor. Provide support. Encourage them to try even if food is spilled.

Visually impaired persons are often very aware of food aromas. They may know the food served. Always tell the person what is on the tray. When feeding a visually impaired person, describe what you are offering. For persons who feed themselves, describe foods and fluids and their place on the tray. Use the numbers on a clock for the location of foods (Fig. 14-4, p. 276).

Many people pray before eating. Allow time and privacy for prayer. This shows respect and that you care about the person.

Meals provide social contact with others. Engage the person in pleasant conversation. However, allow time for chewing and swallowing. Also, sit so that you face the person. Sitting is more relaxing. Standing communicates that you are in a hurry.

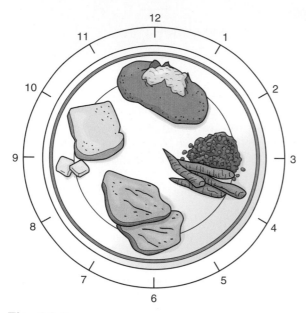

Fig. 14-4 The numbers on a clock are used to help a visually impaired person locate food.

Delegation Guidelines

Feeding the Person

Before feeding a person, you need this information from the nurse and care plan:

- Why the person needs help
- How much help the person needs
- If the person can manage finger foods
- The person's activity limits
- The person's dietary restrictions
- What size portion to feed the person—$\frac{1}{3}$ spoonful or less
- If the person has dysphagia (If so, what safety measures are needed?)
- What observations to report and record:
  —The amount and kind of food eaten
  —Complaints of nausea or dysphagia
  —Signs of dysphagia
  —Signs of aspiration

Safety Alert

Feeding the Person

Remember to check the food temperature. Foods that are very hot can burn the person.

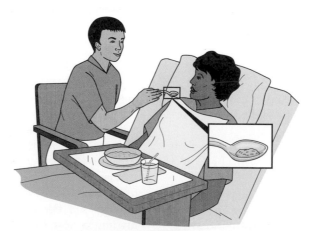

Fig. 14-5 A spoon is used to feed the person. The spoon is no more than one-third full.

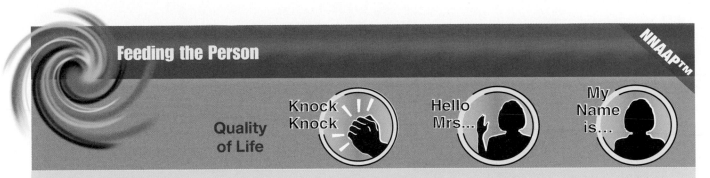

Pre-Procedure

1   Follow *Delegation Guidelines: Feeding the Person.* See *Safety Alert: Feeding the Person.*
2   Explain the procedure to the person.
3   Practice hand hygiene.
4   Position the person in a sitting position.
5   Get the tray. Place it on the overbed table or dining table.

Procedure

6   Identify the person. Check the ID bracelet against the dietary card. Call the person by name.
7   Drape a napkin across the person's chest and underneath the chin.
8   Tell the person what foods and fluids are on the tray.
9   Prepare food for eating. Season food as the person prefers and is allowed on the care plan.
10 Serve foods in the order the person prefers. Alternate between solid and liquid foods. Use a spoon for safety (Fig. 14-5). Allow enough time for chewing. Do not rush the person.
11 Use straws for liquids if the person cannot drink out of a glass or cup. Have one straw for each liquid. Provide short straws for weak persons.
12 Follow the care plan if the person has dysphagia. (Some persons with dysphagia do not use straws.) Give thickened liquid with a spoon.
13 Talk with the person in a pleasant manner. Encourage him or her to eat as much as possible.
14 Wipe the person's mouth with a napkin. Discard the napkin.
15 Note how much and which foods were eaten.
16 Measure and record intake if ordered (Chapter 7).
17 Remove the tray.
18 Assist the person back to his or her room.
19 Assist with oral hygiene and hand washing. Provide for privacy. Decontaminate your hands and put on gloves. Decontaminate your hands after removing the gloves.

Post-Procedure

20 Provide for comfort.
21 Place the signal light within reach.
22 Raise or lower bed rails. Follow the care plan.
23 Complete a safety check of the room. (See inside of front book cover.)
24 Decontaminate your hands.
25 Report and record your observations.

Between-Meal Nourishments

Some diets involve between-meal nourishments. Common nourishments are crackers, milk, juice, a milkshake, cake, wafers, a sandwich, gelatin, and custard. They are served upon arrival on the nursing unit. Provide needed eating utensils, a straw, and a napkin. Follow the same considerations and procedures for serving meal trays and feeding persons.

Providing Drinking Water

Residents need fresh drinking water each shift and whenever the pitcher is empty. Follow the person's fluid orders (p. 273). Some persons cannot have ice. Follow the center's procedure for providing fresh drinking water.

Safety Alert

Providing Drinking Water

Microbes can be spread by water glasses and pitchers. Practice medical asepsis when passing drinking water. Do the following to prevent the spread of microbes:

- Make sure the water pitcher is labeled with the person's name and room and bed number.
- Do not touch the rim or inside of the water glass or pitcher.
- Do not let the ice scoop touch the rim or inside of the water glass or pitcher.
- Do not put the ice scoop in the ice container or dispenser. Place it in the scoop holder or on a towel for the scoop.

MEETING SPECIAL NEEDS

Many people cannot eat or drink because of illness, surgery, or injury. The doctor orders other methods to meet their food and fluid needs.

Enteral Nutrition

Enteral nutrition is giving nutrients through the gastrointestinal tract *(enteral)*. Formula is given through a feeding tube. (**Gavage** is another term for tube feeding.)

- A *nasogastric (NG) tube* is inserted through the nose *(naso)* into the stomach *(gastro)* (Fig. 14-6).
- A *gastrostomy tube* (stomach tube) is inserted into the stomach. A surgically created opening *(stomy)* in the stomach *(gastro)* is needed (Fig. 14-7).

The doctor orders the type and amount of formula. Formula is given through a syringe, a feeding bag, or electronic feeding pump (Fig. 14-8).

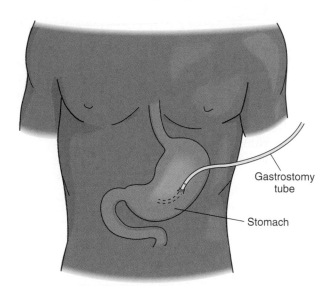

Fig. 14-7 A gastrostomy tube.

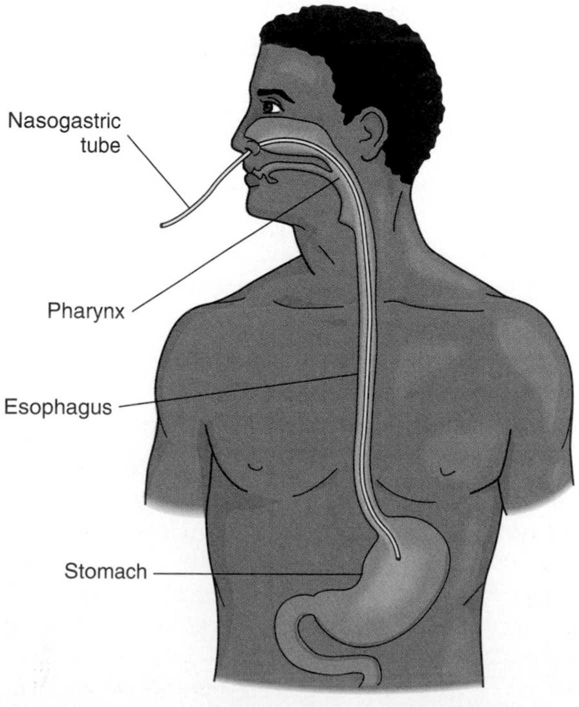

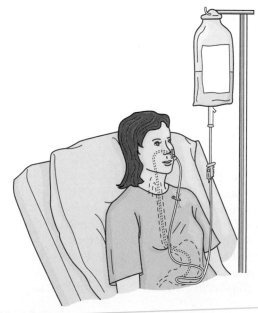

Fig. 14-6 A nasogastric tube is inserted through the nose and esophagus into the stomach.

Fig. 14-8 Formula drips from a feeding bag into the feeding tube.

Preventing Aspiration.

Aspiration is a major risk of enteral nutrition. *Aspiration* is the breathing of fluid or an object into the lungs. It can cause pneumonia and death. Tubes can move out of place from coughing, sneezing, vomiting, suctioning, and poor positioning. A tube can move from the stomach or intestines into the esophagus and then into the airway. *The RN checks tube placement before a feeding. You are never responsible for checking feeding tube placement.*

Aspiration also occurs from regurgitation. **Regurgitation** is the backward flow of food from the stomach into the mouth. Delayed stomach emptying and overfeeding are common causes. To prevent regurgitation:

- Position the person in semi-Fowler's position. Follow the care plan.
- Follow the care plan for how long the person needs to remain in that position. This position may be required for 1 or 2 hours or at all times. Semi-Fowler's position allows formula to move through the gastrointestinal system and prevents aspiration.
- Avoid the left side-lying position. This position prevents the stomach from emptying.

Observations.

Aspiration is a major risk. Report the following to the nurse at once:

- Nausea
- Discomfort during the tube feeding
- Vomiting
- Diarrhea
- Distended (enlarged and swollen) abdomen
- Coughing
- Complaints of indigestion or heartburn
- Redness, swelling, drainage, odor, or pain at the ostomy site
- Elevated temperature
- Signs and symptoms of respiratory distress (Chapter 7)
- Increased pulse rate
- Complaints of flatulence (Chapter 13)

Comfort Measures.

The person with a feeding tube is usually NPO. Dry mouth, dry lips, and sore throat cause discomfort. The person needs frequent oral hygiene, lubricant for the lips, and mouth rinses. These are done every 2 hours while the person is awake. The nose and nostrils are cleaned every 4 to 8 hours. Give care as directed by the nurse and care plan.

Nasogastric tubes can irritate and cause pressure on the nose. Securing the tube helps prevent these problems. Tape or a tube holder secures the tube to the nose. The tube also is secured to the person's gown following center policy.

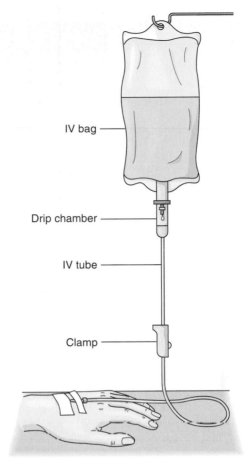

Fig. 14-9 Equipment for IV therapy.

Intravenous Therapy

Intravenous (IV) therapy is giving fluids through a needle or catheter inserted into a vein (Fig. 14-9). *IV* and *IV infusion* also refer to IV therapy. Doctors order IV therapy to:

- Provide fluids
- Replace minerals and vitamins
- Provide sugar for energy
- Give drugs and blood
- Provide hyperalimentation—a solution highly concentrated with proteins, carbohydrates, vitamins, minerals, and sometimes fat

The doctor orders the amount of fluid to give (infuse) per hour and the amount of time to give it in. Electronic pumps often are used to control the flow rate. An alarm sounds if something is wrong. Tell the nurse at once if you hear an alarm. *Never adjust any controls on IV pumps.*

You help meet the hygiene and activity needs of persons with IVs. *You are never responsible for starting or maintaining IV therapy. Nor do you regulate the flow rate or change IV bags. You never give blood or IV drugs.* However, you assist the RN in providing safe care. Follow the measures in Box 14-6, p. 280. Report any of the signs and symptoms in Box 14-7, p. 280 at once.

BOX 14-6   Safety Measures for IV Therapy

- Follow Standard Precautions and the Bloodborne Pathogen Standard.
- Do not move the needle or catheter. Needle or catheter position must be maintained. If the needle or catheter is moved, it may come out of the vein. Then fluid flows into tissues (infiltration), or the flow stops.
- Follow the safety measures for restraints (Chapter 20). The nurse may splint or restrain the extremity to prevent movement. This helps prevent the needle or catheter from moving.
- Protect the IV bag, tubing, and needle or catheter when ambulating the person. Portable IV standards are rolled along next to the person.
- Assist the person with turning and repositioning. Move the IV bag to the side of the bed on which the person is lying. Always allow enough slack in the tubing. The needle dislodges from pressure on the tube.
- Tell the nurse at once if bleeding occurs from the insertion site. Follow Standard Precautions and the Bloodborne Pathogen Standard.
- Tell the nurse at once of any signs and symptoms listed in Box 14-7.

BOX 14-7   Signs and Symptoms of IV Therapy Complications

Local—At the IV site

- Bleeding
- Puffiness or swelling
- Pale or reddened skin
- Complaints of pain at or above the IV site
- Hot or cold skin near the site

Systemic—Involving the Whole Body

- Fever
- Itching
- Drop in blood pressure
- Pulse rate more than 100 beats per minute
- Irregular pulse
- Cyanosis
- Changes in mental function
- Loss of consciousness
- Difficulty breathing
- Shortness of breath
- Decreasing or no urine output
- Chest pain
- Nausea
- Confusion

Review Questions

Circle the **BEST** answer.

1 Nutrition is
   a Fats, proteins, carbohydrates, vitamins, and minerals
   b The processes involved in the ingestion, digestion, absorption, and use of food and fluids by the body
   c The Food Guide Pyramid
   d The balance between calories taken in and used by the body

2 The Food Guide Pyramid encourages
   a A low-fat diet
   b A high-fat diet
   c A low-fiber diet
   d A low-salt diet

3 How many daily servings of the meat group are needed?
   a 6 to 11
   b 3 to 5
   c 2 to 4
   d 2 to 3

4 Which food group contains the *most* fat?
   a Breads, cereal, rice, and pasta
   b Fruits
   c Milk, yogurt, and cheese
   d Meat, poultry, fish, dry beans, eggs, and nuts

5 Protein is needed for
   a Tissue growth and repair
   b The fiber for bowel elimination
   c Body heat and to protect organs from injury
   d Flavor

6 Which provide the *most* protein?
   a Butter and cream
   b Tomatoes and potatoes
   c Meats and fish
   d Corn and lettuce

7 Mr. Bonner is on a sodium-controlled diet. He wants salt for his chicken. You should
   a Bring him the salt
   b Tell the nurse
   c Remind him that added salt is not allowed on his diet
   d Ignore the request

8 Diabetes meal planning involves the following *except*
   a The person's food preferences
   b Eating the same amount of carbohydrates, protein, and fat each day
   c Eating at regular times
   d A high-calorie diet

9 Adult fluid requirements for normal fluid balance are about
   a 1000 to 1500 ml daily
   b 1500 to 2000 ml daily
   c 2000 to 2500 ml daily
   d 2500 to 3000 ml daily

10 A person is NPO. You should
   a Provide a variety of fluids
   b Offer fluids in small amounts
   c Remove the water pitcher and glass
   d Discourage oral hygiene

11 Which statement about feeding a person is *false?*
   a Ask if he or she wants to pray before eating.
   b Use a fork to feed the person.
   c Ask the person the order in which to serve foods.
   d Engage the person in a pleasant conversation.

12 To prevent regurgitation after a tube feeding, the person is positioned in
   a Semi-Fowler's position
   b The prone position
   c In the left side-lying position
   d In the right side-lying position

13 A person with a feeding tube is usually
   a Allowed a regular diet
   b On bed rest
   c NPO
   d In a coma

14 A person is bleeding from an IV site. You should
   a Remove the IV catheter or needle
   b Apply direct pressure
   c Call for the nurse at once
   d Apply a dressing to the site

Answers to these questions are on p. 389.

CHAPTER 15

Skin Care

Objectives

- Define the key terms listed in this chapter
- Describe skin tears and how to prevent them
- Describe pressure ulcers and how to prevent them
- Identify the pressure points in each body position
- Describe circulatory ulcers and how to prevent them
- Explain the purpose of elastic stockings
- Perform the procedure described in this chapter

bedsore A pressure ulcer, pressure sore, or decubitus ulcer

circulatory ulcer An open wound on the lower legs and feet caused by decreased blood flow through the arteries or veins; vascular ulcer

decubitus ulcer A pressure ulcer, pressure sore, or bedsore

friction The rubbing of one surface against another

gangrene A condition in which there is death of tissue

pressure sore A bedsore, decubitus ulcer, or pressure ulcer

pressure ulcer Any injury caused by unrelieved pressure; decubitus ulcer, bedsore, or pressure sore

shearing When skin sticks to a surface while muscles slide in the direction the body is moving

skin tear A break or rip in the skin; the epidermis (top layer) separates from the underlying tissues

vascular ulcer A circulatory ulcer

wound A break in the skin or mucous membrane

A **wound** is a break in the skin or mucous membrane. Good skin care is needed to prevent wounds. Wounds are portals of entry for microbes. Infection is a major threat. It is important to prevent infection and further injury to the wound and nearby tissues.

SKIN TEARS

Older persons have thin and fragile skin. They are at risk for skin tears. A **skin tear** is a break or rip in the skin. The epidermis (top skin layer) separates from the underlying tissues. The hands, arms, and lower legs are common sites for skin tears.

Skin tears are caused by friction and shearing, pulling, or pressure on the skin. Bumping a hand, arm, or leg on any hard surface can cause a skin tear. Beds, bed rails, chairs, wheelchair footplates, and tables are dangers. So is holding the person's arm or leg too tight. Be careful when moving, repositioning, or transferring the person. Bathing, dressing, and other tasks can cause skin tears. So can pulling buttons and zippers across fragile skin. Your jewelry (rings, bracelets, watches) also can cause skin tears.

Skin tears are painful. Tell the nurse at once if you cause or find a skin tear. To prevent skin tears:

- Keep your fingernails short and smoothly filed.
- Keep the persons fingernails short and smoothly filed. Report long and tough toenails to the nurse.
- Do not wear rings with large or raised stones. Do not wear bracelets.
- Dress the person in soft clothing with long sleeves and long pants.
- Follow the care plan and safety rules to lift, move, position, transfer, bathe, and dress the person.
- Prevent shearing and friction.

- Use a lift sheet to lift and turn the person in bed (Chapter 16).
- Provide good lighting. It helps prevent the person from bumping into furniture, walls, and equipment.

PRESSURE ULCERS

A **pressure ulcer** (**decubitus ulcer**, **bedsore**, **pressure sore**) is any injury caused by unrelieved pressure. It usually occurs over a bony area—shoulder blades, elbows, hips, sacrum, knees, ankles, heels, and toes (Fig. 15-1, p. 284).

Causes

Pressure, friction, and shearing are common causes of skin breakdown and pressure ulcers. Other factors include breaks in the skin, poor circulation to an area, moisture, dry skin, and irritation by urine and feces. Older and disabled persons are at great risk for pressure ulcers. Their skin is easily injured. Causes include age-related changes, chronic disease, and general debility.

Pressure occurs when the skin over a bony area is squeezed between hard surfaces. The bone is one hard surface. The other is usually the mattress or chair seat. Squeezing or pressure prevents blood flow to the skin and underlying tissues. Lack of blood flow means oxygen and nutrients cannot get to the cells. Therefore involved skin and tissues die (Fig. 15-2, p. 285).

Friction is the rubbing of one surface against another. Friction scrapes the skin, causing an open area. A poor blood supply or an infection can lead to a pressure ulcer.

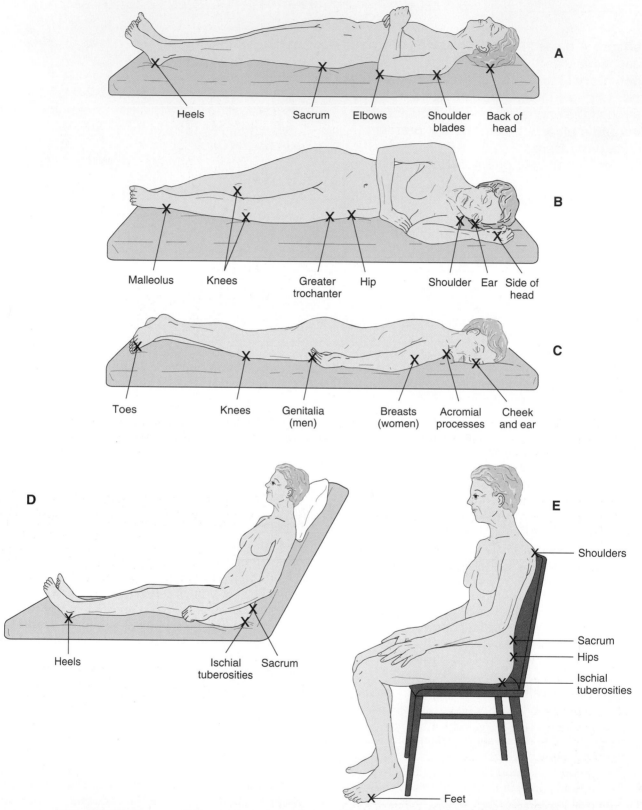

Fig. 15-1 Pressure points. **A,** The supine position. **B,** The lateral position. **C,** The prone position. **D,** Fowler's position. **E,** The sitting position.

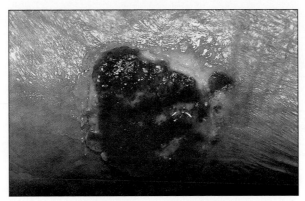

Fig. 15-2 A pressure ulcer.

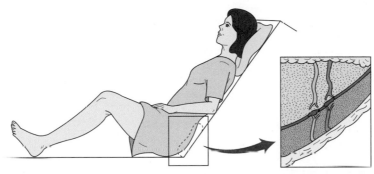

Fig. 15-3 When the head of the bed is raised to a sitting position, skin on the buttocks stays in place. Internal structures move forward as the person slides down in bed. Skin is pinched between the mattress and the hip bones.

Shearing is when the skin sticks to a surface while muscles slide in the direction the body is moving (Fig. 15-3, p. 286). This occurs when the person slides down in the bed or chair. Blood vessels and tissues are damaged. Blood flow to the area is reduced.

Persons at Risk

Persons at risk for pressure ulcers are those who:

- Are confined to bed or chair
- Need some or total help in moving
- Have loss of bowel or bladder control
- Have poor nutrition or fluid balance
- Have altered mental awareness
- Have problems sensing pain or pressure
- Have circulatory problems
- Are older, obese, or very thin

Signs of Pressure Ulcers

The first sign of a pressure ulcer is pale skin or a reddened area. Color changes may be hard to notice in persons with dark skin. The person may complain of pain, burning, or tingling in the area. Some do not feel anything unusual. Box 15-1 describes pressure ulcer stages.

BOX 15-1	**Stages of Pressure Ulcers**
Stage 1	The skin is red. The color does not return to normal when the skin is relieved of pressure (Fig. 15-4, *A*, p. 286). The skin is intact.
Stage 2	The skin cracks, blisters, or peels (Fig. 15-4, *B*, p. 286). There may be a shallow crater.
Stage 3	The skin is gone. Underlying tissues are exposed (Fig. 15-4, *C*, p. 286). The exposed tissue is damaged. There may be drainage from the area.
Stage 4	Muscle and bone are exposed and damaged (Fig. 15-4, *D*). Drainage is likely.

Sites

Pressure ulcers usually occur over bony areas. The bony areas are called *pressure points*. This is because they bear the weight of the body in a certain position (see Fig. 15-1). Pressure from body weight can reduce the blood supply to the area.

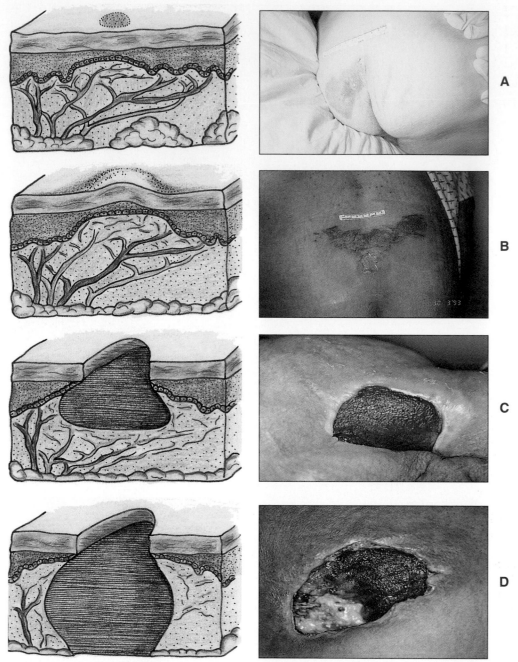

Fig. 15-4 Stages of pressure ulcers. **A,** Stage 1. **B,** Stage 2. **C,** Stage 3. **D,** Stage 4. (Courtesy Laurel Wiersema-Bryant, RN, MSN, Clinical Nurse Specialist, Barnes-Jewish Hospital, St Louis.)

In obese people, pressure ulcers can occur in areas where skin is in contact with skin. Common sites are between abdominal folds, the legs, and the buttocks and under the breasts. Friction occurs in these areas.

Persons who spend a lot of time in bed are at risk for pressure ulcers on the ears. This is from pressure of the ear on the mattress when in the side-lying position.

Prevention and Treatment

Preventing pressure ulcers is much easier than trying to heal them. Good nursing care, cleanliness, and skin care are essential. The measures in Box 15-2 help prevent skin breakdown and pressure ulcers. Follow the person's care plan.

The person at risk for pressure ulcers is placed on a surface that reduces or relieves pressure. Such surfaces include foam, air, alternating air, gel, or water mattresses. The health team decides on the best surface for the person.

BOX 15-2   Measures to Prevent Pressure Ulcers

- Follow the repositioning schedule in the person's care plan. The person is repositioned at least every 2 hours. Some persons are repositioned every 15 minutes.
- Position the person according to the care plan. Use pillows for support as instructed by the nurse. The 30-degree lateral position is recommended (Fig. 15-5).
- Prevent shearing and friction during lifting and moving procedures.
- Prevent shearing. Do not raise the head of the bed more than 30 degrees. Follow the care plan.
- Prevent friction by applying a thin layer of cornstarch to the bottom sheets.
- Provide good skin care. The skin must be clean and dry after bathing. The skin is free of moisture from urine, stools, perspiration, and wound drainage.
- Minimize skin exposure to moisture. Check incontinent persons often (Chapter 13). Also check persons who perspire heavily and those with wound drainage. Change linens and clothing as needed, and provide good skin care.
- Check with the nurse before using soap. Soap can dry and irritate the skin.
- Apply a moisturizer to dry areas such as the hands, elbows, legs, ankles, and heels. The nurse tells you what to use and the areas that need attention.
- Give a back massage when repositioning the person. *Do not massage bony areas.*
- Keep linens clean, dry, and free of wrinkles.
- Apply powder where skin touches skin.
- Do not irritate the skin. Avoid scrubbing or vigorous rubbing when bathing or drying the person.
- Do not massage over pressure points. *Never rub or massage reddened areas.*
- Use pillows and blankets to prevent skin from being in contact with skin. They also reduce moisture and friction.
- Keep the heels off the bed. Use pillows or other devices as the nurse directs. Place the pillows or devices under the lower legs from mid-calf to the ankles.
- Use protective devices as the nurse and care plan direct (p. 288).
- Remind persons sitting in chairs to shift their positions every 15 minutes. This decreases pressure on bony points.
- Report any signs of skin breakdown or pressure ulcers at once.

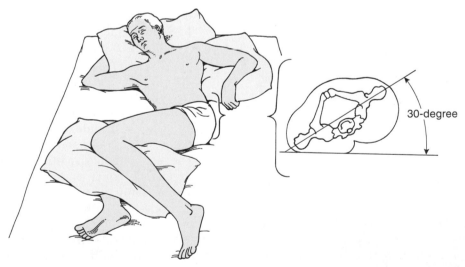

Fig. 15-5 The 30-degree lateral position. Pillows are placed under the head, shoulder, and leg. This position inclines (lifts up) the hip to avoid pressure on the hip. The person does not lie on the hip as in the side-lying position. (From Bryant RA et al: Pressure Ulcers. In Bryant RA, editor: *Acute and chronic wounds: nursing management,* St Louis 1992, Mosby.)

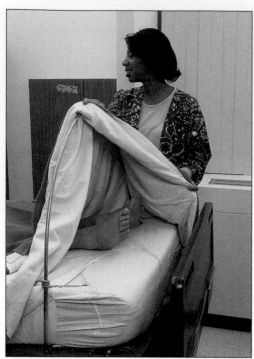

Fig. 15-6 A bed cradle. Linens are brought over the top of the cradle.

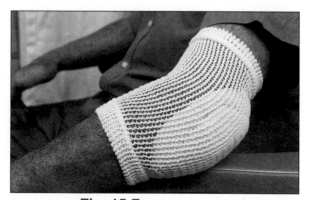

Fig. 15-7 Elbow protector.

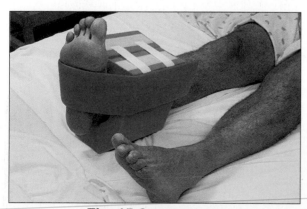

Fig. 15-8 Heel elevator.

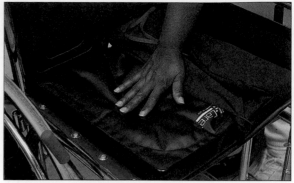

Fig. 15-9 Flotation pad.

The doctor orders wound care products, drugs, treatments, and special equipment to promote healing. The nurse and care plan tell you what to do. These protective devices are often used to prevent and treat pressure ulcers and skin breakdown:

- *Bed cradle*—A bed cradle is placed on the bed. Top linens are brought over the cradle to prevent pressure on the legs and feet (Fig. 15-6).
- *Elbow protectors*—Elbow protectors fit the shape of the elbow (Fig. 15-7). Some have straps to secure them in place.
- *Heel elevators*—Pillows or special cushions are used to raise the heels off the bed (Fig. 15-8). Special braces and splints also are used to keep pressure off the heels.
- *Flotation pads*—Flotation pads or cushions (Fig. 15-9) are made of a gel-like substance. The outer case is heavy plastic. The pad is placed in a pillowcase or special cover. The cover protects the skin.
- *Eggcrate-like mattress*—This is a foam pad that looks like an egg carton (Fig. 15-10). Peaks in the mattress distribute the person's weight more evenly. It is placed on top of the regular mattress. The eggcrate-like mattress is put in a special cover. The cover protects against moisture and soiling. Only a bottom sheet is used to cover the eggcrate-like mattress and cover. No other bottom linens are used.
- *Other equipment*—Trochanter rolls and footboards are also used (Chapter 19).

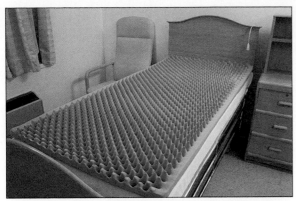

Fig. 15-10 Eggcrate-like mattress on the bed.

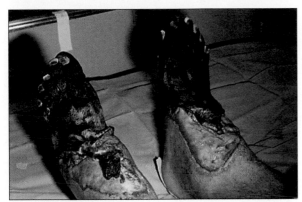

Fig. 15-11 Gangrene. Courtesy Cameron Bangs, MD. (From Auerbach PS: *Wilderness medicine: management of wilderness and environmental emergencies,* ed 3, St Louis, 1995, Mosby.)

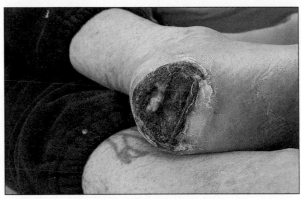

Fig. 15-12 Stasis ulcer.

CIRCULATORY ULCERS

Some people have diseases that affect blood flow to and from the legs and feet. Such poor circulation can lead to pain, open wounds, and swelling of tissues (edema). Infection and gangrene can result from the open wound and poor circulation. **Gangrene** is a condition in which there is death of tissue (Fig. 15-11).

Circulatory ulcers (**vascular ulcers**) are open wounds on the lower legs and feet caused by decreased blood flow through arteries or veins. Persons with diseases affecting the blood vessels are at risk. These wounds are painful and hard to heal.

- *Stasis ulcers (venous ulcers)* are open wounds on the lower legs and feet caused by poor blood return through the veins (Fig. 15-12). The heels and inner aspect of the ankles are common sites. They can occur from skin injury. Scratching is a common cause. Or the ulcers occur spontaneously.
- *Arterial ulcers* are open wounds on the lower legs and feet caused by poor arterial blood flow. They are found between the toes, on top of the toes, and on the outer side of the ankle. The heels are common sites for persons on bedrest. These ulcers can occur from shoes that fit poorly.

BOX 15-3   Measures to Prevent Circulatory Ulcers

- Remind the person not to sit with the legs crossed.
- Position the person according to the care plan.
- Do not use elastic or rubber band–type of garters to hold socks or hose in place.
- Do not dress the person in tight clothes.
- Keep the feet clean and dry. Clean and dry between the toes.
- Do not scrub or rub the skin during bathing and drying.
- Keep linens clean, dry, and wrinkle-free.
- Avoid injury to the legs and feet.
- Make sure shoes fit well.
- Keep pressure off the heels and other bony areas. Use pillows or other devices as the nurse and care plan direct.
- Check the person's legs and feet. Report skin breaks or changes in skin color.
- Do not massage over pressure points. *Never rub or massage reddened areas.*
- Follow the care plan for walking and exercise.

Prevention and Treatment

Circulatory ulcers are hard to heal. Preventing skin breakdown is important. Follow the person's care plan (Box 15-3). The doctor may order elastic stockings to promote circulation.

Elastic Stockings. Elastic stockings are often ordered for persons with circulatory disorders. They also are ordered for persons on bedrest. People on bedrest are at risk for developing blood clots (thrombi). A blood clot is called a *thrombus*.

The elastic exerts pressure on the veins. The pressure promotes venous blood flow to the heart. The stockings also are called *anti-embolism* or *anti-embolic* (*AE*) *stockings.*

Stockings are applied before the person gets out of bed. Otherwise the person's legs can swell from sitting or standing. Stockings are hard to put on when the legs are swollen. They are removed every 8 hours for 30 minutes or according to the care plan. The person lies in bed while they are off. This prevents the legs from swelling.

Safety Alert
Elastic Stockings
Stockings should not have twists, creases, or wrinkles after you apply them. Twists can affect circulation. Creases and wrinkles can cause skin breakdown.

Delegation Guidelines
Elastic Stockings
Before applying elastic stockings, you need this information from the nurse and care plan:
- What size to use—small, medium, or large
- What length to use—thigh-high or knee-high
- When to remove and reapply them
- What observations to report and record:
  —When you applied the stockings
  —Skin color and temperature
  —Leg and foot swelling
  —Signs of skin breakdown
  —Complaints of pain, tingling, or numbness
  —When you removed the stockings and for how long
  —When you reapplied the stockings
  —When you washed the stockings

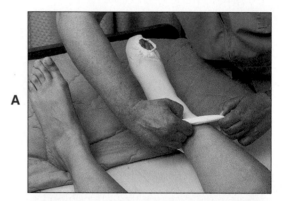

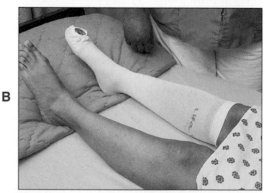

Fig. 15-13 Applying elastic stockings. **A,** The stocking is slipped over the toes, foot, and heel. **B,** The stocking turns right side out as it is pulled up over the leg.

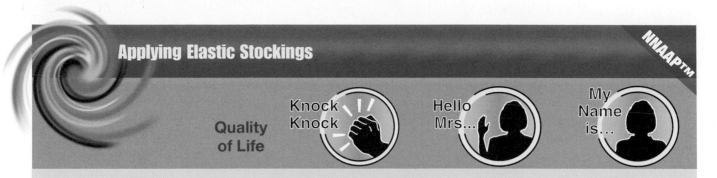

Applying Elastic Stockings

NNAAP™

Quality of Life

Knock Knock

Hello Mrs...

My Name is...

Pre-Procedure

1 Follow *Delegation Guidelines: Elastic Stockings.* See *Safety Alert: Elastic Stockings.*
2 Explain the procedure to the person.
3 Practice hand hygiene.
4 Obtain elastic stockings in the correct size and length.

5 Identify the person. Check the ID bracelet against the assignment sheet. Call the person by name.
6 Provide for privacy.
7 Raise the bed for body mechanics. Bed rails are up if used.

Procedure

8 Lower the bed rail near you if up.
9 Position the person supine.
10 Expose the legs. Fanfold top linens toward the thighs.
11 Turn the stocking inside out down to the heel.
12 Slip the foot of the stocking over the toes, foot, and heel (Fig. 15-13, *A*).

13 Grasp the stocking top. Pull the stocking up the leg. It turns right side out as it is pulled up. The stocking is even and snug (Fig. 15-13, *B*).
14 Remove twists, creases, and wrinkles.
15 Repeat steps 11 through 14 for the other leg.

Post-Procedure

16 Cover the person.
17 Provide for comfort.
18 Lower the bed.
19 Raise or lower bed rails. Follow the care plan.
20 Place the signal light within reach.

21 Unscreen the person.
22 Complete a safety check of the room. (See inside of front book cover.)
23 Decontaminate your hands.
24 Report and record your observations.

Review Questions

Circle the **BEST** answer.

1 Which can cause skin tears?
   a Keeping your nails trimmed and smooth
   b Dressing the person in soft clothing
   c Wearing rings
   d Handling the person gently

2 Pressure ulcers usually occur
   a Between the toes
   b On the lower legs and feet
   c Over bony areas
   d On the chest and abdomen

3 Which can cause pressure ulcers?
   a Repositioning the person every 2 hours
   b Scrubbing and rubbing the skin
   c Applying lotion to dry areas
   d Keeping linens clean, dry, and wrinkle-free

4 To prevent pressure ulcers, the person is positioned in
   a The prone position
   b Fowler's position
   c The 30-degree lateral position
   d The supine position

5 Which are *not* used to treat pressure ulcers?
   a Special beds
   b Waterbeds and flotation pads
   c Plastic drawsheets and waterproof pads
   d Heel elevators and elbow protectors

6 To prevent pressure ulcers, you should do the following *except*
   a Massage bony areas
   b Apply powder where skin touches skin
   c Remind the person to shift positions every 15 minutes
   d Prevent friction and shearing

7 A person has a stasis ulcer. Which measure should you question?
   a Use elastic garters to hold socks in place.
   b Do not cut or trim toenails.
   c Avoid injury to the person's legs.
   d Apply elastic stockings.

8 Which is *not* a common site for arterial ulcers?
   a Between the toes
   b On top of the toes
   c On the outer side of the ankle
   d Behind the knee

9 Elastic stockings
   a Prevent infection
   b Protect bony areas
   c Help venous blood return to the heart
   d Prevent skin tears

10 Elastic stockings are applied
   a In circular turns
   b Before the person gets out of bed
   c When the person is sitting in a chair
   d From top to bottom

Answers to these questions are on p. 389.

CHAPTER 16

Assisting With Moving and Positioning

Objectives

■ Define the key terms listed in this chapter
■ Identify comfort and safety measures for lifting, turning, and moving persons in bed
■ Explain the purpose of a transfer belt (gait belt)
■ Explain how to safely perform transfer procedures
■ Explain why body alignment and position changes are important
■ Identify the comfort and safety measures for positioning a person
■ Position persons in the basic bed positions and in a chair
■ Perform the procedures described in this chapter

dorsal recumbent position The back-lying or supine position

Fowler's position A semi-sitting position; the head of the bed is raised 45 to 90 degrees

gait belt A transfer belt

lateral position The side-lying position

logrolling Turning the person as a unit, in alignment, with one motion

prone position Lying on the abdomen with the head turned to one side

side-lying position The lateral position

Sims' position A left side-lying position in which the upper leg is sharply flexed so it is not on the lower leg and the lower arm is behind the person

supine position The back-lying or dorsal recumbent position

transfer belt A belt used to support persons who are unsteady or disabled; a gait belt

---

You will turn and reposition persons often. You move them in bed. You transfer them to and from chairs, wheelchairs, stretchers, and toilets. During these and other tasks, you must use your body correctly. This protects you and the person from injury.

See Chapter 4 for a review of body mechanics and the musculoskeletal system. Remember to use good body mechanics to protect yourself and others from injury. Do not work alone. Have a co-worker help you lift, move, turn, transfer, or position a person.

LIFTING AND MOVING PERSONS IN BED

Some persons can move and turn in bed. Others need help from at least one person. Those who are weak, unconscious, paralyzed, on complete bed rest, or in casts need help. Sometimes 2 or 3 people or a mechanical lift is needed.

Comfort and Safety

Protect the person's skin during lifting and moving. Friction and shearing injure the skin. Both cause infection and pressure ulcers (Chapter 15).

Reduce friction and shearing by rolling or lifting the person. A cotton drawsheet (Chapter 8) serves as a *lift sheet (turning sheet)* to move the person in bed and reduce friction. Some centers use turning pads for this purpose (p. 297).

Also practice these comfort and safety measures when moving persons:

- Ask co-workers to help *before* starting the procedure.
- Cover and screen the person to protect the right to privacy.
- Protect tubes or drainage containers connected to the person.
- Use caution when moving persons with arthritis or osteoporosis (Chapter 4). Always have help moving them to avoid causing pain or injury.

Delegation Guidelines

Lifting and Moving Persons in Bed

Many delegated tasks involve lifting and moving the person in bed. Before lifting or moving a person, you need this information from the nurse and the care plan:

- Position limits and restrictions
- How far you can lower the head of the bed
- Any limits in the person's ability to move or be repositioned
- What procedure to use
- How many workers are needed to safely lift and move the person
- What equipment is needed—trapeze, lift sheet, mechanical lift
- What pillows can be removed before lifting or turning the person
- How to position the person (p. 319)
- If the person uses bed rails
- What observations to report and record

Safety Alert

Lifting and Moving Persons in Bed

For safety and efficiency, decide how you will move the person before starting the procedure. If you need help from a co-worker, ask someone to help before you begin. Also plan how to protect drainage tubes or containers connected to the person.

Beds are raised horizontally to lift and move persons in bed. This reduces bending and reaching. You must:

- Use the bed correctly
- Protect the person from falling when the bed is raised
- Follow the rules of body mechanics
- Keep the person in good alignment
- Position the person in good alignment after lifting or moving (p. 319)

Moving the Person Up in Bed

When the bed is raised, it is easy to slide down toward the middle and foot of the bed (Fig. 16-1). The person is moved up in bed for good alignment and comfort.

You can sometimes move lightweight adults up in bed alone if they use a trapeze. However, it is best to have help and to use a lift sheet. At least two workers are needed to move heavy, weak, and very old persons up in bed. Always protect the person and yourself from injury.

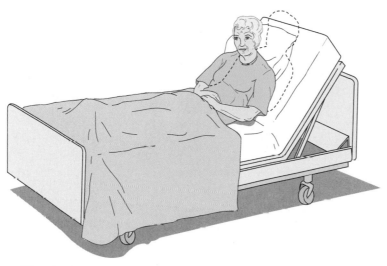

Fig. 16-1 A person in poor alignment after sliding down in bed.

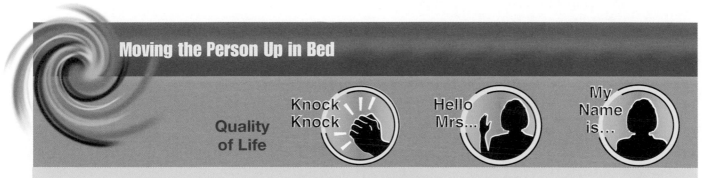

Moving the Person Up in Bed

Quality of Life

Knock Knock

Hello Mrs...

My Name is...

Pre-Procedure

1 Follow *Delegation Guidelines: Lifting and Moving Persons in Bed.* See *Safety Alert: Lifting and Moving Persons in Bed.*
2 Ask a co-worker to assist if you need help.
3 Practice hand hygiene.
4 Identify the person. Check the ID bracelet against the assignment sheet. Call the person by name.
5 Explain what you are going to do.
6 Provide for privacy.
7 Lock the bed wheels.
8 Raise the bed for body mechanics. Bed rails are up if used.

Continued

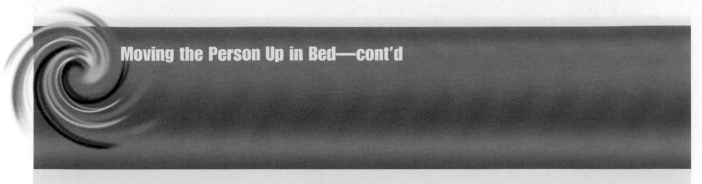

Moving the Person Up in Bed—cont'd

Procedure

9. Lower the head of the bed to a level appropriate for the person. It is as flat as possible.
10. Stand on one side of the bed. Your co-worker stands on the other side.
11. Lower the bed rail near you if up. Your co-worker does the same.
12. Remove pillows as directed by the nurse. Place a pillow against the headboard if the person can be without it. This prevents the person's head from hitting the headboard when being moved up.
13. Stand with a wide base of support. Point the foot near the head of the bed toward the head of the bed. Face the head of the bed.
14. Bend your hips and knees. Keep your back straight.
15. Place one arm under the person's shoulder and one arm under the thighs. Your co-worker does the same. Grasp each other's forearms (Fig. 16-2).
16. Ask the person to grasp the trapeze if he or she has one (Fig. 16-3).
17. Have the person flex both knees.
18. Explain that you will move on the count of "3." The person pushes against the bed with the feet if able.
19. Move the person to the head of the bed on the count of "3." Shift your weight from your rear leg to your front leg (see Figs. 16-2 and 16-3).
20. Repeat steps 13 through 19 if necessary.

Post-Procedure

21. Put the pillow under the person's head and shoulders. Straighten linens.
22. Provide for comfort. Position the person in good alignment (p. 319).
23. Place the signal light within reach.
24. Raise or lower bed rails. Follow the care plan.
25. Raise the head of the bed to a level appropriate for the person.
26. Lower the bed to its lowest position.
27. Unscreen the person.
28. Complete a safety check of the room. (See inside of front book cover.)
29. Decontaminate your hands.
30. Report and record your observations.

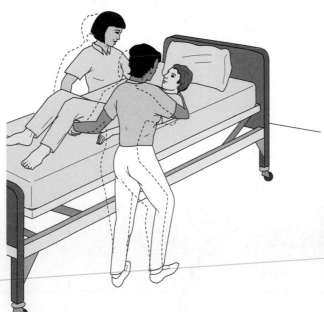

Fig. 16-2 A person is moved up in bed by two nursing assistants. Each has one arm under the person's shoulders and the other under the thighs. They have locked arms under the person. The person's knees are flexed. The nursing assistants shift their weight from the rear leg to the front leg as the person is moved up in bed.

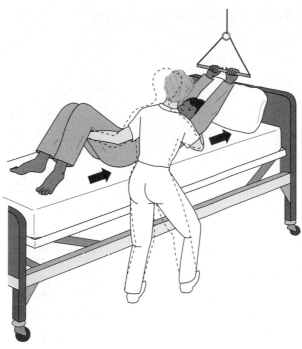

Fig. 16-3 The person grasps a trapeze and flexes the knees. The nursing assistant shifts her body weight from the rear leg to the front leg as she moves the person up in bed. *NOTE:* Although you can move children and lightweight adults alone with this method, it is best to have help.

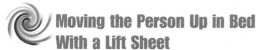

Moving the Person Up in Bed With a Lift Sheet

With a co-worker's help, you can easily and safely move a person up in bed with a *lift sheet*. (It is called a *turning sheet* when used to turn the person. See p. 302.) Friction and shearing are reduced. The person is lifted more evenly. Use a flat sheet folded in half, a drawsheet, or a turning pad (Fig. 16-4). Place it under the person from the head to above the knees.

Use this procedure for:

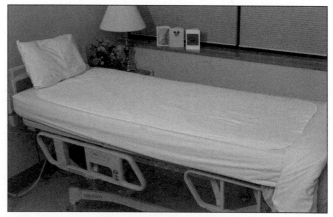

Fig. 16-4 Turning pad.

- Most nursing center residents, particularly those who cannot move themselves
- Persons who are unconscious or paralyzed
- Persons recovering from spinal cord surgery or spinal cord injuries
- Older persons

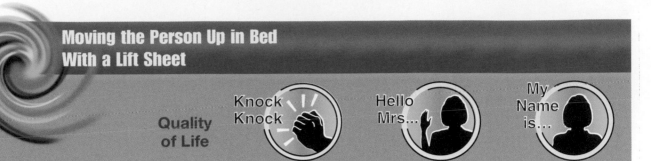

Moving the Person Up in Bed With a Lift Sheet

Quality of Life — Knock Knock — Hello Mrs... — My Name is...

Pre-Procedure

1 Follow *Delegation Guidelines: Lifting and Moving Persons in Bed*, p. 294. See *Safety Alert: Lifting and Moving Persons in Bed*, p. 294.
2 Ask a co-worker to help you.
3 Practice hand hygiene.
4 Identify the person. Check the ID bracelet against the assignment sheet. Call the person by name.
5 Explain what you are going to do.
6 Provide for privacy.
7 Lock the bed wheels.
8 Raise the bed for body mechanics. Bed rails are up if used.

Procedure

9 Lower the head of the bed to a level appropriate for the person. It is as flat as possible.
10 Stand on one side of the bed. Your co-worker stands on the other side.
11 Lower the bed rails if up.
12 Remove pillows as directed by the nurse. Place a pillow against the headboard if the person can be without it.
13 Stand with a broad base of support. Point the foot near the head of the bed toward the head of the bed. Face that direction.
14 Roll the sides of the lift sheet up close to the person.
15 Grasp the rolled-up lift sheet firmly near the person's shoulders and buttocks (Fig. 16-5). Support the head.
16 Bend your hips and knees.
17 Move the person up in bed on the count of "3." Shift your weight from your rear leg to your front leg.
18 Repeat steps 13 through 17 if necessary.
19 Unroll the lift sheet.

Post-Procedure

20 Put the pillow under the person's head and shoulders. Straighten linens.
21 Provide for comfort. Position the person in good alignment (p. 319).
22 Place the signal light within reach.
23 Raise or lower bed rails. Follow the care plan.
24 Raise the head of the bed to a level appropriate for the person.
25 Lower the bed to its lowest position.
26 Unscreen the person.
27 Complete a safety check of the room. (See inside of front book cover.)
28 Decontaminate your hands.
29 Report and record your observations.

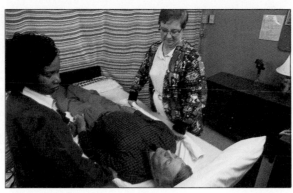

Fig. 16-5 A lift sheet is used to move the person up in bed. The lift sheet extends from the person's head to above the knees. The lift sheet is rolled close to the person and held near the shoulders and buttocks.

Moving the Person to the Side of the Bed

Repositioning and care procedures require moving the person to the side of the bed. The person is moved to the side of the bed before turning. Otherwise, after turning, the person lies on the side of the bed—not in the middle.

Sometimes you have to reach over the person to give care. You reach less if the person is close to you.

One method involves moving the person in segments. One person can sometimes do this. The lift sheet method is used for very old persons, those with arthritis, and those recovering from spinal cord injuries or spinal cord surgery.

Safety Alert

Moving the Person to the Side of the Bed

You need to know which method to use. Get this information from the nurse and the care plan whenever delegated tasks involve moving the person to the side of the bed. Such tasks include repositioning, bedmaking, bathing, and range-of-motion exercises.

The wrong method could seriously injure a person. This is very important for persons who are very old, have arthritis, or have spinal cord involvement.

Using a lift sheet helps prevent pain, skin damage, and injury to the bones, joints, and spinal cord. When using a lift sheet, you need a co-worker to help you.

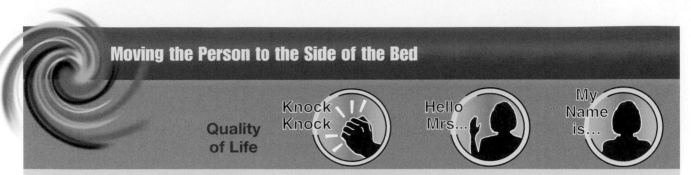

Moving the Person to the Side of the Bed

Quality of Life

Knock Knock

Hello Mrs...

My Name is...

Pre-Procedure

1 Follow *Delegation Guidelines: Lifting and Moving Persons in Bed*. See *Safety Alerts:*
   - *Lifting and Moving Persons in Bed*, p. 294.
   - *Moving the Person to the Side of the Bed*, p. 299.
2 Ask a co-worker to help if using a lift sheet.
3 Practice hand hygiene.
4 Identify the person. Check the ID bracelet against the assignment sheet. Call the person by name.
5 Explain the procedure to the person.
6 Provide for privacy.
7 Lock the bed wheels.
8 Raise the bed for body mechanics. Bed rails are up if used.

Procedure

9 Lower the head of the bed to a level appropriate for the person. It is as flat as possible. Remove all pillows as directed by the nurse.
10 Stand on the side of the bed to which you will move the person.
11 Lower the bed rail near you if bed rails are used. (Both bed rails are lowered for step 15).
12 Stand with your feet about 12 inches apart. One foot is in front of the other. Flex your knees.
13 Cross the person's arms over the person's chest.
14 *Method 1: Moving the person in segments:*
   a Place your arm under the person's neck and shoulders. Grasp the far shoulder.
   b Place your other arm under the mid-back.
   c Move the upper part of the person's body toward you. Rock backward and shift your weight to your rear leg (Fig. 16-6, *A*).
   d Place one arm under the person's waist and one under the thighs.

   e Rock backward to move the lower part of the person toward you (Fig. 16-6, *B*).
   f Repeat the procedure for the legs and feet (Fig. 16-6, *C*). Your arms should be under the person's thighs and calves.
15 *Method 2: Moving the person with a lift sheet:*
   a Roll the lift sheet up close to the person (see Fig. 16-5).
   b Grasp the rolled-up lift sheet near the person's shoulders and hips. Your co-worker does the same. Support the head.
   c Rock backward on the count of "3," moving the person toward you. Your co-worker rocks backward slightly and then forward toward you while keeping the arms straight.
   d Unroll the lift sheet. Remove any wrinkles.

Post-Procedure

16 Provide for comfort.
17 Position the person in good alignment. Follow the nurse's directions and the care plan.
18 Place the signal light within reach.
19 Raise or lower bed rails. Follow the care plan.
20 Lower the bed to its lowest position.
21 Unscreen the person.
22 Complete a safety check of the room. (See inside of front book cover.)
23 Decontaminate your hands.
24 Report and record your observations.

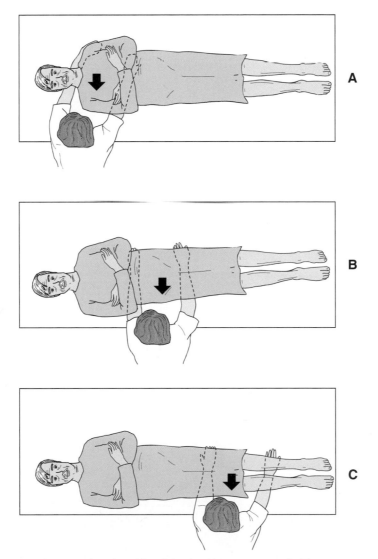

Fig. 16-6 The person is moved to the side of the bed in segments. **A,** The upper part of the body is moved. **B,** The lower part of the body is moved. **C,** The legs and feet are moved.

TURNING PERSONS

Turning persons onto their sides helps prevent complications from bedrest (Chapter 19). Certain procedures require the side-lying position. The person is turned toward or away from you. The direction depends on the person's condition and the situation.

Logrolling with a turning sheet (lift sheet) is used to turn most residents (p. 304). It helps prevent pain in persons with arthritic spines and hips.

Delegation Guidelines

Turning Persons

Before turning and repositioning a person, you need this information from the nurse and the care plan:

* How much help the person needs
* The person's comfort level and what body parts are painful
* Which procedure to use
* What supportive devices are needed for positioning (Chapter 19)
* Where to place pillows
* What observations to report and record

Safety Alert

Turning Persons

Use good body mechanics when turning a person in bed. The person must be in good alignment. Otherwise, musculoskeletal injuries, skin breakdown, or pressure ulcers could occur.

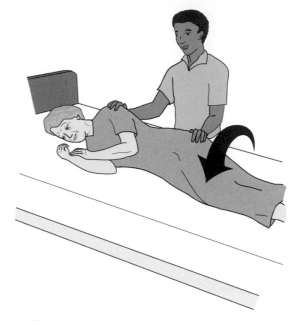

Fig. 16-7 Turning the person away from you.

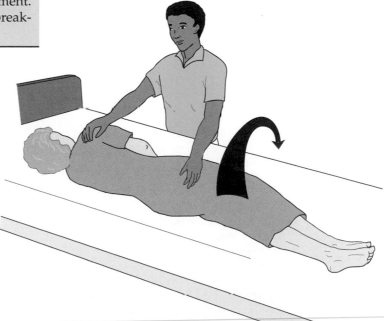

Fig. 16-8 Turning the person toward you.

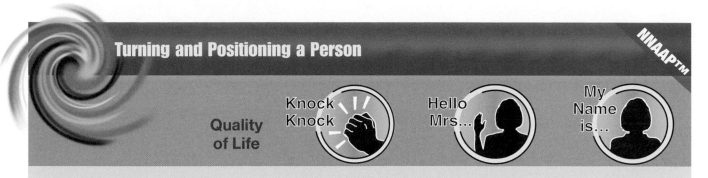

Turning and Positioning a Person

Quality of Life

Knock Knock

Hello Mrs...

My Name is...

Pre-Procedure

1 Follow *Delegation Guidelines: Turning Persons.* See *Safety Alert: Turning Persons.*

2 Practice hand hygiene.

3 Identify the person. Check the ID bracelet against the assignment sheet. Call the person by name.

4 Explain the procedure to the person.

5 Provide for privacy.

6 Lock the bed wheels.

7 Raise the bed for body mechanics. Bed rails are up if used.

Procedure

8 Lower the head of the bed to a level appropriate for the person. It is as flat as possible.

9 Stand on the side of the bed opposite to where you will turn the person. The far bed rail is up if used.

10 Lower the bed rail near you if up.

11 Move the person to the side near you. (See procedure: *Moving the Person to the Side of the Bed,* p. 300.)

12 Cross the person's arms over the person's chest. Cross the leg near you over the far leg.

13 *Turning the person away from you:*

  a Stand with a wide base of support. Flex your knees.

  b Place one hand on the person's shoulder. Place the other on the hip near you.

  c Push the person gently toward the other side of the bed (Fig. 16-7). Shift your weight from your rear leg to your front leg.

14 *Turning the person toward you:*

  a Raise the bed rail if used.

  b Go to the other side. Lower the bed rail if used.

  c Stand with a wide base of support. Flex your knees.

  d Place one hand on the person's far shoulder. Place the other on the far hip.

  e Roll the person toward you gently (Fig. 16-8).

15 Position the person. Follow the nurse's directions and the care plan. The following is common:

  a Place a pillow under the head and neck.

  b Adjust the shoulder. The person should not lie on an arm.

  c Place a small pillow under the upper hand and arm.

  d Position a pillow against the back.

  e Flex the upper knee. Position the upper leg in front of the lower leg.

  f Support the upper leg and thigh on pillows.

Post-Procedure

16 Provide for comfort.

17 Place the signal light within reach.

18 Raise or lower bed rails. Follow the care plan.

19 Lower the bed to its lowest position.

20 Unscreen the person.

21 Complete a safety check of the room. (See inside of front book cover.)

22 Decontaminate your hands.

23 Report and record your observations.

Logrolling

Logrolling is turning the person as a unit, in alignment, with one motion. The spine is kept straight. The procedure is used to turn:

- Older persons with arthritic spines or knees
- Persons recovering from hip fractures
- Persons with spinal cord injuries (the spine is kept straight at all times following spinal cord injury)
- Persons recovering from spinal surgery (the spine is kept straight at all times following spinal surgery)

Two or three staff members are needed for logrolling. Three are needed if the person is tall or heavy. Sometimes a turning sheet is used.

Safety Alert

Logrolling

Following spinal cord injury or surgery, a pillow under the head and neck is usually not allowed. Follow the nurse's directions and the care plan.

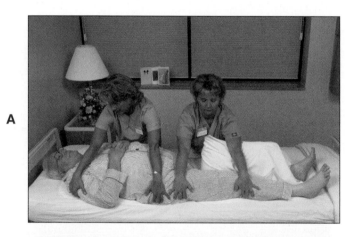

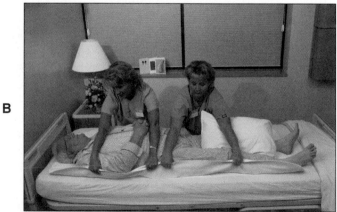

Fig. 16-9 Logrolling. **A,** A pillow is between the person's legs. The arms are crossed on the chest. The person is on the far side of the bed. **B,** A turning sheet is used to logroll a person.

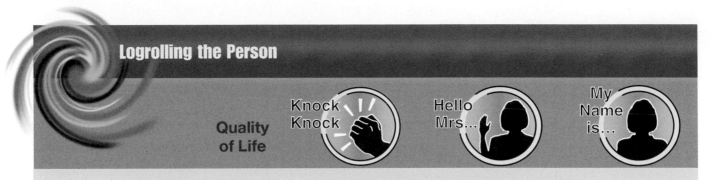

Logrolling the Person

Quality of Life

Knock Knock

Hello Mrs...

My Name is...

Pre-Procedure

1 Follow *Delegation Guidelines: Turning Persons*, p. 302. See *Safety Alerts*:
   • *Turning Persons*, p. 302.
   • *Logrolling*, p. 302.
2 Ask a co-worker to help you.
3 Practice hand hygiene.
4 Identify the person. Check the ID bracelet against the assignment sheet. Call the person by name.
5 Explain the procedure to the person.
6 Provide for privacy.
7 Lock the bed wheels.
8 Raise the bed for body mechanics. Bed rails are up if used.

Procedure

9 Make sure the bed is flat.
10 Stand on the side opposite to which you will turn the person. Your co-worker stands on the other side.
11 Lower the bed rails if used.
12 Move the person as a unit to the side of the bed near you. Use the turning sheet.
13 Place the person's arms across the chest. Place a pillow between the knees.
14 Raise the bed rail if used.
15 Go to the other side.
16 Stand near the shoulders and chest. Your co-worker stands near the buttocks and thighs.
17 Stand with a broad base of support. One foot is in front of the other.
18 Ask the person to hold his or her body rigid.
19 Roll the person toward you (Fig. 16-9, *A*). Or use a turning sheet (Fig. 16-9, *B*). Turn the person as a unit.

Post-Procedure

20 Provide for comfort. Position the person in good alignment. Use pillows as directed by the nurse and care plan. The following is common (unless the person has spinal cord involvement):
   a One pillow against the back for support
   b One pillow under the head and neck if allowed
   c One pillow or folded bath blanket between the legs
   d A small pillow under the arm and hand
21 Place the signal light within reach.
22 Raise or lower bed rails. Follow the care plan.
23 Lower the bed to its lowest position.
24 Unscreen the person.
25 Complete a safety check of the room. (See inside of front book cover.)
26 Decontaminate your hands.
27 Report and record your observations.

⟳ SITTING ON THE SIDE OF THE BED

Residents may become dizzy or faint if they get out of bed too fast. They may need to sit on the side of the bed (*dangle*) for 1 to 5 minutes before walking or transferring. Some increase activity in stages—bedrest, to sitting on the side of the bed, and then to sitting in a chair. Walking is the next step.

While dangling the legs, the person coughs and deep breathes. He or she moves the legs back and forth and in circles. This stimulates circulation.

Two staff members may be needed. The person with balance and coordination problems needs support. If dizziness or fainting occurs, lay the person down.

Safety Alert

Dangling

Problems with sitting and balance often occur after illness, injury, surgery, and bedrest. Some persons who are disabled also have problems sitting and with balance. Provide support when the person is sitting on the side of the bed. This protects the person from falling and other injuries.

Delegation Guidelines

Dangling

The nurse may ask you to help a person sit on the side of the bed. The procedure is part of other tasks—assisting the person to stand, transferring from bed to chair, partial bath, and others. When delegated the dangling procedure or tasks that involve dangling, you need this information from the nurse and the care plan:

- Areas of weakness. For example, if the person's arms are weak, he or she cannot hold onto the side of the mattress for support. If the left side is weak, you need to turn the person onto the stronger right side. The person can use the right arm to help move from the lying to sitting position.
- The amount of help the person needs.
- If you need a co-worker to help you.
- How long the person needs to sit on the side of the bed.
- What exercises the person needs to perform while dangling:
  —Leg and foot exercises (Chapter 19)
  —Range-of-motion exercises (Chapter 19)
- If the person will walk or transfer to a chair after dangling.
- What observations to report and record.

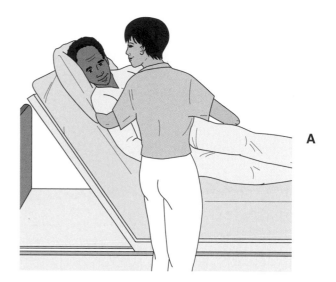

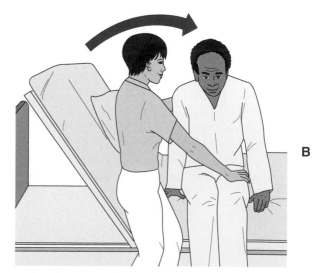

Fig. 16-10 Helping the person sit on the side of the bed. **A,** The person's shoulders and thighs are supported. **B,** The person sits upright as the legs and feet are pulled over the edge of the bed.

Helping the Person Sit on the Side of the Bed (Dangling)

Quality of Life

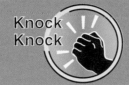
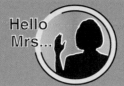
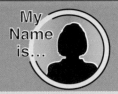

Pre-Procedure

1 Follow *Delegation Guidelines: Dangling.* See *Safety Alert: Dangling.*
2 Explain the procedure to the person.
3 Practice hand hygiene.
4 Identify the person. Check the ID bracelet against the assignment sheet. Call the person by name.
5 Decide what side of the bed to use.
6 Move furniture to provide moving space.
7 Provide for privacy.
8 Position the person in a side-lying position facing you. The person lies on the strong side.
9 Lock the bed wheels.
10 Raise the bed for body mechanics. Bed rails are up if used.

Procedure

11 Raise the head of the bed to a sitting position.
12 Lower the bed rail if up.
13 Stand by the person's hips. Face the foot of the bed.
14 Stand with your feet apart. The foot near the head of the bed is in front of the other foot.
15 Slide one arm under the person's neck and shoulders. Grasp the far shoulder. Place your other hand over the thighs near the knees (Fig. 16-10, *A*).
16 Pivot toward the foot of the bed while moving the person's legs and feet over the side of the bed. As the legs go over the edge of the mattress, the trunk is upright (Fig. 16-10, *B*).
17 Ask the person to hold onto the edge of the mattress. This supports the person in the sitting position.
18 Do not leave the person alone. Provide support if necessary.
19 Check the person's condition:
    a Ask how the person feels. Ask if the person feels dizzy or lightheaded.
    b Check pulse and respirations.
    c Check for difficulty breathing.
    d Note if the skin is pale or bluish in color (cyanosis).
20 Help the person lie down if necessary.
21 Reverse the procedure to return the person to bed.
22 Lower the head of the bed after the person returns to bed. Help him or her move to the center of the bed.

Post-Procedure

23 Provide for comfort. Position the person in good alignment.
24 Place the signal light within reach.
25 Lower the bed to its lowest position.
26 Raise or lower bed rails. Follow the care plan.
27 Return furniture to its proper places.
28 Unscreen the person.
29 Complete a safety check of the room. (See inside of front book cover.)
30 Decontaminate your hands.
31 Report and record your observations.

TRANSFERRING PERSONS

To *transfer* a person means to move the person from one place to another. Persons are often moved from beds to chairs, wheelchairs, shower chairs, commodes, or toilets. Some transfer themselves or need little help. Some persons are transferred by 1, 2, or 3 people.

The rules of body mechanics apply to transfers (Chapter 4). Arrange the room so there is enough space for a safe transfer. Correct chair, wheelchair, commode, or shower chair placement is needed for a safe transfer.

Delegation Guidelines

Transferring Persons

When delegated transferring procedures, you need this information from the nurse and the care plan:

- What procedure to use:
  —Transferring the Person To a Chair or Wheelchair
  —Transferring the Person From a Chair or Wheelchair To Bed
  —Transferring the Person Using a Mechanical Lift
  —Transferring the Person To and From a Toilet
- Areas of weakness. For example, if the person's arms are weak, the person cannot hold the side of the mattress for support. If the person has a weak left side, he or she gets out of bed on the stronger right side. The person can use the right arm to help move from the lying to sitting position.
- What equipment is needed—transfer belt, wheelchair, mechanical lift, positioning devices, wheelchair cushion, and so on.
- The amount of help the person needs.
- How many co-workers need to help you.
- What observations to report and record:
  —Pulse rate before and after the transfer
  —Complaints of lightheadedness, pain, discomfort, difficulty breathing, weakness, or fatigue
  —The amount of help needed to transfer the person
  —How the person helped with the transfer

Safety Alert

Transferring Persons

The person wears nonskid footwear for transfers. Such footwear protects the person from falls. Slipping and sliding are prevented. Remember to securely tie shoelaces. Otherwise the person can trip and fall.

The bed wheels must be locked. And wheelchair and shower chair brakes must be on. Both measures prevent the bed, wheelchair, or shower chair from moving during the transfer. Otherwise, the person can fall. You also are at risk for injury.

Applying Transfer Belts

A **transfer belt** is used to support persons who are unsteady or disabled. It helps prevent falls and other injuries. The belt goes around the person's waist. You grasp underneath the belt to support the person during the transfer. The belt is called a **gait belt** when used for walking with a person. Many centers require staff to use these belts when transferring or walking a person.

Safety Alert

Transfer Belts

Transfer belts are used routinely in nursing centers. If the person needs help, a transfer belt is required. To use one safely, always follow the manufacturer's instructions.

A transfer belt is always applied over clothing. It is never applied over bare skin. Also, it is applied under the breasts. Breasts must not be caught under the belt.

Do not leave excess strap dangling. Tuck the excess strap under the belt.

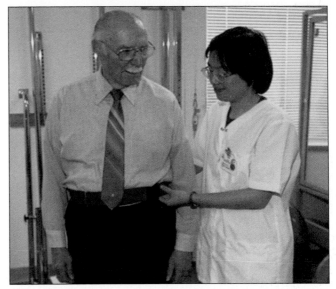

Fig. 16-11 Transfer belt. The belt buckle is positioned off center. The nursing assistant grasps the belt from underneath.

Applying a Transfer Belt

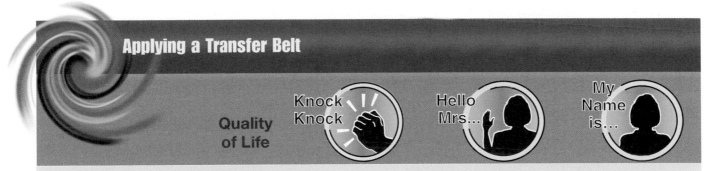

Quality of Life — Knock Knock — Hello Mrs... — My Name is...

Procedure

1   See *Safety Alert: Transfer Belts.*
2   Practice hand hygiene.
3   Identify the person. Check the ID bracelet against the assignment sheet. Call the person by name.
4   Explain the procedure to the person.
5   Provide for privacy.
6   Assist the person to a sitting position.
7   Apply the belt around the person's waist over clothing. Do not apply it over bare skin.

8   Tighten the belt so it is snug. It should not cause discomfort or impair breathing. You should be able to slide 4 fingers (your open, flat hand) under the belt.
9   Make sure that a woman's breasts are not caught under the belt.
10 Place the buckle off center in the front or in the back for the person's comfort (Fig. 16-11). The buckle is not over the spine.

Bed to Chair or Wheelchair Transfers

Safety is important for chair, wheelchair, commode, or shower chair transfers. If the person cannot assist, a mechanical lift is used (p. 315).

Help the person out of bed on his or her strong side. If the left side is weak and the right side strong, get the person out of bed on the right side. In transferring, the strong side moves first. It pulls the weaker side along. Transfers from the weak side are awkward and unsafe. If you must transfer the person from his or her weak side, use a mechanical lift.

Most wheelchairs and bedside chairs have vinyl seats and backs. Vinyl holds body heat. The person becomes warm and perspires more. You can cover the back and seat with a folded bath blanket. This increases the person's comfort in the chair. Some people have wheelchair cushions or positioning devices. Ask the nurse how to use and place the devices.

Safety Alert

Chair or Wheelchair Transfers

The chair or wheelchair must support the person's weight. The number of staff members needed for a transfer depends on the person's abilities, condition, and size.

During the procedure, the person must not put his or her arms around your neck. Otherwise the person can pull you forward or cause you to lose your balance. Neck, back, and other injuries from falls are possible.

Wheelchair wheels are locked for a safe transfer. After the transfer, unlock the wheels to position the wheelchair as the person prefers. After positioning the chair, lock the wheels or keep them unlocked according to the care plan. Locked wheels may be considered to be restraints if the person cannot unlock them to move the wheelchair (Chapter 20). However, falling and other injuries are risks if the person tries to stand when the wheelchair wheels are unlocked.

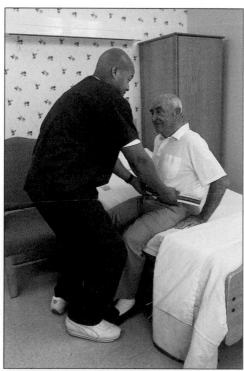

Fig. 16-12 Transferring the person to a chair using a transfer belt. The person's feet and knees are blocked by the nursing assistant's feet and knees. This prevents the person from sliding or falling.

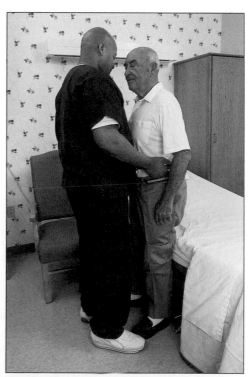

Fig. 16-13 The person is pulled up to a standing position and supported by holding the transfer belt and blocking the person's knees and feet.

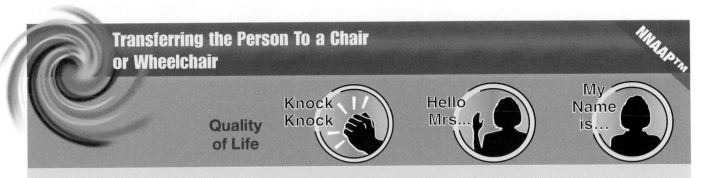

Transferring the Person To a Chair or Wheelchair

Pre-Procedure

1 Follow *Delegation Guidelines: Transferring Persons,* p. 308. See *Safety Alerts:*
   - *Transferring Persons,* p. 308
   - *Transfer Belts,* p. 309
   - *Chair or Wheelchair Transfers,* p. 310
2 Explain the procedure to the person.
3 Collect:
   - Wheelchair or arm chair
   - Bath blanket
   - Lap blanket
   - Robe and nonskid footwear
   - Paper or sheet
   - Transfer belt if needed
   - Seat cushion or positioning device if needed
4 Practice hand hygiene.
5 Identify the person. Check the ID bracelet against the assignment sheet. Call the person by name.
6 Provide for privacy.
7 Decide which side of the bed to use. Move furniture for moving space.

Procedure

8 Place the chair at the head of the bed. The chair is even with the headboard.
9 Place a folded bath blanket, cushion, or positioning device on the seat (if needed).
10 Lock wheelchair wheels. Raise the footplates. Remove or swing front rigging out of the way.
11 Lower the bed to its lowest position. Lock the bed wheels.
12 Fanfold top linens to the foot of the bed.
13 Place the paper or sheet under the person's feet. Put footwear on the person.
14 Help the person sit on the side of the bed. His or her feet touch the floor.
15 Help the person put on a robe.
16 Apply the transfer belt if needed.
17 *Method 1: Using a transfer belt:*
   a Stand in front of the person.
   b Have the person hold onto the mattress.
   c Make sure the person's feet are flat on the floor.
   d Have the person lean forward.
   e Grasp the transfer belt at each side. Grasp the belt from underneath.
   f Brace your knees against the person's knees. Block his or her feet with your feet (Fig. 16-12). Or use the knee and foot of one leg to block the person's weak foot. Place your other foot slightly behind you for balance.

g Ask the person to push down on the mattress and to stand on the count of "3." Pull the person into a standing position as you straighten your knees (Fig. 16-13).
18 *Method 2: No transfer belt:*
   a Follow step 17, a–c.
   b Place your hands under the person's arms. Your hands are around the person's shoulder blades (Fig. 16-14, p. 312).
   c Have the person lean forward.
   d Brace your knees against the person's knees. Block his or her feet with your feet. Or use the knee and foot of one leg to block the person's weak foot. Place your other foot slightly behind you for balance.
   e Ask the person to push down on the mattress and to stand on the count of "3." Pull the person up into a standing position as you straighten your knees.
19 Support the person in the standing position. Hold the transfer belt, or keep your hands around the person's shoulder blades. Continue to block the person's feet and knees with your feet and knees. This helps prevent falling.
20 Turn the person so he or she can grasp the far arm of the chair. The legs will touch the edge of the chair (Fig. 16-15, p. 313).

Continued

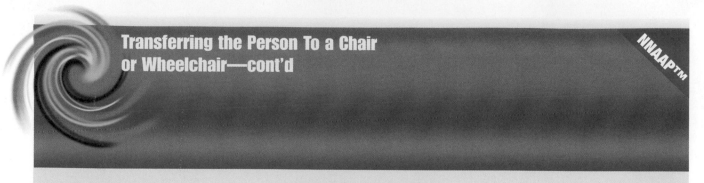

**Transferring the Person To a Chair
or Wheelchair—cont'd**

Procedure—cont'd

21 Continue to turn the person until the other armrest is grasped.

22 Lower him or her into the chair as you bend your hips and knees. The person assists by leaning forward and bending the elbows and knees (Fig. 16-16).

23 Make sure the buttocks are to the back of the seat. Position the person in good alignment.

24 Attach the wheelchair front rigging. Position the person's feet on the footplates.

25 Cover the person's lap and legs with a lap blanket. Keep the blanket off the floor and the wheels.

26 Remove the transfer belt if used.

27 Position the chair as the person prefers. Lock the wheelchair wheels or keep them unlocked according to the care plan.

Post-Procedure

28 Place the signal light and other needed items within reach.

29 Unscreen the person.

30 Complete a safety check of the room. (See inside of front book cover.)

31 Decontaminate your hands.

32 Report and record your observations.

33 See procedure: *Transferring the Person From the Chair or Wheelchair to Bed* (p. 314) to return the person to bed.

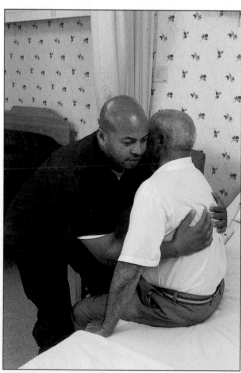

Fig. 16-14 The person is being prepared to stand. The hands are placed under the person's arms and around the shoulder blades.

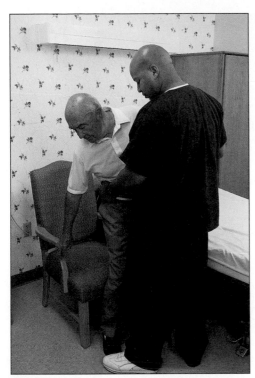

Fig. 16-15 The person is supported as he grasps the far arm of the chair. The legs are against the chair.

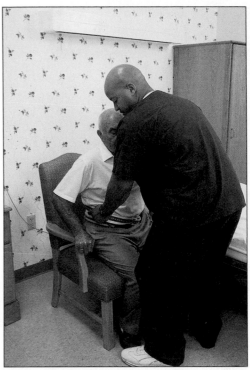

Fig. 16-16 The person holds the armrests, leans forward, and bends the elbows and knees while being lowered into the chair.

Chair or Wheelchair to Bed Transfers

Chair or wheelchair to bed transfers have the same rules as bed to chair transfers. If the person is weak on one side, transfer the person so that the strong side moves first. Therefore the person is transferred to bed on the opposite side from which the person transferred out of bed.

For example, Mrs. Lee's right side is weak. Her left side is strong. To transfer her from bed to chair, the chair was on the left side of the bed. This allowed her left side (strong side) to move first. Now you will transfer Mrs. Lee back to bed. If you leave the chair on the left side of the bed, her right side—the weak side—is near the bed. The weak side will move first. This is unsafe. Therefore you need to move the chair to the other side of the bed. Mrs. Lee's stronger left side will be near the bed. The stronger left side moves first for a safe transfer.

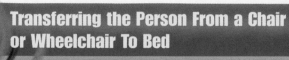

Transferring the Person From a Chair or Wheelchair To Bed

Quality of Life

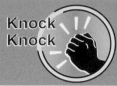 Knock Knock

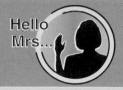 Hello Mrs...

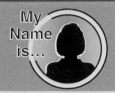 My Name is...

Pre-Procedure

1. Follow *Delegation Guidelines: Transferring Persons*, p. 308. See *Safety Alerts:*
   - *Transferring Persons*, p. 308.
   - *Transfer Belts*, p. 309.
   - *Chair or Wheelchair Transfers*, p. 310.
2. Explain the procedure to the person.
3. Collect a transfer belt (if needed).
4. Practice hand hygiene.
5. Identify the person. Check the ID bracelet against the assignment sheet. Call the person by name.
6. Provide for privacy.

Procedure

7. Move furniture for moving space.
8. Raise the head of the bed to a sitting position. The bed is in the lowest position.
9. Move the signal light so it is on the strong side when the person is in bed.
10. Position the chair or wheelchair so the person's strong side is next to the bed (Fig. 16-17). Have a co-worker help you if necessary.
11. Lock the wheelchair and bed wheels.
12. Remove and fold the lap blanket.
13. Remove the person's feet from the footplates. Raise the footplates. Remove or swing the front rigging out of the way.
14. Apply the transfer belt (if needed).
15. Make sure the person's feet are flat on the floor.
16. Stand in front of the person.
17. Ask the person to hold onto the armrests. Or place your arms under the person's arms. Your hands are around the shoulder blades.
18. Have the person lean forward.
19. Grasp the transfer belt on each side if using it. Grasp underneath the belt.
20. Brace your knees against the person's knees. Block his or her feet with your feet. Or use the knee and foot of one leg to block the person's weak foot. Place your other foot slightly behind you for balance.
21. Ask the person to push down on the armrests on the count of "3." Pull the person into a standing position as you straighten your knees.
22. Support the person in the standing position. Hold the transfer belt, or keep your hands around the person's shoulder blades. Continue to block the person's knees and feet with your knees and feet.
23. Turn the person so he or she can reach the edge of the mattress. The legs will touch the mattress.
24. Continue to turn the person until he or she can reach the mattress with both hands.
25. Lower him or her onto the bed as you bend your hips and knees. The person assists by leaning forward and bending the elbows and knees.
26. Remove the transfer belt.
27. Remove the robe and footwear.
28. Help the person lie down.

Post-Procedure

29. Provide for comfort. Cover the person as needed.
30. Follow the care plan for the use of bed rails.
31. Place the signal light and other needed items within reach.
32. Arrange furniture to meet the person's needs.
33. Unscreen the person.
34. Complete a safety check of the room. (See inside of front book cover.)
35. Decontaminate your hands.
36. Report and record your observations.

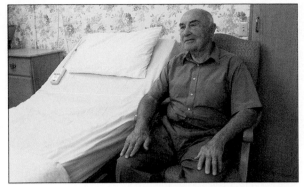

Fig. 16-17 To transfer the person from chair to bed, the chair is positioned so the person's strong side is near the bed.

Using Mechanical Lifts

Persons who cannot help themselves are transferred with mechanical lifts. So are persons too heavy for the staff to transfer. Lifts are used for transfers to chairs, stretchers, tubs, shower chairs, toilets, commodes, whirlpools, or vehicles. Before using a lift:

- Make sure you are trained in its use.
- Make sure the lift works.
- Make sure the sling, straps, hooks, and chains are in good repair.
- Compare the person's weight and the lift's weight limit. Do not use the lift if a person's weight exceeds the lift's capacity.

At least two staff members are needed. The following procedure is used as a guide.

Safety Alert

Mechanical Lifts
Mechanical lifts vary among manufacturers. Also, manufacturers have different models. Knowing how to use one lift does not mean that you know how to use others. Always follow the manufacturer's instructions.

If you have questions, ask the nurse. If you have not used a certain lift before, ask the nurse to show you how to use it safely. Also ask the nurse to help you use it the first time and until you are comfortable using it.

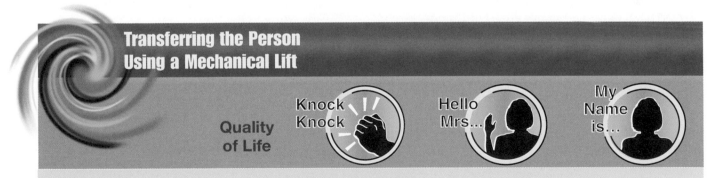

Transferring the Person Using a Mechanical Lift

Pre-Procedure

1 Follow *Delegation Guidelines: Transferring Persons*, p. 308. See *Safety Alerts*:
  - *Transferring Persons*, p. 308.
  - *Mechanical Lifts*, p. 308.
2 Ask a co-worker to help you.
3 Explain the procedure to the person.
4 Collect:
  - Mechanical lift
  - Arm chair or wheelchair
  - Footwear
  - Bath blanket or cushion
  - Lap blanket
5 Practice hand hygiene.
6 Identify the person. Check the ID bracelet against the assignment sheet. Call the person by name.
7 Provide for privacy.

Continued

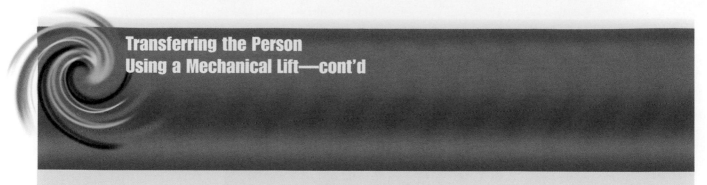

Transferring the Person
Using a Mechanical Lift—cont'd

Procedure

8   Raise the bed for body mechanics. Bed rails are up if used.

9   Lower the head of the bed to a level appropriate for the person. It is flat as possible.

10 Stand on one side of the bed. Your co-worker stands on the other side.

11 Lower the bed rail near you.

12 Center the sling under the person (Fig. 16-18, *A*). To position the sling, turn the person from side to side as if making an occupied bed (Chapter 8). Position the sling according to the manufacturer's instructions.

13 Position the person in semi-Fowler's position.

14 Place the chair at the head of the bed. It should be even with the headboard and about 1 foot away from the bed. Place a folded bath blanket or cushion in the chair.

15 Lock the bed wheels. Lower the bed to its lowest position.

16 Raise the lift so you can position it over the person.

17 Position the lift over the person (Fig. 16-18, *B*).

18 Lock the lift wheels in position.

19 Attach the sling to the swivel bar (Fig. 16-18, *C*).

20 Raise the head of the bed to a sitting position.

21 Cross the person's arms over the chest. He or she can hold onto the straps or chains but not the swivel bar.

22 Raise the lift high enough until the person and sling are free of the bed (Fig. 16-18, *D*).

23 Have your co-worker support the person's legs as you move the lift and person away from the bed (Fig. 16-18, *E*).

24 Position the lift so that the person's back is toward the chair.

25 Position the chair so you can lower the person into it.

26 Lower the person into the chair. Guide the person into the chair (Fig. 16-18, *F*).

27 Lower the swivel bar to unhook the sling. Leave the sling under the person unless otherwise indicated.

28 Put footwear on the person. Position the person's feet on wheelchair footplates.

29 Cover the person's lap and legs with a lap blanket. Keep it off the floor and wheels.

30 Position the chair as the person prefers. Lock the wheelchair wheels or keep them unlocked according to the care plan.

Post-Procedure

31 Place the signal light and other needed items within reach.

32 Unscreen the person.

33 Complete a safety check of the room. (See inside of front book cover.)

34 Decontaminate your hands.

35 Report and record your observations.

36 Reverse the procedure to return the person to bed.

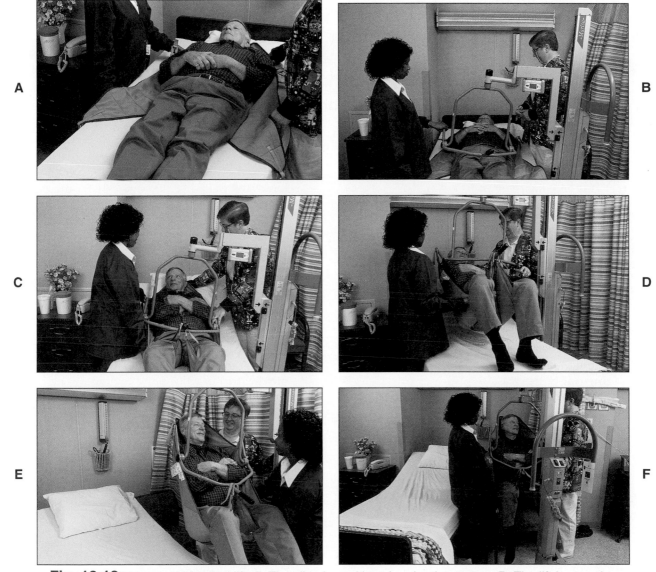

Fig. 16-18 Using a mechanical lift. **A,** The sling is positioned under the person. **B,** The lift is over the person. **C,** The sling is attached to a swivel bar. **D,** The lift is raised until the sling and person are off of the bed. **E,** The person's legs are supported as the person and lift are moved away from the bed. **F,** The person is guided into a chair.

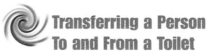

Transferring a Person To and From a Toilet

Getting to the toilet is hard for persons who use wheelchairs. Bathrooms are often small. There is little room for you and a wheelchair. Therefore transfers involving wheelchairs and toilets are often hard. The risk of falls is great.

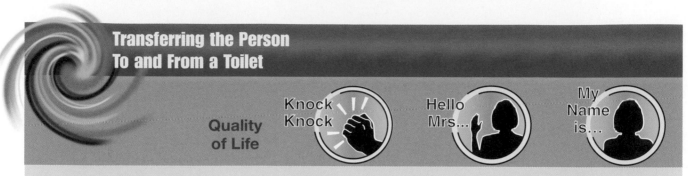

Transferring the Person To and From a Toilet

Quality of Life

Knock Knock

Hello Mrs...

My Name is...

Pre-Procedure

1   Follow *Delegation Guidelines: Transferring Persons,* p. 308. See *Safety Alerts:*
    *   *Transferring Persons,* p. 308.
    *   *Transfer Belts,* p. 309.
    *   *Chair or Wheelchair Transfers,* p. 310.
2   Practice hand hygiene.

3   Make sure the person has an elevated toilet seat. The toilet seat and wheelchair are at the same level.
4   Check the grab bars by the toilet. If they are loose, tell the nurse. Do not transfer the person to the toilet if the grab bars are not secure.

Procedure

5   Have the person wear nonskid footwear.
6   Position the wheelchair next to the toilet if there is enough room. If not, position the wheelchair at a right (90-degree) angle to the toilet (Fig. 16-19). It is best if the person's strong side is near the toilet.
7   Lock the wheelchair wheels.
8   Raise the footplates. Remove or swing the front rigging out of the way.
9   Apply the transfer belt.
10 Help the person unfasten clothing.
11 Use the transfer belt to help the person stand and to turn to the toilet. (See procedure: *Transferring the Person to a Chair or Wheelchair,* p. 311.) The person uses the grab bars to turn to the toilet.
12 Support the person with the transfer belt while he or she lowers clothing. Or have the person hold onto the grab bars for support. Lower the person's pants and undergarments. Or raise the person's skirt or dress and lower undergarments.
13 Use the transfer belt to lower the person onto the toilet seat.
14 Remove the transfer belt.
15 Tell the person you will stay nearby. Remind the person to use the signal light or call for you when help is needed.

16 Close the bathroom door to provide for privacy.
17 Stay near the bathroom. Complete other tasks in the person's room. Or check on the person every 5 minutes.
18 Knock on the bathroom door when the person calls for you.
19 Help with wiping, perineal care (Chapter 11), flushing, and hand washing as needed. Wear gloves, and practice hand hygiene.
20 Apply the transfer belt.
21 Use the transfer belt to help the person stand.
22 Help the person with clothing.
23 Use the transfer belt to transfer the person to the wheelchair. (See procedure: *Transferring the Person to a Chair or Wheelchair,* p. 311.)
24 Make sure the person's buttocks are to the back of the seat. Position the person in good alignment.
25 Position the person's feet on the footplates.
26 Cover the person's lap and legs with a lap blanket. Keep the blanket off the floor and wheels.
27 Position the chair as the person prefers. Lock the wheelchair wheels or keep them unlocked according to the care plan.

Post-Procedure

28 Place the signal light and other needed items within reach.
29 Unscreen the person.
30 Complete a safety check of the room. (See inside of front book cover.)

31 Practice hand hygiene.
32 Report and record your observations.

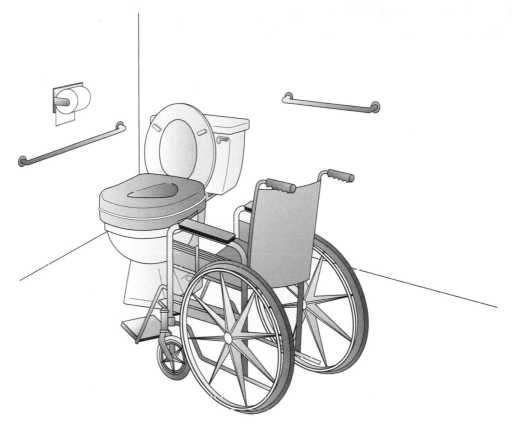

Fig. 16-19 The wheelchair is placed at a right (90-degree) angle to the toilet.

POSITIONING

The person must be properly positioned at all times. Regular position changes and good alignment promote comfort and well-being. Breathing is easier. Circulation is promoted. Proper positioning also helps prevent pressure ulcers and contractures.

Many residents can change their own positions. Some need reminding to do so. Others need help. Still others depend entirely on the nursing team for position changes.

Whether in bed or chair, the person is repositioned at least every 2 hours. Some people are repositioned more often. Follow the nurse's instructions and the care plan. Follow these guidelines to safely position a person:

- Use good body mechanics.
- Ask a co-worker to help you if needed.
- Explain the procedure to the person.
- Be gentle when moving the person.
- Provide for privacy.
- Place the signal light within reach after positioning.
- Use pillows as directed for support and alignment.

Delegation Guidelines

Positioning

Many tasks involve positioning and repositioning. You need this information from the nurse and the care plan:

- Position or positioning limits ordered by the doctor
- How often to turn and reposition the person
- How many co-workers need to help you
- What skin care measures to perform (Chapter 11)
- What range-of-motion exercises to perform (Chapter 19)
- Where to place pillows
- What positioning devices are needed and how to use them
- What observations to report and record

Fowler's Position

Fowler's position is a semi-sitting position. The head of the bed is raised 45 to 90 degrees (Fig. 16-20). For good alignment:

- Keep the spine straight.
- Support the head with a small pillow.
- Support the arms with pillows.

The nurse may ask you to place a small pillow under the lower back, thighs, and ankles. Persons with heart and respiratory disorders usually breathe easier in Fowler's position.

Supine Position

The **supine (dorsal recumbent) position** is the back-lying position (Fig. 16-21). For good alignment:

- Keep the bed flat.
- Support the head and shoulders on a pillow.
- Keep the arms and hands at the sides. You can support the arms with regular pillows. Or you can support the hands on small pillows with the palms down.

The nurse may ask you to place a folded or rolled towel under the lower back and a small pillow under the thighs. A pillow under the lower legs lifts the heels off of the bed. This prevents them from rubbing on the sheets.

Prone Position

Persons in the **prone position** lie on their abdomens with their heads turned to one side. Small pillows are placed under the head, abdomen, and lower legs (Fig. 16-22). Arms are flexed at the elbows with the hands near the head.

You also can position a person with the feet hanging over the end of the mattress (Fig. 16-23). If that is done, a pillow is not needed under the feet.

Lateral Position

A person in the **lateral (side-lying) position** lies on one side or the other (Fig. 16-24):

- Place a pillow under the head and neck.
- Position the upper leg in front of the lower leg. (The nurse may ask you to position the upper leg behind the lower leg, not on top of it.)
- Support the upper leg and thigh with pillows.
- Place a small pillow against the person's back. The person rolls back against the pillow so that his or her back is at 45-degree angle with the mattress.
- Place a small pillow under the upper hand and arm.

See Chapter 15 for the 30-degree side-lying position.

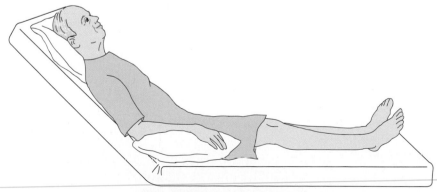

Fig. 16-20 Fowler's position.

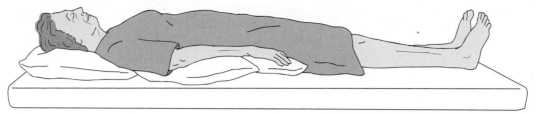

Fig. 16-21 Supine position.

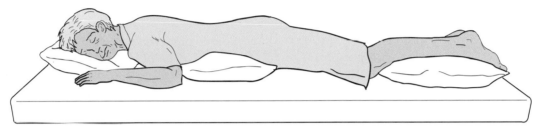

Fig. 16-22 Prone position.

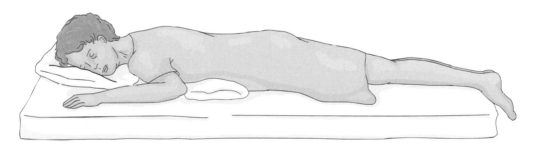

Fig. 16-23 Prone position with the feet hanging over the edge of the mattress.

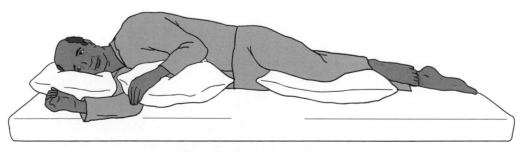

Fig. 16-24 Lateral position.

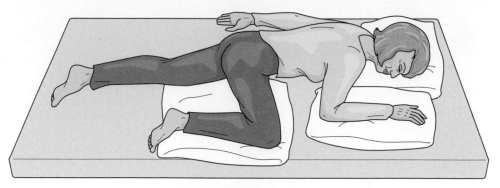

Fig. 16-25 Sims' position.

Sims' Position

The **Sims' position** is a left side-lying position. The upper leg is sharply flexed so it is not on the lower leg. The lower arm is behind the person (Fig. 16-25, p. 322). For good alignment:

- Place a pillow under the person's head and shoulder.
- Support the upper leg with a pillow.
- Place a pillow under the upper arm and hand.

Chair Position

Persons who sit in chairs must hold their upper bodies and heads erect. If not, poor alignment results. For good alignment:

- The person's back and buttocks are against the back of the chair.
- Feet are flat on the floor or wheelchair footplates. Never leave the feet unsupported.
- Backs of the knees and calves are slightly away from the edge of the seat (Fig. 16-26).

The nurse may ask you to put a small pillow between the person's lower back and the chair. This supports the lower back. *A pillow is not used behind the back if restraints are used (Chapter 20).*

Paralyzed arms are supported on pillows. Some residents use positioning aids. Ask the nurse about their proper use.

Repositioning in a Chair or Wheelchair.
The person can slide down into the chair. For good alignment and safety, the person's back and buttocks must be against the back of the chair.

Some persons can help with repositioning. Others need help. Use this method if the person is alert, cooperative, can follow instructions, and has the strength to help:

- Lock the wheelchair wheels.
- Stand in front of the person. Block his or her knees and feet with your knees and feet.
- Apply a transfer belt.
- Remove or swing the front rigging out of the way.
- Position the person's feet flat on the floor.
- Position the person's arms on the armrests.
- Grasp the transfer belt on each side while the person leans forward.
- Ask the person to push with his or her feet and arms on the count of "3."
- Lift the person back into the chair on the count of "3" as the person pushes with his or her feet and arms (Fig. 16-27).

This method is used if the person cannot assist with repositioning. Two staff members are needed (Fig. 16-28):

- Ask a co-worker to help you. Decide who is the tallest. The tallest worker stands behind the wheelchair. The other stands in front of the person.
- Lock the wheelchair wheels.
- Apply a transfer belt.
- Ask the person to place folded hands in his or her lap.
- Remove or swing front rigging out of the way.
- The worker behind the wheelchair grasps the transfer belt on each side.
- The other worker stands in front of the person. He or she places the hands and arms under the person's knees.
- On the count of "3," lift the person to the back of the chair. Support the legs (worker in front) and use the transfer belt (worker in back).

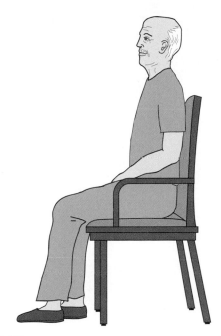

Fig. 16-26 The person is positioned in a chair. The person's feet are flat on the floor, the calves do not touch the chair, and the back is straight and against the back of the chair.

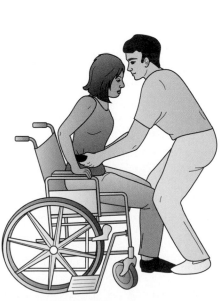

Fig. 16-27 Repositioning the person in a wheelchair. A transfer belt is used to lift the person to the back of the chair.

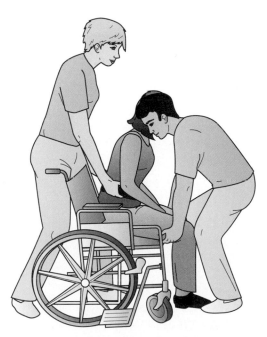

Fig. 16-28 Two workers reposition a person in a wheelchair. The tallest worker stands behind the chair and lifts with the transfer belt. The other worker stands in front of the person. Hands and arms are under the knees to support the legs during repositioning.

Review Questions

Circle the **BEST** answer.

1 Which protects the skin when moving the person in bed?
   a Rolling or lifting the person
   b Sliding the person up in bed
   c Moving the mattress
   d Using positioning aids

2 Whenever you lift, move, turn, transfer, or reposition a person, you must
   a Allow personal choice
   b Protect the person's privacy
   c Use pillows for support
   d Get help from a co-worker

3 You are delegated tasks that involve lifting and moving persons in bed. Which is *true*?
   a The nurse tells you how to position the person.
   b You decide which procedure to use.
   c Bed rails are used at all times.
   d Three workers are needed to complete the task safely.

4 A lift sheet is placed so that it
   a Covers the person's body
   b Is under the person from the head to above the knees
   c Extends from the mid-back to mid-thigh level
   d Covers the entire mattress

5 Before turning a person onto his or her side, you
   a Move the person to the side of the bed
   b Move the person to the middle of the bed
   c Lock arms with the person
   d Position pillows for comfort

6 The logrolling procedure
   a Is used after spinal cord injuries or surgery
   b Requires a transfer belt
   c Requires a mechanical lift
   d Requires a lift sheet

7 When getting ready to dangle a person, you need to know
   a Which side is stronger
   b If bed rails are used
   c If a mechanical lift is needed
   d If a transfer belt is needed

8 Before transferring a person to or from a bed, you must
   a Have the person wear nonskid footwear
   b Lock the bed wheels
   c Apply a transfer belt
   d Position pillows for support

9 A transfer belt is applied
   a To the skin   c Over breasts
   b Over clothing   d Under the robe

10 When transferring a person to bed, a chair, or the toilet
   a The person's strong side moves first
   b The weak side moves first
   c Pillows are used for support
   d The transfer belt is removed

11 You are going to use a mechanical lift. You must do the following *except*
   a Follow the manufacturer's instructions
   b Make sure the lift works
   c Compare the person's weight to the lift's weight limit
   d Use a transfer belt

12 These statements are about transfers to and from a toilet. Which is *false?*
   a The person wears nonskid footwear.
   b Wheelchair wheels must be locked.
   c The person uses the towel bars for support.
   d A transfer belt is used.

13 Residents are repositioned at least every
   a 30 minutes
   b 1 hour
   c 2 hours
   d 3 hours

14 The back-lying position is called
   a Fowler's position
   b The supine position
   c The prone position
   d Sims' position

15 A person is positioned in a chair. The feet
   a Must be flat on the floor
   b Are positioned on footplates
   c Dangle
   d Are positioned on pillows

Answers to these questions are on p. 389.

CHAPTER 17

Mental Health Needs

Objectives

- Define the key terms listed in this chapter
- Identify the developmental tasks for each age-group
- Describe common reactions to the need for nursing center care
- Describe the psychological and social changes that occur with aging
- Describe the common reactions to aging and loss
- Explain how to deal with anger and other behavior issues
- Describe the common mental health disorders

anxiety A vague, uneasy feeling in response to stress

defense mechanisms Unconscious reactions that block unpleasant or threatening feelings

development Changes in mental, emotional, and social function

developmental task A skill that must be completed during a stage of development

growth The physical changes that are measured and that occur in a steady and orderly manner

mental health The person copes with and adjusts to everyday stresses in ways accepted by society

mental illness A disturbance in the ability to cope with or adjust to stress

The whole person is a physical, psychological, social, and spiritual being. To focus only on the physical needs is to ignore the mental parts of the person. *Mental* relates to the mind. It is something that exists in the mind or is done by the mind. It relates to the psychological, social, and spiritual parts of the person.

GROWTH AND DEVELOPMENT

Throughout life, people grow and develop. Changes occur from birth through old age. **Growth** is the physical changes that are measured and that occur in a steady and orderly manner. Growth is measured in height and weight. Changes in appearance and body functions also measure growth.

Development relates to changes in mental, emotional, and social function. A person behaves and thinks in certain ways in each stage of development. A 2-year-old thinks in simple terms. A 40-year-old thinks in complex ways. The entire person is affected.

Growth and development occur in a sequence, order, and pattern. Certain skills must be completed during each stage. A **developmental task** is a skill that must be completed during a stage of development. A stage cannot be skipped. Each stage is the basis for the next stage. Each stage has its own characteristics and developmental tasks (Box 17-1).

Physical Changes

Certain physical changes occur with aging. They happen to everyone. Body processes slow down. Energy level and body efficiency decline. The changes are slow. They occur over many years. Often they are not noticed for a long time. Some people age faster than others. The rate and degree of change vary with each person.

Normal aging does not mean loss of health. Quality of life does not have to decline. The person can adjust to many of the changes.

Some older people are ill, injured, or disabled. Illness, injuries, and disabilities have physical, mental, and social effects. Normal activities—driving, fixing meals, yard work, or hobbies—may be hard or impossible. Daily activities bring pleasure, worth, and contact with others. People often feel angry, upset, and useless when unable to perform them. These feelings may increase if others must perform routine functions for them.

The Need for Nursing Center Care.

Some older persons who are disabled or chronically ill may need nursing center care. They may have many fears and concerns about nursing centers. They may feel lonely and abandoned by family and friends. They may fear depending on strangers. Many may fear increasing loss of function. Some express their fears. Others do not or cannot.

Anger is a common response to needing nursing center care. The person may direct anger at you. However, the person is really angry at the situation. Ask the nurse for help if you have problems dealing with a person's anger (p. 329).

You can help the person feel safe, secure, and loved. Take an extra minute to "visit," to hold a hand, or to give a hug. Show that you are willing to help with personal needs. Respond promptly. Treat each person with respect and dignity.

Hospital patients often are treated as sick, dependent people. Promoting this "sick role" in a nursing center reduces quality of life. The health team focuses on improving the person's quality of life. You must help each person regain or maintain as much physical and mental function as possible.

The person needing nursing center care may suffer some or all of these losses:

- Loss of identify as an active member of a family and community
- Loss of possessions (for example, home, household items, car)
- Loss of independence
- Loss of real-world experiences (for example, shopping, traveling, cooking, driving, hobbies)
- Loss of health and mobility

BOX 17-1 Stages of Growth and Development

Infancy (Birth to 1 year)

- Learning to walk
- Learning to eat solid foods
- Beginning to talk and communicate with others
- Beginning to have emotional relationships with parents, brothers, and sisters
- Developing stable sleep and feeding patterns

Toddlerhood (1 to 3 years)

- Tolerating separation from parents or primary caregivers
- Gaining control of bowel and bladder function
- Using words to communicate
- Becoming less dependent on parents or primary caregivers

Preschool (3 to 6 years)

- Increasing the ability to communicate and understand others
- Performing self-care
- Learning gender differences and developing sexual modesty
- Learning right from wrong and good from bad
- Learning to play with others
- Developing family relationships

School Age (6 to 9 or 10 years)

- Developing social and physical skills needed for playing games
- Learning to get along with children of the same age and background (peers)
- Learning gender-appropriate behaviors and attitudes
- Learning basic reading, writing, and arithmetic skills
- Developing a conscience and morals
- Developing a good feeling and attitude about oneself

Late Childhood (9 or 10 to 12 years)

- Becoming independent of adults and learning to depend on oneself
- Developing and keeping friendships with peers
- Understanding the physical, psychological, and social roles of one's sex
- Developing moral and ethical behavior
- Developing greater muscular strength, coordination, and balance
- Learning how to study

Adolescence (12 to 18 years)

- Accepting changes in the body and appearance
- Developing appropriate relationships with males and females of the same age
- Accepting the male or female role appropriate for one's age
- Becoming independent from parents and adults
- Developing morals, attitudes, and values needed to function in society

Young Adulthood (18 to 40 years)

- Choosing education and a career
- Selecting a partner
- Learning to live with a partner
- Becoming a parent and raising children
- Developing a satisfactory sex life

Middle Adulthood (40 to 65 years)

- Adjusting to physical changes
- Having grown children
- Developing leisure-time activities
- Adjusting to aging parents

Late Adulthood (65 years and older)

- Adjusting to decreased strength and loss of health
- Adjusting to retirement and reduced income
- Coping with a partner's death
- Developing new friends and relationships
- Preparing for one's own death

Such losses may cause the person to feel useless, powerless, and hopeless. Some people try to cope with many losses. They may have a hard time talking to others. Encourage them to talk about the losses. They may find that other residents have similar losses.

Moving to a nursing center can cause feelings of loneliness and isolation. Making new friends helps the person adjust. It also improves quality of life. Some residents cannot visit with friends or get to activities without help. Offer to take them to visit in a friend's room or to an activity. Treat the person with dignity and respect. Also practice good communication skills. Follow the care plan.

Psychological and Social Changes

Social roles change. A parent may depend on an adult child for care. Retirees need activities to replace the work role. Adjusting to the death of a partner, family, and friends is common. The person also faces his or her own death.

People cope with aging in their own way. How they cope depends on:

- Health status
- Life experiences
- Finances
- Education
- Social support systems

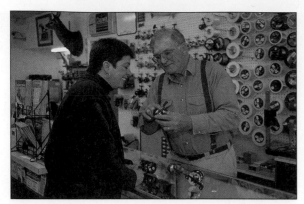

Fig. 17-1 This retired man works at a sports shop.

Retirement. Age 65 is the usual retirement age. Some retire earlier. Others work into their 70s. Retirement is a reward for a lifetime of hard work. The person can relax and enjoy life. Travel, leisure, and doing what one wants are retirement "benefits." Many people enjoy retirement. Poor health and medical bills can make retirement very hard.

Work helps meet love, belonging, and self-esteem needs (Chapter 2). The person feels useful. Friendships develop. Leisure time, recreation, and companionship often involve co-workers. Retirement is hard for some people. Some have part-time jobs (Fig. 17-1). Others do volunteer work. Such activities promote usefulness and well-being.

Reduced Income. Retirement usually means reduced income. Social Security may provide the only income. The retired person still has expenses. Rent or house payments continue. Food, clothing, utility bills, and taxes are other expenses. Car expenses, home repairs, drugs, and health care are other costs. So are entertainment and gifts.

Reduced income may force life-style changes. Examples include:

- Limiting social and leisure events
- Buying cheaper food, clothes, and household items
- Moving to cheaper housing
- Living with children or other family
- Avoiding health care or needed drugs
- Relying on children or other family for money or needed items

Severe money problems can result. Some people plan for retirement. They have savings, investments, retirement plans, and insurance.

Social Relationships. Social relationships change throughout life. (See *Caring About Culture: Foreign-Born Persons.*) Children grow up and leave home. They have their own families. Many live far away from parents. Older family members and friends die, move away, or are disabled. Yet most

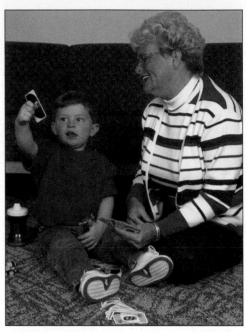

Fig. 17-2 This older woman plays with her grandson.

older people have regular contact with children, grandchildren, family, and friends. Others are lonely. Separation from children is a common cause. So is lack of companionship with people their own age.

Many older people adjust to these changes. Hobbies, church and community events, and new friends help prevent loneliness. Some communities and groups sponsor bus trips to ball games, shopping, plays, and concerts.

Grandchildren can bring great love and joy. Family times help prevent loneliness. They help the older person feel useful and wanted (Fig. 17-2).

Children as Caregivers. Some children care for their older parents. Parents and children change roles. The child now cares for the parent. This helps some older persons feel more secure. Others feel unwanted, in the way, and useless. Some lose dignity and self-respect. Tensions may occur among the child, parent, and other household members. Lack of privacy is a cause. So are disagreements and criticisms about housekeeping, childrearing, cooking, and friends.

BOX 17-2   Dealing With Anger and Behavior Issues

- Recognize frustrating and frightening situations. Put yourself in the person's situation. How would you feel? How would you want to be treated?
- Treat the person with dignity and respect.
- Practice good communication (Chapter 2).
- Answer questions clearly and thoroughly. Ask the nurse to answer questions you cannot answer.
- Keep the person informed. Tell the person what you are going to do and when.
- Do not keep the person waiting. Answer signal lights promptly. If you tell the person that you will do something for him or her, do it promptly.
- Explain the reason for long waits. Ask if you can get or do something to increase the person's comfort.
- Stay calm and professional. Often the person is not angry at you. He or she is angry at another person or situation.
- Do not argue with the person.
- Listen and use silence. The person may feel better if able to express feelings.
- Follow the person's care plan for comfort measures.
- Do the following if the person is becoming agitated or aggressive:
  —Stand away from the person. Judge the length of the person's arms and legs. Stand far enough away so the person cannot hit or kick you.
  —Stand close to the door. Do not become trapped in the room.
  —Know where to find panic buttons, signal lights, alarms, closed-circuit monitors, and other security devices.
  —Keep your hands free.
  —Stay calm. Talk to the person in a calm manner. Do not raise your voice or argue, scold, or interrupt the person.
  —Do not touch the person.
  —Tell the person that you will get the nurse to speak to him or her.
  —Leave the room as soon as you can. Make sure the person is safe.
  —Tell the nurse and security officer about the matter.
  —Complete an incident report according to center policy (Chapter 4).
- Report the person's behavior to the nurse. Discuss how you should deal with the person.

Death of a Partner.   As couples grow older, the chances increase that a partner will die. Women usually live longer than men. Therefore many women become widows.

A person may try to prepare for a partner's death. When death does occur, the loss is still crushing. No amount of preparation is ever enough for the emptiness and changes that result. The person loses a lover, friend, companion, and confidant. Grief can be very great. Serious physical and mental health problems can result. Some lose the will to live. Some attempt suicide.

REACTIONS TO AGING AND LOSS

Illness, injury, and disability affect quality of life. Normal tasks and activities that bring pleasure and contact with others may be hard or impossible. The person will likely face more losses in the future. The person may feel sad and frustrated. The person may also feel helpless and useless. Fear, anger, and anxiety also are common and normal reactions.

Anger

Anger is a common emotion. Causes include fear, pain, and dying and death. Loss of function and loss of control over health and life are causes. Anger also is a symptom of diseases that affect thinking and behavior. Some people are generally angry. Few things please or make them happy. Anger is shown verbally and nonverbally. Verbal outbursts, shouting, raised voices, and rapid speech are common. Some people

are silent. Others are uncooperative. They may refuse to answer questions. Nonverbal signs include rapid movements, pacing, clenched fists, and a red face. Glaring and getting close to you when speaking are other signs. Violent behaviors can occur.

Do not react to the person's anger. Do not avoid the person or lose control. Good communication is needed. Follow the care plan and the guidelines in Box 17-2.

Anxiety

Anxiety is a vague, uneasy feeling in response to stress. The person may not know why or the cause. The person senses danger or harm—real or imagined. The person acts to relieve the unpleasant feeling. Often anxiety occurs when needs are not met.

Some anxiety is normal. However, some people have high levels of anxiety. Signs and symptoms depend on the degree of anxiety (Box 17-3, p. 330).

Coping and defense mechanisms are used to relieve anxiety. Some are healthy. Others are not. Coping mechanisms include eating, drinking, smoking, exercising, fighting, and talking about the problem. Some people play music, go for a walk, take a hot bath, or want to be alone.

Defense mechanisms are unconscious reactions that block unpleasant or threatening feelings (Box 17-4, p. 330). Some use of defense mechanisms is normal. With mental health problems, they are used poorly (p. 331).

BOX 17-3 Signs and Symptoms of Anxiety

- A "lump" in the throat
- "Butterflies" in the stomach
- Rapid pulse
- Rapid respirations
- Increased blood pressure
- Rapid speech
- Voice changes
- Dry mouth
- Sweating
- Nausea
- Diarrhea
- Urinary frequency and urgency
- Poor attention span
- Difficulty following directions
- Difficulty sleeping
- Loss of appetite

BOX 17-4 Defense Mechanisms

Compensation—*Compensate* means to make up for, replace, or substitute. The person makes up for or substitutes a strength for a weakness.
EXAMPLE: A boy is not good in sports. But he learns to play music.

Denial—*Deny* means refusing to accept or believe something that is true. The person refuses to face or accept unpleasant or threatening things.
EXAMPLE: A man had a heart attack. He continues to smoke after being told to quit.

Displacement—*Displace* means to move or take the place of. An individual moves behaviors or emotions from one person, place, or thing to a safe person, place, or thing.
EXAMPLE: You are angry with your boss. You yell at a friend.

Projection—*Project* means to blame another. An individual blames another person or object for unacceptable behavior, emotions, ideas, or wishes.
EXAMPLE: A girl fails a test. She blames a friend for not helping her study.

Rationalization—*Rational* means sensible, reasonable, or logical. An acceptable reason or excuse is given for one's behavior or actions. The real reason is not given.
EXAMPLE: A man is often late for work. He did not get a raise. He says that the boss does not like him.

Regression—*Regress* means to move back or to retreat. The person retreats or moves back to an earlier time or condition.
EXAMPLE: A 3-year-old wants a baby bottle when a new baby comes into the family.

Repression—*Repress* means to hold down or keep back. The person keeps unpleasant or painful thoughts or experiences from the conscious mind. They cannot be recalled or remembered.
EXAMPLE: A child was sexually abused. Now 33 years old, she has no memory of the event.

Behavior Issues

Many people accept illness and disability as part of aging. Others do not adjust well. Besides anger and anxiety, they may have some of the following behaviors. These behaviors are new for some people. For others, the behaviors are lifelong. They are part of one's personality.

- *Demanding behavior*—Nothing seems to please the person. The person is critical of others. He or she wants care given at a certain time and in a certain way. Causes include loss of independence, loss of health, loss of control of life, and unmet needs.
- *Self-centered behavior*—The person cares only about his or her own needs. The needs of others are ignored. The person demands the time and attention of others.
- *Aggressive behavior*—The person may swear, bite, hit, pinch, scratch, or kick. Fear, anger, pain, and dementia (Chapter 18) are causes. Protect the person, others, and yourself from harm (see Box 17-2).
- *Withdrawal*—The person has little or no contact with others. He or she spends time alone and does not take part in social or group events. This may signal physical illness or depression.
- *Inappropriate sexual behavior*—Some people make inappropriate sexual remarks. Or they touch others. Some disrobe or masturbate in public. These behaviors may be on purpose. Or they are caused by disease, confusion, dementia, or drug side effects.

A person's behavior may be unpleasant. You cannot avoid the person or lose control. Good communication is needed. Follow the care plan and the guidelines in Box 17-2.

BOX 17-5 Common Mental Health Disorders

- **Obsessive-compulsive disorder (OCD).** An *obsession* is a recurrent, unwanted thought or idea. *Compulsion* is repeating an act over and over again (a ritual). The act may not make sense, but the person has much anxiety if the act is not done. Common rituals are hand washing, cleaning, and counting to a certain number.
- **Schizophrenia.** *Schizophrenia* means split *(schizo)* mind *(phrenia).* It is a severe, chronic, disabling brain disease. The person with schizophrenia has a severe mental impairment *(psychosis).* Thinking and behavior are disturbed. The person has false beliefs *(delusions).* He or she also has *hallucinations.* That is, the person sees, hears, or feels things that are not real. The person has problems relating to others. He or she may have *paranoia.* That is, the person is suspicious about a person or situation. Responses are inappropriate. Communication is disturbed. The person may ramble or repeat what another says. Sometimes speech cannot be understood. The person may withdraw. That is, the person lacks interest in others. He or she is not involved with people or society. The person may sit for hours alone without moving, speaking, or responding. Some persons *regress.* To regress means to retreat or move back to an earlier time or condition. For example, a 5-year-old wets the bed when there is a new baby. This is normal. Healthy adults do not act like infants or children. However, regression often occurs in schizophrenia.
- **Bipolar disorder.** *Bipolar* means two *(bi)* poles or ends *(polar).* The person with bipolar disorder has severe extremes in mood, energy, and ability to function. There are emotional lows—*depression;* and emotional highs—*mania.* The disorder also is called *manic-depressive illness.* Some people are suicidal. The disorder tends to run in families.
- **Major depression.** Depression involves the body, mood, and thoughts. Symptoms affect sleep, eating, and other activities. The person is very sad. He or she loses interest in daily activities. Depression may

occur just once. It may be caused by a stressful event such as divorce or death of a partner, parent, or child. For some people, episodes of depression occur throughout life. Depression is common in older persons. They have many losses—death of family and friends, loss of health, loss of body functions, loss of independence. Loneliness and the side effects of some drugs also are causes. See Box 17-6 on p. 332 for the signs and symptoms of depression in older persons. Depression in older persons is often overlooked, or a wrong diagnosis is made. Often the person is thought to have a cognitive disorder (Chapter 18). Therefore the depression often is untreated.
- **Personality disorders.** Personality disorders involve rigid and maladaptive behaviors. To *adapt* means to change or adjust. *Mal* means bad, wrong, or ill. *Maladaptive* means to change or adjust in the wrong way. Because of their behaviors, those with personality disorders cannot function well in society. Personality disorders include:
  - —*Abusive personality*—The person copes with anxiety by abusing others. Behavior may be violent.
  - —*Paranoid personality*—The person is very suspicious. He or she distrusts others.
  - —*Antisocial personality*—The person has poor judgment. He or she lacks responsibility and is hostile. The person is not loyal to any person or group. Morals and ethics are lacking. Others are blamed for actions and behaviors. The rights of others do not matter. The person has no guilt. He or she does not learn from experiences or punishment. The person is often in trouble with the police.
- **Substance abuse.** Substance abuse occurs when a person overuses or depends on drugs or alcohol. Dependence may be emotional, psychological, or physical. Legal and illegal drugs are abused. Legal drugs are approved for use in the United States. Doctors prescribe them. Illegal drugs are not approved for use. They are obtained through illegal means.

MENTAL HEALTH DISORDERS

Mental health means that the person copes with and adjusts to everyday stresses in ways accepted by society. **Mental illness** is a disturbance in the ability to cope with or adjust to stress. Behavior and function are impaired. *Mental disorder, emotional illness,* and *psychiatric disorder* also mean *mental illness.*

Causes of mental health disorders include:

- Not being able to cope or adjust to stress
- Chemical imbalances
- Genetics
- Drug or substance abuse
- Social and cultural factors

Some nursing center residents have mental health disorders (Box 17-5). As with physical illnesses and disabilities, mental health disorders can range from mild to severe.

BOX 17-6   Signs and Symptoms of Depression in Older Persons

- Fatigue
- Lack of interest
- Inability to experience pleasure
- Feelings of uselessness
- Feelings of hopelessness
- Feelings of helplessness
- Decreased sexual interest
- Increased dependency
- Anxiety
- Slow or unreliable memory
- Paranoia
- Agitation
- Focus on the past

- Thoughts of death
- Thoughts of suicide
- Difficulty completing activities of daily living
- Changes in sleep patterns
- Lower energy level
- Poor grooming
- Withdrawal from people and interests
- Muscle aches
- Abdominal pain
- Nausea and vomiting
- Dry mouth
- Headaches

Modified from Lueckenotte AG: *Gerontologic nursing,* ed 2, St Louis, 2000, Mosby.

Review Questions

Circle the **BEST** answer.

1   Which is a developmental task of late adulthood?
   a   Adjusting to aging parents
   b   Selecting a partner
   c   Developing new friends and relationships
   d   Developing a good feeling about oneself

2   These statements are about the need for nursing center care. Which is *false?*
   a   Residents often feel lonely.
   b   Residents suffer many losses.
   c   Anger is a common response.
   d   Needing nursing center care is a normal part of aging.

3   You can help new residents adjust to the nursing center by the following *except*
   a   Taking them to a friend's room
   b   Taking them to activities
   c   Treating them with dignity and respect
   d   Keeping the room door closed

4   Retirement usually means
   a   Lowered income
   b   Changes from aging
   c   Companionship and usefulness
   d   Financial security

Review Questions

5 Older people living with their children often feel
- **a** Independent
- **b** Wanted and a part of things
- **c** Useless
- **d** Dignified

6 These statements are about a partner's death. Which is *false?*
- **a** The person loses a lover, friend, companion, and confidante.
- **b** Preparing for the event lessens grief.
- **c** The survivor may develop health problems.
- **d** The survivor's life will likely change.

7 Mr. Porter is angry and agitated. Which is *true?*
- **a** He has a disease that affects thinking and behavior.
- **b** You should stand or sit close to him.
- **c** Listening and silence are important.
- **d** You should use touch to calm him.

8 These statements are about anxiety. Which is *false?*
- **a** Some anxiety is normal.
- **b** The person senses danger or harm.
- **c** Coping and defense mechanisms help relieve anxiety.
- **d** The anxious person has a slow pulse and slow respirations.

9 Mrs. Bolt cares only about her own needs. She does not care about others. Her behavior can be described as
- **a** Demanding
- **b** Self-centered
- **c** Aggressive
- **d** Regressive

10 Which is common in older persons?
- **a** Obsessive-compulsive disorder
- **b** Schizophrenia
- **c** Major depression
- **d** Personality disorder

Answers to these questions are on p. 390.

CHAPTER 18

Care of Cognitively Impaired Residents

Objectives

- Define the key terms listed in this chapter
- Describe confusion, its causes, and related care measures
- Explain the difference between delirium, depression, and dementia
- Describe Alzheimer's disease (AD) and its signs, symptoms, and behaviors
- Explain the care required by persons with AD and other dementias
- Describe the effects of AD on the family

Key Terms

delirium A state of temporary but acute mental confusion

delusion A false belief

dementia The loss of cognitive and social function caused by changes in the brain

hallucination Seeing, hearing, or feeling something that is not real

sundowning Signs, symptoms, and behaviors of AD increase during hours of darkness

---

Changes in the brain and nervous system occur with aging and certain diseases (Box 18-1). Changes in the brain can affect cognitive function. (*Cognitive* relates to knowledge.) Cognitive functioning involves:

- Memory
- Thinking
- Reasoning
- Ability to understand
- Judgment
- Behavior

CONFUSION

Confusion has many causes. Diseases, infections, hearing and vision loss, and drug side effects are some causes. So is brain injury. With aging, blood supply to the brain is reduced. Brain cells are lost. Personality and mental changes can result. Memory and the ability to make good judgments are lost. A person may not know people, the time, or the place. Some people gradually lose the ability to perform daily activities. Behavior changes are common. The person may be angry, restless, depressed, and irritable.

Acute confusion (delirium—p. 336) occurs suddenly. It is usually temporary. Causes include infection, illness, injury, drugs, and surgery. Treatment is aimed at the cause.

Confusion caused by physical changes cannot be cured. Some measures help improve function (Box 18-2). You must meet the person's physical and safety needs.

BOX 18-1 Changes in the Nervous System From Aging

- Brain cells are lost.
- Nerve conduction slows.
- Response and reaction times are slower.
- Reflexes are slower.
- Vision and hearing decrease.
- Taste and smell decrease.
- Touch and sensitivity to pain decrease.
- Blood flow to the brain is reduced.
- Sleep patterns change.
- Memory is shorter.
- Forgetfulness occurs.
- Dizziness can occur.

BOX 18-2 Caring for the Confused Person

- Follow the person's care plan.
- Provide for safety.
- Face the person. Speak clearly and slowly.
- Call the person by name every time you are in contact with him or her.
- State your name. Show your name tag.
- Give the date and time each morning. Repeat as needed during the day or evening.
- Explain what you are going to do and why.
- Give clear, simple directions and answers to questions.
- Ask clear and simple questions. Give the person time to respond.
- Keep calendars and clocks with large numbers in the person's room and in nursing areas (Fig. 18-1, p. 336). Remind the person of holidays, birthdays, and special events.
- Have the person wear eyeglasses and hearing aids as needed.
- Use touch to communicate (Chapter 2).
- Place familiar objects and pictures within the person's view.
- Provide newspapers, magazines, TV, and radio. Read to the person if appropriate.
- Discuss current events with the person.
- Maintain the day-night cycle. Open curtains, shades, and drapes during the day. Close them at night. Use a night-light at night. The person wears regular clothes during the day—not sleepwear.
- Provide a calm, relaxed, and peaceful setting. Prevent loud noises, rushing, and congested hallways and dining rooms.
- Follow the person's routine. Meals, bathing, exercise, TV, and other activities have a schedule. This promotes a sense of order and what to expect.
- Break tasks into small steps when helping the person.
- Do not rearrange furniture or the person's belongings.
- Encourage the person to take part in self-care.
- Be consistent.

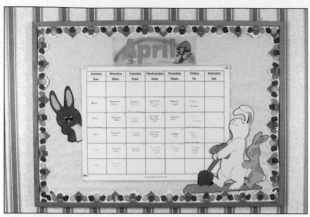

Fig. 18-1 A large calendar can help confused persons.

BOX 18-3	Types and Causes of Dementia

- Alzheimer's disease (AD)
- Alcohol-related dementia and Korsokoff's disease
- AIDS-related dementia
- Cerebrovascular disease—diseased blood vessels (*vascular*) in the brain *(cerebro)*
- Delirium
- Depression
- Drugs that affect brain function
- Nervous system diseases—Huntington's disease, multiple sclerosis, Parkinson's disease, stroke, multi-infarct dementia, brain tumor
- Infection
- Syphilis
- Trauma and head injury

DEMENTIA

Dementia is the loss of cognitive function and social function. It is caused by changes in the brain. (*De* means from. *Mentia* means mind.) Alzheimer's disease (AD) is the most common type of dementia. Other types and causes are listed in Box 18-3.

Dementia is not a normal part of aging. Most older people do not have dementia. Some early warning signs include:

- Recent memory loss that affects job skills
- Problems with common tasks (for example, dressing, cooking, driving)
- Problems with language; forgetting simple words
- Getting lost in familiar places
- Misplacing things and putting things in odd places (for example, putting a watch in the oven)
- Personality changes
- Poor or decreased judgment (for example, going outdoors in the snow without shoes)
- Loss of interest in life

The person needs to see a doctor. The doctor orders many tests. Treatment depends on the cause and problem. Some dementias can be reversed. When the cause is removed, so are the signs and symptoms. Treatable causes include:

- Drugs and alcohol
- Delirium and depression
- Tumors
- Heart, lung, and blood vessel problems
- Head injuries
- Infection
- Vision and hearing problems

Permanent dementias result from changes in the brain. They have no cure. Function declines over time. Parkinson's disease causes changes in the brain. So does cardiovascular disease. Multi-infarct dementia (MID) is caused by many *(multi)* strokes. The stroke leaves an area of damage called an *infarct*. AD is the most common type of permanent dementia.

Delirium and Depression

Delirium and depression can be mistaken for dementia. They occur alone or with dementia. Or the person with dementia suffers from delirium and depression.

Delirium. **Delirium** is a state of temporary but acute mental confusion. Onset is sudden. It is common in older persons with acute or chronic illnesses. Infections, heart and lung diseases, and poor nutrition are common causes. Hypoglycemia is also a cause (Chapter 14). Alcohol and many drugs can cause delirium. Delirium can last for a few hours to as long as 1 month.

Delirium signals physical illness in older persons and in persons with dementia. It is an emergency. The cause must be found and treated. Signs and symptoms of delirium include:

- Anxiety
- Disorientation
- Tremors
- Hallucinations (p. 339)
- Delusions (p. 339)
- Attention problems
- Decline in level of consciousness
- Memory problems

Depression. Depression is the most common mental health problem in older persons. It is often overlooked. A correct diagnosis is needed for proper treatment. Otherwise the person and family have unnecessary emotional, physical, social, and financial discomfort.

Depression, aging, and some drug side effects have similar signs and symptoms. They include:

* Sadness
* Inactivity
* Difficulty thinking
* Problems concentrating
* Feelings of despair
* Problems sleeping
* Changes in appetite
* Fatigue
* Agitation
* Withdrawal

ALZHEIMER'S DISEASE

Alzheimer's disease (AD) is a brain disease. Brain cells that control intellectual and social function are damaged. These functions are affected:

* Memory
* Thinking
* Reasoning
* Judgment
* Language
* Behavior
* Mood
* Personality

The person has problems with work and everyday functions. Problems with family and social relationships occur. There is a steady decline in memory and mental function.

The disease begins slowly. It gets worse and worse over 3 to 20 years. AD occurs in both men and women. Women live longer than men. Therefore more women have AD. Some people in their 40s and 50s have AD. However, it usually occurs after the age of 65. It is often diagnosed around the age of 80. The cause is unknown. A family history of AD is a risk factor.

Signs of AD

The classic sign of AD is *gradual loss of short-term memory*. Other early signs include:

* Problems finding or speaking the right word
* Not recognizing objects
* Forgetting how to use simple, everyday things (like a pencil)
* Forgetting to turn off the stove, close windows, or lock doors
* Mood and personality changes
* Agitation
* Poor judgment (may cause odd behavior)

AD affects the ability to perform complex and simple tasks. Problems with complex tasks appear first. The person has problems using the phone, driving, managing money, planning meals, and working. Over time, problems occur with simple tasks. These include bathing, dressing, eating, using the toilet, and walking. See Box 18-4 for other signs of AD.

BOX 18-4   Other Signs and Symptoms of AD

* Forgets recent events
* Forgets simple directions
* Forgets conversations
* Forgets appointments
* Forgets names (including family members)
* Forgets the names of everyday things (clock, radio, TV, and so on)
* Forgets words
* Substitutes unusual words and names for what is forgotten
* Loses train of thought
* Speaks in a native language
* Curses or swears
* Misplaces things
* Puts things in odd places
* Has problems writing checks or balancing checkbooks
* Gives away large amounts of money
* Does not recognize or understand numbers
* Has problems following conversations
* Has problems reading

* Has problems writing
* Becomes lost in familiar settings
* Forgets where he or she is
* Does not know how to get back home
* Wanders from home
* Cannot tell or understand time
* Cannot tell or understand dates
* Cannot solve everyday problems (iron is left on, stove burners left on, food burning on the stove, and so on)
* Cannot perform everyday tasks (dressing, bathing, brushing teeth, and so on)
* Distrusts others
* Is stubborn
* Withdraws socially
* Is restless
* Becomes suspicious
* Becomes fearful
* Does not want to do things
* Sleeps more than usual

BOX 18-5 Stages of Alzheimer's Disease

Stage 1: Mild

- Memory loss—forgetfulness; forgets recent events
- Problems finding words, finishing thoughts, following directions, and remembering names
- Poor judgment; bad decisions (including when driving)
- Disoriented to time and place
- Lack of spontaneity—less outgoing or interested in things
- Blames others for mistakes, forgetfulness, and other problems
- Moodiness
- Problems performing everyday tasks

Stage 2: Moderate

- Restlessness; increases during the evening hours
- Sleep problems
- Memory loss increases—may not know family and friends
- Dulled senses—cannot tell the difference between hot and cold; cannot recognize dangers
- Fecal and urinary incontinence
- Needs help with activities of daily living (ADL)—bathing, feeding, and dressing self; afraid of bathing; will not change clothes
- Loses impulse control—foul language, poor table manners, sexual aggression, rudeness

- Movement and gait problems—walks slowly, has a shuffling gait
- Communication problems—cannot follow directions; problems with reading, writing, and math; speaks in short sentences or single words; statements may not make sense
- Repeats motions and statements—moves things back and forth constantly; says the same thing over and over again
- Agitation—behavior may be violent

Stage 3: Severe

- Seizures (Chapter 5)
- Cannot speak—may groan, grunt, or scream
- Does not recognize self or family members
- Depends totally on others for all ADL
- Disoriented to person, time, and place
- Totally incontinent of urine and feces
- Cannot swallow—choking and aspiration are risks
- Sleep problems increase
- Becomes bed bound—cannot sit or walk
- Coma
- Death

Stages of AD

AD is often described in terms of 3 stages (Box 18-5). Sometimes it is described as having 7 stages:

- No cognitive decline
- Very mild cognitive decline
- Mild cognitive decline
- Moderate cognitive decline
- Moderately severe cognitive decline
- Severe cognitive decline
- Very severe cognitive decline

Signs and symptoms become more severe with each stage. The disease ends in death.

Behaviors

The following behaviors are common with AD.

Wandering.   Persons with AD are not oriented to person, time, and place. They may wander away and not find their way back. Wandering may be by foot, car, bicycle, or other means. They may be with you one moment and gone the next.

Judgment is poor. They cannot tell what is safe or dangerous. Life-threatening accidents are great risks. They can walk into traffic or into a nearby river, lake, ocean, or forest. If not properly dressed, heat or cold exposure is a risk.

Wandering may have no cause. Or the person may be looking for something or someone—the bathroom, the bedroom, a child, or a partner. Pain, drug side effects, stress, restlessness, and anxiety are possible causes. Sometimes finding the cause prevents wandering.

For persons living at home, the Alzheimer's Association has a Safe Return Program. The program is nationwide. It serves to identify and safely return persons who wander or become lost. A small fee is charged. A family member completes a form and provides a picture. These are entered into a national database. The person receives an ID (wallet card, bracelet or necklace, clothing labels). Anyone finding a person can call the Safe Return number on the ID. Safe Return then calls the family member or caregiver. Some persons are reported missing. Safe Return can provide the person's information and photo to the police.

Sundowning.   With **sundowning,** signs, symptoms, and behaviors of AD increase during hours of darkness. It occurs in the late afternoon and evening hours. As daylight ends and darkness starts, confusion and restlessness increase. So do anxiety, agitation, and other symptoms. Behavior is worse after the sun goes down. It may continue throughout the night.

Sundowning may relate to being tired or hungry. Poor light and shadows may cause the person to see things that are not there. Persons with AD may be afraid of the dark.

Hallucinations.   A **hallucination** is seeing, hearing, or feeling something that is not real. Senses are dulled. Affected persons see animals, insects, or people that are not present. Some hear voices. They may feel bugs crawling or feel that they are being touched.

Sometimes the problem is caused by impaired vision or hearing. The person needs to wear eyeglasses and hearing aids as prescribed.

Delusions.   **Delusions** are false beliefs. People with AD may think they are some other person. Some believe they are in jail, are being killed, or are being attacked. A person may believe that the caregiver is someone else. Many other false beliefs can occur.

Catastrophic Reactions.   These are extreme responses. The person reacts as if there is a disaster or tragedy. The person may scream, cry, or be agitated or combative. These reactions are common from too many stimuli. Eating, music or TV playing, and being asked questions all at once can overwhelm the person.

Agitation and Restlessness.   The person may pace, hit, or yell. Common causes are pain or discomfort, anxiety, lack of sleep, and too many or too few stimuli. Hunger and the need to eliminate also are causes. A calm, quiet setting helps calm the person. So does meeting basic needs.

Caregivers can cause these behaviors. A caregiver may rush the person or be impatient. Or mixed verbal and nonverbal messages are sent. Caregivers always need to look at how their behaviors affect other persons.

Aggression and Combativeness.   These behaviors include hitting, pinching, grabbing, biting, or swearing. They may result from agitation and restlessness. They frighten others.

Sometimes these behaviors are part of the individual's personality. Or pain, fatigue, too much stimulation, caregiver stress, and feeling lost or abandoned are causes. The behaviors can occur during care measures (bathing, dressing) that upset or frighten the person. See Chapter 17 for dealing with the angry person. See Chapter 4 for workplace violence. Also follow the person's care plan.

Screaming.   Persons with AD have communication problems. At first, it is hard to find the right words. As AD progresses, the person speaks in short sentences or in words. Often speech is not understandable.

The person screams to communicate. It is common in persons who are very confused and have poor communication skills. The person may scream a word or a name. Or the person just makes screaming sounds.

Possible causes include hearing and vision problems, pain or discomfort, fear, and fatigue. Too much or not enough stimulation is another cause. The person may react to a caregiver or family member by screaming.

Sometimes these measures are helpful:

- Providing a calm, quiet setting
- Playing soft music
- Having the person wear hearing aids and eyeglasses
- Having a family member or favorite caregiver comfort and calm the person
- Using touch to calm the person

Abnormal Sexual Behaviors.   Sexual behaviors are labeled abnormal because of how and when they occur. Persons with AD are not oriented to person, time, and place. Sexual behaviors may involve the wrong person, the wrong place, and the wrong time. They also cannot control behavior. Healthy persons do not undress or expose themselves in front of others. They do not masturbate or engage in sexual pleasures in public. They know their sexual partners. Persons with AD often mistake someone else for a sexual partner. The person kisses and hugs the other person.

Some behaviors are not sexual. Touching, scratching, and rubbing the genitals can signal infection, pain, or discomfort in the urinary or reproductive systems. Poor hygiene is another cause. So is being wet or soiled from urine or feces.

The nurse encourages the person's sexual partner to show affection. Their normal practices are encouraged. Examples include hand holding, hugging, kissing, and touching. When a person masturbates in public, lead the person to his or her room. Provide for privacy and safety. Good hygiene prevents itching. Clean the person quickly and thoroughly after elimination. Do not let the person stay wet or soiled.

The RN assesses the person for urinary or reproductive system problems. The doctor is contacted as necessary.

Repetitive Behaviors.   *Repetitive* means to repeat over and over again. Persons with AD repeat the same motions over and over again. For example, the person folds the same napkin over and over. Or the person says the same words over and over. Or the same question is asked. Such behaviors do not harm the person. However, they can annoy caregivers and the family.

Harmless acts are allowed. Music, picture books, exercise, and movies are distracting. Taking the person for a walk can help. Such measures also help when words or questions are repeated.

CARE OF THE PERSON WITH AD AND OTHER DEMENTIAS

Usually the person is cared for at home until symptoms are severe. Adult day care may help. Often nursing center care is required. Sometimes hospital care is needed for other illnesses. You may care for persons with AD or other dementias in any of these settings. The person and family need your support and understanding.

People with AD do not choose to be forgetful, incontinent, agitated, or rude. Nor do they choose to have other behaviors, signs, and symptoms of the disease. They cannot control what is happening to them. The disease causes the behaviors. *The disease is responsible, not the person.*

Currently AD has no cure. Symptoms worsen over many years. The rate varies from person to person. Over time, persons with AD depend on others for care. Safety, hygiene, nutrition and fluids, elimination, and activity needs must be met. So must comfort and sleep needs. The person's care plan will include many of the measures listed in Box 18-6.

BOX 18-6 Care of Persons With AD and Other Dementias

Environment

- Follow established routines.
- Avoid changing rooms or roommates.
- Place picture signs on rooms, bathrooms, dining rooms, and other areas (Fig. 18-2, p. 342).
- Keep personal items where the person can see them.
- Stay within the person's sight to the extent possible.
- Place memory aids (large clocks and calendars) where the person can see them.
- Keep noise levels low.
- Play music and show movies from the person's past.
- Select tasks and activities specific to the person's cognitive abilities and interests.

Communication

- Approach the person in a calm, quiet manner.
- Approach the person from the front. Do not approach the person from the side or the back. This can startle the person.
- Call the person by name.
- Identify other people by their names. Avoid pronouns (he, she, them, and so on).
- Follow the rules of communication (Chapter 2).
- Practice measures to promote communication (Chapter 2).
- Use gestures or cues. Point to objects.
- Speak in a calm, gentle voice.
- Speak slowly. Use simple words and sentences.
- Let the person speak. Do not interrupt or rush the person.
- Give the person time to respond.
- Do not criticize, correct, or argue with the person.
- Present one idea, question, or instruction at a time.
- Ask simple questions having simple answers. Do not ask complex questions.
- Do not present the person with many choices.
- Provide simple explanations of all procedures and activities.
- Give consistent responses.

Safety

- Remove harmful, sharp, and breakable objects from the area. This includes knives, scissors, glass, dishes, razors, and tools.
- Provide plastic eating and drinking utensils. This helps prevent breakage and cuts.
- Place safety plugs in electrical outlets.
- Keep cords and electrical equipment out of reach.
- Remove electrical appliances from the bathroom. Examples include hair dryers, curling irons, make-up mirrors, and electric shavers.
- Store personal care items (shampoo, deodorant, lotion, and so on) in a safe place.
- Keep childproof caps on medicine containers and household cleaners.
- Store household cleaners and drugs in locked storage areas.
- Store dangerous equipment and tools in a safe place.
- Remove knobs from stoves, or place childproof covers on the knobs.
- Remove dangerous appliances and power tools from the home.
- Remove firearms from the home.
- Store car keys in a safe place.
- Supervise the person who smokes.
- Store cigarettes, cigars, pipes, matches, and other smoking materials in a safe place.
- Practice safety measures to prevent falls (Chapter 4).
- Practice safety measures to prevent fires (Chapter 4).
- Practice safety measures to prevent burns (Chapter 4).
- Practice safety measures to prevent poisoning (Chapter 4).
- Keep all doors to kitchens, utility rooms, and housekeeping closets locked.

BOX 18-6   Care of Persons With AD and Other Dementias—cont'd

Wandering

- Follow center policy for locking doors and windows. Locks are often placed at the top and bottom of doors (Fig. 18-3, p. 342). The person is not likely to look for a lock in such places.
- Keep door alarms and electronic doors turned on. The alarm goes off when the door is opened.
- Follow center policy for fire exits. Everyone must be able to leave the building if there is a fire.
- Make sure the person wears an ID bracelet or Safe Return ID at all times.
- Exercise the person as ordered. Adequate exercise often reduces wandering.
- Involve the person in activities—folding napkins, dusting a table, sorting socks, rolling yarn, sweeping, sanding blocks of wood, or watering plants.
- Do not use restraints. Restraints require a doctor's order. They also tend to increase confusion and disorientation.
- Do not argue with the person who wants to leave. The person does not understand what you are saying.
- Go with the person who insists on going outside. Make sure he or she is properly dressed. Guide the person inside after a few minutes (Fig. 18-4, p. 342).
- Let the person wander in enclosed areas. Many nursing centers have enclosed areas where residents can walk about (Fig. 18-5, p. 342). They provide a safe place for the person to wander.

Sundowning

- Complete treatments and activities early in the day.
- Provide a calm, quiet setting late in the day.
- Do not restrain the person.
- Encourage exercise and activity early in the day.
- Meet nutrition needs. Hunger can increase restlessness.
- Promote elimination. The need to eliminate can increase restlessness.
- Do not try to reason with the person. He or she cannot understand what you are saying.
- Do not ask the person to tell you what is bothering him or her. Communication is impaired. The person does not understand what you are asking. He or she cannot think or speak clearly.

Hallucinations and Delusions

- Make sure the person wears eyeglasses and hearing aids as needed. Follow the care plan.
- Do not argue with the person. He or she does not understand what you are saying.
- Reassure the person. Tell him or her that you will provide protection from harm.
- Distract the person with some item or activity. Taking the person for a walk may be helpful.
- Use touch to calm and reassure the person.
- Eliminate noises that the person could misinterpret. TV, radio, stereos, furnaces, air conditioners, and other things could affect the person.
- Check lighting. Make sure there are no glares, shadows, or reflections.
- Cover or remove mirrors. The person could misinterpret his or her reflection.

Sleep

- Follow bedtime rituals.
- Use night-lights so the person can see. They help prevent accidents and disorientation.
- Limit caffeine during the day.
- Discourage naps during the day.
- Encourage exercise during the day.
- Reduce noises.

Basic Needs

- Meet food and fluid needs (Chapter 14). Provide finger foods. Cut food and pour liquids as needed.
- Provide good skin care (Chapters 11 and 15). Keep the person's skin free of urine and feces.
- Promote urinary and bowel elimination (Chapter 13).
- Provide incontinence care as needed (Chapter 13).
- Promote exercise and activity during the day (Chapter 19). This helps reduce wandering and sundowning behaviors. The person may also sleep better.
- Reduce intake of coffee, tea, and cola drinks. These contain caffeine. Caffeine is a stimulant. It can increase restlessness, confusion, and agitation.
- Provide a quiet, restful setting. Soft music is better than loud TV programs.
- Play music during care activities such as bathing and during meals.
- Promote personal hygiene (Chapter 11). Do not force the person into a shower or tub. People with AD are often afraid of bathing. Try bathing the person when he or she is calm. Use the person's preferred bathing method (tub bath, shower, bed bath). Provide privacy, and keep the person warm. Do not rush the person.
- Provide oral hygiene (Chapter 11).
- Choose clothing that is comfortable and simple to put on. Front-opening garments are easy to put on. Pullover tops are harder to put on. And the person may become frightened when his or her head is inside the pullover top.
- Select clothing that closes with Velcro. Such items are easy to put on and take off. Buttons, zippers, snaps, and other closures can frustrate the person.
- Offer simple clothing choices (Fig. 18-6, p. 342). Let the person choose between two shirts or two blouses, two pants or two slacks, and so on.
- Lay clothing out in the order it will be put on. Hand the person one clothing item at a time. Tell or show the person what to do. Do not rush him or her.
- Have equipment ready for any procedure. This reduces the amount of time the person is involved in care measures.
- Observe for signs and symptoms of health problems (Chapter 9).
- Prevent infection (Chapter 3).

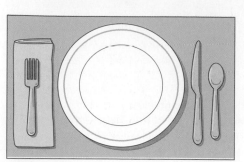

Fig. 18-2 Signs give cues to persons with dementia.

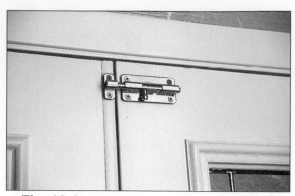

Fig. 18-3 A slide lock is at the top of the door.

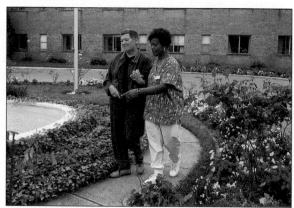

Fig. 18-4 Walk outside with the person who wanders. Then guide the person back inside after a few minutes.

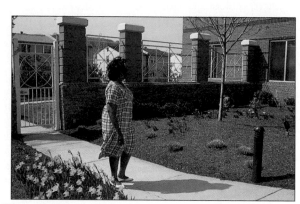

Fig. 18-5 An enclosed garden allows persons with AD to wander in a safe setting.

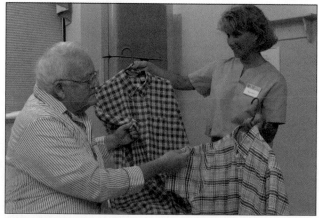

Fig. 18-6 The person with AD is offered simple clothing choices.

Comfort and safety are important. Good skin care and alignment prevent skin breakdown and contractures. You must take special care to treat these persons with dignity and respect. They have the same rights as persons who are alert and active. Talk to them in a calm voice. Always explain what you are going to do. Massage, soothing touch, music, and aroma therapy are comforting and relaxing. The person may need hospice care as death nears (Chapter 1).

The person can have other health problems and injuries. However, the person may not know there is pain, fever, constipation, incontinence, or other signs and symptoms. Carefully observe the person. Report any change in the person's usual behavior to the nurse.

Infection is a major risk. The person cannot fully tend to self-care. Infection can occur from poor hygiene. This includes poor skin care, oral hygiene, and perineal care after bowel and bladder elimination. Inactivity and immobility can cause pneumonia and pressure ulcers.

The person needs to feel useful, worthwhile, and active. This promotes self-esteem. Therapists work with one person, a small group, or a large group. Therapies and activities focus on the person's strengths and past successes. For example:

- A woman used to cook. She helps clean fruit.
- A man was a good dancer. Activities are planned so he can dance.
- A man likes to clean. He helps with dusting.

Supervised activities meet the person's needs and cognitive abilities. The person's interests are considered. Activities are based on what the person enjoys and can do. Some people like crafts, exercise, gardening, and listening and moving to music. Others like sing-alongs, reminiscing, and board games. Some like to string beads, fold towels, or roll dough. Massage, range-of-motion exercises, and touch are also important therapies.

The Family

The person may live at home or with a partner, children, or other family members. The family gives care. Or someone stays with the person. Health care is sought when the family cannot deal with the situation or meet the person's needs. Home health care may help for a while. Adult day care is an option. Long-term care is needed when:

- The person cannot meet his or her own needs
- Family members cannot meet the person's needs
- The person no longer knows the caregiver
- Family members have health problems
- Money problems occur
- The person's behaviors present dangers to self or others

Diagnostic tests, doctor's visits, drugs, and home care are costly. So is long-term care. The person's medical care can drain family finances.

The family has special needs. Caring for the person at home or in a nursing center is stressful. There are physical, emotional, social, and financial stresses. Adult children are in the *sandwich generation.* They are caught between their own children who need attention and an ill parent who needs care. Caring for two families is stressful. Often adult children have jobs too.

Caregivers can suffer from anger, anxiety, depression, and sleeplessness. Some cannot concentrate or are irritable. They can develop health problems. They need to take care of their own health. A healthy diet, exercise, and plenty of rest are needed. Asking for help is important. The caregiver needs to feel free to ask family and friends for help.

Caregivers need much support and encouragement. Many join AD support groups. The groups are sponsored by hospitals, nursing centers, and the Alzheimer's Association. The Alzheimer's Association has chapters in cities and towns across the country. Support groups offer encouragement and advice. People in similar situations share their feelings, anger, frustration, guilt, and other emotions. They also share coping and caregiving ideas.

The family often feels helpless. No matter what is done, the person only gets worse. Much time, money, energy, and emotion are needed to care for the person. Anger and resentment may result. Guilt feelings are common. The family also knows that the person did not choose the disease. They know that the person does not choose to have its signs, symptoms, and behaviors. Sometimes behaviors are embarrassing. The family may be upset and angry that the loved one cannot show love or affection.

The family is an important part of the health team. They help plan the person's care whenever possible. They need to learn how to bathe, feed, dress, and give oral hygiene to the person. They also need to learn how to provide a safe setting. The nurse and support group will help the family learn to give necessary care.

Special Care Units

Many nursing centers have special care units for persons with AD and other dementias. Some units are secured. This means that entrances and exits are locked. Persons in these units have a safe setting to move about it. They cannot wander away. Some persons have aggressive behaviors that disrupt or threaten others. They may need a secured unit.

At some point, the secured unit is no longer needed for safe care. For example, the person's condition progresses from stage 2 to stage 3. The person cannot sit or walk. Wandering is not a concern. The person is transferred to another unit.

Quality of Life

Quality of life is important for all persons with confusion and dementia. Nursing center residents have rights under OBRA. They may not know or be able to exercise their rights. However, the family knows the person's rights. They want those rights protected. They want respect and dignity for the loved one.

The person has the right to privacy and confidentiality. Protect the person from exposure. Only those involved in the person's care are present for care and procedures. The person is allowed to visit in private. Space is provided for a private visit. Protect confidentiality. Do not share information about the person's care and condition with others.

Personal choice is important. If the person is able, encourage simple choices. For example, a person chooses to wear a dress or slacks. Watching or not watching TV may be a simple choice. The family makes choices if the person cannot. They choose bath times, menus, clothing, activities, and other care.

The person has the right to keep and use personal items. Some items provide comfort. A pillow, blanket, afghan, or sweater may have meaning to the person. The person may not know why or even recognize the item. Still, it is important. Keep personal items safe. Protect the person's property from loss or damage.

These persons must be kept free from abuse, mistreatment, and neglect. Caring for persons with confusion and dementia is often very frustrating. Some behaviors are hard to deal with. Family and staff can become short-tempered and angry. Protect the person from abuse (Chapter 1). Report any signs of abuse to the nurse at once. Be patient and calm when caring for these persons. Talk with the nurse if you are becoming upset. Sometimes an assignment change is needed for a while.

All persons have the right to be free from restraints (Chapter 20). Restraints require a doctor's order. They are used only if it is the best way to protect the person. They are not used for staff convenience. Restraints can make confusion and demented behaviors worse. The nurse tells you when to use restraints.

Activity and a safe setting promote quality of life (see Box 18-6). Safe, calm, and quiet activities are needed. The recreational therapist and other health team members will find activities that are best for each person. These are part of the person's care plan.

Validation Therapy

Validation therapy may be part of the person's care plan. The therapy is based on these principles:

- All behavior has meaning.
- Development occurs in a sequence, order, and pattern. Certain tasks must be completed during a stage of development. A stage cannot be skipped. Each stage is the basis for the next stage.
- If a person does not successfully complete a stage of development, unresolved issues and emotions may surface later in life.
- A person may return to the past to resolve such issues and emotions.
- Caregivers need to listen and provide empathy.
- Attempts are not made to correct the person's thoughts or bring the person back to reality. For example:
  —While going from room to room, Mrs. Bell calls for her babies. In reality, her babies died shortly after birth. The caregiver does not tell Mrs. Bell that her babies died after they were born. Instead, the caregiver says: "Tell me about your babies."
  —Mrs. Brown sits all day on a bench by the window. She says that she is at the train station waiting to meet her husband. In reality, her husband was killed during World War II. Buried in England, he never returned home. The caregiver does not remind Mrs. Brown of what happened. Instead, the caregiver encourages Mrs. Brown to talk about her husband.
  —Mr. Garcia was 3 years old when his father died. He holds a ball constantly. He is very upset when anyone tries to remove it from his hand. He calls for his father and repeats "play ball, play ball." The caregiver does not remind Mr. Garcia that he is 80 years old and that his father died many years ago. Instead, the caregiver says "Tell me about playing ball."

The health team decides if validation therapy might help a person. If so, it will be part of the person's care plan. Proper use of validation therapy requires special training. If the therapy is used in your center, you will receive the training needed to use it correctly.

Review Questions

Circle the **BEST** answer.

1. Cognitive function relates to the following *except*
   a. Memory loss and personality
   b. Thinking and reasoning
   c. Ability to understand
   d. Judgment and behavior

2. A person is confused after surgery. The confusion is likely to be
   a. Permanent
   b. Temporary
   c. Caused by an infection
   d. Caused by brain injury

3. The confused person is
   a. Restrained in bed at night
   b. Given many tasks to keep busy
   c. Easily distracted
   d. Never a danger to self or others

4. Joe Dunn has delusions. A delusion is
   a. A false belief
   b. An illness caused by changes in the brain
   c. Seeing, hearing, or feeling something that is not real
   d. Alzheimer's disease

5. Joe Dunn has AD. Which is *true?*
   a. AD occurs only in older persons.
   b. Diet and drugs can cure the disease.
   c. AD and delirium are the same.
   d. AD ends in death.

6. The following are common in persons with AD *except*
   a. Memory loss, poor judgment, and sleep disturbances
   b. Loss of impulse control and the ability to communicate
   c. Wandering, delusions, and hallucinations
   d. Paralysis, dyspnea, and pain

7. Sundowning means that
   a. The person becomes sleepy when the sun sets
   b. Behaviors become worse in the late afternoon and evening hours
   c. Behavior improves at night
   d. The person is in the third stage of the disease

8. Joe Dunn is screaming. You know that this is
   a. An agitated reaction
   b. His way of communicating
   c. Caused by a delusion
   d. A repetitive behavior

9. AD support groups do the following *except*
   a. Provide care
   b. Offer encouragement and care ideas
   c. Provide support for the family
   d. Promote the sharing of feelings and frustrations

10. Joe Dunn tends to wander. You should do the following *except*
    a. Make sure door alarms are turned on
    b. Make sure he wears an ID bracelet
    c. Help him with exercise as ordered
    d. Tell him where to wander safely

11. Safety is important for Joe Dunn. Which is *false?*
    a. Safety plugs are placed in electrical outlets.
    b. Cleaners and drugs are kept locked up.
    c. He can keep smoking materials.
    d. Sharp and breakable objects are removed from his environment.

12. You are caring for Joe Dunn. Which is *false?*
    a. You can reason with him.
    b. Touch can calm and reassure him.
    c. A calm, quiet setting is important.
    d. Help is needed with ADL.

Answers to these questions are on p. 390.

CHAPTER 19

Basic Restorative Care

Objectives

- Define the key terms listed in this chapter
- Describe how aging and common health problems affect the nervous system
- Describe how rehabilitation and restorative care involve the whole person
- Identify the complications to prevent
- Describe the physical, psychological, and social aspects of rehabilitation and restorative care
- Describe common self-help and positioning devices
- Explain the rules for performing range-of-motion exercises
- Describe four walking aids
- Explain your role in rehabilitation and restorative care
- Explain how to promote quality of life
- Perform the procedures described in this chapter

Key Terms

abduction Moving a body part away from the midline of the body

activities of daily living (ADL) The activities usually done during a normal day in a person's life

adduction Moving a body part toward the midline of the body

ambulation The act of walking

atrophy The decrease in size or a wasting away of tissue

contracture The lack of joint mobility caused by abnormal shortening of a muscle

disability Any lost, absent, or impaired physical or mental function

dorsiflexion Bending the toes and foot up at the ankle

extension Straightening a body part

external rotation Turning the joint outward

flexion Bending a body part

footdrop The foot falls down at the ankle; permanent plantar flexion

hyperextension Excessive straightening of a body part

internal rotation Turning the joint inward

plantar flexion The foot *(plantar)* is bent *(flexion)*; bending the foot down at the ankle

pronation Turning the joint downward

prosthesis An artificial replacement for a missing body part

range of motion (ROM) The movement of a joint to the extent possible without causing pain

rehabilitation The process of restoring the person to the highest possible level of physical, psychological, social, and economic function

restorative aide A nursing assistant with special training in restorative nursing and rehabilitation skills

restorative nursing care Care that helps persons regain their health, strength, and independence

rotation Turning the joint

supination Turning the joint upward

Disease, injury, surgery, and aging can affect body function. Often more than one function is lost. A **disability** is any lost, absent, or impaired physical or mental function. Losses are temporary or permanent. Eating, bathing, dressing, and walking are hard or seem impossible. Disabilities are short-term or long-term. The person may depend totally or in part on others for basic needs. The degree of disability affects how much function is possible. Nervous system problems are common causes of disabilities (Box 19-1, p. 348).

REHABILITATION AND RESTORATIVE NURSING CARE

Rehabilitation is the process of restoring the person to the highest possible level of physical, psychological, social, and economic function. The focus is on improving abilities. Sometimes improved function is not possible. Then the goal is to prevent further loss of function. This helps the person maintain the best possible quality of life.

Some persons are weak. Many cannot perform daily activities. **Restorative nursing care** is care that helps persons regain their health, strength, and independence. Some people have more progressive illnesses. They become more and more disabled. Rehabilitation and restorative nursing programs do the following:

* Help maintain the highest level of function
* Prevent unnecessary decline in function

A disability has physical, psychological, and social effects. The person with a disability needs to adjust physically, psychologically, socially, and economically. Abilities—what the person can do—are stressed. Complications are prevented. They can lead to further disability.

Restorative nursing care and rehabilitation focus on the whole person. The process starts when the person first seeks health care. The goals are to regain health, strength, and independence. This may involve measures and assistive devices that promote:

* Self-care—hygiene, grooming, eating
* Elimination—urinary and bowel
* Positioning
* Pressure ulcer prevention
* Mobility—exercise and ambulation (p. 355)
* Communication
* Cognitive function

Text continued on p. 352

BOX 19-1   The Nervous System

Structure and Function

The nervous system controls, directs, and coordinates body functions. Its two main divisions are:

- The *central nervous system* (CNS). It consists of the *brain* and *spinal cord* (Fig. 19-1, p. 350).
- The *peripheral nervous system*. It involves the *nerves* throughout the body (Fig. 19-2, p. 350).

Nerves carry messages or impulses to and from the brain. Nerves connect to the spinal cord. They are easily damaged and take a long time to heal. Some nerve fibers have a protective covering called a *myelin sheath.* The myelin sheath also insulates the nerve fiber. Nerve fibers covered with myelin conduct impulses faster than those fibers without it.

The Central Nervous System

The brain is covered by the skull. The cerebrum is the largest part of the brain. It is the center of thought and intelligence. The cerebrum is divided into two halves called the right and left *hemispheres.* The right hemisphere controls movement and activities on the body's left side. The left hemisphere controls the right side.

The outside of the cerebrum is called the *cerebral cortex* (Fig. 19-3, p. 350). It controls reasoning, memory, consciousness, speech, voluntary muscle movement, vision, hearing, sensation, and other activities.

The cerebellum regulates and coordinates body movements. It controls balance and the smooth movements of voluntary muscles. Injury to the cerebellum results in jerky movements, loss of coordination, and muscle weakness.

The brainstem connects the cerebrum to the spinal cord. The brainstem contains the *midbrain, pons,* and *medulla.* The midbrain and pons relay messages between the medulla and the cerebrum. The medulla controls heart rate, breathing, blood vessel size, swallowing, coughing, and vomiting. The brain connects to the spinal cord at the lower end of the medulla.

The spinal cord lies within the spinal column. The cord is about 18 inches long. It contains pathways that conduct messages to and from the brain.

The brain and spinal cord are covered and protected by three layers of connective tissue called *meninges.* The space between the middle and inner layers is filled with *cerebrospinal fluid.* Cerebrospinal fluid cushions shocks that could injure brain and spinal cord structures.

The Peripheral Nervous System

The peripheral nervous system has *cranial nerves* and *spinal nerves.* Cranial nerves conduct impulses between the brain and the head, neck, chest, and abdomen. They conduct impulses for smell, vision, hearing, pain, touch, temperature, and pressure. They also conduct impulses for voluntary and involuntary muscles. Spinal nerves carry impulses from the skin, extremities, and the internal structures not supplied by cranial nerves.

Changes With Aging

Nerve cells are lost. Nerve conduction and reflexes slow. Responses are slower. For example, an older person slips. The message telling the brain of the slip travels slowly. The message from the brain to prevent the fall also travels slowly. The person falls.

Blood flow to the brain is reduced. Dizziness may occur. It increases the risk for falls. Practice measures to prevent falls (Chapter 4). Remind the person to get up slowly from the bed or chair. This helps prevent dizziness.

Brain cells are lost over time. This affects personality and mental function. So does reduced blood flow to the brain. Memory is shorter. Forgetfulness increases. Responses slow. Confusion, dizziness, and fatigue may occur. Older people often remember events from long ago better than recent events. Many older people are mentally active and involved in current events. They show fewer personality and mental changes. (See Chapter 18 for confusion and dementia.)

Common Disorders

Nervous system disorders can affect mental and physical functions. They can affect the ability to speak, understand, feel, see, hear, touch, think, control bowels and bladder, or move.

- *Stroke*—is a disease affecting the blood vessels that supply blood to the brain. It also is called a *cerebrovascular accident (CVA).* Blood flow in the brain is affected. Brain cells in the area affected do not get oxygen and nutrients. Brain cells die. Brain damage occurs. Functions controlled by that part of the brain are lost or impaired. If the person survives, some brain damage is likely. Functions lost depend on the area of brain damage (Fig. 19-4, p. 351). The effects of a stroke include:
  - —Loss of face, hand, arm, leg, or body control
  - —Hemiplegia (paralysis on one side of the body)
  - —Changing emotions—crying easily or mood swings, sometimes for no reason
  - —Difficulty swallowing (Chapter 14)
  - —Dimmed vision
  - —Aphasia (Chapter 2)
  - —Slow or slurred speech
  - —Changes in sight, touch, movement, and thought
  - —Impaired memory
  - —Urinary frequency, urgency, or incontinence
  - —Depression
  - —Frustration
- *Parkinson's disease*—is a slow, progressive disorder with no cure. Degeneration of a part of the brain occurs. Signs and symptoms become worse over time (Fig. 19-5, p. 351). Swallowing and chewing problems, constipation, and bladder problems also develop. So do sleep problems, depression, memory

BOX 19-1   The Nervous System—cont'd

loss, slow thinking, and emotional changes (fear and insecurity). Speech changes occur. They include slurred, monotone, and soft speech. Some people talk too fast or repeat what they say.

- *Multiple sclerosis (MS)*—is a chronic disease. *Multiple* means many. *Sclerosis* means hardening or scarring. The myelin (which covers nerve fibers) in the brain and spinal cord is destroyed. Nerve impulses are not sent to and from the brain in a normal manner. Functions are impaired or lost. There is no cure. Symptoms usually start between the ages of 20 and 40. Women are affected more often than men. Symptoms depend on the damaged area. Vision problems may occur. Muscle weakness and balance problems affect standing and walking. Paralysis can occur. Tremors, numbness and tingling, loss of feeling, speech problems, dizziness, and poor coordination are common. Problems with concentration, attention, memory, judgment, and behavior may occur. Fatigue increases such problems. Bowel, bladder, and sexual function problems occur. Respiratory muscle weakness is common. So are anger and depression.

- *Head injuries*—can involve the scalp, skull, and brain tissue. Some injuries are minor. They cause temporary loss of consciousness. Others are more serious. Brain tissue is bruised or torn. Bleeding can occur in the brain or nearby structures. Permanent brain damage or death may result. Causes include falls, vehicle crashes, and sports injuries. Often there are other injuries. Spinal cord injuries are likely. If the person survives, some permanent damage is likely. Paralysis, mental retardation, and personality changes may be permanent. The same is true for speech, breathing, bowel, and bladder problems.

- *Spinal cord injuries*—can permanently damage the nervous system. Common causes are stab or bullet wounds, vehicle crashes, falls, and sports injuries. Problems depend on the level of injury. The higher the level of injury, the more functions lost (Fig. 19-6, p. 351). With lumbar injuries, leg function is lost. Injuries at the thoracic level cause loss of muscle function below the chest. Injuries at the lumbar or thoracic levels cause paraplegia. Cervical injuries cause quadriplegia—loss of function to the arms, chest, and below the chest.

- *Developmental disabilities*—are disabilities that occur before 22 years of age. Causes can occur before, during, or after birth. The disability is severe and permanent. Function is limited in three or more life skills: self-care, understanding and expressing language, learning, mobility, self-direction, capacity for independent living, and the ability to support oneself financially. Developmentally disabled children become adults. They need life-long assistance, support, and special services. These conditions are common:
    —*Mental retardation*—involves low intellectual function (learning, thinking, and reasoning). Adaptive behavior is impaired. (*Adapt* means to change or adjust.) Mental retardation ranges from mild to severe.
    —*Down syndrome (DS)*—is caused by an extra 21st chromosome. It occurs at fertilization. Normally each sex cell (male and female) has 23 chromosomes. When they unite, the cell has 46 chromosomes. In DS, there are 47 chromosomes. DS causes some level of mental retardation. Many children have heart defects and vision and hearing problems. They need speech, language, physical, and occupational therapies. Most learn self-care skills.
    —*Cerebral palsy (CP)*—is a term applied to a group of disorders involving muscle weakness or poor muscle control *(palsy)*. The defect is in the motor region of the brain *(cerebral)*. Abnormal movements, posture, and coordination result. The defect results from brain damage. It occurs before, during, or within a few months after birth. Lack of oxygen to the brain is the usual cause. Congenital brain defects (faulty brain development) are other causes. Brain damage in infancy and early childhood also can result in CP. There is no cure. Body movements and body parts are affected. The person with CP can have many other impairments. They include:
- Mental retardation
- Learning disabilities
- Hearing, speech, and vision impairments
- Bladder and bowel control problems
- Seizures
- Difficulty swallowing
- Attention deficit hyperactivity disorder (short attention span, poor concentration, and increased activity)

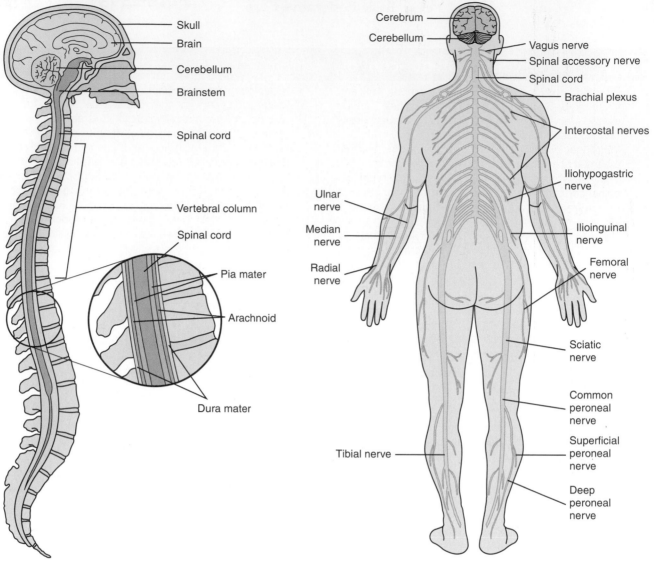

Fig. 19-1 Central nervous system.

Fig. 19-2 Peripheral nervous system.

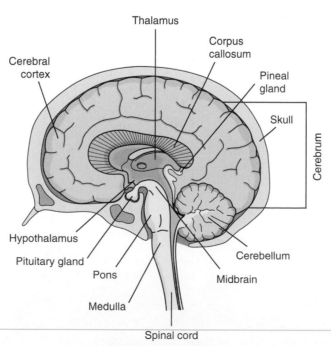

Fig. 19-3 The brain.

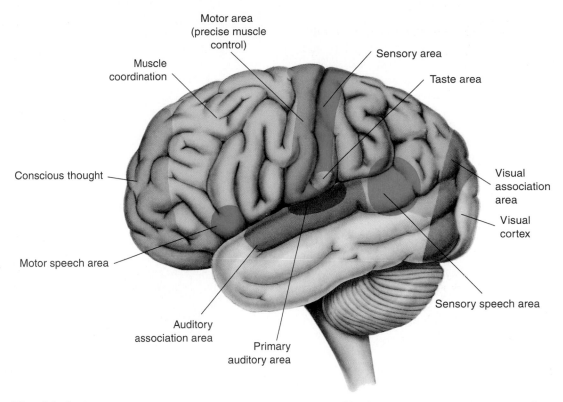

Motor area (precise muscle control)

Muscle coordination

Sensory area

Taste area

Conscious thought

Visual association area

Visual cortex

Motor speech area

Sensory speech area

Auditory association area

Primary auditory area

Fig. 19-4 Functions lost from a stroke depend on the area of brain damage. (From Thibodeau GA, Patton KT: *The human body in health & disease,* ed 3, St Louis, 2002, Mosby.)

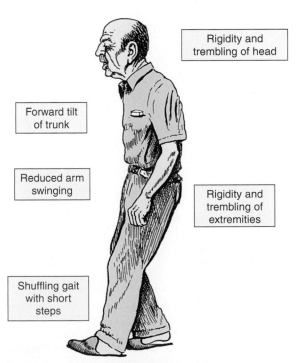

Rigidity and trembling of head

Forward tilt of trunk

Reduced arm swinging

Rigidity and trembling of extremities

Shuffling gait with short steps

Fig. 19-5 Signs of Parkinson's disease. (From Thibodeau GA, Patton KT: *The human body in health & disease,* ed 3, St Louis, 2002, Mosby.)

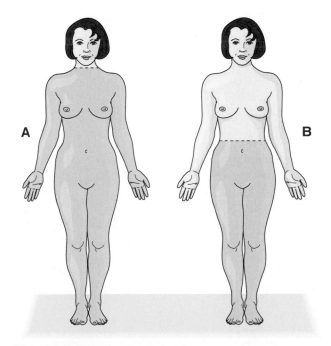

A

B

Fig. 19-6 The *shaded areas* show the areas of paralysis. **A,** Quadriplegia. **B,** Paraplegia.

Restorative Aides

Some centers have restorative aides. A **restorative aide** is a nursing assistant with special training in restorative nursing and rehabilitation skills. These aides assist the nursing and health teams as needed.

Usually nursing assistants are promoted to restorative aide positions. Those chosen have excellent work ethics, job performance, and skills. Required training varies among states. If there are no state requirements, the center provides any needed training.

PHYSICAL ASPECTS

Complications must be prevented. They can occur from bedrest, prolonged illness, or recovery from surgery or injury. Bowel and bladder problems are prevented. So are pressure ulcers.

Self-care is a major goal. **Activities of daily living (ADL)** are the activities usually done during a normal day in a person's life. ADL include bathing, oral hygiene, dressing, eating, elimination, and moving about. The health team evaluates the person's ability to perform ADL. They decide if self-help devices are needed.

Sometimes the hands, wrists, and arms are affected. Equipment is changed, made, or bought to meet the person's needs. Eating devices include glass holders, plate guards, and silverware with curved handles or cuffs (Chapter 14). Some persons cannot perform back-and-forth brushing motions for oral hygiene. Electric toothbrushes are helpful. Longer handles attach to combs, brushes, and sponges (Fig. 19-7). There are self-help devices for cooking, dressing, writing, phone calls, and other tasks (Fig. 19-8).

Some people need wheelchairs. If possible, they learn wheelchair transfers. Such transfers include to and from the bed, toilet, bathtub, sofa, and chair and in and out of cars (Fig. 19-9, p. 354).

A **prosthesis** is an artificial replacement for a missing body part. The person learns how to use an artificial arm or leg (Fig. 19-10, p. 354). The goal is for the prosthesis to be like the missing body part in function and appearance.

Difficulty swallowing (dysphagia) may occur after a stroke. The person may need a dysphagia diet (Chapter 14). When possible, exercises are taught to improve swallowing. Persons who cannot swallow need enteral nutrition (Chapter 14). Aphasia (difficulty speaking) may occur from a stroke (Chapter 2). Speech therapy and communication devices (Chapter 2) are helpful.

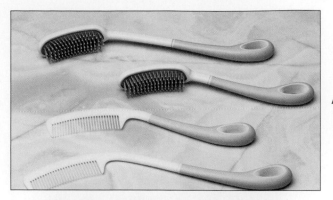

A

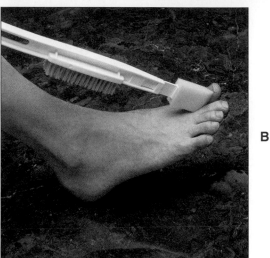

B

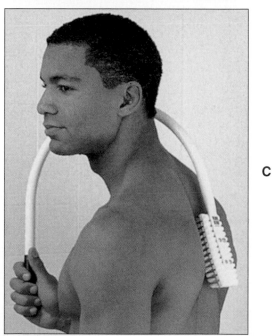

C

Fig. 19-7 A, Long-handled combs and brushes for hair care. **B,** Long-handled brush for bathing. **C,** Brush with a curved handle. (**A** and **B,** Courtesy Northcoast Medical, Inc., Morgan Hill, Calif.; **C,** Courtesy Sammons Preston: An AbilityOne Company, Bolingbrook, Ill.)

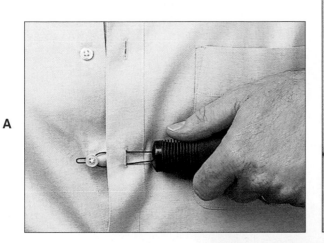

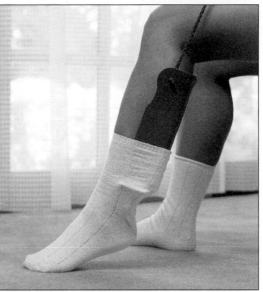

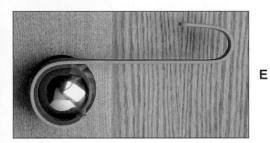

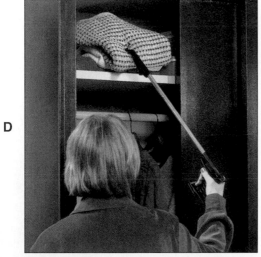

Fig. 19-8 A, A button hook is used to button and zip clothing. **B,** A sock assist is used to pull on socks and stockings. **C,** A shoe remover is used to take off shoes. **D,** Reachers are helpful to remove items from high shelves. **E,** A door knob turner increases leverage to help turn the knob. (**A, B, C,** and **E,** Courtesy Northcoast Medical, Inc., Morgan Hill, Calif.; **D,** Courtesy Sammons Preston, An AbilityOne Company, Bolingbrook, Ill.)

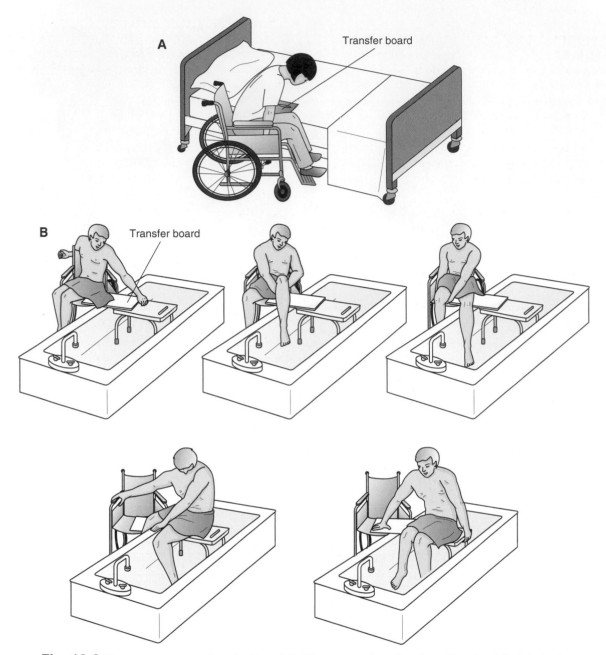

Fig. 19-9 The person uses a transfer board. **A,** The person transfers from the wheelchair to bed. **B,** The person transfers from the wheelchair to the bathtub.

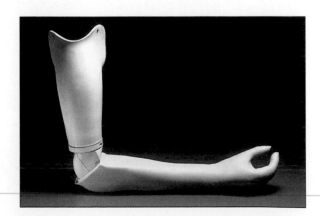

Fig. 19-10 Arm prosthesis. (Courtesy Motion Control, Subsidiary of Fillauer, Salt Lake City, Utah.)

Mobility

Illness, surgery, injury, pain, and aging cause weakness and some activity limits. Inactivity, whether mild or severe, affects every body system. It also affects mental well-being. Residents are encouraged to be as active as possible. The care plan includes the person's activity level and needed exercises.

Bedrest. Doctors order bedrest to reduce physical activity and pain, promote rest, increase strength, and promote healing. These types of bedrest are common:

- *Bedrest*—Some ADL are allowed. Self-feeding, oral hygiene, bathing, shaving, and hair care are often allowed.
- *Strict bedrest*—Everything is done for the person. No ADL are allowed. In some centers this is called *complete bedrest.*
- *Bedrest with commode privileges*—The person uses the commode for elimination.
- *Bedrest with bathroom privileges (bedrest with BRP)*—The person can use the bathroom for elimination.

Bedrest and lack of exercise and activity can cause serious complications. Every system is affected. Pressure ulcers, constipation, and fecal impaction can result. Urinary tract infections and renal calculi (kidney stones) can occur. So can thrombi (blood clots) and pneumonia (infection of the lung).

The musculoskeletal system is also affected. A **contracture** is the lack of joint mobility caused by abnormal shortening of a muscle. The contracted muscle is fixed into position, is deformed, and cannot stretch (Fig. 19-11). Common sites are the fingers, wrists, elbows, toes, ankles, knees, and hips. They can also occur in the neck and spine. The person is permanently deformed and disabled. **Atrophy** is the decrease in size or the wasting away of tissue. Tissues shrink in size. Muscle atrophy is a decrease in size or a wasting away of muscle (Fig. 19-12). These complications must be prevented for normal movement.

Good nursing care prevents complications from bedrest. Good alignment, range-of-motion exercises, and frequent position changes are needed. These are part of the care plan.

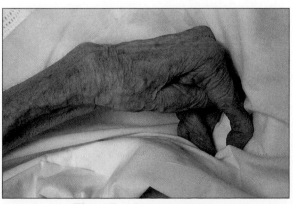

Fig. 19-11 A contracture.

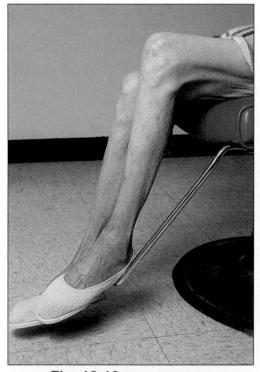

Fig. 19-12 Muscle atrophy.

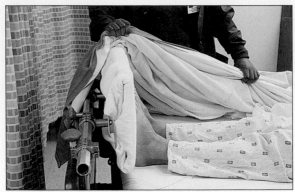

Fig. 19-13 A footboard. Feet are flush with the board to keep them in normal alignment.

Positioning.   Positioning is discussed in Chapter 16. These devices are often used to support and maintain the person in a certain position:

- *Footboards*—are placed at the foot of mattresses (Fig. 19-13). They prevent plantar flexion that can lead to footdrop. In **plantar flexion** the foot *(plantar)* is bent *(flexion)*. **Footdrop** is when the foot falls down at the ankle (permanent plantar flexion). The footboard is placed so the soles of the feet are flush against it. The feet are in good alignment as when standing. Footboards also serve as bed cradles. They prevent pressure ulcers by keeping the top linens off the feet and toes.
- *Trochanter rolls*—prevent the hips and legs from turning outward (external rotation) (Fig. 19-14). A bath blanket is folded to the desired length and rolled up. The loose end is placed under the person from the hip to the knee. Then the roll is tucked along the body.
- *Hip abduction wedges*—keep the hips abducted (Fig. 19-15). The wedge is placed between the person's legs. These are common after hip replacement surgery.
- *Hand rolls or hand grips*—prevent contractures of the thumb, fingers, and wrist (Fig. 19-16). Foam rubber sponges, rubber balls, and finger cushions also are used (Fig. 19-17).
- *Splints*—keep the elbows, wrists, thumbs, fingers, ankles, and knees in normal position. They are usually secured in place with Velcro. Some have foam padding (Fig. 19-18).
- *Bed cradles*—keep the weight of top linens off the feet and toes (Chapter 15). The weight of top linens can cause footdrop and pressure ulcers.

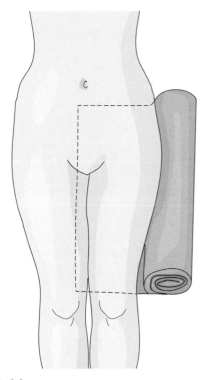

Fig. 19-14 A trochanter roll is made from a bath blanket. It extends from the hip to the knee.

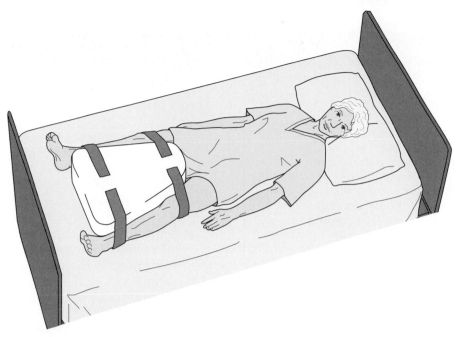

Fig. 19-15 Hip abduction wedge.

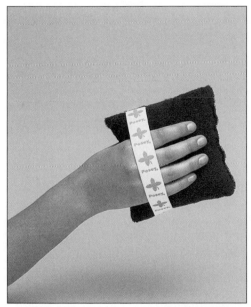

Fig. 19-16 Hand grip. (Courtesy J.T. Posey Co., Arcadia, Calif.)

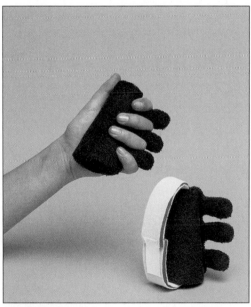

Fig. 19-17 Finger cushion. (Courtesy J.T. Posey Co., Arcadia, Calif.)

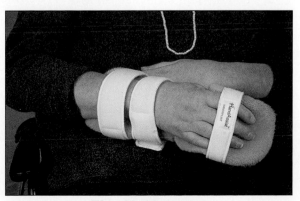

Fig. 19-18 A splint.

BOX 19-2   Joint Movements

Abduction—moving a body part away from the midline of the body

Adduction—moving a body part toward the midline of the body

Extension—straightening a body part

Flexion—bending a body part

Hyperextension—excessive straightening of a body part

Dorsiflexion—bending the toes and foot up at the ankle

Rotation—turning the joint

Internal rotation—turning the joint inward

External rotation—turning the joint outward

Plantar flexion—bending the foot down at the ankle

Pronation—turning the joint downward

Supination—turning the joint upward

Range-of-Motion Exercises. The movement of a joint to the extent possible without causing pain is the **range of motion (ROM)** of that joint. Range-of-motion exercises involve moving the joints through their complete range of motion (Box 19-2). They are usually done at least 2 times a day:

- *Active* range-of-motion exercises—The person does the exercise.
- *Passive* range-of-motion exercises—Someone moves the joints through their range of motion.
- *Active-assistive* range-of-motion exercises—The person does the exercises with help.

ADL involve joint movements. The doctor or nurse orders range-of-motion exercises for persons on bedrest. They also order them for persons who cannot walk, turn, or transfer themselves because of illness or injury.

Text continued on p. 364

Delegation Guidelines

Range-of-Motion Exercises

When delegated range-of-motion exercises, you need this information from the nurse and the care plan:

- The kind of range-of-motion exercises ordered—active, passive, active-assistive
- Which joints to exercise
- How often the exercises are done
- How many times to repeat each exercise
- What observations to report and record:
  —The time the exercises were performed
  —The joints exercised
  —The number of times the exercises were performed on each joint
  —Complaints of pain or signs of stiffness or spasm
  —The degree to which the person took part in the exercises

Safety Alert

Range-of-Motion Exercises

Range-of-motion exercises can cause injury if not done properly. Muscle strain, joint injury, and pain are possible. Practice the rules in Box 19-3 when performing or assisting with range-of-motion exercises.

Range-of-motion exercises to the neck can cause serious injury if not done properly. In some centers, nursing assistants must have special training before doing such exercises. Other centers do not let nursing assistants do them. Know your center's policy. Perform range-of-motion exercises to the neck only if allowed by your center and the RN instructs you to do so.

BOX 19-3   Performing Range-of-Motion Exercises

- Exercise only the joints the nurse tells you to exercise.
- Expose only the body part being exercised.
- Use good body mechanics.
- Support the part being exercised.
- Move the joint slowly, smoothly, and gently.
- Do not force a joint beyond its present range of motion or to the point of pain.
- *Perform range-of-motion exercises to the neck only if allowed by center policy.* In some centers, only physical or occupational therapists do neck exercises. This is because of the danger of neck injuries.

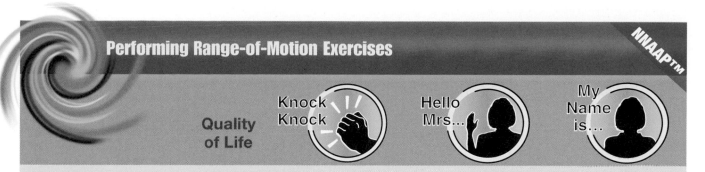

Performing Range-of-Motion Exercises

Quality of Life
- Knock Knock
- Hello Mrs...
- My Name is...

Pre-Procedure

1 Follow *Delegation Guidelines: Range-of-Motion Exercises*. See *Safety Alert: Range-of-Motion Exercises*.
2 Practice hand hygiene.
3 Identify the person. Check the ID bracelet against the assignment sheet. Call the person by name.
4 Explain the procedure to the person.
5 Obtain a bath blanket.
6 Provide for privacy.
7 Raise the bed for body mechanics. Bed rails are up if used.

Procedure

8 Lower the bed rail near you if up.
9 Position the person supine.
10 Cover the person with a bath blanket. Fanfold top linens to the foot of the bed.
11 Exercise the neck *if allowed by your center and if the RN instructs you to do so* (Fig. 19-19, p. 361):
  a Place your hands over the person's ears to support the head. Support the jaws with your fingers.
  b Flexion—bring the head forward. The chin touches the chest.
  c Extension—straighten the head.
  d Hyperextension—bring the head backward until the chin points up.
  e Rotation—turn the head from side to side.
  f Lateral flexion—move the head to the right and to the left.
  g Repeat flexion, extension, hyperextension, rotation, and lateral flexion 5 times—or the number of times stated on the care plan.
12 Exercise the shoulder (Fig. 19-20, p. 361):
  a Grasp the wrist with one hand. Grasp the elbow with the other hand.
  b Flexion—raise the arm straight in front and over the head.
  c Extension—bring the arm down to the side.
  d Hyperextension—move the arm behind the body. (Do this if the person sits in a straight-backed chair or is standing.)
  e Abduction—move the straight arm away from the side of the body.
  f Adduction—move the straight arm to the side of the body.
  g Internal rotation—bend the elbow. Place it at the same level as the shoulder. Move the forearm down toward the body.

  h External rotation—move the forearm toward the head.
  i Repeat flexion, extension, hyperextension, abduction, adduction, and internal and external rotation 5 times—or the number of times stated on the care plan.
13 Exercise the elbow (Fig. 19-21, p. 362):
  a Grasp the person's wrist with one hand. Grasp the elbow with your other hand.
  b Flexion—bend the arm so the same-side shoulder is touched.
  c Extension—straighten the arm.
  d Repeat flexion and extension 5 times—or the number of times stated on the care plan.
14 Exercise the forearm (Fig. 19-22, p. 362):
  a Pronation—turn the hand so the palm is down.
  b Supination—turn the hand so the palm is up.
  c Repeat pronation and supination 5 times—or the number of times stated on the care plan.
15 Exercise the wrist (Fig. 19-23, p. 362):
  a Hold the wrist with both of your hands.
  b Flexion—bend the hand down.
  c Extension—straighten the hand.
  d Hyperextension—bend the hand back.
  e Radial flexion—turn the hand toward the thumb.
  f Ulnar flexion—turn the hand toward the little finger.
  g Repeat flexion, extension, hyperextension, and radial and ulnar flexion 5 times—or the number of times stated on the care plan.

Continued

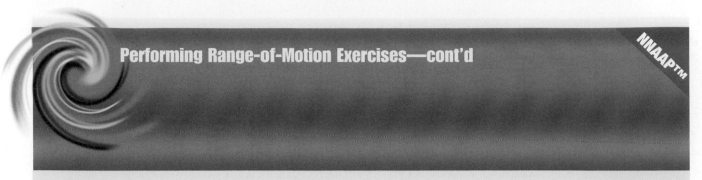

Performing Range-of-Motion Exercises—cont'd

Procedure—cont'd

16   Exercise the thumb (Fig. 19-24, p. 362):
    a   Hold the person's hand with one hand. Hold the thumb with your other hand.
    b   Abduction—move the thumb out from the inner part of the index finger.
    c   Adduction—move the thumb back next to the index finger.
    d   Opposition—touch each fingertip with the thumb.
    e   Flexion—bend the thumb into the hand.
    f   Extension—move the thumb out to the side of the fingers.
    g   Repeat abduction, adduction, opposition, flexion, and extension 5 times—or the number of times stated on the care plan.

17   Exercise the fingers (Fig. 19-25, p. 362):
    a   Abduction—spread the fingers and the thumb apart.
    b   Adduction—bring the fingers and thumb together.
    c   Extension—straighten the fingers so the fingers, hand, and arm are straight.
    d   Flexion—make a fist.
    e   Repeat abduction, adduction, extension, and flexion 5 times—or the number of times stated on the care plan.

18   Exercise the hip (Fig. 19-26, p. 362):
    a   Support the leg. Place one hand under the knee. Place your other hand under the ankle.
    b   Flexion—raise the leg.
    c   Extension—straighten the leg.
    d   Abduction—move the leg away from the body.
    e   Adduction—move the leg toward the other leg.
    f   Internal rotation—turn the leg inward.
    g   External rotation—turn the leg outward.
    h   Repeat flexion, extension, abduction, adduction, and internal and external rotation 5 times—or the number of times stated on the care plan.

19   Exercise the knee (Fig. 19-27, p. 363):
    a   Support the knee. Place one hand under the knee. Place your other hand under the ankle.
    b   Flexion—bend the leg.
    c   Extension—straighten the leg.
    d   Repeat flexion and extension of the knee 5 times—or the number of times stated on the care plan.

20   Exercise the ankle (Fig. 19-28, p. 363):
    a   Support the foot and ankle. Place one hand under the foot. Place your other hand under the ankle.
    b   Dorsiflexion—pull the foot forward. Push down on the heel at the same time.
    c   Plantar flexion—turn the foot down. Or point the toes.
    d   Repeat dorsiflexion and plantar flexion 5 times—or the number of times stated on the care plan.

21   Exercise the foot (Fig. 19-29, p. 363):
    a   Continue to support the foot and ankle.
    b   Pronation—turn the outside of the foot up and the inside down.
    c   Supination—turn the inside of the foot up and the outside down.
    d   Repeat pronation and supination 5 times—or the number of times stated on the care plan.

22   Exercise the toes (Fig. 19-30, p. 363):
    a   Flexion—curl the toes.
    b   Extension—straighten the toes.
    c   Abduction—spread the toes apart.
    d   Adduction—pull the toes together.
    e   Repeat flexion, extension, abduction, and adduction 5 times—or the number of times stated on the care plan.

23   Cover the leg. Raise the bed rail if used.

24   Go to the other side. Lower the bed rail near you if up.

25   Repeat steps 12 through 23.

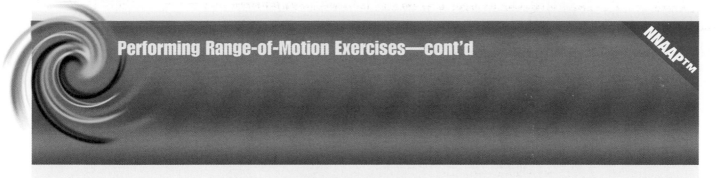

Performing Range-of-Motion Exercises—cont'd

NNAAP™

Post-Procedure

26 Provide for comfort.

27 Cover the person. Remove the bath blanket.

28 Raise or lower bed rails. Follow the care plan.

29 Lower the bed to its lowest level.

30 Place the signal light within reach.

31 Unscreen the person.

32 Return the bath blanket to its proper place.

33 Complete a safety check of the room. (See inside of front book cover.)

34 Decontaminate your hands.

35 Report and record your observations.

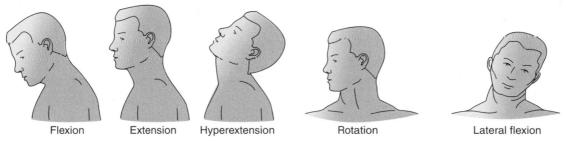

Flexion   Extension   Hyperextension   Rotation   Lateral flexion

Fig. 19-19 Range-of-motion exercises for the neck.

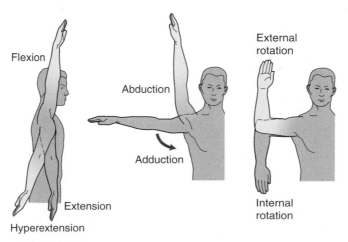

Flexion

Abduction

External rotation

Adduction

Extension

Hyperextension

Internal rotation

Fig. 19-20 Range-of-motion exercises for the shoulder.

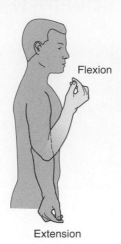

Flexion

Extension

Fig. 19-21 Range-of-motion exercises for the elbow.

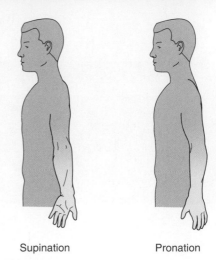

Supination   Pronation

Fig. 19-22 Range-of-motion exercises for the forearm.

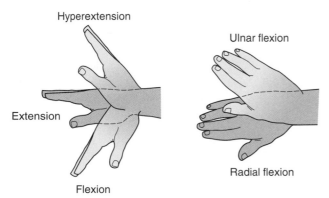

Hyperextension

Ulnar flexion

Extension

Flexion

Radial flexion

Fig. 19-23 Range-of-motion exercises for the wrist.

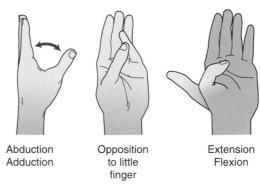

Abduction   Opposition   Extension
Adduction   to little   Flexion
                finger

Fig. 19-24 Range-of-motion exercises for the thumb.

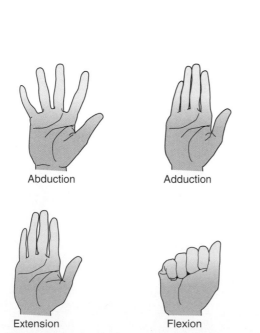

Abduction   Adduction

Extension   Flexion

Fig. 19-25 Range-of-motion exercises for the fingers.

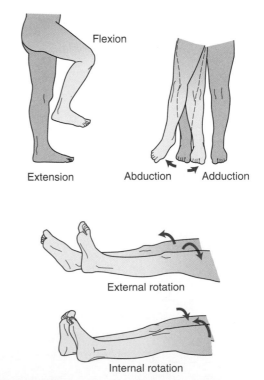

Flexion

Extension   Abduction   Adduction

External rotation

Internal rotation

Fig. 19-26 Range-of-motion exercises for the hip.

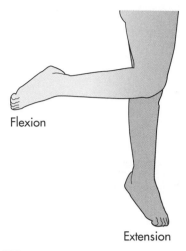

Flexion

Extension

Fig. 19-27 Range-of-motion exercises for the knee.

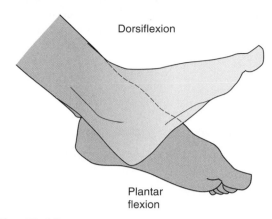

Dorsiflexion

Plantar
flexion

Fig. 19-28 Range-of-motion exercises for the ankle.

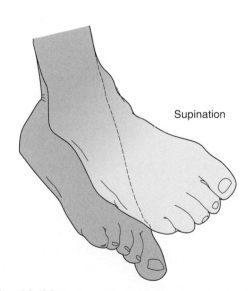

Supination

Fig. 19-29 Range-of-motion exercises for the foot.

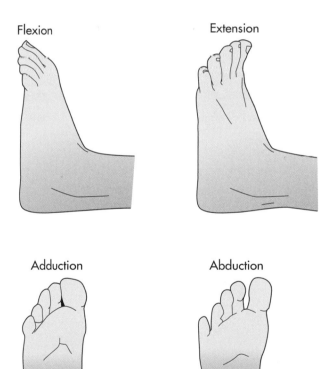

Flexion

Extension

Adduction

Abduction

Fig. 19-30 Range-of-motion exercises for the toes.

Ambulation.   After bedrest, activity increases slowly and in steps. First the person dangles (sits on the side of the bed). Sitting in a bedside chair follows. Next the person walks in the room and then in the hallway. **Ambulation,** the act of walking, is not a problem if contractures and muscle atrophy were prevented.

Delegation Guidelines

Ambulation

Before helping with ambulation, you need this information from the nurse and the care plan:

- How much help the person needs
- If the person uses a cane, walker, crutches, or a brace
- Areas of weakness—right arm or leg, left arm or leg
- How far to walk the person
- What observations to report and record:
    —How well the person tolerated the activity
    —Complaints of pain or discomfort
    —The distance walked

Safety Alert

Ambulation

Practice the safety measures to prevent falls (Chapter 4). Use a gait belt (transfer belt) when helping a person with ambulation. Also use it to help the person stand.

If a person starts to fall, do not try to prevent the fall. Ease the person to the floor. See Chapter 4.

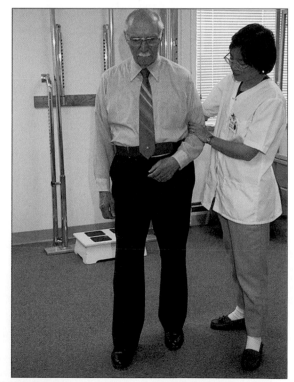

Fig. 19-31 Assist with ambulation by walking to the side and slightly behind the person. Use a gait belt for the person's safety.

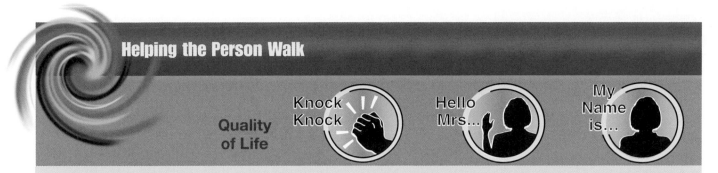

Helping the Person Walk

Pre-Procedure

1 Follow *Delegation Guidelines: Ambulation.* See *Safety Alert: Ambulation.*
2 Explain the procedure to the person.
3 Practice hand hygiene.
4 Collect the following:
- Robe and nonskid shoes
- Paper or sheet to protect bottom linens
- Gait (transfer) belt

5 Identify the person. Check the ID bracelet against the assignment sheet. Call the person by name.
6 Provide for privacy.

Procedure

7 Lower the bed to its lowest position. Lock the bed wheels. Lower the bed rail if up.
8 Fanfold top linens to the foot of the bed.
9 Place the paper or sheet under the person's feet. Put the shoes on the person.
10 Help the person to dangle. (See procedure: *Helping the Person Sit on the Side of the Bed (Dangle),* p. 307.)
11 Help the person put on the robe.
12 Apply the gait belt. (See procedure: *Applying a Transfer Belt,* p. 309.)
13 Help the person stand. (See procedure: *Transferring the Person To a Chair or Wheelchair,* p. 311.) Grasp the gait belt at each side. Or place your arms under the person's arms around to the shoulder blades.
14 Stand at the person's side while he or she gains balance. Hold the belt at the side and back. Or have one arm around the back to support the person.

15 Encourage the person to stand erect with the head up and back straight.
16 Help the person walk. Walk to the side and slightly behind the person. Provide support with the gait belt (Fig. 19-31). Or have one arm around the back to support the person. Encourage the person to use the hand rail on his or her strong side.
17 Encourage the person to walk normally. The heel strikes the floor first. Discourage shuffling, sliding, or walking on tiptoes.
18 Walk the required distance if the person tolerates the activity. Do not rush the person.
19 Help the person return to bed. (See procedure: *Transferring the Person From a Chair or Wheelchair To Bed,* p. 314.)
20 Lower the head of the bed. Help the person to the center of the bed.
21 Remove the shoes. Remove the paper or sheet over the bottom sheet.

Post-Procedure

22 Provide for comfort. Cover the person.
23 Place the signal light within reach.
24 Raise or lower bed rails. Follow the care plan.
25 Return the robe and shoes to their proper place.
26 Unscreen the person.

27 Complete a safety check of the room. (See inside of front book cover.)
28 Decontaminate your hands.
29 Report and record your observations.

Walking Aids.   Walking aids support the body. The physical therapist or RN measures and teaches the person to use the device.

Crutches.   Crutches are used when the person cannot use one leg or when one or both legs need to gain strength. Some persons with permanent leg weakness can use crutches.

Falls are a risk. Follow these safety measures:

*   Check the crutch tips. They must not be worn down, torn, or wet. Replace worn or torn crutch tips. Dry wet tips with a towel or paper towels.
*   Check crutches for flaws. Check wooden crutches for cracks and metal crutches for bends.
*   Tighten all bolts.
*   Street shoes are worn. They must be flat and have nonskid soles.
*   Clothes must fit well. Loose clothes may get caught between the crutches and underarms. Loose clothes and long skirts can hang forward and block the person's view of the feet and crutch tips.
*   Practice safety rules to prevent falls (Chapter 4).
*   Keep crutches within the person's reach. Put them by the person's chair or against a wall.

Canes.   Canes are used for weakness on one side of the body. They help provide balance and support (Fig. 19-32). A cane is held on the strong side of the body. (If the left leg is weak, the cane is held in the right hand.) The cane tip is about 6 to 10 inches to the side of the foot. It is about 6 to 10 inches in front of the foot on the strong side. The grip is level with the hip. The person walks as follows:

*   *Step 1:* The cane is moved forward 6 to 10 inches (Fig. 19-33, *A*).
*   *Step 2:* The weak leg (opposite the cane) is moved forward even with the cane (Fig. 19-33, *B*).
*   *Step 3:* The strong leg is moved forward and ahead of the cane and the weak leg (Fig. 19-33, *C*).

Walkers.   A walker gives more support than a cane (Fig. 19-34). The walker is picked up and moved about 6 to 8 inches in front of the person. The person then moves the weak leg and foot and then the strong leg and foot up to the walker (Fig. 19-35).

Wheeled walkers have wheels on the front legs and rubber tips on the back legs. The person pushes the walker ahead about 6 to 8 inches and then walks up to it. Rubber tips on the back legs prevent the walker from moving while the person is walking or standing. Some have a braking action when weight is applied to the walker's back legs.

Baskets, pouches, and trays attach to the walker (see Fig. 19-34). They are used for needed items. This allows more independence. They also free the hands to grip the walker.

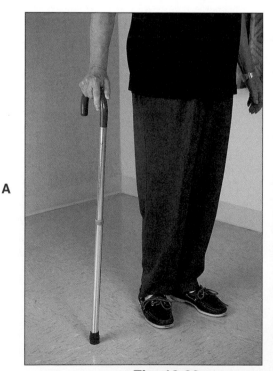
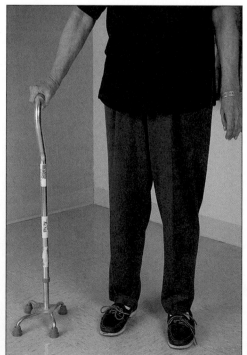

Fig. 19-32 A, Single-tip cane. **B,** Four-point cane.

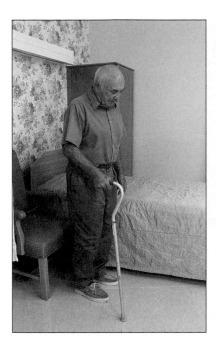 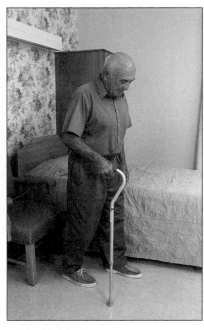 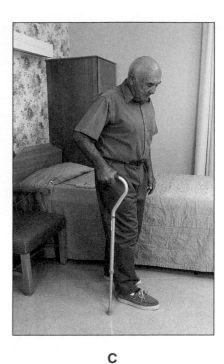

A   B   C

Fig. 19-33 Walking with a cane. **A,** The cane is moved forward about 6 to 10 inches. **B,** The leg opposite the cane (weak leg) is brought forward even with the cane. **C,** The leg on the cane side (strong side) is moved ahead of the cane and the weak leg.

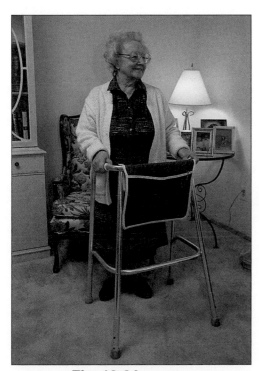

Fig. 19-34 A walker.

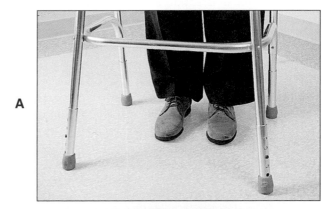

A

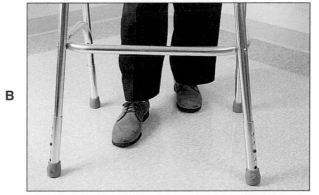

B

Fig. 19-35 Walking with a walker. **A,** The walker is moved about 6 inches in front of the person. **B,** Both feet are moved up to the walker.

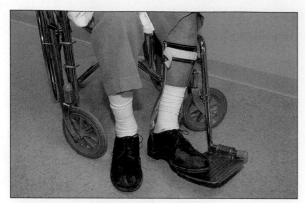

Fig. 19-36 Leg brace.

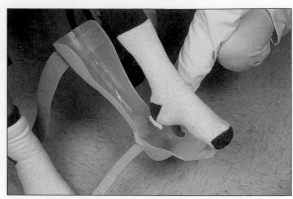

Fig. 19-37 Ankle-foot orthosis (AFO).

Braces. Braces support weak body parts. They also prevent or correct deformities or prevent joint movement. A brace is applied over the ankle, knee, or back (Fig. 19-36). An ankle-foot orthosis (AFO) is placed in the shoe (Fig. 19-37). Then the foot is inserted. The device is secured in place with a Velcro strap.

Skin and bony points under braces are kept clean and dry. This prevents skin breakdown. Report redness or signs of skin breakdown at once (Chapter 15). Also report complaints of pain or discomfort. The nurse assesses the skin under braces every shift. The care plan tells you when to apply and remove a brace.

PSYCHOLOGICAL AND SOCIAL ASPECTS

A disability can affect function and appearance. Self-esteem and relationships may suffer. The person may feel unwhole, useless, unattractive, unclean, or undesirable. The person may deny the disability. The person may expect therapy to correct the problem. He or she may be depressed, angry, and hostile.

Successful rehabilitation depends on the person's attitude. The person must accept his or her limits and be motivated. The focus is on abilities and strengths. Despair and frustration are common. Progress may be slow. Learning a new task is a reminder of the disability. Old fears and emotions may recur.

Remind persons of their progress. They need help accepting disabilities and limits. Give support, reassurance, and encouragement. Meeting psychological and social needs is part of the care plan. Spiritual support helps some persons.

THE REHABILITATION AND RESTORATIVE CARE TEAM

Rehabilitation and restorative care are a team effort. The person is the key member of the team. The family, doctor, nursing team, and other health team members assist the person in setting goals and planning care. All help the person regain function and independence.

The team meets often to discuss the person's progress. Changes in the care plan are made as needed. The person and family attend the meetings when possible. Family members are a key part of the team. They provide support and encouragement. Often they help with care when the person returns home.

Your Role

Every part of your job focuses on promoting the person's independence. Preventing decline in function also is a goal. The many procedures, care measures, and rules in this book apply. Safety, communication, legal, and ethical aspects apply. So do the measures in Box 19-4.

QUALITY OF LIFE

Successful rehabilitation and restorative care improve the person's quality of life. A hopeful and winning outlook is helpful. Often the process is slow and

BOX 19-4   Assisting With Rehabilitation and Restorative Care

- Follow the nurse's instructions carefully.
- Follow the person's care plan.
- Follow the person's daily routine.
- Provide for safety (Chapter 4).
- Protect the person's rights (Chapter 6). Privacy and personal choice are very important.
- Report early signs and symptoms of complications. They include pressure ulcers, contractures, and bowel and bladder problems.
- Keep the person in good alignment at all times.
- Use safe transfer methods (Chapter 16).
- Practice measures to prevent pressure ulcers (Chapter 15).
- Turn and reposition the person as directed.
- Perform range-of-motion exercises as instructed.
- Apply assistive devices as ordered.
- Do not pity the person or give sympathy.
- Encourage the person to perform ADL to the extent possible.
- Allow time for the person to complete tasks. Do not rush the person.
- Give praise when even a little progress is made.
- Provide emotional support and reassurance.
- Try to understand and appreciate the person's situation, feelings, and concerns.
- Provide for spiritual needs.
- Practice the methods described in the care plan when assisting the person.
- Practice the task that the person must do. This helps you guide and direct the person.
- Know how to apply the person's self-help devices.
- Know how to use and operate special equipment used by the person.
- Stress what the person can do. Focus on abilities and strengths, not disabilities and weaknesses.
- Remember that muscles will atrophy if not used.
- Have a hopeful outlook.

frustrating. Promoting quality of life helps the person's attitude. The more the person can do alone, the better his or her quality of life. To promote quality of life:

- *Protect the right to privacy.* The person relearns old or practices new skills in private. No one needs to watch. They do not need to see mistakes, falls, spills, or clumsiness. Nor do they need to see anger or tears. Privacy protects dignity and promotes self-respect.
- *Encourage personal choice.* This gives the person control. Not being able to control body movements or functions is very frustrating. Persons are allowed and encouraged to control their lives to the extent possible. Persons who are sad and depressed may not want to make choices. Encourage them to do so. It can help them feel in control of those things that affect them. Personal choice is important in planning care.
- *Protect the right to be free from abuse and mistreatment.* Sometimes improvement is not seen for weeks. Learning to use a self-help device takes time. Learning to speak after a stroke can take a long time. So can learning how to dress when there is paralysis. What seems simple is often very hard for the person. Repeated explanations and demonstrations may have no or little effect. You may become upset and short-tempered. Or other staff or the family may have such behaviors. Protect the person from physical and mental abuse and mistreatment. No one can shout, scream, or yell at the person. Nor can they call the person names. They cannot hit or strike the person. Unkind remarks are not allowed. Report signs of abuse or mistreatment to the nurse.

- *Learn to deal with your anger and frustration.* The person does not choose loss of function. If the process upsets you, think how the person must feel. Discuss your feelings with the nurse. The nurse can suggest ways to help you control or express your feelings. Perhaps you can assist other persons for a while.
- *Encourage activities.* Encourage the person to join in group activities. There may be concern about how others view the disability. Provide support and reassurance. Remind the person that others have disabilities. They can give support and understanding. Allow personal choice. The person should do what interests him or her. The person usually chooses activities that he or she can do.
- *Provide a safe setting.* It must meet the person's needs. Needed changes are made. The overbed table and bedside stand are moved to the person's strong side. The person may need a special chair. If unable to use the signal light, another way is needed to communicate with the staff. The rehabilitation team suggests these and other changes. They explain the need and purpose to the person and family.
- *Show patience, understanding, and sensitivity.* Progress may be slow and hard to see. The person may be upset and discouraged. Give support, encouragement, and praise when needed. Stress the person's abilities and strengths. Do not give pity or sympathy.

Review Questions

Circle the **BEST** answer.

1. Rehabilitation and restorative care focus on
   a. What the person cannot do
   b. What the person can do
   c. The whole person
   d. The person's rights

2. Rehabilitation begins with preventing
   a. Angry feelings
   b. Contractures and pressure ulcers
   c. Illness and injury
   d. Loss of self-esteem

3. A person is on bedrest. Which is *false?*
   a. The commode is used for elimination.
   b. Bedrest helps reduce pain and promotes healing.
   c. Complications of bedrest include pressure ulcers, constipation, and blood clots.
   d. Contractures and muscle atrophy can occur.

4. Which helps prevent plantar flexion?
   a. An eggcrate-like mattress
   b. A footboard
   c. A trochanter roll
   d. Hand rolls

5. Which prevents the hip from turning outward?
   a. An eggcrate-like mattress
   b. A footboard
   c. A trochanter roll
   d. A leg brace

6. A contracture is
   a. The loss of muscle strength from inactivity
   b. The lack of joint mobility from shortening of a muscle
   c. A decrease in the size of a muscle
   d. A blood clot in the muscle

7. Passive range-of-motion exercises are performed by
   a. The person
   b. Someone else
   c. The person with the help of another
   d. The person with the use of a footboard

8. ROM exercises are ordered. You do the following *except*
   a. Support the part being exercised
   b. Move the joint slowly, smoothly, and gently
   c. Force the joint through full range of motion
   d. Exercise only the joints indicated by the nurse

9. Flexion involves
   a. Bending the body part
   b. Straightening the body part
   c. Moving the body part toward the body
   d. Moving the body part away from the body

10. Which statement about ambulation is *false?*
    a. A gait belt is used if the person is weak or unsteady.
    b. The person can shuffle or slide when walking after bedrest.
    c. Walking aids may be needed.
    d. Crutches, canes, walkers, and braces are common walking aids.

11. You are getting a person ready to crutch walk. You should do the following *except*
    a. Check the crutch tips
    b. Have the person wear nonskid shoes
    c. Get a pair of crutches from physical therapy
    d. Tighten the bolts on the crutches

Review Questions

12 A single-tip cane is used
  a At waist level
  b On the strong side
  c On the weak side
  d On either side

13 Mr. Olson has weakness on his right side. ADL are
  a Done by him to the extent possible
  b Done by you
  c Postponed until he can use his right side
  d Supervised by a therapist

14 Persons with disabilities are likely to feel the following *except*
  a Undesirable
  b Angry and hostile
  c Depressed
  d Relief

15 Which statement is *false?*
  a Sympathy and pity help the person adjust to the disability.
  b You should know how to apply self-help devices.
  c You should know how to use equipment used in the person's care.
  d You need to convey hopefulness to the person.

16 Mr. Olson is learning to use a walker. He asks to have music played. You should
  a Tell him music is not allowed
  b Choose some music
  c Ask him to choose some music
  d Ask a therapist to choose some music

17 Mr. Olson's right side is weak. The signal light is on his right side. You move it to the left side. You have promoted his quality of life by
  a Protecting him from abuse and mistreatment
  b Allowing personal choice
  c Providing for his safety
  d Taking part in his activities

Circle **T** if the statement is true or **F** if the statement is false.

18 **T F** A person's speech therapy should be done in private.
19 **T F** You tell Mr. Olson that he cannot have dessert until he does his exercises. This is abuse and mistreatment.
20 **T F** You need to stress the person's abilities and strengths.
21 **T F** A single-tip cane and a four-point cane give the same support.
22 **T F** When using a cane, the feet are moved first.
23 **T F** Mrs. Parker uses a walker. She moves the walker first and then her feet.
24 **T F** A person has a brace. Bony areas need protection from skin breakdown.

Answers to these questions are on p. 390.

CHAPTER 20

Restraint Alternatives and Safe Restraint Use

Objectives

- Define the key terms listed in this chapter
- Describe the purpose and complications of restraints
- Identify restraint alternatives
- Explain how to use restraints safely
- Perform the procedure described in this chapter

active physical restraint A restraint attached to the person's body and to a fixed (non-movable) object; it restricts movement or body access

passive physical restraint A restraint near but not directly attached to the person's body; it does not totally restrict freedom of movement and allows access to certain body parts

restraint Any item, object, device, garment, material, or drug that limits or restricts a person's freedom of movement or access to one's body

---

Many safety measures are presented in Chapter 4. However, some persons need extra protection. They may present dangers to themselves or others. For example:

- Mrs. Perez forgets to call for help when getting up and with walking. Falling is a risk.
- Mrs. Wilson tries to pull out her feeding tube. The tube is part of her treatment.
- Ms. Walsh scratches and picks at a wound. This can damage the skin or the wound.
- Mr. Ross wanders. He may wander into traffic or get lost in neighborhoods, parks, forests, or other areas. Exposure to hot or cold weather presents other dangers.
- Mr. Winters tries to hit, pinch, and bite the staff. They are at risk for harm.

Every attempt is made to protect the person without using restraints. Sometimes they are needed. A **restraint** is any item, object, device, garment, material, or drug that limits or restricts a person's freedom of movement or access to one's body. Restraints are used only as a *last resort* to protect persons from harming themselves or others.

HISTORY OF RESTRAINT USE

Until the late 1980s, restraints were thought to *prevent* falls. Research shows that restraints *cause* falls. Falls occur when persons try to get free of the restraints. Injuries are more serious from falls in restrained persons than in those not restrained.

Restraints also were used to prevent wandering or interfering with treatment. They were often used for persons who showed confusion, poor judgment, or behavior problems. Their purpose was to protect a person. However, they can cause serious harm, even death (Box 20-1).

OBRA, the Centers for Medicare & Medicaid Services (CMS), and the Federal Food and Drug Administration (FDA) have guidelines about restraint use. So do states and accrediting agencies. They do not forbid restraint use. *However, all other appropriate alternatives must be tried first.*

BOX 20-1	Risks of Restraint Use	
• Agitation	• Fractures
• Anger	• Humiliation
• Bruises	• Mistrust
• Cuts	• Nerve injuries
• Constipation	• Pneumonia
• Dehydration	• Pressure ulcers
• Depression	• Strangulation
• Embarrassment	• Urinary incontinence
• Fecal incontinence	• Urinary tract infection

RESTRAINT ALTERNATIVES

Often there are causes and reasons for harmful behaviors. Knowing and treating the cause can prevent restraint use. The nurse tries to find out what the behavior means:

- Is the person in pain?
- Is the person ill or injured?
- Is the person short of breath? Are cells getting enough oxygen?
- Is the person afraid in a new setting?
- Does the person need to urinate or have a bowel movement?
- Is a dressing or bandage tight or causing other discomfort?
- Is clothing tight or causing other discomfort?
- Is the person's position uncomfortable?
- Is the person too hot or too cold?
- Is the person hungry?
- Is the person thirsty?
- Are body fluids, secretions, or excretions causing skin irritation?
- Is the person seeing, hearing, or feeling things that are not real (Chapter 18)?
- Is the person confused or disoriented (Chapter 18)?
- Are drugs causing the behaviors?

Restraint alternatives for the person are identified (Box 20-2, p. 374). They become part of the care plan. Care plan changes are made as needed. Restraint alternatives may not protect the person. Then the doctor may need to order restraints.

BOX 20-2   Alternatives to Restraints

- Diversion is provided. This includes TV, videos, music, games, books, relaxation tapes, and so on.
- Lifelong habits and routines are in the care plan. For example, showers before breakfast; reads in the bathroom; walks outside before lunch; watches TV after lunch; and so on.
- Family and friends make videos of themselves for the person to watch.
- Videos are made of visits with family and friends for the person to watch.
- Time is spent in supervised areas (dining room, lounge, near nurses' station).
- Pillows, wedge cushions, posture, and positioning aids are used.
- The signal light is within reach.
- Signal lights are answered promptly.
- Food, fluid, and elimination needs are met.
- The bedpan, urinal, or commode is within the person's reach.
- Back massages are given.
- Family, friends, and volunteers visit.
- The person has companions and sitters.
- Time is spent with the person.
- Extra time is spent with a person who is restless.
- Reminiscing is done with the person.
- A calm, quiet setting is provided.
- The person wanders in safe areas.
- The entire staff is aware of persons who tend to wander. This includes staff in housekeeping, maintenance, business office, dietary, and so on.
- Exercise programs are provided.
- Outdoor time is planned during nice weather.
- The person does jobs or tasks he or she consents to.
- Warning devices are used on beds, chairs, and doors.
- Knob guards are used on doors.
- Padded hip protectors are worn under clothing (Fig. 20-1).
- Floor cushions are placed next to beds (Fig. 20-2).
- Roll guards are attached to the bed frame (Fig. 20-3).
- Falls are prevented.
- The person's furniture meets his or her needs (lower bed, reclining chair, rocking chair).
- Walls and furniture corners are padded.
- Observations and visits are made at least every 15 minutes.
- The person is moved closer to the nurses' station.
- Procedures and care measures are explained.
- Frequent explanations are given about required equipment or devices.
- Persons who are confused are oriented to person, time, and place. Calendars and clocks are provided.
- Light is adjusted to meet the person's needs and preferences.
- Staff assignments are consistent.
- Uninterrupted sleep is promoted.
- Noise levels are reduced.

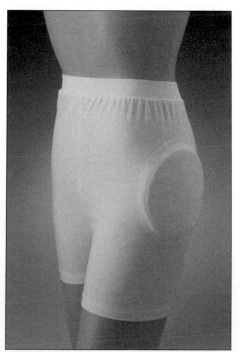

Fig. 20-1 Hip protector. (Courtesy J. T. Posey Co., Arcadia, Calif.)

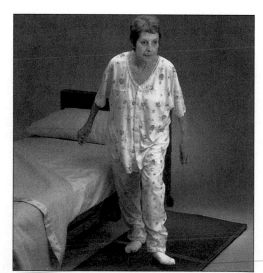

Fig. 20-2 Floor cushion. (Courtesy J. T. Posey Co., Arcadia, Calif.)

SAFE RESTRAINT USE

Restraints can cause serious injury and even death. They are not used to discipline a person or for staff convenience. *Discipline* is any action that punishes or penalizes a person. *Convenience* is any action that:

- Controls the person's behavior
- Requires less effort by the center
- Is not in the person's best interests

Restraints are used only when necessary to treat a person's medical symptoms. Symptoms may be physical, emotional, or behavioral. Sometimes restraints are needed to protect the person or others. That is, residents may behave in ways that are harmful to themselves or others (p. 373).

Imagine what it is like to be restrained:

- Your nose itches. But your hands and arms are restrained. You cannot scratch your nose.
- You need to use the bathroom. Your hands and arms are restrained. You cannot get up. You cannot reach your signal light. You soil yourself with urine or a bowel movement.
- Your phone is ringing. You cannot answer it because your hands and arms are restrained.
- You are thirsty. You cannot reach the water glass because your wrists are restrained.
- You hear the fire alarm. You have on a restraint. You cannot get up to move to a safe place. You must wait until someone rescues you.

What would you try to do? Would you calmly lie or sit there? Would you try to get free from the restraint? Would you cry out for help? What would the nursing staff think? Would they think that you are uncomfortable? Or would they think that you are agitated and uncooperative? Would they think your behavior is improving or getting worse? Would you feel anger, embarrassment, or humiliation?

Put yourself in the person's situation. That will help you understand how the person feels. Treat the person like you would want to be treated—with kindness, caring, respect, and dignity.

Physical and Drug Restraints

According to OBRA and CMS, *physical restraints* include these points:

- May be any manual method, physical or mechanical device, material, or equipment
- Is attached to or next to the person's body
- Cannot be easily removed by the person
- Restricts freedom of movement or access to one's body

Physical restraints are applied to the chest, waist, elbows, wrists, or ankles. They confine the person to a bed or chair. Or they prevent movement of a body part. Some furniture or barriers also prevent free movement:

- Geriatric chairs (Geri-chairs) or chairs with attached trays (Fig. 20-4). Such chairs are often used for persons needing support to sit up.
- Placing any chair so close to a wall that the person cannot move.
- Bed rails.
- Sheets tucked in so tightly that they restrict movement.

Drugs are restraints if they:

- Control behavior or restrict movement
- Are not standard treatment for the person's condition

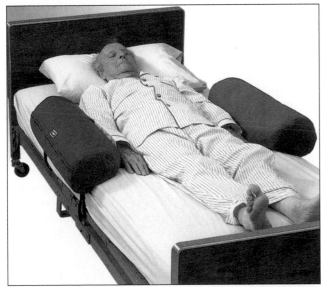

Fig. 20-3 Roll guard. (Courtesy J. T. Posey Co., Arcadia, Calif.)

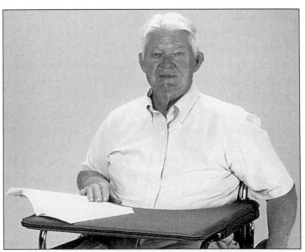

Fig. 20-4 This lap-top tray is a restraint alternative. It is considered a restraint when used to prevent freedom of movement. (Courtesy J. T. Posey Co., Arcadia, Calif.)

Sometimes drugs can help persons who are confused or disoriented. They may become anxious, agitated, or aggressive. The doctor may order drugs to control these behaviors. The goal is to control the behavior without making the person sleepy and unable to function at his or her highest level.

Complications of Restraint Use

Box 20-1 lists complications from restraints. Injuries occur as the person tries to get free of the restraint. Cuts, bruises, and fractures are common. Injuries also occur from using the wrong restraint, applying it wrong, or keeping it on too long. *The most serious risk is death from strangulation.*

There are also mental effects. Restraints affect dignity and self-esteem. Depression, anger, and agitation are common. So are embarrassment, humiliation, and mistrust.

Restraints are medical devices. The Safe Medical Device Act applies if a restraint causes illness, injury, or death. Also, CMS requires that the center report any death that occurs while a person is in restraints.

Safety Guidelines

If a restraint is used, the least restrictive method is used. While providing protection, it allows the greatest amount of movement or body access possible. Follow the safety measures listed in Box 20-3. Also remember the following:

- *Restraints are used to protect the person. They are not used for staff convenience or to discipline a person.* Restraining someone is not easier than properly supervising and observing the person. A restrained person requires more staff time for care, supervision, and observation.
- *Restraints require a written doctor's order.* The doctor gives the reason for the restraint, what body part to restrain, what to use, and how long to use it. This information is on the care plan and your assignment sheet.
- *The least restrictive method is used.* An **active physical restraint** attaches to the person's body and to a fixed (non-movable) object. It restricts movement or body access. Vest, jacket, ankle, wrist, and some belt restraints are active physical restraints. A **passive physical restraint** is near but not directly attached to the person's body (bed rails or wedge cushions). It does not totally restrict freedom of movement. It allows access to certain body parts. Passive physical restraints are the least restrictive.

- *Restraints are used only after trying other ways to protect the person.* Some people can harm themselves or others. The care plan must include measures to protect the person and prevent harm to others. Restraints are allowed only after other measures fail to protect the person (see Box 20-2). See fall prevention measures in Chapter 4.
- *Unnecessary restraint is false imprisonment (Chapter 1).* If told to apply a restraint, you must clearly understand the need. If not, politely ask about its use. If you apply a restraint that is not needed, you could face false imprisonment charges.
- *Informed consent is required.* The person must understand the reason for the restraint. The person is told about risks of restraint use. If the person cannot give informed consent, his or her legal representative is given the information. Restraints cannot be used without consent. The doctor or nurse provides the necessary information and obtains the consent.
- *The manufacturer's instructions are followed.* The manufacturer gives instructions about applying and securing the restraint. Failure to follow them could affect the person's safety. You could be negligent for improperly applying or securing a restraint.
- *The person's basic needs must be met.* The restraint must be snug and firm but not tight. Tight restraints affect circulation and breathing. The person must be comfortable and able to move the restrained part to a limited and safe extent. The person is checked at least every 15 minutes or as often as required by the person's needs. Food, fluid, comfort, safety, exercise, hygiene, and elimination needs must be met.
- *Restraints are applied with enough help to protect the person and staff from injury.* Combative and agitated people can hurt themselves and the staff when restraints are applied. Enough staff members are needed to complete the task safely and quickly.
- *Restraints can increase confusion and agitation.* Whether confused or alert, people are aware of restricted movements. They may try to get out of the restraint or struggle or pull at it. Some restrained persons beg others to free or to help release them. These behaviors often are viewed as signs of confusion. Confusion increases in some persons because they do not understand what is happening to them. Restrained persons need repeated explanations and reassurance. Spending time with them has a calming effect.

- *Quality of life must be protected.* Restraints are used for as short a time as possible. The care plan must show how restraint use is reduced. The goal is to meet the person's needs with as little restraint as possible. You must meet the person's physical and psychosocial needs. Visit with the person and explain the reason for restraints.
- *The person is observed at least every 15 minutes or more often as required by the care plan.* Restraints are dangerous. Injuries and deaths can occur from improper restraint use and poor observation.

Complications from restraints are prevented. Interferences with breathing and circulation are examples. Practice the safety measures in Box 20-3.

- *The restraint is removed, the person repositioned, and basic needs met at least every 2 hours.* This includes food, fluid, hygiene, and elimination needs and giving skin care. Range-of-motion exercises are done. Or you help the person walk according to the care plan.

Text continued on p. 381

BOX 20-3   Safety Measures for Using Restraints

- Use the restraint noted in the care plan. The least restrictive device is used.
- Apply a restraint only after being instructed about its proper use.
- Demonstrate proper application of the restraint to the nurse before applying it.
- Use the correct size. The nurse and care plan tell you what size to use. Small restraints are tight. They cause discomfort and agitation. They also restrict breathing and circulation. Strangulation is a risk from big or loose restraints.
- Use only restraints that have manufacturer instructions and warning labels.
- Read the manufacturer's warning labels. Note the front and back of the restraint.
- Follow the manufacturer's instructions. Some restraints are safe for bed, chair, and wheelchair use. Others are used only with certain equipment.
- Do not use sheets, towels, tape, rope, straps, bandages, or other items to restrain a person.
- Use intact restraints. Look for tears, cuts, or frayed fabric or straps. Look for missing or loose hooks, loops, or straps or other damage.
- Do not use restraints to position a person on a toilet.
- Do not use restraints to position a person on furniture that does not allow for correct application. Follow the manufacturer's instructions.
- Follow center policies and procedures.
- Position the person in good alignment before applying the restraint.
- Pad bony areas and skin. This prevents pressure and injury from the restraint.
- Secure the restraint. It should be snug but allow some movement of the restrained part.
  - *If applied to the chest:* Make sure that the person can breathe easily. A flat hand should slide between the restraint and the person's body (Fig. 20-5, p. 378).
  - *For wrist and mitt restraints:* You should be able to slide one or two fingers under the restraint.
- Follow the manufacturer's instructions to check for snugness.

- Criss-cross vest restraints in front (Fig. 20-6, p. 378). Do not criss-cross restraints in the back unless part of the manufacturer's instructions (Fig. 20-7, p. 379). Criss-crossing vests in the back can cause death from strangulation.
- Tie restraints according to center policy. The policy should follow the manufacturer's instructions. Quick-release buckles or airline-type buckles are used (Fig. 20-8, p. 379). So are quick-release ties (Fig. 20-9, p. 379).
- Secure straps out of the person's reach.
- Leave 1 to 2 inches of slack in the straps. This allows some movement of the part.
- Secure the restraint to the movable part of the bed frame at waist level (see Fig. 20-9). For chairs, secure straps to the wheelchair or the chair frame (Fig. 20-10, p. 379).
- Make sure that straps will not slide in any direction. If straps slide, they change the restraint's position. The person can get suspended off the mattress or chair (Figs. 20-11, p. 379 and 20-12, p. 380). Strangulation can result.
- Never secure restraints to the bed rails. The person can reach bed rails to release knots or buckles. Also, injury to the person is likely when raising or lowering bed rails.
- Use bed rail covers or gap protectors according to the nurse's instructions (Fig. 20-13). They prevent entrapment between the rails or the bed rail bars (see Fig. 20-11). Entrapment can occur between:
  - The bars of a bed rail
  - The space between half-length (split) bed rails
  - The bed rail and mattress
  - The headboard or footboard and mattress
- Keep full bed rails up when using a vest, jacket, or belt restraint. Also use bed rail covers or gap protectors. Otherwise the person could fall off the bed and strangle on the restraint. If half-length bed rails are used, the person can get caught between them.
- Position the person in semi-Fowler's position when using a vest, jacket, or belt restraint.

Continued

BOX 20-3   Safety Measures for Using Restraints—cont'd

- Position the person in a chair so the hips are well to the back of the chair.
- Apply a belt restraint at a 45-degree angle over the hips (Fig. 20-14, p. 381).
- Do not use back cushions when a person is restrained in a chair. If the cushion moves out of place, slack occurs in the straps. Strangulation could result if the person slides forward or down from the extra slack (see Fig. 20-12, p. 380).
- Do not cover the restraint with a sheet, blanket, bedspread, or other covering. The restraint must be within plain view at all times.
- Check the person's circulation at least every 15 minutes if mitt, wrist, or ankle restraints are applied. You should feel a pulse at a pulse site below the restraint. Fingers or toes should be warm and pink. Tell the nurse at once if:
  - —You cannot feel a pulse
  - —Fingers or toes are cold, pale, or blue in color
  - —The person complains of pain, numbness, or tingling in the restrained part
  - —The skin is red or damaged
- Check the person at least every 15 minutes if a belt, jacket, or vest restraint is used. The person should be able to breathe easily. Also check the position of the restraint, especially in the front and back.
- Check the person at least every 15 minutes for safety and comfort.
- Monitor persons in the supine position constantly. They are at great risk for aspiration if vomiting occurs (Chapter 14). Call for the nurse at once.
- Do not use a restraint near a fire, flame, or smoking materials. Restraint fabrics may ignite easily.
- Keep scissors in your pocket. In an emergency, cutting the tie may be faster than untying the knot. Never leave scissors at the bedside or where the person can reach them.
- Remove the restraint and reposition the person every 2 hours. Meet the person's basic needs:
  - —Meet elimination needs.
  - —Offer food and fluids.
  - —Meet hygiene needs.
  - —Give skin care.
  - —Perform range-of-motion exercises, or ambulate the person. Follow the care plan.
  - —Chart what was done, the care given, your observations, and when and what you reported to the nurse.
- Keep the signal light within the person's reach.
- Report to the nurse every time you checked the person and released the restraint. Report your observations and the care given. Follow center policy for recording.

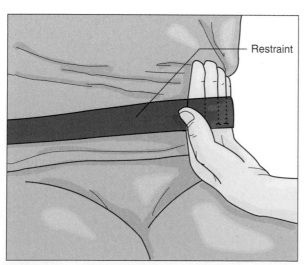

Fig. 20-5 A flat hand slides between the restraint and the person.

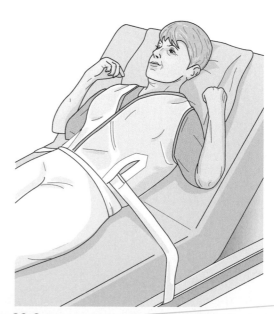

Fig. 20-6 Vest restraint criss-crosses in front. (NOTE: Bed rails are raised after the restraint is applied and secured.)

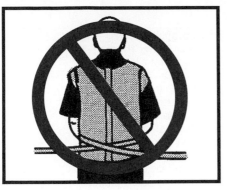

Fig. 20-7 Never criss-cross vest or jacket straps in back. (Courtesy J. T. Posey Co., Arcadia, Calif.)

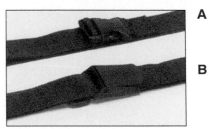

Fig. 20-8 A, Quick-release buckle. **B,** Airline-type buckles. (Courtesy J. T. Posey Co., Arcadia, Calif.)

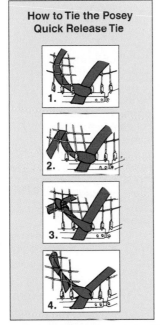

How to Tie the Posey Quick Release Tie

1.
2.
3.
4.

Fig. 20-9 The Posey quick-release tie. (Courtesy J. T. Posey Co., Arcadia, Calif.)

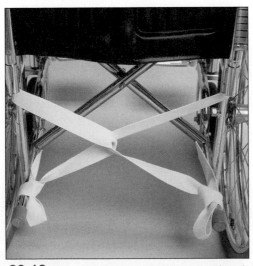

Fig. 20-10 The restraint straps are secured to the wheelchair frame with quick-release ties. (Courtesy J. T. Posey Co., Arcadia, Calif.)

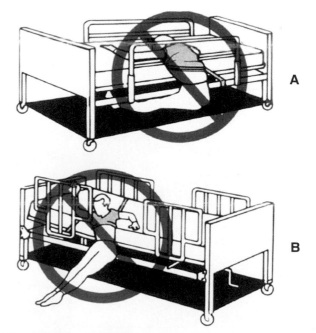

Fig. 20-11 A, A person can get suspended and caught between bed rail bars. **B,** The person can get suspended and caught between half-length bed rails. (Courtesy J. T. Posey Co., Arcadia, Calif.)

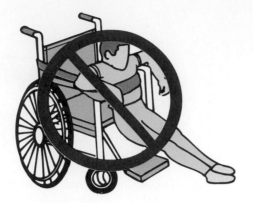

Straps to prevent sliding should always be over the thighs—NOT around the waist or chest. Straps should be at a 45° angle and secured to the chair under the seat, not behind the back. They should be snug but comfortable and not restrict breathing. If a belt or vest is too loose or applied around the waist, the person may slide partially off the seat— resulting in possible suffocation and death.

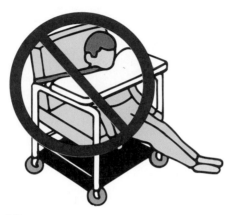

Tray tables (with or without a belt or vest) pose potential danger if the person should slide partly under the table and become caught. This could result in suffocation and death. Make sure the person's hips are positioned at the back of the chair— this may necessitate the use of an anti-slide material (Posey Grip), a pommel cushion, or a restrictive device if the person shows any tendency to slide forward.

Fig. 20-12 Strangulation could result if the person slides forward or down because of extra slack in the restraint. (Courtesy J. T. Posey Co., Arcadia, Calif.)

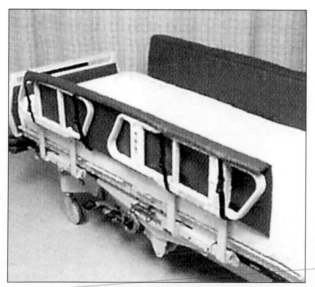

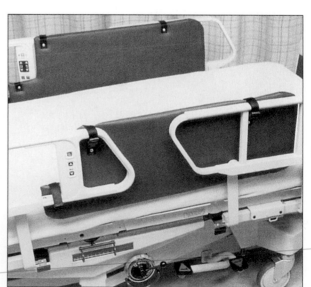

Fig. 20-13 A, Bed rail covers. **B,** Gap protectors. (Courtesy J. T. Posey Co., Arcadia, Calif.)

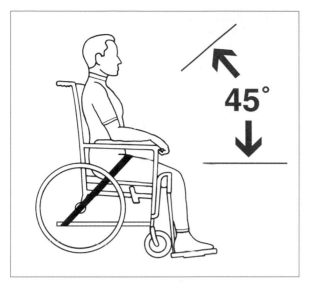

Fig. 20-14 The safety belt is at a 45-degree angle over the hips. (Courtesy J. T. Posey Co., Arcadia, Calif.)

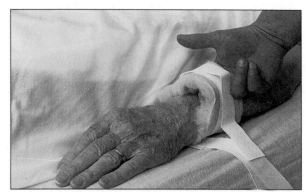

Fig. 20-15 Wrist restraint. The soft part is toward the skin. Note that 2 fingers fit between the restraint and the wrist.

Reporting and Recording

You might apply restraints or care for a restrained person. Report the following to the nurse. If you are allowed to chart, include this information:

- The type of restraint applied
- The body part or parts restrained
- The reason for the application
- Safety measures taken (for example, bed rails padded and up)
- The time you applied the restraint
- The time you removed the restraint
- The care given when the restraint was removed
- Skin color and condition
- The pulse felt in the restrained part
- Changes in the person's behavior
- Complaints of a tight restraint, difficulty breathing, and pain, numbness, or tingling in the restrained part (report these complaints to the nurse at once)

Applying Restraints

Restraints are made of cloth or leather. Cloth restraints are mitts, belts, straps, jackets, and vests. They are applied to the wrists, ankles, hands, waist, and chest. Leather restraints are applied to the wrists and ankles. They are used for extreme agitation and combativeness.

Wrist Restraints.   Wrist restraints (limb holders) limit arm movement (Fig. 20-15). They may be used when a person continually tries to pull out tubes used for treatment (IV, feeding tube, catheter, or wound drainage tubes). Or the person tries to scratch, pick at, pull at, or peel the skin, a wound, or a dressing. This can damage the skin or the wound.

Mitt Restraints.   Hands are placed in mitt restraints. They prevent finger use. They do not prevent hand, wrist, or arm movements. They are used for the same reasons as wrist restraints. Most mitts are padded (Fig. 20-16, p. 382).

Belt Restraints.   The belt restraint (Fig. 20-17, p. 382) is used when injuries from falls are risks. The person cannot get out of bed or out of a chair. However, the person can turn from side to side or sit up in bed.

The belt is applied around the waist and secured to the bed or chair. It is applied over a garment. The person can release the quick-release type. It is less restrictive than those that only staff members can release.

Vest Restraints and Jacket Restraints.   Vest and jacket restraints are applied to the chest. They may be used to prevent injuries from falls. And they may be used for persons who need positioning for a medical treatment. The person cannot turn in bed or get out of bed or a chair.

A jacket restraint is applied with the opening in the back. For a vest restraint, the vest crosses in front (see Fig. 20-6). *The straps of vest and jacket restraints always cross in the front.* They must never cross in the back. Vest and jacket restraints are never worn backwards. Strangulation or other injury could occur if the person slides down in the bed or chair. The restraint is always applied over a garment. (*NOTE: A vest or jacket restraint may have a positioning slot in the back. Criss-cross the straps following the manufacturer's instructions.*)

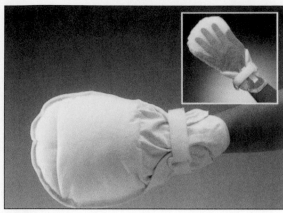

Fig. 20-16 Mitt restraint. (Courtesy J. T. Posey Co., Arcadia, Calif.)

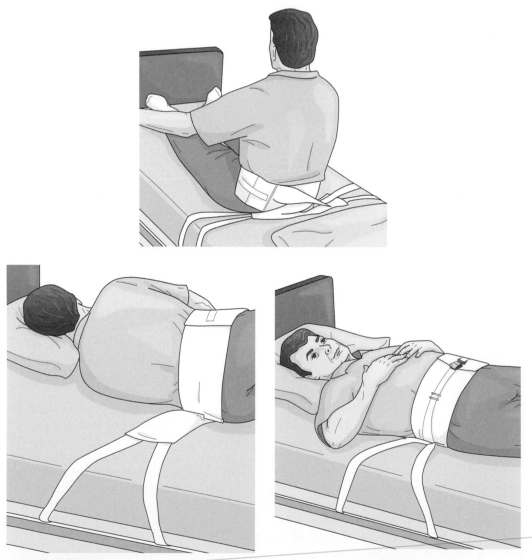

Fig. 20-17 Belt restraint. (NOTE: Bed rails are raised after the restraint is applied and secured.)

Vest and jacket restraints have life-threatening risks. Death can occur from strangulation. If the person gets caught in the restraint, it can become so tight that the person's chest cannot expand to inhale air. The person quickly suffocates and dies. Restraints must be applied correctly. For vest and jacket restraints, this is critical. You are advised to only assist the nurse in applying them. The nurse should assume full responsibility for applying a vest or jacket restraint.

Delegation Guidelines

Applying Restraints

Before applying a restraint, you need this information from the nurse and the care plan:

- Why the doctor ordered the restraint
- What type and size to use
- Where to apply the restraint
- How to safely apply the restraint (Have the nurse show you how to apply it. Then demonstrate correct application back to the nurse.)
- How to correctly position the person
- What bony areas to pad and how to pad them
- If bed rail covers or gap protectors are needed
- If bed rails are up or down
- What special equipment is needed
- If the person needs to be checked more often than every 15 minutes
- When to apply and release the restraint

Safety Alert

Applying Restraints

Restraints can cause serious harm, even death. Always follow the manufacturer's instructions. Check the person at least every 15 minutes or more often as instructed by the nurse and the care plan.

Never use force to apply a restraint. Always ask a co-worker to help apply a restraint to a person who is confused and agitated. Report any problems to the nurse at once.

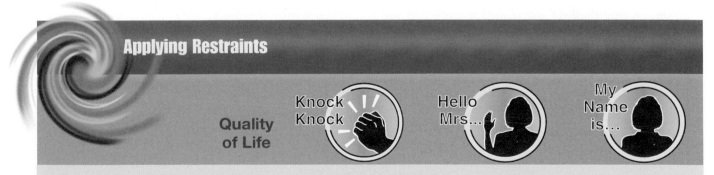

Applying Restraints

Quality of Life

Knock Knock

Hello Mrs...

My Name is...

Pre-Procedure

1 Follow *Delegation Guidelines: Applying Restraints.* See *Safety Alert: Applying Restraints.*
2 Collect the following as instructed by the nurse:
   - Correct type and size of restraints
   - Padding for bony areas
   - Bed rail pads or gap protectors

3 Practice hand hygiene.
4 Identify the person. Check the ID bracelet against the assignment sheet. Call the person by name.
5 Explain the procedure to the person.
6 Provide for privacy.

Continued

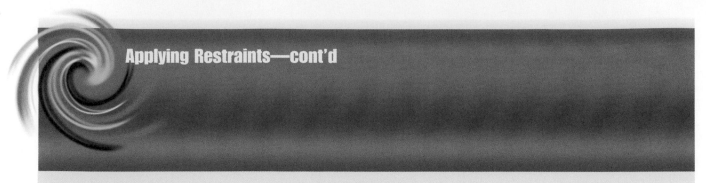

Applying Restraints—cont'd

Procedure

7   Make sure the person is comfortable and in good alignment.

8   Put the bed rail pads or gap protectors on the bed if the person is in bed, if needed. Follow the manufacturer's instructions.

9   Pad bony areas according to the nurse's instructions.

10   Read the manufacturer's instructions. Note the front and back of the restraint.

11   *For wrist restraints:*

    a   Apply the restraint following the manufacturer's instructions. Place the soft part toward the skin.

    b   Secure the restraint so it is snug but not tight. Make sure you can slide 1 or 2 fingers under the restraint (see Fig. 20-15). Follow the manufacturer's instructions.

    c   Tie the straps to the movable part of the bed frame out of the person's reach. Use a center-approved tie. Leave 1 to 2 inches of slack in the straps.

    d   Repeat steps 11, a, b, and c for the other wrist.

12   *For mitt restraints:*

    a   Make sure the person's hands are clean and dry.

    b   Apply the mitt restraint. Follow the manufacturer's instructions.

    c   Tie the straps to the movable part of the bed frame. Use a center-approved tie. Leave 1 to 2 inches of slack in the straps.

    d   Make sure the restraint is snug. Slide in 2 fingers between the restraint and the wrist. Follow the manufacturer's instructions. Adjust the straps if it is too loose or too tight. Check for snugness again.

    e   Repeat steps 12, b, c, and d for the other hand.

13   *For a belt restraint:*

    a   Assist the person to a sitting position.

    b   Apply the restraint with your free hand. Follow the manufacturer's instructions.

    c   Remove wrinkles or creases from the front and back of the restraint.

    d   Bring the ties through the slots in the belt.

    e   Help the person lie down if he or she is in bed.

    f   Make sure the person is comfortable and in good alignment.

    g   Secure the straps to the movable part of the bed frame out of the person's reach or to the chair or wheelchair. Use a center-approved tie. Leave 1 to 2 inches of slack in the straps.

14   *For a vest restraint:*

    a   Assist the person to a sitting position.

    b   Apply the restraint with your free hand. Follow the manufacturer's instructions. The "V" part of the vest crosses in front.

    c   Make sure the vest is free of wrinkles in the front and back.

    d   Help the person lie down if he or she is in bed.

    e   Bring the straps through the slots.

    f   Make sure the person is comfortable and in good alignment.

    g   Secure the straps to the chair or to the movable part of the bed frame. If secured to the bed frame, the straps are secured at waist level out of the person's reach. Use a center-approved tie. Leave 1 to 2 inches of slack in the straps.

    h   Make sure the vest is snug. Slide an open hand between the restraint and the person. Adjust the restraint if it is too loose or too tight. Check for snugness again.

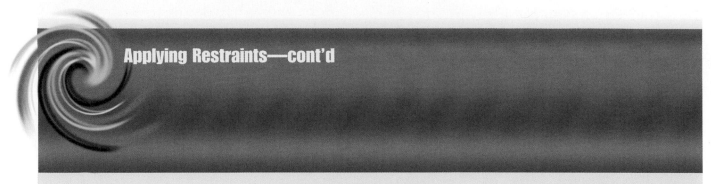

Applying Restraints—cont'd

Procedure—cont'd

15 *For a jacket restraint:*

  a Assist the person to a sitting position.

  b Apply the restraint with your free hand. Follow the manufacturer's instructions. Remember, the jacket opening goes in the back.

  c Close the back with the zipper, ties, or hook-and-loop closures.

  d Make sure the side seams are under the arms. Remove any wrinkles in the front and back.

  e Help the person lie down if he or she is in bed.

  f Make sure the person is comfortable and in good alignment.

  g Secure the straps to the chair or to the movable part of the bed frame. If secured to the bed frame, the straps are secured at waist level out of the person's reach. Use a center-approved knot. Leave 1 to 2 inches of slack in the straps.

  h Make sure the jacket is snug. Slide an open hand between the restraint and the person. Adjust the restraint if it is too loose or too tight. Check for snugness again.

Post-Procedure

16 Position the person as the nurse directs. Provide for comfort.

17 Place the signal light within the person's reach.

18 Raise or lower bed rails. Follow the care plan and the manufacturer's instructions for the restraint.

19 Unscreen the person.

20 Complete a safety check of the room. (See inside of front book cover.)

21 Decontaminate your hands.

22 Check the person and the restraints at least every 15 minutes. Report and record your observations:

  a For wrist and mitt restraints: check the pulse, color, and temperature of the restrained parts.

  b For vest, jacket, and belt restraints: check the person's breathing. *Call for the nurse at once if the person is not breathing or is having difficulty breathing.* Make sure the restraint is properly positioned in the front and back.

23 Do the following at least every 2 hours:

- Remove the restraint.
- Reposition the person.
- Meet food, fluid, hygiene, and elimination needs.
- Give skin care.
- Perform range-of-motion exercises or ambulate the person. Follow the care plan.
- Reapply the restraints.
- Provide for comfort.

24 Complete a safety check of the room. (See inside of front book cover.)

25 Report and record your observations and the care given.

Review Questions

Circle **T** if the statement is true or **F** if the statement is false.

1. **T F** Restraint alternatives fail to protect a person. The nurse can order a restraint.
2. **T F** Restraints can be used for staff convenience.
3. **T F** A device is a restraint only if it is attached to the person's body.
4. **T F** Bed rails are restraints.
5. **T F** Restraints are used only for specific medical symptoms.
6. **T F** Restraints can be used to protect the person from harming others.
7. **T F** Unnecessary restraint is false imprisonment.
8. **T F** Informed consent is needed for restraint use.
9. **T F** You can apply restraints when you think they are needed.
10. **T F** Restraint straps are secured within the person's reach.
11. **T F** You can use a vest restraint to position a person on the toilet.
12. **T F** Restraints are removed every 2 hours to reposition the person and give skin care.
13. **T F** Restraint straps are tied to bed rails.
14. **T F** Some drugs are restraints.
15. **T F** A vest restraint crosses in front.
16. **T F** Bed rails are left down when vest restraints are used.

Circle the **BEST** answer.

17. These statements are about restraints. Which is *false*?
    a A restraint can be an object, device, garment, or material.
    b A restraint limits or restricts a person's movement.
    c Some drugs are restraints.
    d A restraint is used when the nurse thinks it is needed.

18. Which is *not* a restraint alternative?
    a Positioning the person's chair close to a wall.
    b Answering signal lights promptly
    c Taking the person outside in nice weather
    d Padding walls and corners of furniture

19. Physical restraints
    a Control mental function
    b Control a behavior
    c Confine a person to a bed or chair
    d Decrease care needs

20. The following can occur because of restraints. Which is the *most* serious?
    a Fractures
    b Strangulation
    c Pressure ulcers
    d Urinary tract infection

Review Questions

21 A belt restraint is applied to a person in bed. Where should you tie the straps?
   a To the bed rails
   b To the head board
   c To the movable part of the bed frame
   d To the foot board

22 Mrs. Hall has a restraint. You should check her and the position of the restraint at least
   a Every 15 minutes
   b Every 30 minutes
   c Every hour
   d Every 2 hours

23 Mrs. Hall has mitt restraints. Which of these is especially important to report to the nurse?
   a Her heart rate
   b Her respiratory rate
   c Why the restraints were applied
   d If you felt a pulse in the restrained extremities

24 Which are *not* used to prevent falls?
   a Wrist restraints
   b Jacket restraints
   c Belt restraints
   d Vest restraints

25 The doctor ordered mitt restraints for Mrs. Hall. You need the following information from the nurse *except*
   a What size to use
   b What other equipment is needed
   c What drugs Mrs. Hall is taking
   d When to apply and release the restraints

26 A person has a vest restraint. It is not too tight or too loose if you can slide
   a A fist between the vest and the person
   b One finger between the vest and the person
   c An open hand between the vest and the person
   d Two fingers between the vest and the person

27 The correct way to apply any restraint is to follow the
   a Nurse's directions
   b Doctor's orders
   c Care plan
   d Manufacturer's instructions

Answers to these questions are on p. 390.

Review Question Answers

Chapter 1: Working in Long-Term Care

1. a
2. b
3. a
4. b
5. c
6. b
7. a
8. a
9. b
10. a
11. c
12. b
13. c
14. a
15. d
16. a
17. d
18. a
19. b
20. a
21. a
22. c
23. c
24. d
25. c
26. a
27. b
28. c
29. d
30. a
31. c

Chapter 2: Communication and Interpersonal Skills

1. d
2. c
3. d
4. c
5. d
6. d
7. a
8. c
9. d
10. b
11. a
12. d
13. b
14. d
15. c
16. a

17. d
18. c
19. c
20. b
21. a
22. b
23. b
24. c
25. c
26. b

Chapter 3: Preventing Infection

1. T
2. F
3. F
4. F
5. F
6. b
7. d
8. d
9. d
10. c
11. a
12. d
13. c
14. d
15. d
16. c

Chapter 4: Safety

1. F
2. T
3. T
4. T
5. F
6. T
7. F
8. T
9. T
10. T
11. F
12. a
13. a
14. c
15. d
16. d
17. a
18. b
19. d
20. b
21. d

22. d
23. a
24. c
25. b
26. c
27. b
28. d
29. d
30. b
31. c
32. d

Chapter 5: Basic Emergency Care

1. a
2. b
3. c
4. b
5. c
6. b
7. c
8. b
9. c
10. b
11. a
12. a
13. b
14. b

Chapter 6: Promoting Residents' Rights and Independence

1. a
2. c
3. b
4. a
5. d
6. b
7. a
8. b
9. a
10. c
11. c
12. c
13. d
14. b
15. b
16. d
17. b
18. a
19. c
20. b
21. c
22. a

Review Question Answers

Chapter 7: Measurements

1. c
2. b
3. c
4. c
5. a
6. a
7. d
8. b
9. c
10. a
11. b
12. c
13. c
14. b
15. c
16. d

Chapter 8: Care of the Resident's Environment

1. c
2. d
3. b
4. a
5. b
6. b
7. c
8. b
9. b
10. a
11. b
12. a
13. T
14. F
15. T
16. T
17. T

Chapter 9: Observing, Reporting, and Recording

1. c
2. d
3. c
4. d
5. d
6. d
7. c
8. c
9. d
10. c

Chapter 10: The Dying Person

1. b
2. b
3. a
4. b
5. a
6. d
7. c
8. a
9. b
10. b

Chapter 11: Oral Hygiene and Bathing

1. T
2. F
3. F
4. F
5. F
6. F
7. F
8. F
9. T
10. T
11. T
12. d
13. c
14. c
15. d

Chapter 12: Grooming

1. d
2. b
3. c
4. d
5. d
6. b
7. d
8. b
9. F
10. T
11. T
12. F

Chapter 13: Elimination

1. b
2. d
3. a
4. b

5. b
6. a
7. a
8. c
9. d
10. a
11. b
12. a
13. a
14. d
15. b

Chapter 14: Nutrition

1. b
2. a
3. d
4. d
5. a
6. c
7. c
8. d
9. c
10. c
11. b
12. a
13. c
14. c

Chapter 15: Skin Care

1. c
2. c
3. b
4. c
5. c
6. a
7. a
8. d
9. c
10. b

Review Question Answers

Chapter 16: Assisting With Moving and Positioning

1 a
2 b
3 a
4 b
5 a
6 a
7 a
8 b
9 b
10 a
11 d
12 c
13 c
14 b
15 a

Chapter 17: Mental Health Needs

1 c
2 d
3 d
4 a
5 c
6 b
7 c
8 d
9 b
10 c

Chapter 18: Care of Cognitively Impaired Residents

1 a
2 b
3 c
4 a
5 d
6 d
7 b
8 b
9 a
10 d
11 c
12 a

Chapter 19: Basic Restorative Care

1 c
2 b
3 a
4 b
5 c
6 b
7 b
8 c
9 a
10 b
11 c
12 b
13 a
14 d
15 a
16 c
17 c
18 T
19 T
20 T
21 F
22 F
23 T
24 T

Chapter 20: Restraint Alternatives and Safe Restraint Use

1 F
2 F
3 F
4 T
5 T
6 T
7 T
8 T
9 F
10 F
11 F
12 T
13 F
14 T
15 T
16 F
17 d
18 a
19 c
20 b
21 c
22 a
23 d
24 a
25 c
26 c
27 d

Appendix A

National Nurse Aide Assessment Program (NNAAP™)
Written (or Oral) Exam Content Outline

The NNAAP Written Examination is comprised of seventy (70) multiple choice questions. Ten (10) of these questions are pre-test (non-scored) questions on which statistical information will be collected.

The English or Spanish Oral Examination is comprised of sixty (60) multiple-choice questions and ten (10) word recognition (or reading comprehension) questions.

I. PHYSICAL CARE SKILLS

A. Activities of Daily Living ......7% of exam
1. Hygiene
2. Dressing and Grooming
3. Nutrition and Hydration
4. Elimination
5. Rest/Sleep/Comfort

B. Basic Nursing Skills ....37% of exam
1. Infection Control
2. Safety/Emergency
3. Therapeutic/Technical Procedures
4. Data Collection and Reporting

C. Restorative Skills ....5% of exam
1. Prevention
2. Self Care/Independence

II. PSYCHOSOCIAL CARE SKILLS

A. Emotional and Mental Health Needs ....10% of exam
B. Spiritual and Cultural Needs ....3% of exam

III. ROLE OF THE NURSE AIDE

A. Communication ....10% of exam
B. Client Rights ....15% of exam
C. Legal and Ethical Behavior ....5% of exam
D. Member of the Health Care Team ....8% of exam

National Nurse Aide Assessment Program (NNAAP™)
Skills Evaluation

LIST OF SKILLS

1. Washes hands
2. Measures and records weight of ambulatory client
3. Provides mouth care
4. Dresses client with affected right arm
5. Transfers client from bed to wheelchair
6. Assists client to ambulate
7. Cleans and stores dentures
8. Performs passive range-of-motion (ROM) for one shoulder
9. Performs passive range-of-motion (ROM) for one knee and one ankle
10. Measures and records urinary output
11. Assists clients with use of bedpan
12. Provides perineal care for incontinent client
13. Provides catheter care
14. Takes and records oral temperature
15. Takes and records radial pulse, and counts and records respirations
16. Takes and records client's blood pressure (one-step procedure)
17. Takes and records client's blood pressure (two-step procedure)
18. Puts one knee-high elastic stocking on client
19. Makes an occupied bed
20. Provides foot care
21. Provides fingernail care
22. Feeds client who cannot feed self
23. Positions client on side
24. Gives modified bed bath (face, and one arm, hand, and underarm)
25. Shampoos client's hair in bed

Numeric Identifier_____

MINIMUM DATA SET (MDS) — *VERSION 2.0*
FOR NURSING HOME RESIDENT ASSESSMENT AND CARE SCREENING

BASIC ASSESSMENT TRACKING FORM

SECTION AA. IDENTIFICATION INFORMATION

1.	RESIDENT NAME⊙	
		a. (First)　　b. (Middle Initial)　　c. (Last)　　d. (Jr/Sr)
2.	GENDER⊙	1. Male　　　　2. Female
3.	BIRTHDATE⊙	☐☐ — ☐☐ — ☐☐☐☐
		Month　　Day　　Year
4.	RACE/ ETHNICITY	1. American Indian/Alaskan Native　　4. Hispanic
		2. Asian/Pacific Islander　　5. White, not of
		3. Black, not of Hispanic origin　　Hispanic origin
5.	SOCIAL SECURITY⊙ AND MEDICARE NUMBERS⊙ [C in 1st box if non med. no.]	a. Social Security Number
		☐☐☐ — ☐☐ — ☐☐☐☐
		b. Medicare number (or comparable railroad insurance number)
		☐☐☐☐☐☐☐☐☐☐
6.	FACILITY PROVIDER NO.⊙	a. State No.
		☐☐☐☐☐☐☐☐☐☐☐
		b. Federal No.
		☐☐☐☐☐☐☐☐☐☐☐
7.	MEDICAID NO. ["+" if pending, "N" if not a Medicaid recipient]⊙	☐☐☐☐☐☐☐☐☐☐☐
8.	REASONS FOR ASSESS- MENT	[Note—Other codes do not apply to this form]

8. REASONS FOR ASSESSMENT

a. Primary reason for assessment
1. Admission assessment (required by day 14)
2. Annual assessment
3. Significant change in status assessment
4. Significant correction of prior full assessment
5. Quarterly review assessment
10. Significant correction of prior quarterly assessment
0. *NONE OF ABOVE*

b. *Codes for assessments required for Medicare PPS or the State*
1. *Medicare 5 day assessment*
2. *Medicare 30 day assessment*
3. *Medicare 60 day assessment*
4. *Medicare 90 day assessment*
5. *Medicare readmission/return assessment*
6. *Other state required assessment*
7. *Medicare 14 day assessment*
8. *Other Medicare required assessment*

9. Signatures of Persons who Completed a Portion of the Accompanying Assessment or Tracking Form

I certify that the accompanying information accurately reflects resident assessment or tracking information for this resident and that I collected or coordinated collection of this information on the dates specified. To the best of my knowledge, this information was collected in accordance with applicable Medicare and Medicaid requirements. I understand that this information is used as a basis for ensuring that residents receive appropriate and quality care, and as a basis for payment from federal funds. I further understand that payment of such federal funds and continued partici- pation in the government-funded health care programs is conditioned on the accuracy and truthful- ness of this information, and that I may be personally subject to or may subject my organization to substantial criminal, civil, and/or administrative penalties for submitting false information. I also certify that I am authorized to submit this information by this facility on its behalf.

Signature and Title	Sections	Date
a.		
b.		
c.		
d.		
e.		
f.		
g.		
h.		
i.		
j.		
k.		
l.		

GENERAL INSTRUCTIONS

Complete this information for submission with all full and quarterly assessments (Admission, Annual, Significant Change, State or Medicare required assessments, or Quarterly Reviews, etc.)

⊙ = Key items for computerized resident tracking

☐ = When box blank, must enter number or letter　　[a.] = When letter in box, check if condition applies

MDS 2.0 September, 2000

(From Centers for Medicare and Medicaid Services, http://cms.hhs.gov/medicaid/mds20)

Resident _____ Numeric Identifier _____

MINIMUM DATA SET (MDS) — *VERSION 2.0*
FOR NURSING HOME RESIDENT ASSESSMENT AND CARE SCREENING

BACKGROUND (FACE SHEET) INFORMATION AT ADMISSION

SECTION AB. DEMOGRAPHIC INFORMATION

1.	DATE OF ENTRY	*Date the stay began. Note — Does not include readmission if record was closed at time of temporary discharge to hospital, etc. In such cases, use prior admission date*

☐☐ — ☐☐ — ☐☐☐☐
Month — Day — Year

2.	ADMITTED FROM (AT ENTRY)	1. Private home/apt. with no home health services 2. Private home/apt. with home health services 3. Board and care/assisted living/group home 4. Nursing home 5. Acute care hospital 6. Psychiatric hospital, MR/DD facility 7. Rehabilitation hospital 8. Other	
3.	LIVED ALONE (PRIOR TO ENTRY)	0. No 1. Yes 2. In other facility	

4.	ZIP CODE OF PRIOR PRIMARY RESIDENCE	☐☐☐☐☐

5.	RESIDEN-TIAL HISTORY 5 YEARS PRIOR TO ENTRY	(*Check all settings* resident **lived in** during 5 years prior to date of entry given in item AB1 above)	
		Prior stay at this nursing home	a.
		Stay in other nursing home	b.
		Other residential facility—board and care home, assisted living, group home	c.
		MH/psychiatric setting	d.
		MR/DD setting	e.
		NONE OF ABOVE	f.

6.	LIFETIME OCCUPA-TION(S) [Put "/" between two occupations]	☐☐☐☐☐☐☐☐☐☐☐☐☐☐☐☐☐☐

7.	EDUCATION (*Highest Level Completed*)	1. No schooling 2. 8th grade/less 3. 9-11 grades 4. High school	5. Technical or trade school 6. Some college 7. Bachelor's degree 8. Graduate degree	
8.	LANGUAGE	(*Code for correct response*) **a.** Primary Language 0. English 1. Spanish 2. French 3. Other **b.** If other, specify		
9.	MENTAL HEALTH HISTORY	Does resident's RECORD indicate any history of mental retardation, mental illness, or developmental disability problem? 0. No 1. Yes		

10.	CONDITIONS RELATED TO MR/DD STATUS	(*Check all conditions* that are related to MR/DD status that were manifested before age 22, and are likely to continue indefinitely)	
		Not applicable—no MR/DD (Skip to AB11)	a.
		MR/DD with organic condition	
		Down's syndrome	b.
		Autism	c.
		Epilepsy	d.
		Other organic condition related to MR/DD	e.
		MR/DD with no organic condition	f.

11.	DATE BACK-GROUND INFORMA-TION COMPLETED	☐☐ — ☐☐ — ☐☐☐☐ Month — Day — Year

SECTION AC. CUSTOMARY ROUTINE

1.	CUSTOMARY ROUTINE	(*Check all that apply.* If all information UNKNOWN, check last box only.)	

(*In year prior to DATE OF ENTRY to this nursing home, or year last in community if now being admitted from another nursing home*)

CYCLE OF DAILY EVENTS

Stays up late at night (e.g., after 9 pm)	a.
Naps regularly during day (at least 1 hour)	b.
Goes out 1+ days a week	c.
Stays busy with hobbies, reading, or fixed daily routine	d.
Spends most of time alone or watching TV	e.
Moves independently indoors (with appliances, if used)	f.
Use of tobacco products at least daily	g.
NONE OF ABOVE	h.

EATING PATTERNS

Distinct food preferences	i.
Eats between meals all or most days	j.
Use of alcoholic beverage(s) at least weekly	k.
NONE OF ABOVE	l.

ADL PATTERNS

In bedclothes much of day	m.
Wakens to toilet all or most nights	n.
Has irregular bowel movement pattern	o.
Showers for bathing	p.
Bathing in PM	q.
NONE OF ABOVE	r.

INVOLVEMENT PATTERNS

Daily contact with relatives/close friends	s.
Usually attends church, temple, synagogue (etc.)	t.
Finds strength in faith	u.
Daily animal companion/presence	v.
Involved in group activities	w.
NONE OF ABOVE	x.
UNKNOWN—Resident/family unable to provide information	y.

SECTION AD. FACE SHEET SIGNATURES

SIGNATURES OF PERSONS COMPLETING FACE SHEET:

a. Signature of RN Assessment Coordinator	Date

I certify that the accompanying information accurately reflects resident assessment or tracking information for this resident and that I collected or coordinated collection of this information on the dates specified. To the best of my knowledge, this information was collected in accordance with applicable Medicare and Medicaid requirements. I understand that this information is used as a basis for ensuring that residents receive appropriate and quality care, and as a basis for payment from federal funds. I further understand that payment of such federal funds and continued participation in the government-funded health care programs is conditioned on the accuracy and truthfulness of this information, and that I may be personally subject to or may subject my organization to substantial criminal, civil, and/or administrative penalties for submitting false information. I also certify that I am authorized to submit this information by this facility on its behalf.

Signature and Title	Sections	Date
b.		
c.		
d.		
e.		
f.		
g.		

☐ = When box blank, must enter number or letter   ☐a. = When letter in box, check if condition applies

MDS 2.0 September, 2000

Resident _____ Numeric Identifier _____

MINIMUM DATA SET (MDS) — VERSION 2.0
FOR NURSING HOME RESIDENT ASSESSMENT AND CARE SCREENING
FULL ASSESSMENT FORM
(Status in last 7 days, unless other time frame indicated)

SECTION A. IDENTIFICATION AND BACKGROUND INFORMATION

1.	RESIDENT NAME	
		a. (First) **b.** (Middle Initial) **c.** (Last) **d.** (Jr/Sr)

2.	ROOM NUMBER	☐☐☐☐☐

3.	ASSESS-MENT REFERENCE DATE	**a.** Last day of MDS observation period
		☐☐ — ☐☐ — ☐☐☐☐
		Month Day Year
		b. Original (0) or corrected copy of form (enter number of correction)

4a.	DATE OF REENTRY	Date of reentry from most recent temporary discharge to a hospital in last 90 days (or since last assessment or admission if less than 90 days)
		☐☐ — ☐☐ — ☐☐☐☐
		Month Day Year

5.	MARITAL STATUS	1. Never married 3. Widowed 5. Divorced
		2. Married 4. Separated

6.	MEDICAL RECORD NO.	☐☐☐☐☐☐☐☐☐☐

7.	CURRENT PAYMENT SOURCES FOR N.H. STAY	(Billing Office to indicate; **check all that apply in last 30 days**)
		Medicaid per diem **a.**	VA per diem **f.**
		Medicare per diem **b.**	Self or family pays for full per diem **g.**
		Medicare ancillary part A **c.**	Medicaid resident liability or Medicare co-payment **h.**
		Medicare ancillary part B **d.**	Private insurance per diem (including co-payment) **i.**
		CHAMPUS per diem **e.**	Other per diem **j.**

8.	REASONS FOR ASSESS-MENT [Note—If this is a discharge or reentry assessment, only a limited subset of MDS items need be completed]	**a.** Primary reason for assessment
		1. Admission assessment (required by day 14)
		2. Annual assessment
		3. Significant change in status assessment
		4. Significant correction of prior full assessment
		5. Quarterly review assessment
		6. Discharged—return not anticipated
		7. Discharged—return anticipated
		8. Discharged prior to completing initial assessment
		9. Reentry
		10. Significant correction of prior quarterly assessment
		0. NONE OF ABOVE
		b. Codes for assessments required for Medicare PPS or the State
		1. Medicare 5 day assessment
		2. Medicare 30 day assessment
		3. Medicare 60 day assessment
		4. Medicare 90 day assessment
		5. Medicare readmission/return assessment
		6. Other state required assessment
		7. Medicare 14 day assessment
		8. Other Medicare required assessment

9.	RESPONSI-BILITY/ LEGAL GUARDIAN	(**Check all that apply**)
		Legal guardian **a.**	Durable power attorney/financial **d.**
		Other legal oversight **b.**	Family member responsible **e.**
		Durable power of attorney/health care **c.**	Patient responsible for self **f.**
			NONE OF ABOVE **g.**

10.	ADVANCED DIRECTIVES	(For those items with supporting **documentation** in the medical record, check all that apply)
		Living will **a.**	Feeding restrictions **f.**
		Do not resuscitate **b.**	Medication restrictions **g.**
		Do not hospitalize **c.**	Other treatment restrictions **h.**
		Organ donation **d.**	
		Autopsy request **e.**	NONE OF ABOVE **i.**

SECTION B. COGNITIVE PATTERNS

1.	COMATOSE	(Persistent vegetative state/no discernible consciousness)
		0. No 1. Yes (If yes, skip to Section G)

2.	MEMORY	(Recall of what was learned or known)
		a. Short-term memory OK—seems/appears to recall after 5 minutes
		0. Memory OK 1. Memory problem
		b. Long-term memory OK—seems/appears to recall long past
		0. Memory OK 1. Memory problem

3.	MEMORY/ RECALL ABILITY	(Check all that resident was **normally able to recall during last 7 days**)
		Current season **a.**	That he/she is in a nursing home **d.**
		Location of own room **b.**	
		Staff names/faces **c.**	NONE OF ABOVE are recalled **e.**

4.	COGNITIVE SKILLS FOR DAILY DECISION-MAKING	(Made decisions regarding tasks of daily life)
		0. INDEPENDENT—decisions consistent/reasonable
		1. MODIFIED INDEPENDENCE—some difficulty in new situations only
		2. MODERATELY IMPAIRED—decisions poor; cues/supervision required
		3. SEVERELY IMPAIRED—never/rarely made decisions

5.	INDICATORS OF DELIRIUM— PERIODIC DISOR-DERED THINKING/ AWARENESS	(Code for behavior in the **last 7 days**.) [Note: Accurate assessment requires conversations with staff and family who have direct knowledge of resident's behavior over this time].
		0. Behavior not present
		1. Behavior present, not of recent onset
		2. Behavior present, over last 7 days appears different from resident's usual functioning (e.g., new onset or worsening)
		a. EASILY DISTRACTED—(e.g., difficulty paying attention; gets sidetracked)
		b. PERIODS OF ALTERED PERCEPTION OR AWARENESS OF SURROUNDINGS—(e.g., moves lips or talks to someone not present; believes he/she is somewhere else; confuses night and day)
		c. EPISODES OF DISORGANIZED SPEECH—(e.g., speech is incoherent, nonsensical, irrelevant, or rambling from subject to subject; loses train of thought)
		d. PERIODS OF RESTLESSNESS—(e.g., fidgeting or picking at skin, clothing, napkins, etc; frequent position changes; repetitive physical movements or calling out)
		e. PERIODS OF LETHARGY—(e.g., sluggishness; staring into space; difficult to arouse; little body movement)
		f. MENTAL FUNCTION VARIES OVER THE COURSE OF THE DAY—(e.g., sometimes better, sometimes worse; behaviors sometimes present, sometimes not)

6.	CHANGE IN COGNITIVE STATUS	Resident's cognitive status, skills, or abilities have changed as compared to status of **90 days ago** (or since last assessment if less than 90 days)
		0. No change 1. Improved 2. Deteriorated

SECTION C. COMMUNICATION/HEARING PATTERNS

1.	HEARING	(With hearing appliance, if used)
		0. HEARS ADEQUATELY—normal talk, TV, phone
		1. MINIMAL DIFFICULTY when not in quiet setting
		2. HEARS IN SPECIAL SITUATIONS ONLY—speaker has to adjust tonal quality and speak distinctly
		3. HIGHLY IMPAIRED/absence of useful hearing

2.	COMMUNI-CATION DEVICES/ TECH-NIQUES	(**Check all that apply** during last 7 days)
		Hearing aid, present and used **a.**
		Hearing aid, present and not used regularly **b.**
		Other receptive comm. techniques used (e.g., lip reading) **c.**
		NONE OF ABOVE **d.**

3.	MODES OF EXPRESSION	(**Check all used** by resident to make needs known)
		Speech **a.**	Signs/gestures/sounds **d.**
		Writing messages to express or clarify needs **b.**	Communication board **e.**
			Other **f.**
		American sign language or Braille **c.**	NONE OF ABOVE **g.**

4.	MAKING SELF UNDER-STOOD	(Expressing information content—however able)
		0. UNDERSTOOD
		1. USUALLY UNDERSTOOD—difficulty finding words or finishing thoughts
		2. SOMETIMES UNDERSTOOD—ability is limited to making concrete requests
		3. RARELY/NEVER UNDERSTOOD

5.	SPEECH CLARITY	(Code for speech in the **last 7 days**)
		0. CLEAR SPEECH—distinct, intelligible words
		1. UNCLEAR SPEECH—slurred, mumbled words
		2. NO SPEECH—absence of spoken words

6.	ABILITY TO UNDER-STAND OTHERS	(Understanding verbal information content—however able)
		0. UNDERSTANDS
		1. USUALLY UNDERSTANDS—may miss some part/intent of message
		2. SOMETIMES UNDERSTANDS—responds adequately to simple, direct communication
		3. RARELY/NEVER UNDERSTANDS

7.	CHANGE IN COMMUNI-CATION/ HEARING	Resident's ability to express, understand, or hear information has changed as compared to status of **90 days ago** (or since last assessment if less than 90 days)
		0. No change 1. Improved 2. Deteriorated

☐ = When box blank, must enter number or letter ☐a. = When letter in box, check if condition applies

MDS 2.0 September, 2000

Resident _____ Numeric Identifier _____

SECTION D. VISION PATTERNS

1.	VISION	*(Ability to see in adequate light and with glasses if used)* 0. *ADEQUATE*—sees fine detail, including regular print in newspapers/books 1. *IMPAIRED*—sees large print, but not regular print in newspapers/books 2. *MODERATELY IMPAIRED*—limited vision; not able to see newspaper headlines, but can identify objects 3. *HIGHLY IMPAIRED*—object identification in question, but eyes appear to follow objects 4. *SEVERELY IMPAIRED*—no vision or sees only light, colors, or shapes; eyes do not appear to follow objects	
2.	VISUAL LIMITATIONS/ DIFFICULTIES	Side vision problems—decreased peripheral vision (e.g., leaves food on one side of tray, difficulty traveling, bumps into people and objects, misjudges placement of chair when seating self)	a.
		Experiences any of following: sees halos or rings around lights; sees flashes of light; sees "curtains" over eyes	b.
		NONE OF ABOVE	c.
3.	VISUAL APPLIANCES	Glasses; contact lenses; magnifying glass 0. No 1. Yes	

SECTION E. MOOD AND BEHAVIOR PATTERNS

| 1. | INDICATORS OF DEPRES- SION, ANXIETY, SAD MOOD | *(Code for indicators observed in last 30 days, Irrespective of the assumed cause)*
0. Indicator not exhibited in last 30 days
1. Indicator of this type exhibited up to five days a week
2. Indicator of this type exhibited daily or almost daily (6, 7 days a week) |

VERBAL EXPRESSIONS OF DISTRESS

a. Resident made negative statements—e.g., "*Nothing matters; Would rather be dead; What's the use; Regrets having lived so long; Let me die*"

b. Repetitive questions—e.g., "*Where do I go; What do I do?*"

c. Repetitive verbalizations—e.g., calling out for help, ("*God help me*")

d. Persistent anger with self or others—e.g., easily annoyed, anger at placement in nursing home; anger at care received

e. Self deprecation—e.g., "*I am nothing; I am of no use to anyone*"

f. Expressions of what appear to be unrealistic fears—e.g., fear of being abandoned, left alone, being with others

g. Recurrent statements that something terrible is about to happen—e.g., believes he or she is about to die, have a heart attack

h. Repetitive health complaints—e.g., persistently seeks medical attention, obsessive concern with body functions

i. Repetitive anxious complaints/concerns (non-health related) e.g., persistently seeks attention/reassurance regarding schedules, meals, laundry, clothing, relationship issues

SLEEP-CYCLE ISSUES

j. Unpleasant mood in morning

k. Insomnia/change in usual sleep pattern

SAD, APATHETIC, ANXIOUS APPEARANCE

l. Sad, pained, worried facial expressions—e.g., furrowed brows

m. Crying, tearfulness

n. Repetitive physical movements—e.g., pacing, hand wringing, restlessness, fidgeting, picking

LOSS OF INTEREST

o. Withdrawal from activities of interest—e.g., no interest in long standing activities or being with family/friends

p. Reduced social interaction

2.	MOOD PERSIS- TENCE	**One or more indicators** of depressed, sad or anxious mood **were not easily altered by attempts to "cheer up", console, or reassure the resident over last 7 days** 0. No mood 1. Indicators present, 2. Indicators present, indicators easily altered not easily altered	
3.	CHANGE IN MOOD	Resident's mood status has changed as compared to status of **90 days ago** (or since last assessment if less than 90 days) 0. No change 1. Improved 2. Deteriorated	
4.	BEHAVIORAL SYMPTOMS	**(A)** *Behavioral symptom **frequency in last 7 days*** 0. Behavior not exhibited in last 7 days 1. Behavior of this type occurred 1 to 3 days in last 7 days 2. Behavior of this type occurred 4 to 6 days, but less than daily 3. Behavior of this type occurred daily **(B)** *Behavioral symptom **alterability in last 7 days*** 0. Behavior not present OR behavior was easily altered 1. Behavior was not easily altered	(A) (B)
		a. WANDERING (moved with no rational purpose, seemingly oblivious to needs or safety)	
		b. VERBALLY ABUSIVE BEHAVIORAL SYMPTOMS (others were threatened, screamed at, cursed at)	
		c. PHYSICALLY ABUSIVE BEHAVIORAL SYMPTOMS (others were hit, shoved, scratched, sexually abused)	
		d. SOCIALLY INAPPROPRIATE/DISRUPTIVE BEHAVIORAL SYMPTOMS (made disruptive sounds, noisiness, screaming, self-abusive acts, sexual behavior or disrobing in public, smeared/threw food/feces, hoarding, rummaged through others' belongings)	
		e. RESISTS CARE (resisted taking medications/ injections, ADL assistance, or eating)	

| 5. | CHANGE IN BEHAVIORAL SYMPTOMS | Resident's behavior status has changed as compared to **status of 90 days ago** (or since last assessment if less than 90 days)
0. No change   1. Improved   2. Deteriorated | |

SECTION F. PSYCHOSOCIAL WELL-BEING

1.	SENSE OF INITIATIVE/ INVOLVE- MENT	At ease interacting with others	a.
		At ease doing planned or structured activities	b.
		At ease doing self-initiated activities	c.
		Establishes own goals	d.
		Pursues involvement in life of facility (e.g., makes/keeps friends; involved in group activities; responds positively to new activities; assists at religious services)	e.
		Accepts invitations into most group activities	f.
		NONE OF ABOVE	g.
2.	UNSETTLED RELATION- SHIPS	Covert/open conflict with or repeated criticism of staff	a.
		Unhappy with roommate	b.
		Unhappy with residents other than roommate	c.
		Openly expresses conflict/anger with family/friends	d.
		Absence of personal contact with family/friends	e.
		Recent loss of close family member/friend	f.
		Does not adjust easily to change in routines	g.
		NONE OF ABOVE	h.
3.	PAST ROLES	Strong identification with past roles and life status	a.
		Expresses sadness/anger/empty feeling over lost roles/status	b.
		Resident perceives that daily routine (customary routine, activities) is very different from prior pattern in the community	c.
		NONE OF ABOVE	d.

SECTION G. PHYSICAL FUNCTIONING AND STRUCTURAL PROBLEMS

1. **(A)** ADL SELF-PERFORMANCE—(**Code** for resident's **PERFORMANCE OVER ALL SHIFTS during last 7 days**—Not including setup)

   0. *INDEPENDENT*—No help or oversight —OR— Help/oversight provided only 1 or 2 times during last 7 days

   1. *SUPERVISION*—Oversight, encouragement or cueing provided 3 or more times during last 7 days —OR— Supervision (3 or more times) plus physical assistance provided only 1 or 2 times during last 7 days

   2. *LIMITED ASSISTANCE*—Resident highly involved in activity; received physical help in guided maneuvering of limbs or other nonweight bearing assistance 3 or more times —OR—More help provided only 1 or 2 times during last 7 days

   3. *EXTENSIVE ASSISTANCE*—While resident performed part of activity, over last 7-day period, help of following type(s) provided 3 or more times:
—Weight-bearing support
—Full staff performance during part (but not all) of last 7 days

   4. *TOTAL DEPENDENCE*—Full staff performance of activity during entire 7 days

   8. *ACTIVITY DID NOT OCCUR* during entire 7 days

   (B) ADL SUPPORT PROVIDED—(**Code** for **MOST SUPPORT PROVIDED OVER ALL SHIFTS during last 7 days**; code **regardless** of resident's self-performance classification)

   0. No setup or physical help from staff
   1. Setup help only
   2. One person physical assist   8. ADL activity itself did not
   3. Two+ persons physical assist   occur during entire 7 days

			(A) SELF-PERF	(B) SUPPORT
a.	BED MOBILITY	How resident moves to and from lying position, turns side to side, and positions body while in bed		
b.	TRANSFER	How resident moves between surfaces—to/from: bed, chair, wheelchair, standing position (EXCLUDE to/from bath/toilet)		
c.	WALK IN ROOM	How resident walks between locations in his/her room		
d.	WALK IN CORRIDOR	How resident walks in corridor on unit		
e.	LOCOMO- TION ON UNIT	How resident moves between locations in his/her room and adjacent corridor on same floor. If in wheelchair, self-sufficiency once in chair		
f.	LOCOMO- TION OFF UNIT	How resident moves to and returns from off unit locations (e.g., areas set aside for dining, activities, or treatments). **If facility has only one floor**, how resident moves to and from distant areas on the floor. If in wheelchair, self-sufficiency once in chair		
g.	DRESSING	How resident puts on, fastens, and takes off all items of **street clothing**, including donning/removing prosthesis		
h.	EATING	How resident eats and drinks (regardless of skill). Includes intake of nourishment by other means (e.g., tube feeding, total parenteral nutrition)		
i.	TOILET USE	How resident uses the toilet room (or commode, bedpan, urinal); transfer on/off toilet, cleanses, changes pad, manages ostomy or catheter, adjusts clothes		
j.	PERSONAL HYGIENE	How resident maintains personal hygiene, including combing hair, brushing teeth, shaving, applying makeup, washing/drying face, hands, and perineum (EXCLUDE baths and showers)		

Resident _____

2.	BATHING	How resident takes full-body bath/shower, sponge bath, and transfers in/out of tub/shower (EXCLUDE washing of back and hair.) **Code for most dependent** in self-performance and support. (A) BATHING SELF-PERFORMANCE codes appear below		(A)	(B)
		0. Independent—No help provided			
		1. Supervision—Oversight help only			
		2. Physical help limited to transfer only			
		3. Physical help in part of bathing activity			
		4. Total dependence			
		8. Activity itself did not occur during entire 7 days (*Bathing support codes are as defined in* **Item 1, code B above**)			

3.	TEST FOR BALANCE (see training manual)	(*Code for ability during test in the* **last 7 days**) 0. Maintained position as required in test 1. Unsteady, but able to rebalance self without physical support 2. Partial physical support during test; or stands (sits) but does not follow directions for test 3. Not able to attempt test without physical help	
		a. Balance while standing	
		b. Balance while sitting—position, trunk control	

4.	FUNCTIONAL LIMITATION IN RANGE OF MOTION (see training manual)	(*Code for limitations during* **last 7 days** *that interfered with daily functions or placed resident at risk of injury*) (A) *RANGE OF MOTION* (B) *VOLUNTARY MOVEMENT* 0. No limitation 0. No loss 1. Limitation on one side 1. Partial loss 2. Limitation on both sides 2. Full loss		(A)	(B)
		a. Neck			
		b. Arm—Including shoulder or elbow			
		c. Hand—Including wrist or fingers			
		d. Leg—Including hip or knee			
		e. Foot—Including ankle or toes			
		f. Other limitation or loss			

5.	MODES OF LOCOMOTION	(**Check all that apply** during **last 7 days**)		
		Cane/walker/crutch	a.	
		Wheeled self	b.	
		Other person wheeled	c.	
		Wheelchair primary mode of locomotion	d.	
		NONE OF ABOVE	e.	

6.	MODES OF TRANSFER	(**Check all that apply** during **last 7 days**)		
		Bedfast all or most of time	a.	
		Bed rails used for bed mobility or transfer	b.	
		Lifted manually	c.	
		Lifted mechanically	d.	
		Transfer aid (e.g., slide board, trapeze, cane, walker, brace)	e.	
		NONE OF ABOVE	f.	

7.	TASK SEGMENTATION	Some or all of ADL activities were broken into subtasks during **last 7 days** so that resident could perform them 0. No 1. Yes	

8.	ADL FUNCTIONAL REHABILITATION POTENTIAL	Resident believes he/she is capable of increased independence in at least some ADLs	a.
		Direct care staff believe resident is capable of increased independence in at least some ADLs	b.
		Resident able to perform tasks/activity but is very slow	c.
		Difference in ADL Self-Performance or ADL Support, comparing mornings to evenings	d.
		NONE OF ABOVE	e.

9.	CHANGE IN ADL FUNCTION	Resident's ADL self-performance status has changed as compared to status of **90 days ago** (or since last assessment if less than 90 days) 0. No change 1. Improved 2. Deteriorated	

SECTION H. CONTINENCE IN LAST 14 DAYS

1.	CONTINENCE SELF-CONTROL CATEGORIES (**Code for resident's PERFORMANCE OVER ALL SHIFTS**)
	0. *CONTINENT*—Complete control [*includes use of indwelling urinary catheter or ostomy device that does not leak urine or stool*]
	1. *USUALLY CONTINENT*—BLADDER, incontinent episodes once a week or less; BOWEL, less than weekly
	2. *OCCASIONALLY INCONTINENT*—BLADDER, 2 or more times a week but not daily; BOWEL, once a week
	3. *FREQUENTLY INCONTINENT*—BLADDER, tended to be incontinent daily, but some control present (e.g., on day shift); BOWEL, 2-3 times a week
	4. *INCONTINENT*—Had inadequate control BLADDER, multiple daily episodes; BOWEL, all (or almost all) of the time

a.	BOWEL CONTINENCE	Control of bowel movement, with appliance or bowel continence programs, if employed	
b.	BLADDER CONTINENCE	Control of urinary bladder function (if dribbles, volume insufficient to soak through underpants), with appliances (e.g., foley) or continence programs, if employed	

2.	BOWEL ELIMINATION PATTERN	Bowel elimination pattern regular—at least one movement every three days	a.	Diarrhea	c.
				Fecal impaction	d.
		Constipation	b.	NONE OF ABOVE	e.

Numeric Identifier _____

3.	APPLIANCES AND PROGRAMS	Any scheduled toileting plan	a.	Did not use toilet room/ commode/urinal	f.
		Bladder retraining program	b.	Pads/briefs used	g.
		External (condom) catheter	c.	Enemas/irrigation	h.
		Indwelling catheter	d.	Ostomy present	i.
		Intermittent catheter	e.	*NONE OF ABOVE*	j.

4.	CHANGE IN URINARY CONTINENCE	Resident's urinary continence has changed as compared to status of **90 days ago** (or since last assessment if less than 90 days) 0. No change 1. Improved 2. Deteriorated	

SECTION I. DISEASE DIAGNOSES

Check only those diseases that have a relationship to current ADL status, cognitive status, mood and behavior status, medical treatments, nursing monitoring, or risk of death. (Do not list inactive diagnoses)

1.	DISEASES	(*If none apply,* CHECK the NONE OF ABOVE box)			
		ENDOCRINE/METABOLIC/ NUTRITIONAL		Hemiplegia/Hemiparesis	v.
				Multiple sclerosis	w.
		Diabetes mellitus	a.	Paraplegia	x.
		Hyperthyroidism	b.	Parkinson's disease	y.
		Hypothyroidism	c.	Quadriplegia	z.
		HEART/CIRCULATION		Seizure disorder	aa.
		Arteriosclerotic heart disease (ASHD)	d.	Transient ischemic attack (TIA)	bb.
		Cardiac dysrhythmias	e.	Traumatic brain injury	cc.
		Congestive heart failure	f.	**PSYCHIATRIC/MOOD**	
		Deep vein thrombosis	g.	Anxiety disorder	dd.
		Hypertension	h.	Depression	ee.
		Hypotension	i.	Manic depression (bipolar disease)	ff.
		Peripheral vascular disease	j.	Schizophrenia	gg.
		Other cardiovascular disease	k.	**PULMONARY**	
		MUSCULOSKELETAL		Asthma	hh.
		Arthritis	l.	Emphysema/COPD	ii.
		Hip fracture	m.	**SENSORY**	
		Missing limb (e.g., amputation)	n.	Cataracts	jj.
		Osteoporosis	o.	Diabetic retinopathy	kk.
		Pathological bone fracture	p.	Glaucoma	ll.
		NEUROLOGICAL		Macular degeneration	mm.
		Alzheimer's disease	q.	**OTHER**	
		Aphasia	r.	Allergies	nn.
		Cerebral palsy	s.	Anemia	oo.
		Cerebrovascular accident (stroke)	t.	Cancer	pp.
				Renal failure	qq.
		Dementia other than Alzheimer's disease	u.	*NONE OF ABOVE*	rr.

2.	INFECTIONS	(*If none apply,* CHECK the NONE OF ABOVE box)			
		Antibiotic resistant infection (e.g., Methicillin resistant staph)	a.	Septicemia	g.
				Sexually transmitted diseases	h.
		Clostridium difficile (c. diff.)	b.	Tuberculosis	i.
		Conjunctivitis	c.	Urinary tract infection **in last 30 days**	j.
		HIV infection	d.	Viral hepatitis	k.
		Pneumonia	e.	Wound infection	l.
		Respiratory infection	f.	NONE OF ABOVE	m.

3.	OTHER CURRENT OR MORE DETAILED DIAGNOSES AND ICD-9 CODES	a. _____	| | | • | |
		b. _____	| | | • | |
		c. _____	| | | • | |
		d. _____	| | | • | |
		e. _____	| | | • | |

SECTION J. HEALTH CONDITIONS

1.	PROBLEM CONDITIONS	(**Check all problems present** in **last 7 days** unless other time frame is indicated)			
		INDICATORS OF FLUID STATUS		Dizziness/Vertigo	f.
				Edema	g.
		Weight gain or loss of 3 or more pounds within a 7 day period	a.	Fever	h.
				Hallucinations	i.
				Internal bleeding	j.
		Inability to lie flat due to shortness of breath	b.	Recurrent lung aspirations in **last 90 days**	k.
		Dehydrated; output exceeds input	c.	Shortness of breath	l.
				Syncope (fainting)	m.
		Insufficient fluid; did **NOT** consume all/almost all liquids provided during **last 3 days**	d.	Unsteady gait	n.
				Vomiting	o.
		OTHER		*NONE OF ABOVE*	p.
		Delusions	e.		

Resident ______________________ Numeric Identifier ______________________

2.	PAIN SYMPTOMS	(*Code the **highest level of pain** present in the **last 7 days***) **a. FREQUENCY** with which resident complains or shows evidence of pain 0. No pain (***skip to J4***) 1. Pain less than daily 2. Pain daily **b. INTENSITY** of pain 1. Mild pain 2. Moderate pain 3. Times when pain is horrible or excruciating
3.	PAIN SITE	(*If pain present, **check all sites** that apply in **last 7 days***) Back pain a. Bone pain b. Chest pain while doing usual activities c. Headache d. Hip pain e. Incisional pain f. Joint pain (other than hip) g. Soft tissue pain (e.g., lesion, muscle) h. Stomach pain i. Other j.
4.	ACCIDENTS	(***Check all that apply***) Fell in **past 30 days** a. Fell in **past 31-180 days** b. Hip fracture in **last 180 days** c. Other fracture in **last 180 days** d. *NONE OF ABOVE* e.
5.	STABILITY OF CONDITIONS	Conditions/diseases make resident's cognitive, ADL, mood or behavior patterns unstable—(fluctuating, precarious, or deteriorating) a. Resident experiencing an acute episode or a flare-up of a recurrent or chronic problem b. End-stage disease, 6 or fewer months to live c. *NONE OF ABOVE* d.

SECTION K. ORAL/NUTRITIONAL STATUS

1.	ORAL PROBLEMS	Chewing problem a. Swallowing problem b. Mouth pain c. *NONE OF ABOVE* d.
2.	HEIGHT AND WEIGHT	*Record (**a.**) **height in inches** and (**b.**) **weight in pounds**. Base weight on most recent measure in **last 30 days**; measure weight consistently in accord with standard facility practice—e.g., in a.m. after voiding, before meal, with shoes off, and in nightclothes* a. HT (in.) b. WT (lb.)
3.	WEIGHT CHANGE	**a. Weight loss**—5 % or more in **last 30 days**; or 10 % or more in **last 180 days** 0. No 1. Yes **b. Weight gain**—5 % or more in **last 30 days**; or 10 % or more in **last 180 days** 0. No 1. Yes
4.	NUTRITIONAL PROBLEMS	Complains about the taste of many foods a. Regular or repetitive complaints of hunger b. Leaves 25% or more of food uneaten at most meals c. *NONE OF ABOVE* d.
5.	NUTRITIONAL APPROACHES	(***Check all that apply in last 7 days***) Parenteral/IV a. Feeding tube b. Mechanically altered diet c. Syringe (oral feeding) d. Therapeutic diet e. Dietary supplement between meals f. Plate guard, stabilized built-up utensil, etc. g. On a planned weight change program h. *NONE OF ABOVE* i.
6.	PARENTERAL OR ENTERAL INTAKE	(***Skip to Section L if neither 5a nor 5b is checked***) **a.** Code the proportion of **total calories** the resident received through parenteral or tube feedings in the **last 7 days** 0. None 3. 51% to 75% 1. 1% to 25% 4. 76% to 100% 2. 26% to 50% **b.** Code the average **fluid intake** per day by IV or tube in **last 7 days** 0. None 3. 1001 to 1500 cc/day 1. 1 to 500 cc/day 4. 1501 to 2000 cc/day 2. 501 to 1000 cc/day 5. 2001 or more cc/day

SECTION L. ORAL/DENTAL STATUS

1.	ORAL STATUS AND DISEASE PREVENTION	Debris (soft, easily movable substances) present in mouth prior to going to bed at night a. Has dentures or removable bridge b. Some/all natural teeth lost—does not have or does not use dentures (or partial plates) c. Broken, loose, or carious teeth d. Inflamed gums (gingiva); swollen or bleeding gums; oral abcesses; ulcers or rashes e. Daily cleaning of teeth/dentures or daily mouth care—by resident or staff f. *NONE OF ABOVE* g.

SECTION M. SKIN CONDITION

1.	ULCERS (Due to any cause)	(*Record the number of ulcers at each ulcer stage—regardless of cause. If none present at a stage, record "0" (zero). Code all that apply during **last 7 days**. Code 9 = 9 or more.*) ***[Requires full body exam.]***	Number at Stage
		a. Stage 1. A persistent area of skin redness (without a break in the skin) that does not disappear when pressure is relieved.	
		b. Stage 2. A partial thickness loss of skin layers that presents clinically as an abrasion, blister, or shallow crater.	
		c. Stage 3. A full thickness of skin is lost, exposing the subcutaneous tissues - presents as a deep crater with or without undermining adjacent tissue.	
		d. Stage 4. A full thickness of skin and subcutaneous tissue is lost, exposing muscle or bone.	
2.	TYPE OF ULCER	(*For each type of ulcer, **code for the highest stage in the last 7 days** using scale in item M1—i.e., 0=none; stages 1, 2, 3, 4*) a. Pressure ulcer—any lesion caused by pressure resulting in damage of underlying tissue b. Stasis ulcer—open lesion caused by poor circulation in the lower extremities	
3.	HISTORY OF RESOLVED ULCERS	Resident had an ulcer that was resolved or cured **in LAST 90 DAYS** 0. No 1. Yes	
4.	OTHER SKIN PROBLEMS OR LESIONS PRESENT	(***Check all that apply** during **last 7 days***) Abrasions, bruises a. Burns (second or third degree) b. Open lesions other than ulcers, rashes, cuts (e.g., cancer lesions) c. Rashes—e.g., intertrigo, eczema, drug rash, heat rash, herpes zoster d. Skin desensitized to pain or pressure e. Skin tears or cuts (other than surgery) f. Surgical wounds g. *NONE OF ABOVE* h.	
5.	SKIN TREATMENTS	(***Check all that apply** during **last 7 days***) Pressure relieving device(s) for chair a. Pressure relieving device(s) for bed b. Turning/repositioning program c. Nutrition or hydration intervention to manage skin problems d. Ulcer care e. Surgical wound care f. Application of dressings (with or without topical medications) other than to feet g. Application of ointments/medications (other than to feet) h. Other preventative or protective skin care (other than to feet) i. *NONE OF ABOVE* j.	
6.	FOOT PROBLEMS AND CARE	(***Check all that apply** during **last 7 days***) Resident has one or more foot problems—e.g., corns, callouses, bunions, hammer toes, overlapping toes, pain, structural problems a. Infection of the foot—e.g., cellulitis, purulent drainage b. Open lesions on the foot c. Nails/calluses trimmed during **last 90 days** d. Received preventative or protective foot care (e.g., used special shoes, inserts, pads, toe separators) e. Application of dressings (with or without topical medications) f. *NONE OF ABOVE* g.	

SECTION N. ACTIVITY PURSUIT PATTERNS

1.	TIME AWAKE	(***Check appropriate time periods over last 7 days***) Resident awake all or most of time (i.e., naps no more than one hour per time period) in the: Morning a. Afternoon b. Evening c. *NONE OF ABOVE* d.
(If resident is comatose, skip to Section O)		
2.	AVERAGE TIME INVOLVED IN ACTIVITIES	**(When awake and not receiving treatments or ADL care)** 0. Most—more than 2/3 of time 2. Little—less than 1/3 of time 1. Some—from 1/3 to 2/3 of time 3. None
3.	PREFERRED ACTIVITY SETTINGS	(***Check all settings** in which activities are **preferred***) Own room a. Day/activity room b. Inside NH/off unit c. Outside facility d. *NONE OF ABOVE* e.
4.	GENERAL ACTIVITY PREFERENCES (adapted to resident's current abilities)	(***Check all PREFERENCES** whether or not activity is currently available to resident*) Cards/other games a. Crafts/arts b. Exercise/sports c. Music d. Reading/writing e. Spiritual/religious activities f. Trips/shopping g. Walking/wheeling outdoors h. Watching TV i. Gardening or plants j. Talking or conversing k. Helping others l. *NONE OF ABOVE* m.

Resident_____   Numeric Identifier_____

5.	PREFERS CHANGE IN DAILY ROUTINE	Code for resident preferences in daily routines 0. No change 1. Slight change 2. Major change	
		a. Type of activities in which resident is currently involved	
		b. Extent of resident involvement in activities	

SECTION O. MEDICATIONS

1.	NUMBER OF MEDICA-TIONS	(*Record the number of different* medications used in the **last 7 days**; enter "0" if none used)	
2.	NEW MEDICA-TIONS	(*Resident currently receiving medications that were initiated during the* **last 90 days**) 0. No 1. Yes	
3.	INJECTIONS	(***Record the number of DAYS*** injections of any type received during the **last 7 days**; enter "0" if none used)	
4.	DAYS RECEIVED THE FOLLOWING MEDICATION	(***Record the number of DAYS*** during **last 7 days**; enter "0" if not used. Note—enter "1" for long-acting meds used less than weekly)	

a. Antipsychotic		d. Hypnotic
b. Antianxiety		e. Diuretic
c. Antidepressant		

SECTION P. SPECIAL TREATMENTS AND PROCEDURES

1.	SPECIAL TREAT-MENTS, PROCE-DURES, AND PROGRAMS	a. SPECIAL CARE—**Check** treatments or programs received during the **last 14 days**

TREATMENTS		PROGRAMS	
		Ventilator or respirator	l.
Chemotherapy	a.	**PROGRAMS**	
Dialysis	b.	Alcohol/drug treatment program	m.
IV medication	c.		
Intake/output	d.	Alzheimer's/dementia special care unit	n.
Monitoring acute medical condition	e.	Hospice care	o.
Ostomy care	f.	Pediatric unit	p.
Oxygen therapy	g.	Respite care	q.
Radiation	h.	Training in skills required to return to the community (e.g., taking medications, house work, shopping, transportation, ADLs)	r.
Suctioning	i.		
Tracheostomy care	j.		
Transfusions	k.	NONE OF ABOVE	s.

b. **THERAPIES** - Record the number of days and total minutes each of the following therapies was administered (for at least 15 minutes a day) in the **last 7 calendar days** (Enter 0 if none or less than 15 min. daily) [Note—count only post admission therapies]

(A) = # of days administered for **15 minutes or more** (B) = total # of minutes provided in **last 7 days**	DAYS (A)	MIN (B)
a. Speech - language pathology and audiology services		
b. Occupational therapy		
c. Physical therapy		
d. Respiratory therapy		
e. Psychological therapy (by any licensed mental health professional)		

2.	INTERVEN-TION PROGRAMS FOR MOOD, BEHAVIOR, COGNITIVE LOSS	(Check all interventions or strategies used in last 7 days—no matter where received)	
		Special behavior symptom evaluation program	a.
		Evaluation by a licensed mental health specialist in **last 90 days**	b.
		Group therapy	c.
		Resident-specific deliberate changes in the environment to address mood/behavior patterns—e.g., providing bureau in which to rummage	d.
		Reorientation—e.g., cueing	e.
		NONE OF ABOVE	f.

3.	NURSING REHABILITA-TION/RESTOR-ATIVE CARE	Record the NUMBER OF DAYS each of the following rehabilitation or restorative techniques or practices was **provided to the resident for more than or equal to 15 minutes per day in the last 7 days** (Enter 0 if none or less than 15 min. daily.)

a. Range of motion (passive)		f. Walking	
b. Range of motion (active)		g. Dressing or grooming	
c. Splint or brace assistance		h. Eating or swallowing	
TRAINING AND SKILL PRACTICE IN:		i. Amputation/prosthesis care	
d. Bed mobility		j. Communication	
e. Transfer		k. Other	

4.	DEVICES AND RESTRAINTS	(*Use the following codes for **last 7 days**:*) 0. Not used 1. Used less than daily 2. Used daily	
		Bed rails	
		a. — Full bed rails on all open sides of bed	
		b. — Other types of side rails used (e.g., half rail, one side)	
		c. Trunk restraint	
		d. Limb restraint	
		e. Chair prevents rising	
5.	HOSPITAL STAY(S)	Record number of times resident was admitted to hospital with an overnight stay **in last 90 days** (or since last assessment if less than 90 days). (*Enter 0 if no hospital admissions*)	
6.	EMERGENCY ROOM (ER) VISIT(S)	Record number of times resident visited ER without an overnight stay **in last 90 days** (or since last assessment if less than 90 days). (*Enter 0 if no ER visits*)	
7.	PHYSICIAN VISITS	In the **LAST 14 DAYS** (or since admission if less than 14 days in facility) how many days has the physician (or authorized assistant or practitioner) examined the resident? (*Enter 0 if none*)	
8.	PHYSICIAN ORDERS	In the **LAST 14 DAYS** (or since admission if less than 14 days in facility) how many days has the physician (or authorized assistant or practitioner) changed the resident's orders? *Do not include order renewals without change.* (*Enter 0 if none*)	
9.	ABNORMAL LAB VALUES	Has the resident had any abnormal lab values during the **last 90 days** (or since admission)? 0. No 1. Yes	

SECTION Q. DISCHARGE POTENTIAL AND OVERALL STATUS

1.	DISCHARGE POTENTIAL	a. Resident expresses/indicates preference to return to the community 0. No 1. Yes	
		b. Resident has a support person who is positive towards discharge 0. No 1. Yes	
		c. Stay projected to be of a short duration— discharge projected **within 90 days** (do not include expected discharge due to death) 0. No 2. Within 31-90 days 1. Within 30 days 3. Discharge status uncertain	

2.	OVERALL CHANGE IN CARE NEEDS	Resident's overall self sufficiency has changed significantly as compared to status of **90 days ago** (or since last assessment if less than 90 days)
		0. No change 1. Improved—receives fewer 2. Deteriorated—receives
		               supports, needs less more support
		               restrictive level of care	

SECTION R. ASSESSMENT INFORMATION

1.	PARTICIPA-TION IN ASSESS-MENT	a. Resident: 0. No 1. Yes	
		b. Family: 0. No 1. Yes 2. No family	
		c. Significant other: 0. No 1. Yes 2. None	

2. **SIGNATURE OF PERSON COORDINATING THE ASSESSMENT:**

a. Signature of RN Assessment Coordinator (sign on above line)

b. Date RN Assessment Coordinator signed as complete

	—	—	
Month		Day	Year

Resident _____   Numeric Identifier _____

SECTION T. THERAPY SUPPLEMENT FOR MEDICARE PPS

1.	SPECIAL TREAT-MENTS AND PROCE-DURES	**a. RECREATION THERAPY**—*Enter number of days and total minutes of recreation therapy administered (**for at least 15 minutes a day**) in the last 7 days* (*Enter 0 if none*)

		DAYS (A)	MIN (B)
(A) = # of days administered for 15 minutes or more			
(B) = total # of minutes provided in last 7 days			

Skip unless this is a Medicare 5 day or Medicare readmission/ return assessment.

b. ORDERED THERAPIES—*Has physician ordered any of following therapies to begin in FIRST 14 days of stay—physical therapy, occupational therapy, or speech pathology service?*
0. No   1. Yes

If not ordered, skip to item 2

c. Through day 15, provide an estimate of the number of days when at least 1 therapy service can be expected to have been delivered.

d. Through day 15, provide an estimate of the number of therapy minutes (across the therapies) that can be expected to be delivered?

2.	WALKING WHEN MOST SELF SUFFICIENT	*Complete item 2 if ADL self-performance score for TRANSFER (G.1.b.A) is 0,1,2, or 3 AND at least one of the following are present:*

- Resident received physical therapy involving gait training (P.1.b.c)
- Physical therapy was ordered for the resident involving gait training (T.1.b)
- Resident received nursing rehabilitation for walking (P.3.f)
- Physical therapy involving walking has been discontinued within the past 180 days

Skip to item 3 if resident did not walk in last 7 days

(FOR FOLLOWING FIVE ITEMS, BASE CODING ON THE EPISODE WHEN THE RESIDENT WALKED THE FARTHEST WITHOUT SITTING DOWN. INCLUDE WALKING DURING REHABILITATION SESSIONS.)

a. Furthest distance walked without sitting down during this episode.

0. 150+ feet   3. 10-25 feet
1. 51-149 feet   4. Less than 10 feet
2. 26-50 feet

b. Time walked without sitting down during this episode.

0. 1-2 minutes   3. 11-15 minutes
1. 3-4 minutes   4. 16-30 minutes
2. 5-10 minutes   5. 31+ minutes

c. Self-Performance in walking during this episode.

0. *INDEPENDENT*—No help or oversight
1. *SUPERVISION*—Oversight, encouragement or cueing provided
2. *LIMITED ASSISTANCE*—Resident highly involved in walking; received physical help in guided maneuvering of limbs or other nonweight bearing assistance
3. *EXTENSIVE ASSISTANCE*—Resident received weight bearing assistance while walking

d. Walking support provided associated with this episode (code regardless of resident's self-performance classification).

0. No setup or physical help from staff
1. Setup help only
2. One person physical assist
3. Two+ persons physical assist

e. Parallel bars used by resident in association with this episode.

0. No   1. Yes

3.	CASE MIX GROUP	Medicare						State					

MDS 2.0 September, 2000

SECTION V. RESIDENT ASSESSMENT PROTOCOL SUMMARY   Numeric Identifier _____

Resident's Name:	Medical Record No.:

1. Check if RAP is triggered.

2. For each triggered RAP, use the RAP guidelines to identify areas needing further assessment. Document relevant assessment information regarding the resident's status.

   • Describe:
   — Nature of the condition (may include presence or lack of objective data and subjective complaints).
   — Complications and risk factors that affect your decision to proceed to care planning.
   — Factors that must be considered in developing individualized care plan interventions.
   — Need for referrals/further evaluation by appropriate health professionals.

   • Documentation should support your decision-making regarding whether to proceed with a care plan for a triggered RAP and the type(s) of care plan interventions that are appropriate for a particular resident.

   • Documentation may appear anywhere in the clinical record (e.g., progress notes, consults, flowsheets, etc.).

3. Indicate under the Location of RAP Assessment Documentation column where information related to the RAP assessment can be found.

4. For each triggered RAP, indicate whether a new care plan, care plan revision, or continuation of current care plan is necessary to address the problem(s) identified in your assessment. The Care Planning Decision column must be completed within 7 days of completing the RAI (MDS and RAPs).

A. RAP PROBLEM AREA	(a) Check if triggered	Location and Date of RAP Assessment Documentation	(b) Care Planning Decision—check if addressed in care plan
1. DELIRIUM			
2. COGNITIVE LOSS			
3. VISUAL FUNCTION			
4. COMMUNICATION			
5. ADL FUNCTIONAL/ REHABILITATION POTENTIAL			
6. URINARY INCONTINENCE AND INDWELLING CATHETER			
7. PSYCHOSOCIAL WELL-BEING			
8. MOOD STATE			
9. BEHAVIORAL SYMPTOMS			
10. ACTIVITIES			
11. FALLS			
12. NUTRITIONAL STATUS			
13. FEEDING TUBES			
14. DEHYDRATION/FLUID MAINTENANCE			
15. DENTAL CARE			
16. PRESSURE ULCERS			
17. PSYCHOTROPIC DRUG USE			
18. PHYSICAL RESTRAINTS			

B.

1. Signature of RN Coordinator for RAP Assessment Process _____   2. ☐☐ — ☐☐ — ☐☐☐☐
   Month   Day   Year

3. Signature of Person Completing Care Planning Decision _____   4. ☐☐ — ☐☐ — ☐☐☐☐
   Month   Day   Year

MDS 2.0 September, 2000

RESIDENT ASSESSMENT PROTOCOL TRIGGER LEGEND FOR REVISED RAPS (FOR MDS VERSION 2.0)

Key:
- ● = One item required to trigger
- ❷ = Two items required to trigger
- ★ = One of these three items, plus at least one other item required to trigger
- @ = When both ADL triggers present, maintenance takes precedence

Proceed to RAP Review once triggered

MDS ITEM		CODE	Delirium	Cognitive Loss/Dementia	Visual Function	Communication	ADL-Rehabilitation Trigger A @	ADL-Maintenance Trigger B @	Urinary Incontinence and Indwelling Catheter	Psychosocial Well-Being	Mood State	Behavioral Symptoms	Activities Trigger A	Activities Trigger B	Falls	Nutritional Status	Feeding Tubes	Dehydration/Fluid Maintenance	Dental Care	Pressure Ulcers	Psychotropic Drug Use	Physical Restraints	MDS ITEM
B2a	Short term memory	1		●																			B2a
B2b	Long term memory	1		●																			B2b
B4	Decision making	1,2,3		●																			B4
B4	Decision making	3					●																B4
B5a to B5f	Indicators of delirium	2	●																		●		B5a to B5f
B6	Change in cognitive status	2	●																		●		B6
C1	Hearing	1,2,3				●																	C1
C4	Understood by others	1,2,3				●																	C4
C6	Understand others	1,2,3		●		●																	C6
C7	Change in communication	2																			●		C7
D1	Vision	1,2,3			●																		D1
D2a	Side vision problem	√			●																		D2a
E1a to E1p	Indicators of depression, anxiety, sad mood	1,2									●												E1a to E1p
E1n	Repetitive movement	1,2																			●		E1n
E1o	Withdrawal from activities	1,2								●													E1o
E2	Mood persistence	1,2									●												E2
E3	Change in mood	2	●																		●		E3
E4aA	Wandering	1,2,3											●										E4aA
E4aA - E4eA	Behavioral symptoms	1,2,3										●											E4aA - E4cA
E5	Change in behavioral symptoms	1										●											E5
E5	Change in behavioral symptoms	2	●																		●		E5
F1d	Establishes own goals	√								●													F1d
F2a to F2d	Unsettled relationships	√								●													F2a to F2d
F3a	Strong id, past roles	√								●													F3a
F3b	Lost roles	√								●													F3b
F3c	Daily routine different	√								●													F3c
G1aA - G1jA	ADL self-performance	1,2,3,4					●																G1aA - G1jA
G1aA	Bed mobility	2,3,4,8																		●			G1aA
G2A	Bathing	1,2,3,4					●																G2A
G3b	Balance while sitting	1,2,3																		●			G3b
G6a	Bedfast	√																		●			G6a
G8a,b	Resident, staff believe capable	√					●																G8a,b
H1a	Bowel incontinence	1,2,3,4																		●			H1a
H1b	Bladder incontinence	2,3,4							●														H1b
H2b	Constipation	√																			●		H2b
H2d	Fecal impaction	√																			●		H2d
H3c,d,e	Catheter use	√							●														H3c,d,e
H3g	Use of pads/briefs	√							●														H3g
I1i	Hypotension	√																			●		I1i
I1j	Peripheral vascular disease	√																		●			I1j
I1ee	Depression	√																			●		I1ee
I1jj	Cataracts	√			●																		I1jj
I1ll	Glaucoma	√			●																		I1ll
I2j	UTI	√																●					I2j
I3	Dehydration diagnosis	276.5																●					I3
J1a	Weight fluctuation	√																●					J1a
J1c	Dehydrated	√																●					J1c
J1d	Insufficient fluid	√																●					J1d
J1f	Dizziness	√													●						●		J1f
J1h	Fever	√																●					J1h
J1i	Hallucinations	√																			●		J1i
J1j	Internal bleeding	√																●					J1j
J1k	Lung aspirations	√																			●		J1k
J1m	Syncope	√																			●		J1m

RESIDENT ASSESSMENT PROTOCOL TRIGGER LEGEND FOR REVISED RAPS (FOR MDS VERSION 2.0)

Key:
- ● = One item required to trigger
- ❷ = Two items required to trigger
- ★ = One of these three items, plus at least one other item required to trigger
- @ = When both ADL triggers present, maintenance takes precedence

Proceed to RAP Review once triggered

MDS ITEM		CODE	Delirium	Cognitive Loss/Dementia	Visual Function	Communication	ADL-Rehabilitation Trigger A @	ADL-Maintenance Trigger B @	Urinary Incontinence and Indwelling Catheter	Psychosocial Well-Being	Mood State	Behavioral Symptoms	Activities Trigger A	Activities Trigger B	Falls	Nutritional Status	Feeding Tubes	Dehydration/Fluid Maintenance	Dental Care	Pressure Ulcers	Psychotropic Drug Use	Physical Restraints	
J1n	Unsteady gait	√																				●	J1n
J4a,b	Fell	√													●							●	J4a,b
J4c	Hip fracture	√													●							●	J4c
K1b	Swallowing problem	√																				●	K1b
K1c	Mouth pain	√																	●				K1c
K3a	Weight loss	1														●							K3a
K4a	Taste alteration	√														●							K4a
K4c	Leave 25% food	√														●							K4c
K5a	Parenteral/IV feeding	√														●		●					K5a
K5b	Feeding tube	√															●	●					K5b
K5c	Mechanically altered	√														●							K5c
K5d	Syringe feeding	√														●							K5d
K5e	Theraputic diet	√														●							K5e
L1a,c,d,e	Dental	√																	●				L1a,c,d,e
L1f	Daily cleaning teeth	Not √																	●				L1f
M2a	Pressure ulcer	2,3,4													●								M2a
M2a	Pressure ulcer	1,2,3,4																		●			M2a
M3	Previous pressure ulcer	1																		●			M3
M4e	Impaired tactile sense	√																		●			M4e
N1a	Awake morning	√								❷													N1a
N2	Involved in activities	0								❷													N2
N2	Involved in activities	2,3										●											N2
N5a,b	Prefers change in daily routine	1,2										●											N5a,b
O4a	Antipsychotics	1-7																			★		O4a
O4b	Antianxiety	1-7													●						★		O4b
O4c	Antidepressants	1-7													●						★		O4c
O4e	Diuretic	1-7																●					O4e
P4c	Trunk restraint	1,2													●							●	P4c
P4c	Trunk restraint	2																		●			P4c
P4d	Limb restraint	1,2																				●	P4d
P4e	Chair prevents rising	1,2																				●	P4e

Appendix C

USEFUL SPANISH VOCABULARY AND PHRASES*

CHAPTER 1: WORKING IN LONG-TERM CARE

Miss	señorita.
	(seh-nyoh-ree-tah)
Mrs.	señora
	(seh-nyoh-rah)
Mr.	señor
	(seh-nyohr)
Hello!	¡Hola!
	(Oh-lah)
I am going to cover you.	Lo voy acubrir
	(Loh boy ah-koo-breer)
Excuse me.	Con permiso.
	(kohn pehr-mee-soh)
Good morning, sir.	Buenos días, señor.
	(Boo-eh-nohs dee-ahs, seh-nyohr)
Good afternoon.	¡Buenas tardes!
	(Boo-eh-nahs tahr-dehs)
How may I help you?	¿En qué puedo servirle?
	(Ehn keh poo-eh-doh sehr-beer-leh)
Thank you for talking to me!	¡Gracias por hablar conmigo!
	(Grah-see-ahs pohr ah-blahr kohn-mee-goh)
Good morning, doctor!	!Buenos días, doctor!
	(Boo-eh-nohs dee-ahs, dohk-tohr)
You are welcome.	De nada.
	(Deh nah-dah)
employ	emplear
	(ehm-pleh-ahr)
My name is . . .	Mi nobres es . . ./Me llamo . . .
	(Mee nohm-breh ehs/Meh yah-moh)
Please!	¡Por favor!
	(Pohr fah-bohr)
Thank you!	¡Gracias!
	(Grah-see-ahs)

---

* This appendix is presented for your convenience. Please note: This listing does not include all chapters; only those for which vocabulary and phrases directly relate to the content in this textbook.

Translations taken from Joyce EV, Villanueva ME: *Say it in Spanish: A Guide for Health Care Professionals*, ed 3, Philadelphia, 2000, WB Saunders.

Thank you very much!	¡Muchas gracias!
	(Moo-chahs grah-see-ahs)
What can I help you with?	¿En qué puedo ayudarlo?
	(Ehn keh poo-eh-doh ah-yoo-dahr-loh)
Yes, sir.	Sí, señor.
	(See, seh-nyohr)

CHAPTER 2: COMMUNICATION AND INTERPERSONAL SKILLS

Number	English	Spanish	Pronunciation
1	one	uno	(oo-noh)
2	two	dos	(dohs)
3	three	tres	(trehs)
4	four	cuatro	(koo-ah-troh)
5	five	cinco	(seen-koh)
6	six	seis	(seh-ees)
7	seven	siete	(see-eh-teh)
8	eight	ocho	(oh-choh)
9	nine	nueve	(noo-eh-beh)
10	ten	diez	(dee-ehs)
11	eleven	once	(ohn-seh)
12	twelve	doce	(doh-seh)
13	thirteen	trece	(treh-seh)
14	fourteen	catorce	(kah-tohr-seh)
15	fifteen	quince	(keen-seh)
16	sixteen	dieciséis	(dee-ehs-ee-seh-ees)
17	seventeen	diecisiete	(dee-ehs-ee-see-eh-teh)
18	eighteen	dieciocho	(dee-ehs-ee-oh-choh)
19	nineteen	diecinueve	(dee-ehs-ee-noo-eh-beh)
20	twenty	veinte	(beh-een-teh)
30	thirty	treinta	(treh-een-tah)
40	forty	cuarenta	(koo-ah-rehn-tah)
50	fifty	cincuenta	(seen-koo-ehn-tah)
60	sixty	sesenta	(seh-sehn-tah)
70	seventy	setenta	(seh-tehn-tah)
80	eighty	ochenta	(oh-chehn-tah)
90	ninety	noventa	(noh-behn-tah)
100	one hundred	cien	(see-ehn)

abdomen	abdomen
	(ahb-doh-mehn)
communication	comunicación
	(koh-moo-nee-kah-see-ohn)
black	negro
	(neh-groh)
blue	azul
	(ah-sool)
clear	claro
	(klah-roh)
green	verde
	(behr-deh)
red	rojo
	(roh-hoh)
yellow	amarillo
	(ah-mah-ree-yoh)
white	blanco
	(blahn-koh)
Monday	lunes
	(loo-nehs)
Tuesday	martes
	(mahr-tehs)
Wednesday	miércoles
	(mee-ehr-koh-lehs)
Thursday	jueves
	(hoo-eh-behs)
Friday	viernes
	(bee-ehr-nehs)
Saturday	sábado
	(sah-bah-doh)
Sunday	domingo
	(doh-meen-goh)
what?	¿qué?/¿qué tal?
	(keh/keh tahl)
when?	¿cuándo?
	(koo-ahn-doh)
where?	¿dónde?
	(dohn-deh)

why?	¿por qué?
	(pohr keh)
for whom?	¿para quién?
	(pah-rah kee-ehn)
for what?	¿para qué?
	(pah-rah keh)
which?	¿cuál?
	(koo-ahl)
who?	¿quién?
	(kee-ehn)
how many?	¿cuántos?
	(koo-ahn-tohs)
how much?	¿cuánto?
	(koo-ahn-toh)
no, not	no
	(noh)
no one, nobody	nadie
	(nah-dee-eh)
nothing	nada
	(nah-dah)
never, not ever	nunca, jamás
	(noon-kah, hah-mahs)
neither	tampoco
	(tahm-poh-koh)
neither . . . nor	ni . . . ni
	(nee . . . nee)
not one, not any	ninguno
	(neen-goo-noh)
without	sin
	(seen)
Every two hours.	Cada dos horas.
	(Kah-dah dohs oh-rahs)
Hello, I'm John Goodguy.	Hola, soy John Goodguy.
	(Oh-lah, soh-ee John Goodguy)
Hello, Mrs. Mora.	Hola, señora Mora.
	(Oh-lah, seh-nyoh-rah Moh-rah)
How are you?	¿Cómo está?
	(Koh-moh ehs-tah)

How do you feel?	¿Cómo te sientes?
	(Koh-moh teh see-ehn-tehs)
How do you feel now?	¿Cómo se siente ahora?
	(Koh-moh seh see-ehn-teh ah-oh-rah)
Let me know how you feel.	Dígame cómo se siente.
	(Dee-gah-meh koh-moh seh see-ehn-teh)
My name is . . .	Mi nombre es . . ./Me llamo . . .
	(Mee nohm-breh ehs/Meh yah-moh)s
Good-bye!	¡Hasta luego!
	(Ahs-tah loo-eh-goh)
Hi!	!Hola!
	(Oh-lah)
Good morning.	Buenos días.
	(Boo-eh-nohs dee-ahs)
Good afternoon.	Buenas tardes.
	(Boo-eh-nahs tahr-dehs)
Good evening.	Buenas noches.
	(Boo-ch-nahs noh-chehs)
Do you speak English?	¿Habla inglés?
	(Ah-blah een-glehs)
Thank you!	¡Gracias!
	(Grah-see-ahs)
Thank you very much!	¡Muchas gracias!
	(Moo-chahs grah-see-ahs)
You are welcome.	De nada.
	(Deh nah-dah)
respect	respeto
	(rehs-peh-toh)
the family	la familia
	(lah fah-mee-lee-ah)
father	padre
	(pah-dreh)
dad	papá
	(pah-pah)
mother	madre
	(mah-dreh)
mom	mamá
	(mah-mah)

husband	esposo
	(ehs-poh-soh)
wife	esposa
	(ehs-poh-sah)
sister	hermana
	(ehr-mah-nah)
brother	hermano
	(ehr-mah-noh)
son	hijo
	(ee-hoh)
daughter	hija
	(ee-hah)
niece	sobrina
	(soh-bree-nah)
nephew	sobrino
	(soh-bree-noh)
grandmother	abuela
	(ah-boo-eh-lah)
grandfather	abuelo
	(ah-boo-eh-loh)
grandparents	abuelos
	(ah-boo-eh-lohs)
aunt	tía
	(tee-ah)
uncle	tío
	(tee-oh)
stepfather	padrastro
	(pah-drahs-troh)
stepmother	madrastra
	(mah-drahs-trah)
stepson	hijastro
	(ee-hahs-troh)
stepdaughter	hijastra
	(ee-hahs-trah)
children	hijos
	(eeh-hohs)
great-grandparents	bisabuelos
	(bee-sah-boo-eh-lohs)

mother-in-law	suegra (soo-eh-grah)
father-in-law	suegro (soo-eh-grah)
sister-in-law	cuñada (koo-nyah-dah)
brother-in-law	cuñado (koo-nyah-doh)
cousins	primos (pree-mohs)
cousin (female)	prima (pree-mah)
cousin (male)	primo (pree-moh)
grandchildren	nietos (nee-eh-tohs)
godparents	padrinos (pah-dree-nohs)
godfather	padrino (pah-dree-noh)
godmother	madrina (mah-dree-nah)
Do you understand?	¿Comprende?/¿Entiende? (Kohm-prehn-deh/ Ehn-tee-ehn-deh)
Are you cold?	¿Tiene frío? (Tee-eh-neh free-oh)
Are you hot?	¿Tiene calor? (tee-eh-neh kah-lohr)
Are you hungry?	¿Tiene hambre? (Tee-eh-neh ahm-breh)
Are you sleepy?	¿Tiene sueño? (Tee-eh-neh soo-eh-nyoh)
Are you thirsty?	¿Tiene sed? (Tee-eh-neh sehd)
Is that enough?	¿Es suficiente? (Ehs soo-fee-see-ehn-teh)
Is that a lot?	¿Es mucho? (Ehs moo-choh)

Is that too much?	¿Es demasiado?
	(Ehs deh-mah-see-ah-doh)
Are you comfortable?	¿Está cómoda?
	(Ehs tah koh-moh-dah)
A nurse will see you.	Una enfermera la atenderá.
	(Ooh-nah ehn-fehr-meh-rah lah ah-tehn-deh-rah)
Good!	¡Bueno!
	(Boo-eh-noh)
Good afternoon, Miss González.	Buenas tardes, señorita González.
	(Boo-eh-nahs tahr-dehs, seh-nyoh-ree-tah Gohn-sah-lehs)
Good luck!	¡Buena suerte!
	(Boo-eh-nah soo-ehr-teh)
Have a good day!	¡Pase un buen día!
	(Pah-seh oon boo-ehn dee-ah)
Hello.	Hola
	(Oh-lah)
I am through.	Ya terminé.
	(Yah tehr-mee-neh)
I will see you tomorrow.	Le veré mañana.
	(Lah beh-reh mah-nyah-nah)
I will return shortly.	Regresaré en seguida.
	(Reh-greh-sah-reh ehn seh-ghee-dah)
If you don't understand, please let me know.	Si no entiende, dígame por favor.
	(See noh ehn-tee-ehn-deh, dee-gah-meh pohr fah-bohr)

CHAPTER 3: PREVENTING INFECTION

Wash well all fruits and vegetables.	Lave bien frutas y verduras.
	(Lah-beh bee-ehn froo-tahs ee behr-doo-rahs)
Wash hands before eating.	Lave las manos antes de comer.
	(Lah-beh lahs mah-nohs ahn-tehs deh koh-mehr)
bacteria	Bacteria
	(bahk-teh-ree-ah)
inflammation	Inflamación
	(een-flah-mah-see-ohn)
pathogen	Patogénico
	(pah-toh-heh-nee-koh)

What causes AIDS?

¿Qué causa el SIDA?

(Keh kah-oo-sah ehl see-dah)

A virus known as HIV

El virus causal del SIDA se conoce como VIH . . .

(Ehl bee-roos kah-oo-sahl dehl see-dah seh koh-noh-seh koh-moh beh-ee-ah- cheh[VIH])

Who is at risk of getting AIDS?

¿Quién está en riesgo de contraer el SIDA?

(Kee-ehn ehs-tah ehn ree-ehs- goh deh kohn-trah-ehr ehl see-dah)

sexually active homosexual and
  bisexual males or females

homosexuales activos y hombres o mujeres
  bisexuales

(oh-moh-sehx-oo-ah-lehs ahk-tee-bohs ee ohm-brehs oh moo-heh-rehs bee-sehx- oo-ah-lehs)

intravenous drug abusers

los que abusan de las drogas intravenosas

(lohs keh ah-boo-sah deh lahs droh-gahs een-trah- beh-noh-sahs)

hemophiliacs and recipients of blood/
  blood components

hemofílicos, donadores de sangre o transfusión con
  sangre contaminada

(eh-moh-fee-lee-kohs, doh- nah-doh-rehs deh sahn-greh oh trahns-foo-see-ohn kohn sahn-greh kohn-tah- mee-nah-dah)

fetus of infected mothers

fetos de madres contamnadas

(feh-tohs deh mah-drehs kohn-tah-mee-nah-dahs)

Infected persons can transmit the virus.

Las personas infectadas pueden transmitir el virus

(Lahs pehr-soh-nahs een fehk-tah-dahs poo-ehdehn-trahns-mee-teer ehl bee-roos)

Can casual contact cause AIDS?

¿Los contactos eventaules puden causar SIDA?

(Lohs kohn-tahk-tohs eh- behn-too-ah-lehspoo-eh-dehn kah-oo-sahr see-dah)

HIV is not transmissible by casual contact, nor . . .

El VIH no es transmitido en forma casual, ni por . . .

(Ehl VIH noh ehs trahns-mee-tee-doh ehn fohr-mah kah-soo-ahl, nee pohr:)

living in the same house as infected persons

vivir en la misma casa con personas infectadas

(bee-beer ehn lah mees-mah kah-sah kohn pehr-soh-nahs een-fehk-tah-dahs)

eating food handled by persons with AIDS

comer comida preparada por personas infectadas
  con SIDA

(koh-mehr koh-mee-dah preh-pah-rah-dah pohr pehr-soh-nahs een-fehk- tah-dahs kohn see-dah)

coughing, sneezing, kissing, or swimming
  with infected persons

tos, estornudo, besar, o nadar con personas
  infectadas

(tohs, ehs-tohr-noo-doh, beh-sahr oh nah-dahr kohn pehr-soh-nahs een-fehk-tah-dahs)

How serious is AIDS?

¿Qué tan serio es el SIDA?

(Keh tahn seh-ree-oh ehs- ehl see-dah)

Is there a danger from donated blood?

¿Qué peligro hay por sangre donada?

(Keh peh-lee-groh ah-ee pohr sahn-greh doh-nah-dah)

The risk of contracting HIV is not high.

Blood banks and other centers use sterile equipment and disposable needles.

El riesgo de contraer VIH no es alto. Los bancos de sangre y otros centros usan equipos estériles y agujas desechables.

(Ehl ree-ehs-goh deh kohn-trah-ehr VIH noh ehs ahl-toh. Lohns bahn-kohs deh sahn-greh ee oh-trohs sehn-trohs oo-sahn eh-kee- pohs ehs-teh-ree-lehs ee ah-goo-hahs deh-seh-chah- blehs)

The U.S. Public Health Service recommends:

El Departamento de Salud Pública de los Estados Unidos recomienda:

(Ehl Deh-pahr-tah-mehn-toh deh Sah-lood Poo-blee-kah deh lohs Ehs-tah-dohs Oo- nee-dohs reh-koh-mee- ehn-dah)

1. Know sexual background/habits of partners.

1. Conozca los hábitos sexuales de su pareja.

(Koh-nohs-kah lohs ah-bee-tohs sex-oo-ah-lehs deh soo pah-reh-hah)

2. Use a condom or prophylactic.

2. Use un condón o profiláctico.

(Oo-seh oon kohn-dohn oh proh-fee-lahk-tee-koh)

3. If your partner is in a high-risk group, cease sexual relations.

3. Si su compañera está en el grupo de alto riesgo, suspenda las relaciones sexuales.

(See soo kohm-pah-nyeh-rah ehs-tah ehn ehl groo-pah deh ahl-toh ree-ehs-goh, soos-pehn-dah lahs reh- lah-see-ohn-ehs sehx-oo- ahl-ehs)

4. Eliminate multiple sexual partners.

4. Elimine múltiples compa—eros sexuales.

(Eh-lee-mee-neh mool-tee- plehs kohm-pha-nyeh-rohs sehx-oo-ah-lehs)

5. Don't use intravenous drugs with contaminated needles; don't share needles or syringes.

5. No use drogas intravenosas con agujas contami-nadas; no comparta aguijas o jeringas.

(Noh oos-eh droh-gahs een-trah-veh-noh-sahs kohn ah-goo-hahs kohn-tah- mee-nah-dahs; noh kohm-pahr-tah ah-goo-hahs oh hehr-een-gahs)

hepatitis

hepatits

(eh-pah-tee-tees)

CHAPTER 4: SAFETY

What can I help you with?

¿En qué puedo ayudarlo?

(Ehn keh poo-eh-doh ah-yoo-dahr-loh)

This is the call bell.

Este es el timbre.

(Ehs-teh ehs ehl teem-breh)

coma

coma

(koh-mah)

comatose	comatoso
	(koh-mah-toh-soh)
Call if you need help.	Llame si necesita ayuda.
	(Yah-meh see neh-seh-see-tah ah-yoo-dah)
No smoking.	No se permite fumar.
	(Noh seh pehr-mee-teh foo-mahr)
Wear this bracelet all the time.	Use esta pulsera todo el tiempo.
	(Oo-seh ehs-tah pool-seh-rah toh-doh ehl tee-ehm-poh)
You cannot smoke here.	No puede fumar aquí.
	(Noh poo-eh-deh foo-mahr ah-kee)
You cannot smoke in your room.	No puede fumar en el cuatro.
	(Noh poo-eh-deh foo-mahr ehn ehl koo-ahr-toh)

CHAPTER 5: BASIC EMERGENCY CARE

We are going to the hospital.	Vamos al hospital.
	(Bah-mohs ahl ohs-pee-tahl)
We are going in the ambulance.	Vamos en la ambulancia.
	(Bah-mohs ehn lah ahm-boo-lahn-see-ah)
cardiac	cardíaco
	(kahr-dee-ah-koh)

CHAPTER 6: PROMOTING RESIDENT'S RIGHTS AND INDEPENDENCE

sex	sexo
	(sehx-oh)
sexual	sexual
	(sehx-oo-ahl)

CHAPTER 7: MEASUREMENTS

I will start by taking vital signs.	Voy a empezar por tomar los signos vitales.
	(Boy ah ehm-peh-sahr pohr toh-mahr lohs seeg-nohs bee-tah-lehs)
Take the temperature rectally.	Tome la temperatura por el recto.
	(Toh-meh lah tehm-peh-rah-too-rah pohr ehl rehk-toh)
bradycardia	bradicardia
	(brah-dee-kahr-dee-ah)
fever	fatal
	(fah-tahl)
pulse	pulso
	(pool-soh)

rectal

rectal

(rehk-tahl)

stethoscope

estetoscopio

(ehs-teh-tohs-koh-pee-oh)

systole

sístole

(sees-toh-leh)

thermometer

termómetro

(tehr-moh-meh-troh)

I will take the radial pulse.

Voy a tomar su pulso radial.

(Boy ah toh-mahr soo pool- soh rah-dee-ahl)

I will take your blood pressure.

Voy a tomar tu presión de sangre.

(Boy ah toh-mahr too preh- see-ohn deh sahn-greh)

asthma

asma

(ahs-mah)

CHAPTER 8: CARE OF THE RESIDENT'S ENVIRONMENT

These buttons move the bed up/down.

Estos botones mueven la cama arriba/abajo.

(Ehs-tohs boh-tah-nehs moo-eh-behn lah kay-mah ah-ree-bah/ah-bah-hoh)

You can raise the head.

Puede levantar la cabeza.

(Poo-eh-deh leh-bahn-tahr lah kah-beh-sah)

You can raise the feet.

Puede levantar los pies.

(Poo-eh-deh leh-bahn-tahr lohs pee-ehs)

The rails lower down.

El barandal se baja.

(Ehl bah-rahn-dahl seh bah-hah)

Your towels are in the bathroom.

Sus toallas están en el baño.

(Soos too-ahyahs ehs-tahn ehn ehl bah-nyoh)

There is an emergency light.

Hay una luz para emergencias.

(Ah-ee oo-nah loos pah-rah eh-mehr-hehn-see-ahs)

Pull the cord in the bathroom.

Jale el cordón en el baño.

(Hah-leh ehl kohr-dohn ehn ehl bah-nyoh)

The bell will sound.

La campana sonará.

(Lah kahm-pah-nah soh-nah-rah)

This button lowers (raises) the headboard.

Este botón baha (sube) la cabecera de la cama.

(Ehs-teh boh-tohn bah-hah (soo-beh) lah kah-beh-seh-rah deh lah kah-mah)

The chair turns into a bed.

Esta silla se hace cama.

(Ehs-tah see-yah seh ah-seh kah-mah)

This is the radio.	Este es el radio.
	(Ehs-teh ehs ehl rah-dee-oh)
This is the call bell/buzzer.	Este es la campana/el timbre.
	(Ehs-teh ehs lah kahm- pah-nah/ehl teem-breh)
You have a private bathroom.	Tiene un baño/inodoro privado.
	(Tee-eh-neh oon bah-nyoh/ee-noh-doh-roh pree-bah-doh)
linen	Lino
	(lee-noh)
Do you need more pillows?	¿Necesita más almohadas?
	(Neh-seh-see-tah mahs ahl-moh-ah-dahs)

CHAPTER 9: OBSERVING, REPORTING, AND RECORDING

Do you know where we are?	¿Sabe dónde está?
	(Sah-beh dohn-deh ehs-tah)
Do you know the day?	¿Qué día es hoy?
	(Keh dee-ah ehs oh-ee)
Where does it hurt?	¿Dónde le duele?
	(Don-deh leh doo-eh-leh)
Point.	Apunte./Señale.
	(Ah-poon-teh/Seh-nyah-leh)
Did you fall?	¿Se cayó?
	(Seh kah-yoh)
Do you have any symptoms: nausea, dizziness, other unusual feelings?	¿Tiene algún síntoma como náuseas, vértigo, otra sensación rara?
	(Tee-eh-neh ahl-goon seen-toh-mah koh-moh nah-oo-seh-ahs, behr-tee- goh, oh-trah sehn-sah- see-ohn rah-rah)
Does the pain move from one place to another?	¿El dolor se mueve de un lugar a otro?
	(Ehl doh-lohr seh moo-eh-beh deh oon loo-gahr ah oh-trah)
Does the pain get better if you stop and rest?	¿Se mejora el dolor si se detiene y descansa?
	(Seh meh-hoh-rah ehl doh-lohr see seh deh-tee- eh-neh ee dehs-kahn-sah)
Has the pain gotten worse or gotten better?	¿Se ha puesto el dolor peor o mejor?
	(Seh ah poo-ehs-toh ehl doh-lohr peh-ohr oh meh-hohr)
How often do you have the pain?	¿Qué tan seguido tiene el dolor?
	(Keh tahn seh-gee-doh tee-eh-neh ehl doh-lohr)
How severe is the pain?	¿Qué tan severo es el dolor?
	(Keh tahn seh-beh-roh ehs ehl doh-lohr)

On a scale from 1 [insignificant] to 10 [unbearable]	En una escala del 1 [insignificante] al 10 [intolerable]:
	(Ehn oo-nah ehs-kah-lah dehl oo-noh [een-seeg-nee-fee-kahn-teh] ahl deeehs [een- toh-leh-rah-bleh])
Is the pain there all the time, or does it come and go?	¿Está el dolor allí todo el tiempo, o va y viene?
	(Ehs-tah ehl doh-lohr ah- yee toh-doh ehl tee-ehm-poh, oh bah ee bee- ehn-eh?)
What caused the pain?	¿Qué causó el dolor?
	(Keh kah-oo-soh ehl doh-lohr)
What did you do that caused the pain?	¿Qué hacía cuando apareció el dolor?
	(Keh ah-see-ah koo-ahn-doh ah-pah-reh-see-oh ehl doh-lohr)
What makes the pain better?	¿Qué hace mejorar el dolor?
	(Keh ah-seh meh-hoh-rahr ehl doh-lohr)
What is wrong?	¿Qué pasa?
	(Keh pah-sah)
Is there any pain?	¿Tiene algún dolor?
	(Tee-eh-neh ahl-goon doh-lohr)
What is hurting you?	¿Qué le duele?
	(Keh leh doo-eh-leh)
How are you?	¿Cómo está?
	(Koh-moh ehs-tah)
Do you have vision problems?	¿Tienes problemas con la visión?
	(Tee-eh-nehs proh-bleh-mahs kohn lah bee-see-ohn)
Do you wear glasses?	¿Usas anteojos/lentes?
	(Oo-sahs ahn-teh-ohhohs/lehn-tehs)
Do you have problems with your teeth?	¿Tienes promblemas con los dientes?
	(Tee-eh-nehs prog-bleh-mahs kohn lohs dee-ehn-tehs)
At what time do you go to sleep?	¿A qué hora te acuestas a dormir?
	(Ah keh oh-rah teh ah-koo- ehs-tahs ah dohr-meer)
How many hours do you sleep?	¿Cuantás horas duermes?
	(Koo-ahn-tahs oh-rahs doo-ehr-mehs)
Do you wake up at night?	¿Te despiertas en la noche?
	(Teh dehs-pee-ehr-tahs ehn lah noh-che)
Have you had headaches?	¿Ha tenido dolor de cabeza?
	(Ah teh-nee-doh doh-lohr deh kah-beh-sah)
Do you have dizzy spells?	¿Tiene mareos?
	(Tee-eh-neh mah-reh-ohs)
Swelling of the ankles?	¿Hinchazón en los tobillos?
	(Een-chah-sohn ehn lohs toh-bee-yohs)

nausea	náusea
	(nah-oo-seh-ah)
normal	normal
	(nohr-mahl)
Are you nauseated?	¿Está nauseado?/¿Tiene náuseas?
	(Ehs-tah nah-oo-seh-ah-doh/Tee-eh-neh nah-oo-seh-ahs)
Are you okay?	¿Está bien?/¿Se siente bien?
	(Ehs-tah bee-ehn/Seh see-ehn-teh bee-ehn)
Do you feel nauseated?	¿Se siente nauseado?
	(Seh see-ehn-teh nah-oo- seh-ah-doh)
Do you feel weak?	¿Se siente débril?
	(Seh see-ehn-teh deh-beel)
Do you have pain?	¿Tiene dolor?
	(Tee-eh-neh doh-lohr)
Is there any pain?	¿Tiene algún dolor?
	(Tee-eh-neh ahl-goon doh-lohr)
Is there anything that worries you?	¿Hay algo que le preocupa?
	(Ah-ee ahl-goh keh leh preh-oh-koo-pah)
Is there anything else bothering you?	¿Hay otra cosa que le moleste?
	(Ah-ee oh-trah koh-sah keh-leh moh-lehs-teh)
Is there numbness/a tingling sensation/burning in your leg/arm/foot/hand?	¿Está entumecido/adormecido/tiene ardor en su pierna/brazo/pie/mano?
	(Ehs-tah ehn-too-meh-see- doh/ah-dohr-meh-see-do/ tee-eh-neh ahr-dohr chn soo pee-ehr-nah/brah-soh/pee-eh/mah-noh)
Tell me if there is pain.	Dime si duele.
	(Dee-meh see doo-eh-leh)
Tell me if it hurts.	Dime si esto te duele.
	(Dee-meh see ehs-toh teh doo-eh-leh)
The pain is in one place?	¿El dolor es fijo?
	(Ehl doh-lohr ehs fee-hoh)
The pain is localized, sharp.	El dolor está fijo, agudo.
	(Ehl doh-lohr ehs-tah ehn ehl lah-dohl kohs-tah-doh)
The pain is on the side.	El dolor está en el lado/costado.
	(Ehl doh-lohr ehs-tah ehn ehl lah-dohl kohs-tah-doh)
The pain is sharp?	¿El dolor es agudo?
	(Ehl doh-lohr ehs ah-goo-doh)
What brought you to the hospital?	¿Qué lo trajo al hospital?
	(Keh loh trah-hoh ahl ohs-pee-tahl)

What is the matter?	¿Qué le pasa/sucede?
	(Keh leh pah-sah/soo-seh-deh)
What is the pain like?	¿Qué tipo de dolor tiene?
	(Keh tee-oh deh doh-lohr tee-eh-neh)
What other discomfort do you have?	¿Qué otra molestia tiene?
	(Keh oh-trah moh-lehs-tee-ah tee-eh-neh)
What symptoms do you have?	¿Qué síntomas tiene?
	(Keh seen-toh-mahs tee-eh-neh)
When you have pain, do you get nauseated?	Cuando tiene dolor, ¿le dan náuseas?
	(Koo-ahn-doh tee-eh-neh doh-lohr, leh dahn nah-oo-seh-ahs)

Time	Standard	Military (hours P.M.)
one o'clock	la una	las trece horas
	(la oo-nah)	(lahs treh-seh oh-rahs)
two o'clock	las dos	las catorce horas
	(lahs dohs)	(lahs kah-tohr-seh oh-rahs)
three o'clock	las tres	las quince horas
	(lahs trehs)	(lahs keen-seh oh-rahs)
four o'clock	las cuatro	las dieciséis horas
	(lahs koo-ah-troh)	(lahs dee-ehs-ee-seh-ees oh-rahs)
five o'clock	las cinco	las diecisiete horas
	(lahs seen-koh)	(lahs dee-ehs-ee-see-eh-teh oh-rahs)
six o'clock	las seis	las dieciocho horas
	(lahs seh-ees)	(lahs dee-ehs-ee-oh-choh oh-rahs)
seven o'clock	las siete	las diecinueve horas
	(lahs see-eh-teh)	(lahs dee-ehs-ee-noo-eh-beh oh-rahs)
eight o'clock	las ocho	las veinte horas
	(lahs oh-choh)	(lahs beh-een-teh oh-rahs)
nine o'clock	las nueve	las veintiuna horas
	(lahs noo-eh-beh)	(lahs beh-een-tee-oo-nah oh-rahs)
ten o'clock	las diez	las veintidós horas
	(lahs dee-ehs)	(lahs beh-een-tee-dohs oh-rahs)
eleven o'clock	las once	las veintitrés horas
	(lahs ohn-seh)	(lahs beh-een-tee-trehs oh-rahs)
twelve o'clock/midnight	las doce/la media noche	las cero horas
	(lahs doh-seh/lah meh-dee-ah non-cheh)	(lahs seh-roh-oh-rahs)
		las veinticuatro horas
		(lahs beh-een-tee-koo-ah-troh oh-rahs)

CHAPTER 10: THE DYING PERSON

cancer

cáncer

(kahn-sehr)

CHAPTER 11: ORAL HYGIENE AND BATHING

I am going to clean your teeth.

Voy a limpairle los dientes.

(Boy ah leem-pee-ahr-leh lohs dee-ehn-tehs)

Rinse your mouth.

Enjuague su boca.

(Ehn-hoo ah-geh soo boh-kah)

Here is a glass of water to rinse with.

Aquí está un vaso de agua para que se enjuague.

(Ah-kee-ehs-tah oon bah-soh deh ah-goo-ah pah-rah keh seh ehn-hoo-ah-geh)

Open your mouth, please.

Abra la boca, por favor.

(Ah-brah lah boh-kah, pohr fah-bohr)

I am going to insert your dentures.

Voy a ponerle la dentadura.

(Boh-ee ah poh-hehr-leh lah dehn-tah-doo-rah)

There is a shower.

Hay una ducha/regadera.

(Ah-ee oo-nah doo-chah/reh-gah-deh-rah)

There is also a bathtub/tub.

También hay una bañera/tina.

(Tahm-bee-ehn ah-ee oo-nah bah-nych-rah/tee-nah)

Use dental floss.

Use hilo dental.

(Oo-seh ee-loh dehn-tahl)

CHAPTER 12: GROOMING

Mrs. . . ., I need to help you change clothes.

Señora . . ., necesito ayudarle a cambiar su ropa.

(Se–ora . . ., neh-seh-see-toh ah-yoo-dahr-leh ah kahm-bee-ahr soo roh-pah)

CHAPTER 13: ELIMINATION

When was the last time you used the toilet?

¿Cuándo fue la última vez gue hizo del baño/que obró?

(Koo-ahn doh foo-eh lah ool-tee-mah behs keh ee-soh dehl bah-nyoh/ keh oh-broh)

How often do you urinate?

¿Cuántas veces ornia?

(Koo-ahn-tahs beh-sehs oh-ree-nah)

Do you want the bedpan?

¿Quiere el pato/el bacín?

(Kee-eh-reh ehl pah-toh/ehl bah-seen)

Do you have problems with starting to urinate?

¿Tiene dificultad para empezar a orinar?

(Tee-eh-neh dee-fee-kool-tahd pah-rah ehm-peh-sahr ah oh-ree-nahr)

Do you want to pass urine?

¿Quiere orinar?

(Kee-eh-reh oh-ree-nahr)

Everytime you go to the bathroom to void, you must place the urine in the container.

Cada vez que vaya al baño a orinar, debe poner la orina en el recipiente.

(Kah-dah behs keh bah-yah ahl bah-nyoh ah oh-ree-nahr, deh-beh poh-nehr lah oh-ree-nah ehn ehl reh-see- pee-ehn-teh)

I will ask you to void.

Le diré que orine.

(Leh dee-reh keh oh-ree-neh)

Are you constipated?

¿Está esterñido?

(Ehs-tah ehs-treh-nyee-doh)

Do you have diarrhea?

¿Tiene diarrea?

(Tee-eh-neh dee-ah-reh-ah)

Do you wish to have a bowel movement?

¿Quiere evacuar/hacer del baño?

(Kee-eh-reh eh-bah-koo-ahr/ah-sehr dehl bah-nyoh)

A bowel movement.

Hacer del baño.

(Ah-sehr dehl bah-nyoh)

Do you want to have a bowel movement?

¿Quiere evacuar?¿Quiere obrar?

(Kee-eh-reh eh-bah-koo-ahr/Kee-eh-reh oh-brahr)

I will collect a sample of feces.

Voy a recoger una muestra de excremento.

(Boy ah reh-koh-hehr oo-nah moo-ehs-trah deh ehx-kreh-mehn-toh)

CHAPTER 14: NUTRITION

Have you eaten?

¿Ha comido?

(Ah koh-mee-doh)

What did you eat?

¿Qué comido?

(Keh koh-mee-doh)

Do you take a special diet?

¿Toma dieta especial?

(Toh-mah dee-eh-tah ehs- peh-see-ah-lehs)

What foods do you like?

¿Qué alimentos le gustan?

(Keh ah-lee-mehn-tohs leh goos-tahn)

What foods do you dislike?

¿Qué alimentos le disgustan?

(Keh ah-lee-mehn-tohs leh dees-goos-tahn)

How many times do you eat per day?

¿Cuántas veces come por día?

(Koo-ahn-tahs beh-sehs koh- meh pohr dee-ah)

What did you eat for breakfast?

¿Qué comió en el desayuno?

(Keh koh-mee-oh ehn ehl deh-sah-yoo-noh)

I am going to give you a list.

Voy a darle una lista.

(Boy ah dahr-leh oo-nah lees-tah)

For breakfast:	Para el desayuno:
	(Pah-rah ehl deh-sah- yoo-noh)
eggs	huevos (oo-eh-bohs)
toast	pan tostado
	(pahn tohs-tah-doh)
coffee	café
	(kah-feh)
milk	leche
	(leh-cheh)
juice	jugo
	(joo-goh)
fruit	fruta
	(froo-tah)
How do you like your coffee?	¿Comó le gusta el café?
	(Koh-moh leh goos-tah ehl kah-feh)
black	negro
	(neh-groh)
with cream	con crema
	(kohn kreh-mah)
with sugar	con azúcar
	(kohn ah-soo-kahr)
What kind of coffee?	¿Qué clase de café?
	(Keh klah-seh deh kah-feh)
regular	regular
	(reh-goo-lahr)
decaffeinated	descafeinado
	(dehs-kah-feh-ee-nah-doh)
instant	instantáneo
	(eens-tahn-tah-neh-oh)
What kind of juices?	¿Qué clase de jugos?
	(Keh klah-seh deh joo-gohs)
orange	naranja
	(nah-rah-hah)
grape	uva
	(oo-bah)
apple	manzana
	(mahn-sah-nah)
grapefruit	toronja
	(toh-rohn-hah)

prune	ciruela
	(see-roo-eh-lah)
tomato	tomate
	(toh-mah-teh)
How do you like the eggs fixed?	¿Cómo le gustan los huevos?
	(Koh-moh leh goos-tahn lohs oo-eh-bohs)
scrambled	revueltos
	(reh-boo-ehl-tohs)
over-easy	volteados
	(bohl-teh-ah-dohs)
fried	fritos
	(free-tohs)
hard-boiled	duros
	(doo-rohs)
with ham	con jamón
	(kohn hah-mahn)
We have cereals.	Tenemos cereales.
	(Teh-neh-mohs seh-reh-ah-lehs)
oatmeal	avena
	(ah-beh-nah)
cream of wheat	crema de trigo
	(kreh-mah deh tree-goh)
corn flakes	hojitas de maíz/corn flakes
	(oh-hee-tahs de mah-ees/hohrn fleh-ee-ks)
Do you like them hot/cold?	¿Le gustan calientes/fríos?
	(Leh goos-tahn kah-lee-ehn-tehs/free-ohs)
We have meats:	Tenemos carnes:
	(Teh-nehmohs kahr-nehs)
beef	res
	(rehs)
hamburger	hamburguesa
	(ahm-boor-geh-sah)
steak	bistec
	(bees-tehk)
roast	rostizado
	(rohs-tee-sah-doh)
pork	puerco
	(poo-ehr-koh)

chops	chuletas
	(choo-leh-tahs)
ribs	costillas
	(kohs-tee-yahs)
chicken	pollo
	(poh-yoh)
fried chicken	pollo frito
	(poh-yoh free-toh)
baked chicken	pollo asado
	(poh-yoh ah-sah-doh)
breast	pechuga
	(peh-choo-gah)
leg	pierna
	(pee-ehr-nah)
wings	alas
	(ah-lahs)
fish	pescado
	(pehs-kah-doh)
breaded	empanizado
	(ehm-pah-nee-sah-doh)
broiled fish	pescado al horno
	(pehs-kah-doh ahl ohr-noh)
Among the vegetables that we serve are:	Entre los vegetales que servimos hay:
	(Ehn-treh lohs beh-heh-tah-lehs keh sehr-bee-mohs ah-ee)
potatoes	papas
	(pah-pahs)
baked potatoes	papas asadas
	(pah-pahs ah-sah-dahs)
french fries	papas fritas
	(pah-pahs free-tahs)
mashed potatoes	puré de papas
	(poo-reh deh pah-pahs)
green beans	ejotes/habichuelas
	(eh-hoh-tehs/ah-bee-choo- eh-lahs)
peas	chícharos
	(chee-chah-rohs)
corn	maíz/elote
	(mah-ees/eh-loh-teh)

beans	frijoles/habas
	(free-hoh-lehs/ah-bahs)
pinto beans	frijol pinto
	(free-hohl peen-toh)
refried	refritos
	(reh-free-tohs)
salad	ensalada
	(ehn-sah-lah-dah)
lettuce	lechuga
	(leh-choo-gah)
We also have desserts:	También tenemos postres:
	(Tahm-bee-ehn teh-neh-mohs pohs-trehs)
ice cream	nieve/helado
	(nee-eh-beh/eh-lah-doh)
vanilla	vainilla
	(bah-ee-nee-yah)
chocolate	chocolate
	(choh-koh-lah-teh)
strawberry	fresa
	(freh-sah)
pies	pasteles
	(pahs-teh-lehs)
pecan	nuez
	(noo-ehs)
apple	manzana
	(mahn-sah-nah)
cookies	galletas
	(gah-yeh-tahs)
candy	dulces
	(dool-sehs)
The water is in the glass/pitcher.	El aqua están en el vaso/la jarra.
	(Ehl ah-goo-ah ehs-tah ehn ehl bah-soh/lah hah-rah)
Do you want water?	¿Quere agua?
	(Kee-eh-reh ah-goo-ah)
Do you need ice?	¿Necesita hielo?
	(Neh-seh-see-tah ee-eh-loh)

The fork, spoon, and knife are wrapped in the napkin.

El tenedor, cuchara y cuchillo están envueltos en la servilleta.

(Ehl teh-neh-dohr, koo-chah-rah ee koo-chee-yoh ehs-tahn ehn-boo-ehl-tohs ehn lah sehr-bee-yeh-tah)

There is a straw.

Hay un popote.

(Ah-ee oon poh-poh-teh)

The salt and pepper are in these packets.

La sal y pimienta están en estos paquetes.

(Lah sahl ee pee-mee-ehn-tah ehs-tahn ehn ehs-tohn pah-keh-tehs)

The cover is hot.

La cubeirta está caliente.

(Lah koo-bee-ehr-tah ehs-tah kah-lee-ehn-teh)

It keeps the food warm.

Guarda la comida tibia.

(Goo-ahr-dah lah koh-mee-dah tee-bee-ah)

Select your foods from the menu after breakfast.

Seleccione las comidas del menú después del de sayuno.

(Seh-lehk-see-oh-neh lahs koh-mee-dahs dehl meh-noo dehs-poo-chs dehl deh-sah-yoo-noh)

dehydration

deshidratación

(deh-see-drah-tah-see-ohn)

nutrition

nutrición

(noo-tree-see-ohn)

salt

sal

(sahl)

Do you want:

¿Quiere:

(Kee-eh-reh)

a glass of water?

un vaso de agua?

(oon bah-soh deh ah-goo-ah)

a glass of juice?

un vaso de jugo?

(oon bah-soh deh hoo-goh)

Do you want:

¿Quiere:

(Kee-eh-reh)

something to eat?

algo de comer?

(ahl-goh deh koh-mehr)

something to drink?

algo de tomar/beber?

(ahl-goh deh toh-mahr/beh-behr)

After meals.

Después de las comidas.

(Dehs-poo-ehs deh lahs koh-mee-dahs)

Are you hungry?

¿Tiene hambre?

(Tee-eh-neh ahm-breh)

Difficulty in swallowing . . .	Diffcultad al tragar . . .
	(Dee-fee-kool-tahd ahl-trah-gahr)
Do you want a cup of coffee?	¿Quiere una taza de café?
	(Kee-eh-reh oo-nah tah-sah deh-kah-feh)
Do you want a glass of juice?	¿Quiere un vaso con jugo?
	(Kee-eh-reh oon bah-soh kohn hoo-goh)
Do you want a glass of water?	¿Quiere un vaso con agua?
	(Kee-eh-reh oon bah-soh kohn ah-goo-ah)
Do you want something to drink?	¿Quiere algo de tomar/beber?
	(Kee-eh-reh ahl-goh deh toh-mahr/beh-behr)
How do you like your eggs fixed?	¿Comó le gustan los huevos?
	(Koh-moh leh goos-tahn lohs oo-eh-bohs)
How do you like your coffee?	¿Cómo le gusta el café?
	(Koh-moh leh goos-tah ehl kah-feh)
How many glasses of water do you drink?	¿Cuántos vasos de agua toma?
	(Koo-ahn-tohs bah-sohs de ah-goo-ah toh-mah)
The meals are served at. . . .	Los alimentos se sirven a. . .
	(Lohs ah-lee-mehn-tohs seh seer-behn ah)
When was the last time you ate?	¿Cuándo fue la última vez que comió?
	(Koo-ahn-doh foo-eh lah ool-tee-mah behs keh koh-mee-oh)
You have to choose three meals a day.	Tiene que escoger tres comidas diarias.
	(Tee-eh-neh keh ehs-koh-hehr trehs koh-mee-dahs dee-ah-ree-ahs)

CHAPTER 15: SKIN CARE

ulcer	úlcera
	(ool-seh-rah)

CHAPTER 16: ASSISTING WITH MOVING AND POSITIONING

Sit in the chair.	Siéntese en la silla.
	(See-ehn-teh-seh ehn lah see-yah)
spinal	espinal
	(ehs-pee-nahl)
Do you need the headboard up?	¿Necesita levantar más la cabecera?
	(Neh-seh-see-tah leh-bahn- tahr mahs lah kah-beh-seh-rah)
I am going to help you lie down.	Voy a ayudarlo a acostarse.
	(Boy ah ah-yoo-dahr-loh ah ah-kohs-tahr-seh)

I will help you sit.	Le ayudaré a sentarse.
	(Leh ah-yoo-dah-reh ah sehn-tahr-seh)
Turn on your side.	Voltéese de lado.
	(Bhol-teh-eh-seh deh lah-doh)
Turn to your side.	Voltéate de lado.
	(Bhol-teh-ah-teh deh lah-doh)

CHAPTER 18: CARE OF COGNITVELY IMPAIRED RESIDENTS

delirious	delirio
	(deh-lee-ree-oh)

CHAPTER 19: BASIC RESTORATIVE CARE

Please stay/remain in bed.	Por favor, quédeses en la cama.
	(Pohr fah-bohr, keh-deh-seh ehn lah kan-mah)
Lift your arm.	Levanta tu brazo.
	(leh-bahn-tah too brah-soh)
Extend it.	Extiéndelo.
	(Ehx-tee-ehn-deh-loh)
Flex it.	Dóblalo.
	(Doh-blah-loh)
Rotate it.	Gíralo./Dale vuelta.
	(Hee-rah-loh/Dah-leh boo-ehl-tah)
Bend your elbow.	Dobla el codo.
	(doh-blah ehl koh-doh)
Turn your forearm.	Voltea el antebrazo.
	(Bohl-teh-ah ehl ahn-teh brah-soh)
Open your hand.	Abre tu mano.
	(Ah-breh too mah-noh)
Close it.	Ciérrala.
	(See-eh-rah-lah)
Open the fingers wide.	Separa bien los dedos.
	(Seh-pah-rah bee-ehn lohs deh-dohs)
Bend the wrist.	Dobla la muñeca.
	(Doh-blah lah moo-nyeh-kah)
Extend your wrist.	Extiende tu muñeca.
	(Ehx-tee-ehn-deh too moo-nyeh-kay)

Lift your leg.	Levanta la pierna.
	(Leh-bahn-tah lah pee- ehr-nah)
Bend it.	Dóblala.
	(Doh-blah-lah)
Bend your hip.	Dobla tu Cadera.
	(Doh-blah too kah-deh-rah)
Straighten your knee.	Endereza la rodilla.
	(Ehn-deh-reh-sah lah roh-dee-yah)
Move your leg.	Mueve tu pierna.
	(Moo-eh-beh too pee- ehr-nah)
Forward.	Adelante.
	(Ah-deh-lahn-teh)
Backward.	Atrás.
	(Ah-trahs)
Turn it to the left.	Voltéalo hacia la izquierda.
	(Bohl-teh-ah-loh ah-see-ah lah ees-kee-ehr-dah)
Turn it to the right.	Voltéalo hacia la derecha.
	(Bohl-teh-ah-loh ah-see-ah lah deh-reh-chah)
Lift your foot.	Levanta tu pie.
	(Leh-bahn-tah too pee-eh)
Bend your toes.	Dobla tus dedos (del pie).
	(Doh-blah toos deh-dohs (dehl pee-eh)
Lower your foot.	Baja el pie.
	(Bah-hah ehl pee-eh)
Flex the foot upward.	Dobla el pie hacia arriba.
	(Doh-blah ehl pee-eh ah-see- ah ah-ree-bah)
Straighten your leg.	Endereza tu pierna.
	(Ehn-deh-reh-sah too pee- ehr-nah)
Please walk.	Camina, por favor.
	(Kah-mee-nah, pohr fah-bohr)
exercise	ejercicio
	(eh-hehr-see-see-oh)
syncope	síncope
	(seen-koh-peh)
Activities are part of the plan.	Las actividades son parte del plan.
	(Lahs ahk-tee-bee-dah-dehs sohn pahr-teh dehl plahn)
Are you dizzy?	¿Tiene mareos?
	(Tee-eh-neh mah-reh-ohs)

Do you feel dizzy?	¿Se siente mareado?
	(Seh see-ehn-teh mah-reh- ah-doh)
Extend your arm.	Extiende tu brazo.
	(Ehx-tee-ehn-deh too brah-soh)
Extend your leg and foot.	Extiende tu pierna y pie.
	(Ehx-tee-ehn-deh too pee- ehr-nah ee pee-eh)
Flex your foot upward.	Dobla el pie para arriba.
	(Doh-blah ehl pee-eh pah-rah ah-ree-bah)
Flex your arm.	Dobla tu brazo.
	(Doh-blah too brah-soh)
Now raise the left arm.	Ahora levante el brazo izquierdo.
	(Ah-oh-rah leh-bahn-teh ehl brah-soh ees-kee-ehr-doh)
Turn the forearm.	Voltea el antebrazo.
	(Bhol-teh-ah ehl ahn-teh-brah-soh)

Glossary

abduction Moving a body part away from the midline of the body

abuse The intentional mistreatment or harm of another person

active physical restraint A restraint attached to the person's body and to a fixed (non-movable) object; it restricts movement or body access

activities of daily living (ADL) The activities usually done during a normal day in a person's life

adduction Moving a body part toward the midline of the body

advance directive A document stating a person's wishes about health care when that person cannot make his or her own decisions

alopecia Hair loss

ambulation The act of walking

anorexia Loss of appetite

anxiety A vague, uneasy feeling in response to stress

aphasia The inability (a) to speak (phasia)

asepsis Being free of disease-producing microbes

aspiration Breathing fluid or an object into the lungs

assault Intentionally attempting or threatening to touch a person's body without the person's consent

atrophy The decrease in size or a wasting away of tissue

base of support The area on which an object rests

battery Touching a person's body without his or her consent

bedsore A pressure ulcer, pressure sore, or decubitus ulcer

biohazardous waste Items contaminated with blood, body fluids, secretions, and excretions; *bio* means life, and *hazardous* means dangerous or harmful

blood pressure The amount of force exerted against the walls of an artery by the blood

body alignment The way the head, trunk, arms, and legs are aligned with one another; posture

body language Messages sent through facial expressions, gestures, posture, hand and body movements, gait, eye contact, and appearance

body mechanics Using the body in an efficient and careful way

body temperature The amount of heat in the body that is a balance between the amount of heat produced and the amount lost by the body

calorie The amount of energy produced when the body burns food

cardiac arrest The heart and breathing stop suddenly and without warning

carrier A human or animal that is a reservoir for microbes but does not have signs and symptoms of infection

catheter A tube used to drain or inject fluid through a body opening

chart The medical record

circulatory ulcer An open wound on the lower legs and feet caused by decreased blood flow through the arteries or veins; vascular ulcer

civil laws Laws concerned with relationships between people

clean technique Medical asepsis

colostomy A surgically created opening (*stomy*) between the colon (*colo*) and abdominal wall

coma A state of being unaware of one's surroundings and being unable to react or respond to people, places, or things

communicable disease A disease caused by pathogens that spread easily; a contagious disease

communication The exchange of information—a message sent is received and interpreted by the intended person

confidentiality Trusting others with personal and private information

constipation The passage of a hard, dry stool

contagious disease Communicable disease

contamination The process of becoming unclean

contracture The lack of joint mobility caused by abnormal shortening of a muscle

convulsion A seizure

crime An act that violates a criminal law

criminal laws Laws concerned with offenses against the public and against society

culture The characteristics of a group of people—language, values, beliefs, habits, likes, dislikes, customs—passed from one generation to the next

dandruff Excessive amount of dry, white flakes from the scalp

decubitus ulcer A pressure ulcer, pressure sore, or bedsore

defamation Injuring a person's name and reputation by making false statements to a third person

defecation The process of excreting feces from the rectum through the anus; a bowel movement

defense mechanisms Unconscious reactions that block unpleasant or threatening feelings

delegate To authorize another person to perform a task

delirium A state of temporary but acute mental confusion

delusion A false belief

dementia The loss of cognitive and social function caused by changes in the brain

development Changes in mental, emotional, and social function

developmental task A skill that must be completed during a stage of development

diarrhea The frequent passage of liquid stools

diastolic pressure The pressure in the arteries when the heart is at rest

disability Any lost, absent, or impaired physical or mental function

disinfection The process of destroying pathogens

dorsal recumbent position The back-lying or supine position

dorsiflexion Bending the toes and foot up at the ankle

dysphagia Difficulty (*dys*) swallowing (*phagia*)

dysuria Painful or difficult (*dys*) urination (*uria*)

enema The introduction of fluid into the rectum and lower colon

enteral nutrition Giving nutrients through the gastrointestinal tract (*enteral*)

ethics Knowledge of what is right conduct and wrong conduct

expressive aphasia Difficulty expressing or sending out thoughts

expressive-receptive aphasia Difficulty expressing or sending out thoughts and difficulty receiving information

extension Straightening a body part

external rotation Turning the joint outward

fainting The sudden loss of consciousness from an inadequate blood supply to the brain; syncope

false imprisonment Unlawful restraint or restriction of a person's movement

fecal impaction The prolonged retention and buildup of feces in the rectum

fecal incontinence The inability to control the passage of feces and gas through the anus

feces The semisolid mass of waste products in the colon that are expelled through the anus

flatulence The excessive formation of gas in the stomach and intestines

flatus Gas or air passed through the anus

flexion Bending a body part

footdrop The foot falls down at the ankle; permanent plantar flexion

Fowler's position A semi-sitting position; the head of the bed is raised 45 to 90 degrees

fraud Saying or doing something to trick, fool, or deceive a person

friction The rubbing of one surface against another

full visual privacy Having the means to be completely free from public view while in bed

gait belt A transfer belt

gangrene A condition in which there is death of tissue

gavage Tube feeding

geriatrics The care of aging people

gerontology The study of the aging process

growth The physical changes that are measured and that occur in a steady and orderly manner

hallucination Seeing, hearing, or feeling something that is not real

harassment To trouble, torment, offend, or worry a person by one's behavior or comments

hazardous substance Any chemical in the workplace that can cause harm

hematuria Blood (*hemat*) in the urine (*uria*)

hemorrhage The excessive loss of blood in a short time

hirsutism Excessive body hair in women and children

hospice An agency or program for persons who are dying

hyperextension Excessive straightening of a body part

hypertension Systolic pressures that remain above *(hyper)* 140 mm Hg and diastolic pressures that remain above 90 mm Hg

hypotension When the systolic blood pressure is below *(hypo)* 90 mm Hg and the diastolic pressure is below 60 mm Hg

ileostomy A surgically created opening *(stomy)* between the ileum *(small intestine; ileo)* and the abdominal wall

incident Any event that has harmed or could harm a resident, staff member, or visitor

infection A disease resulting from the invasion and growth of microbes in the body

infection control Methods to prevent the spread of infection

interdisciplinary health care team A variety of health workers who work together to provide for the person's total care

internal rotation Turning the joint inward

intravenous (IV) therapy Giving fluids through a needle or catheter inserted into a vein; IV, IV therapy, and IV infusion

invasion of privacy Violating a person's right not to have his or her name, picture, or private affairs exposed or made public without giving consent

lateral position The side-lying position

law A rule of conduct made by a government body

libel Making false statements in print or writing or through pictures or drawings

licensed practical nurse (LPN) A nurse who has completed a 1-year nursing program and has passed a licensing test; called licensed vocational nurse (LVN) in some states

licensed vocational nurse (LVN) Licensed practical nurse

logrolling Turning the person as a unit, in alignment, with one motion

malpractice Negligence by a professional person

medical asepsis Practices used to remove or destroy pathogens and to prevent their spread from one person or place to another person or place; clean technique

medical record A written account of a person's condition and response to treatment and care; chart

mental health The person copes with and adjusts to everyday stresses in ways accepted by society

mental illness A disturbance in the ability to cope with or adjust to stress

microbe A microorganism

microorganism A small *(micro)* living plant or animal *(organism)* seen only with a microscope; a microbe

need Something necessary or desired for maintaining life and mental well-being

negligence An unintentional wrong in which a person did not act in a reasonable and careful manner and causes harm to a person or to a person's property

nocturia Frequent urination *(uria)* at night *(noct)*

non-pathogen A microbe that does not usually cause an infection

nonverbal communication Communication that does not use words

nursing assistant A person who gives basic nursing care under the supervision of a licensed nurse.

nursing center A facility that provides medical, nursing, dietary, recreational, rehabilitative, and social services; nursing facility or nursing home

nutrient A substance that is ingested, digested, absorbed, and used by the body

nutrition The processes involved in the ingestion, digestion, absorption, and use of foods and fluids by the body

objective data Information that is seen, heard, felt, or smelled; signs

observation Using the senses of sight, hearing, touch, and smell to collect information

oliguria Scant amount *(olig)* of urine *(uria)*; less than 500 ml in 24 hours

ombudsman Someone who supports or promotes the needs and interests of another person

Omnibus Budget Reconciliation Act of 1987 (OBRA) A federal law concerned with the quality of life, health, and safety of residents

oral hygiene Mouth care

ostomy A surgically created opening

passive physical restraint A restraint near but not directly attached to the person's body; it does not totally restrict freedom of movement and allows access to certain body parts

pathogen A microbe that is harmful and can cause an infection

perineal care Cleaning the genital and anal areas; pericare

plantar flexion The foot *(plantar)* is bent *(flexion)*; bending the foot down at the ankle

polyuria Abnormally large amounts *(poly)* of urine *(uria)*

postmortem After *(post)* death *(mortem)*

pressure sore A bedsore, decubitus ulcer, or pressure ulcer

pressure ulcer Any injury caused by unrelieved pressure; decubitus ulcer, bedsore, or pressure sore

pronation Turning the joint downward

prone position Lying on the abdomen with the head turned to one side

prosthesis An artificial replacement for a missing body part

pulse The beat of the heart felt at an artery as a wave of blood passes through the artery

pulse rate The number of heartbeats or pulses felt in 1 minute

range of motion (ROM) The movement of a joint to the extent possible without causing pain

receptive aphasia Difficulty receiving information

recording The written account of care and observations; charting

registered nurse (RN) A nurse who has completed a 2-, 3-, or 4-year nursing program and has passed a licensing test

regurgitation The backward flow of food from the stomach into the mouth

rehabilitation The process of restoring the person to the highest possible level of physical, psychological, social, and economic function

religion Spiritual beliefs, needs, and practices

reporting The oral account of care and observations

respiration Breathing air into (inhalation) and out of (exhalation) the lungs

restorative aide A nursing assistant with special training in restorative nursing and rehabilitation skills

restorative nursing care Care that helps persons regain their health, strength, and independence

restraint Any item, object, device, garment, material, or drug that limits or restricts a person's freedom of movement or access to one's body

reverse Trendelenburg's position The head of the bed is raised, and the foot of the bed is lowered

rigor mortis The stiffness or rigidity *(rigor)* of skeletal muscles that occurs after death *(mortis)*

rotation Turning the joint

seizure Violent and sudden contractions or tremors of muscle groups; convulsion

semi-Fowler's position The head of the bed is raised 30 degrees; or the head of the bed is raised 30 degrees and the knee portion is raised 15 degrees

sexuality The physical, psychological, social, cultural, and spiritual factors that affect a person's feelings and attitudes about his or her sex

shearing When skin sticks to a surface while muscles slide in the direction the body is moving

shock Results when organs and tissues do not get enough blood

side-lying position The lateral position

signs Objective data

Sims' position A left side-lying position in which the upper leg is sharply flexed so it is not on the lower leg and the lower arm is behind the person

skilled nursing facility (SNF) A facility that provides nursing care for residents who need complex care but do not need hospital services; may be part of a nursing center or a hospital

skin tear A break or rip in the skin; the epidermis (top layer) separates from the underlying tissues

slander Making false statements orally

sphygmomanometer A cuff and measuring device used to measure blood pressure

sterile The absence of *all* microbes

sterilization The process of destroying *all* microbes

stoma An opening; see *colostomy* and *ileostomy*

stool Excreted feces

subjective data Things a person tells you about that you cannot observe through your senses; symptoms

sundowning Signs, symptoms, and behaviors of AD increase during hours of darkness

supination Turning the joint upward

supine position The back-lying or dorsal recumbent position

symptoms Subjective data

systolic pressure The amount of force needed to pump blood out of the heart into the arterial circulation

task A function, procedure, activity, or work that does not require an RN's professional knowledge or judgment

terminal illness An illness or injury for which there is no reasonable expectation of recovery

transfer belt A belt used to support persons who are unsteady or disabled; a gait belt

Trendelenburg's position The head of the bed is lowered, and the foot of the bed is raised

urinary frequency Voiding at frequent intervals

urinary incontinence The loss of bladder control

urinary urgency The need to void at once

urination The process of emptying urine from the bladder; voiding

vascular ulcer A circulatory ulcer

verbal communication Communication that uses written or spoken words

vital signs Temperature, pulse, respirations, and blood pressure

voiding Urination

work ethics Behavior in the workplace

workplace violence Violent acts directed toward persons at work or while on duty

wound A break in the skin or mucous membrane

Index